Newly Expanded!

The World's Greatest Treasury of
HEALTH
SECRETS

Bottom Line
Books
www.BottomLineSecrets.com

The World's Greatest Treasury of Health Secrets...Newly Expanded

Copyright © 2008 Boardroom® Inc.

10 9 8 7 6 5 4 3

All rights reserved, including the right to reproduce
this material or parts thereof in any form.

ISBN 0-88723-501-8

Bottom Line Books® publishes the advice of expert authorities in
many fields. The information in this book is not a substitute for
personal medical advice. Before making any decision regarding your
health, please consult a physician or another health-care practitioner.

Telephone numbers, prices, offers and Web sites listed in this book are accurate
at the time of publication, but they are subject to frequent change.

p.cm.
Includes index.

Bottom Line Books® is an imprint of
Boardroom® Inc.
281 Tresser Blvd., Stamford, CT 06901

Printed in the United States of America

Contents

1 • BEST OF BESTS

The Time/Health Connection.....................................1
How to Stop Worrying About Disease 3
Creating Your Medical Family Tree to Save Your Life...............4
Secrets to Staying Healthy—and Happy—While Traveling 5
How to Read Your Body's Messages.........................7
Dr. Joyce Brothers's Secrets of Winning the
    Ever-Changing Game of Life...................................9
Use It…or Lose It Physically…Mentally.....................11
12 Quick and Easy Things You Can Do
    To Improve Your Health.......................................13
Advice on How to Give Advice to Others................14
How to Survive Natural Disasters…Hurricanes…
    Earthquakes…Floods, etc. 16
How to Avoid the All-Too-Common Common Cold..............17
How to Stop Sinusitis..19
Indigestion…How to Be Rid of It Forever! 20
Cosmetic Surgery…The Best Solutions...................22
All About Dizziness...23
How to Win the Chronic-Pain War 25
Beating Arthritis Pain 27
Beating Joint Pain...29
Beating Migraines...31
Best Ways to Prevent Colon Cancer.......................33
Aspirin Therapy Reduces Colon Cancer Risk 34
Prostate Cancer: What Every Man Must Know Now...............34
Colon Cancer Self-Defense Essentials.....................36
Often-Overlooked Causes of Chronic Fatigue..........38
High Blood Pressure…The Silent Killer...................40
Lifesaving Breakthroughs in Stroke Treatment..................41

For Serious Medical Emergencies.............................43
Easy Ways to Save Big Money on Prescription Drugs............44
The Importance of Support Groups for Chronic Illness.........45

2 • EVERYDAY REMEDIES

The Ultimate Guide to Infectious Disease.................47
Everything You Need to Know About Bacteria!.........49
How to Stay Healthy on Your Next Airplane Flight................49
Water Therapy for Common Ailments......................50
How to Feel and Look Younger...............................51
How to Break Bad Habits.......................................51
Simple Solutions for Incontinence..........................52
Hemorrhoid Self-Defense.......................................53
Prevention and Treatment of Common Foot Problems...........53
Heel Pain Relief..55
Medicine Cabinet Must-Haves.................................56
Extend the Life of Athletic Shoes...........................56
Emergency Ice Packs...56
CPR to the Rescue..56
Music Fights Insomnia 56
How to Reduce Your Risk of Cancer........................57
Can't Sleep?...57
Help for People Who Can't Fall Asleep....................57
Elevation and Breathing...57
Control Pet Allergies...57
Feeling Forgetful?...58
Does Drinking Coffee Help Control Hay Fever?.......58
All About Home Testing 58
Bee Sting First Aid 58
A Shot to Relieve Constipation 58

Drink Up!..59
Three Quick Massages..59
Headache Prevention...59
Avoiding Headache Triggers 59
Headache Relief...59
Beat Heartburn Without Drugs............................60
For Better Driving with Arthritis…......................60
Arthritis in the Kitchen......................................60
Homemade Heating Pad.......................................60
To Stop a Nosebleed…...60
Better Dandruff Shampoo Use.............................61
Tongue Scraping..61
Better Toothbrushing..61
Avoid Bad Breath..61
Jaw Pain Relief...62
Bike Helmet Fact...62
Quick Cures..62
Painless Adhesive Bandage Removal....................62
Neck Pain Relief...62
Natural Air Filters..62

3 • HEART MATTERS

It's Never Too Late to Start Taking Care of Your Heart 63
Preventing Heart Disease.....................................65
Eating Right for a Healthy Heart and Long Life......................67
Heart Disease and Weight 68
How to Survive a Heart Attack 68
A Benefit of Having Friends.................................70
Heart Trouble Predictor.......................................70
Longer Life 70
Symptoms of Angina Pectoris..............................70
Hypertension…What You Need to Know..............71
High Blood Pressure Mistakes Can Easily Be Avoided............72
Borderline Blood Pressure Risk...........................74
Best Place to Take Your Blood Pressure................74
Angioplasty Trap...74
How Effective Are Implantable Defibrillators?......................75
Beating Heart Disease: When Surgery Is Necessary…
    And When It's Not...75
What to Do When the Doctor Says Bypass Surgery..................77
Better Bypass Surgery..78
New Surgical Procedure for Heart Failure Sufferers 78
Open-Heart Surgery Breakthrough.......................79
Saving Your Heart Without Bypass Surgery…
    Without Angioplasty......................................79
Bypass Surgery Dangers Are Real........................81
New and Better Ways to Keep Cholesterol Under Control......81
For a Better Echocardiogram................................82
Aspirin and Anger...83
Better than Aspirin..83
Heart Health Trap..83
Work Hours May Be Hazardous...........................83
Cholesterol Drug Benefits 83
Helping Blood Vessels Work Properly...................84
Best Heart Disease Treatment..............................84
Easy Disease Risk Reducer...................................84
A Smoke-Free World..84
Timing Is Critical..85
Height and Heart Disease.....................................85
Even a Little Is Too Much 85
Test Results Can Vary..85
Exercise and Heart Attack....................................85
More Harm than Good?..86
Hooray! Heart Help!...86
Hunting Danger...86
Personality Danger...86
Mother's Diet and Heart Disease Link..................87
Fish Oil and Heart Attacks..................................87
Cutting Heart Attack Death Risks........................87
Beta-Blockers and Heart Attacks.........................87
Garlic and Cholesterol Link.................................87
Psychological Stress Danger.................................88
Triglyceride Levels...88
Stroke Risk Reduction...88
Early Treatment Is Best..88

4 • YOUR DOCTOR AND YOU

The Smart Way to Pick a Physician 89
How to Get the Most from Your
    Doctor–Patient Relationship...........................90
How to Get the Best Care from Your Doctor..........91
How to Get the Most from Your HMO...................93
How to Get the Very Best Possible Medical Care 94
Questions to Ask When Your Doctor
    Recommends a Specialist................................95
How to Find a Doctor of Alternative Medicine 96
Is Your Doctor Listening?....................................96
Better Doctor–Patient Communications.................97
The Right Way to Talk to Your Doctor..................97
Is There Something Your Doctor Isn't Telling You?...............98
Protect Yourself from Your Doctor's
    Financial Interests...99
To Take Charge of Your Medical Care..................100
To Control Your Medical Costs….........................100
GPs Often Err When Prescribing Psychiatric Drugs..............101
To Prevent High Blood Pressure in the Doctor's Office 101
Dirty Hands and Doctors...................................101
Medical Hygiene..101
Is Your Doctor Up-to-Date?...............................101
MDs and Continuing Education..........................102
Plan Ahead for Medical Emergencies..................102
Prescription Danger...102
When to Look for a New Doctor.........................102
Women and Their Doctors..................................102
Easier Dental Visits...103
How to Tell a Good Dentist from a Bad One........103

5 • THE TRUTH ABOUT MEDICINES

Where to Get Information on the Drugs You Take...............105
These Cholesterol Drugs Prevent Cancer,
    Alzheimer's and More 106
Marijuana Can Be Effective Medicine..................107
Antibiotics: Too Much of a Good Thing?.............107
Medication Errors Can Be Avoided…Easily..........108
How to Measure Dosages....................................110
The Eight Most Common Medication Mistakes…
    And How to Avoid Them..............................110
Dangerous Drug Interactions..............................112
Over-the-Counter vs. Prescription Drugs.............114
Finish All Prescriptions......................................114
Expiration Date Alert...114
Kids' Medication Overuse...................................114
Prescription Drug Self-Defense I.........................115
Prescription Drug Self-Defense II........................115
How to Save on Your Medicines.........................115
Aspirin? Tylenol? Advil? None of the Above?.......115
Painkiller Danger...116
Insomnia and Painkillers....................................116
Tablets vs. Liquids...117
Economical Cholesterol Control..........................117
Cholesterol Controversy.....................................117

Aspirin Reduces Colon Cancer Risk.......................................117
Drug Scare Reality..117
Testosterone Patch Is Available...118
Daily Headache Syndrome...118
All About Rebound Headaches..118
Don't Self-Medicate...118
Antidepressant Danger..118
Attention Arthritis Sufferers..119
Break the Strep-Throat Cycle...119
Ulcerative Colitis and Nicotine Therapy.................................119
Former Smokers and Nicotine Gum... 119
Seizure Relief...120
Aspirin Therapy and Stomach Problems..................................120
Grapefruit Juice Danger..120
Channel Blockers and Cancer Link.......................................120
Asthmatics and Inhalers..120
Asthma Trap...121
Shingles Treatment..121
Who Should Get the Hepatitis A Vaccine?..............................121
Cut Your Risk of Getting an Ulcer.......................................121
Statins vs. Depression...121
Better Bowel Movements..122
Magnesium Poisoning...122
Medical History Danger..122

6 • HEALTH SECRETS FOR WOMEN

The Secrets of a Happy, Healthy Menopause.........................123
The Great Hormone Debate...124
Estrogen Trap...126
Wrinkle Remover...126
Strategies for Avoiding Troublesome Breast Cysts....................127
Easy Relief for Hot Flashes...128
Breast Cancer and Abortions...128
Evaluating Breast Lumps...128
Breakthroughs in Breast Cancer Screening..............................128
Milk and Breast Cancer Connection......................................130
Surprising High Heels Benefit..130
A Bra/Breast Cancer Connection?...130
Smart Sports Bra Buying...131
Most Breast Lumps Are Normal...131
Breast Implant Trap...132
When to Schedule a Mammogram...132
Large Women and Mammograms..132
Antiperspirants and Mammograms..132
Incontinence and Exercise Connection...................................133
Urinary Incontinence Advance...133
Osteoporosis Advance..133
A Mile a Day..133
Cancer and Chemotherapy..133
Weight Loss May Not Be Good for Some...............................134
Hot Summer Days and Premature Labor.................................134
Depression–Osteoporosis Link...134
Breast-Feeding Benefit...134
Pregnancy and Smoking...134
Folic Acid's Role in Pregnancy..135
Morning Sickness Self-Defense..135
Pregnancy and Thinking...135
The Truth About "Post-Baby Blues"......................................135
Bladder Pain Relief..135
How Reliable Are Pregnancy Ultrasound Exams?.....................136
Anorexia and Older Women...136
Female Athletes and Knee Injuries.......................................136
Bone Density Study..136
Women and Calcium...136
Getting Enough Minerals..137
Incontinence and Smoking..137
How Women Can Outwit the Sneaky Malignancy
    That Killed Gilda Radner...137
Weight-Loss Health Trap..139
Stretch Mark Help...139
Risky Surgery...139
Cervix-Sparing Hysterectomy..139
Vaginal Douching Danger..140
Unfaithful Husbands and Cancer Link....................................140
Sex and Urinary Tract Infections..140
UTI Warning..140
Emergency Birth Control..140
Safest Birth Control Pills..141
Yeast Infection Relief...141
Ease Menstrual Cramps..141
Diaphragms and Cystitis Risk..141
More on Fertility Treatment..141
Treatment for Ovarian Cancer...142
Powder Risk...142
Fertility Drugs and Ovarian Cancer......................................142
Ovary Removal Danger...142

7 • THE HEALTHY FAMILY

What You Need to Know About Your Child's Health Care ...143
Are Your Immunizations Up-to-Date?....................................144
Healthy Toll-Free Calls...145
The Highest Life Expectancy..146
Flu Self-Defense..146
Remedy for Low Back Pain..146
Preventing Back Injuries...146
Declaring War on Asthma..146
Can't Stomach a Roller Coaster Ride?....................................148
Easier Ways to Get Dressed...148
GERD: A New Name for an Old Problem...............................149
Test Your Knowledge About the Common Cold........................150
How to Avoid Irregularity...151
Mosquito Prevention..152
Cuts and Scrapes...152
No More Snoring...152
Children and Sex...153
No More Mumbling..153
Spring Allergies?...153
Hepatitis B Vaccine and Preteens...155
Kids Get Ulcers, Too..155
Young Children Don't Need Pillows.......................................155
Music and Babies...155
Your Baby's Diet...155
What Never to Feed Young Children......................................155
Exercise Benefits...156
Prevent Infant Tooth Decay...156
Lead and Obesity...156
SIDS Fact..156
Getting Kids to Eat Fruits and Vegetables...............................156
Kids and Sunglasses Safety..156
The Value of Imaginary Friends..157
Sleep and Behavior..157
Poison Alert..157
Kids and Caffeine..157
Secondhand Smoke and Kids..157
Kids and Dehydration...158
Skin Care for Kids in Puberty..158
Don't Forget This Person..158
Balloon Danger...158
Children and Choking...158
How to Help Your Child Have a Great Time at Camp.............159
Safety Standards for Children's Camps....................................160

Warts and Children 160
Helping Your Kids Relax 161
Anxiety Disorders in the Family..............................161
How to Stop a Child's Bed-Wetting........................161
Bed-Wetting Prevention Alert.................................161
ADHD Relief..161
Ear Infections...162
Childhood Ear Infection?...162
Restless Legs Syndrome…Almost Five Million
  Sufferers…How to Tell if You're One and What to
  Do About It..162
Puberty Fact...163
Drawstring Danger..163
Three Common Misconceptions About
  The Two Kinds of Diabetes...................................163
Cold Sore Relief...165
Kegel Exercises Beat Incontinence in Women 165
How to Stop Recurring Hemorrhoids.....................165
Keeping Wounds from Scarring 166
Pediatrician's Home Remedies 166

8 • REDUCE STRESS, LENGTHEN LIVES

You Can Make Stress Work for You.........................167
Stress Avoidance Secrets: Proven Strategies.........168
How to Turn Stress into Strengths 170
Cut Stress Now…16 Quick Relaxation Techniques 172
Just Relax!..173
Relaxation Can Control Seizures.............................173
Quick Stress Buster 173
Sleep vs. Stress 173
Cholesterol Levels Are Affected by Stress.............173
Good for Your Heart...173
Fight Stress Anytime, Anywhere.............................174
Plants and Stress...174
Top Stress Reducer..174
Music and Stress...174
Writing Helps 174
Wonderfully Simple Stress-Busters........................175

9 • HOSPITAL AND SURGERY AWARENESS

How to Have a Healthier, Happier Hospitalization..............177
Signs of a Good Hospital 179
Hospital Rankings 179
Shrewder Hospital Stays..179
How to Win the Hospital Game 179
How to Survive a Hospital Stay...............................181
What I Learned About Doctors and Hospitals
  On My Way to Recovery 182
Don't Let Them Throw You Out of the Hospital 184
Cold Rooms and Heart Attacks...............................185
Common Hospital Billing Errors.............................186
The Truth About Hospitals and Medication Mistakes............186
Shorter Recovery Time...186
Questions to Ask if Considering Heart Surgery.....187
How to Prepare for Outpatient Surgery..................188
Secrets of Rapid Healing After Surgery.................189
Heart Surgery Recovery Fact...................................190
Common Procedure May Be Unsafe 190
Shop Around First 190
Heel Surgery Danger...190
Transfusion Trap..190
Anesthesia and Operations......................................191
Predicting Laser Eye Surgery Success....................191
LASIK Surgery Warning 191
Endoscopy…Is Your Doctor Competent?...............191
To Reduce Blood Transfusion Risk 191
All About the Latest Fat-Removal Technique.........192
The Major Hospital Hazards and How to Avoid Them.........192
Safer Surgery...193
Best Hernia Surgery Option.....................................194
Coffee Drinker and Surgery Trap............................194
Cataract Breakthrough 194

10 • HEALTH SECRETS FOR MEN

Hair Loss Prevention…Replacement…Regrowth 195
Make the Most of Less Hair......................................197
Domineering Men Die Sooner..................................197
Men and Their Metabolism......................................197
Potbelly Risk..197
Almost All Men Can Become Fathers 197
Infertility Factors..198
Infertility and Infections..198
Tight Underwear and Male Infertility.....................198
Premature Ejaculation Help 198
Safer Alternative to Vasectomy Reversals..............198
Impotence Drug News..199
Snoring and Impotence..199
Curved Penis Help 199
Strategies for Overcoming Impotence 199
Treatments for Male Impotence 200
Better Approach to Impotence 202
Impotence Predicts Heart Disease 202
Hormones and Men's Health....................................203
Saw Palmetto Benefits..203
Treatment for Prostate Problems 203
For the Enlarged Prostate...204
Best Time for Prostate Test.......................................204
Prostate Test Schedule..204
Best Treatments for Prostate Enlargement 204
Prostate Cancer Drug...206
What's Better for Early-Stage Prostate Cancer—
  Radiation or Surgery?...206
More Prostate News...206
Testicular Cancer Self-Defense................................207
Divorce and Men..208
Breast Cancer Strikes Men, Too...............................208
Low-Fat Diets and Men...208

11 • FOOD AND NUTRITION TIPS
FOR A HEALTHIER YOU

The New Superfoods 209
The "Healthy" Diet Can Actually Be Bad for You...............211
Curative Curry?..212
Grapefruit and Oranges Protect the Heart 213
Better than Butter..213
Eggs Can Be Part of a Healthful Diet......................213
A Most Expensive Hamburger.................................213
Protein and Kidney Disease.....................................213
Two Are Better than One..213
Foods Can Change Your Moods...............................214
Food Danger Zones...214
Salt-Watchers...214
We Are What We Eat...214
Better Pasta Buying..216
Added Fiber Helps...216
Tomatoes and Prostate Cancer Link........................217
Red Meat and Non-Hodgkin's Lymphoma 217
Vegetarianism Can Mask Anorexia.........................217

Prevent Asthma, Cataracts, Gallstones and Heart Failure by
    Eating the Right Foods 217
Finish Your Cereal 218
Nonfat Pancake Recipe 219
Sparkling Waters May Be Sugary 219
Lactose Intolerance 219
Antioxidants and Fewer Health Problems 219
A Good-for-You Frozen Treat 220
Control Your Cholesterol Without Drugs 220
Better Breakfasts 222
Creamy Dishes Without Cream 222
What You Should Know About Caffeine 222
Liquid Nutritional Supplements Are No
    Substitute for Real Food 223
Distilled Water Is Safe to Drink 223
All About Food Allergies 223
Spinach Pasta Contains Very Little Spinach 225
Power Eating...Foods to Make
    You More Productive 225
Cancer Self-Defense 226
Wasted Food Statistics 226
Little-Known Blood Clot Buster 226
Counting Calories 227
The Ultimate Summer Barbecue 227
Dangerous Diets 228
Simple Dieting Trick 228
If You Need to Use Eggs 228
More About Flavonoids 228
Arthritic Knee? 228
Cut Kidney Stone Recurrence 229
Safer Meat Marinating 229
Cut the Fat 229
Proven Diet for Arthritis Pain Relief 229
Fruit Juice Trap 231
Eat Less Fat...Easy Ways 231
Other Calcium Sources 231
Eat Healthier 231
Ales, Beer and Alcohol 231
Healthy Cheese Cooking 232
Medication Trap 232
More Fat-Free Food Traps 232
Treatments for Nail Fungus 232
Reducing Heart Attack Risk 232
Hidden Allergies...How to Identify the Causes 233
Diet and Alzheimer's Connection 234
Social Drinking Facts 234
The Rest of the Story About Diet and Cancer...
    Fat vs. Fiber...and the Best Sources of
    Cancer-Fighting Phytonutrients 235
Best Low-Fat Nut 236
Your Diet and Your Immune System 236
Super Fat-Blocker 238
Anticholesterol Supplement 238
Which Fruit Contains the Most Antioxidants? 238

12 • VITAMINS AND MINERALS SAVVY

All You Ever Really Wanted to Know...Almost...
    About Vitamins and Minerals 239
Which Mineral Supplements Should You Take? 241
The Value of Herbal Ingredients 242
Nutritional Supplements: What You Really Need
    For Optimal Health 242
Which Vitamins? Which Minerals? Here's What I Do 244
Timed-Release Vitamin Alert 245
Where Never to Store Your Vitamins 245
Depression and Vitamin B Connection 245

Calcium Is Inexpensive 245
Vitamin B-12 Alert 245
Vitamin C to the Rescue 246
Vitamin C and Arthritis 246
Possible Ulcer Protection 246
Relief from Colds 246
Vitamin C Danger 246
Cold-Weather Wellness 247
Bladder Cancer and Vitamin C 247
Vitamin C and Artery Link 247
Vitamin D and Diabetes 247
Adults and Vitamin D 247
Vitamin E Protects the Lungs 248
Vitamins vs. Birth Defects 248
Vitamin E, Aspirin and Stroke Connection 248
Vitamin E and Cuts 248
Vitamin E and Exercise 248
Beta-Carotene Update 249
Folic Acid Danger 249
Folic Acid Benefits 249
Magnesium Fights Migraines 249
Selenium vs. Cancer Facts 250
More Good Things About Selenium 250
Chromium Picolinate Danger 250

13 • FOR A HEALTHY SEX LIFE

The Healing Power of Good Sex 251
How to Have Great Sex Every Time 253
Herpes Update 254
How to Perk Up Your Sex Life 254
Love and Sex After 60 256
Exercises May Relieve Impotence 258
Prescription Drugs that Affect Sex 258
Better Sex, Better Sleep 259
Women Are Just as Likely as Men
    To Initiate Sexual Contact 259
Saying No to Sex 259
Sex and Heart Attacks 259
Sex Can Relieve Arthritis Pain 260
Premature Ejaculation Drug 260
Lovemaking Is More than Sex 260
Drug for Genital Herpes 260
Dr. Ruth's Secrets of Great Sex 260
Sex Isn't Only for the Healthy 260
Better Communication 261
Sex and Headaches 261
Hysterectomies and Sex 261
Sexual Frequency 261
Home HIV Test Kits 261
Sensual Massage Made Easy 262
How to Find the Best Egg or Sperm Donor 262
Questions that Keep Love Alive 262
Eminent Sex Therapist Reveals Her Secret
    Weapon Against Sexual Problems 262
Get in Sync 264
Sleep Positions and Relationships 264

14 • GROWING OLDER—HEALTHIER

The Key to Successful Aging 265
Alzheimer's Self-Defense 267
On Healthy Aging 268
Latest Findings on How to Live Longer 269
Mistakes Doctors Make When Treating Older Patients 270
Treatments for Parkinson's Disease 271
Vitamin Deficiency and Memory 272

Vitamins Do Help...272
Colon Cancer Detection...272
Stronger Seniors...273
Owning a Dog Can Extend Your Life.....................273
Safer Lifting Now..273
How to Maintain Peak Mental Ability as You Get Older......273
Estrogen and Dementia...275
Vitamin E and Aging...275
Consider Nursing Home Transfer Policies...............275
Fever Danger..275
Blood Pressure Pill Benefit....................................275
Exercise Improves Hearing....................................276
Exercise vs. Alzheimer's..276
The Mind/Body Approach to Arthritis....................276
Risk Reducers..278
Fainting Danger..278
Best Shoes for Senior Citizens...............................278
How to Guard Against Macular Degeneration..........278
Congestive Heart Failure and Blood Pressure Link...280
Alzheimer's Relief...280
PSA Testing: More Harm than Good?.....................280
Avoiding Disabling Falls..281
Free Eldercare..281
Dentist May Hold Key to Stroke Risk......................281
Stroke Sufferer Fact...282
Alcohol and Disease...Stroke...Diabetes...and Cancer......282
How Effective Is Colon Cancer Drug?.....................283
Smoking Kills 400,000 Americans Each Year...
    Here's How Not to Be One of Them.....................283
Getting the Right Treatment..................................284
Rural Living and Longevity Link.............................285
Medical Care Self-Defense.....................................285
Antiaging Supplements: Dr. Ken Cooper Explains
    What Works...and What Doesn't.........................286
Osteoporosis Risk Indicator...................................287
To Minimize Osteoporosis Risk...............................287
How to Stay Safe in This Crazy, Crazy World...........287
Harry Lorayne's Cures for Absentmindedness..........289
Pessimism Can Kill...290
Curing Aggression..291
Hip Fracture Reduction...291
How to Boost a Flagging Memory............................291

15 • TAKING CARE OF THE OUTER YOU— YOUR SKIN

Make Your Skin Look Young Again Without Surgery...........293
Low-Fat Diets May Reduce Skin Cancer Risk.........................295
Help for Unsightly Scars..295
Does Your Hair Protect You from the Sun?...............295
Vitamin C vs. Wrinkles..295
Skin Cancer—How to Protect Yourself.....................295
A Day Without Sunshine?.......................................297
Sunscreens Are Effective for Three Years After Purchase......297
Our Skin Would Change Very Little Over Time...........297
Melanoma Watch...299
Sunlight Is Not the Only Threat to Skin..................299
Rosacea Sufferers...300
Dandruff Shampoo Delay.......................................300
The Big Mistake Shingles Sufferers Make................300
An Itch May Be More than Skin Deep.....................301
How to Tell When the Sun Is Dangerous.................301
All-Year Sun Defense..302
Much...Much Younger Looking Skin in 15 Minutes a Day....302
Acne Drug..304
UVB Rays Are Everywhere.....................................304
Skin Cancer Sufferer Risk......................................304
Repairing Skin Damage...304
Sunscreen Danger..304
Sun Protection..305
What Keeps Skin Young…and What Doesn't...............305
The Dangers of Ultraviolet Light.............................306
Diabetic's Foot Ulcer Danger.................................306
Foot Pain Relief...307
Melanoma: What Your Doctor Isn't Telling You..........307
More Skin Cancer Facts...308
A Word About Surgery...308
What Causes Tiny Red Lines on the Cheeks?............308

16 • HEALTH ALERTS

All About Leg Cramps...309
Diabetes Alert..310
Disinfectant Danger..310
Rodent Danger...310
Another Danger in the Kitchen...............................311
The Scary Truth About Blood Transfusions..............311
Lead Danger...313
Drinking Danger..313
Underwear Danger...313
Boating Danger...313
Allergy Attacks and Food.......................................314
Ear Thermometer Danger.......................................314
Get a Tetanus Booster Shot Every 10 Years.............314
Drinking Unfiltered Coffee May Raise Your
    Blood Cholesterol Level.....................................314
Another Secondhand-Smoke Danger........................314
Yikes! Another Measles Shot?................................314
In-Line Skating Injuries on the Rise.......................315
Stroke Diagnosis Danger..315
Don't Cut Back on Caffeine Suddenly.....................315
Hidden Dangers in Household Products...
    In Everyday Foods, Too.....................................315
Meningitis Warning...317
Even the Best Medical Labs Can Make Mistakes…....317
Asthma Attacks Can Be Triggered by Thunderstorms.....317
Nose Piercing Is Dangerous...................................317
Glucose Level Alert...317
Cigar Dangers..318
Even Moderately High Blood Pressure
    Can Damage Kidneys..318
Smokers' Sleep Trap...318
Shoveling Snow Stresses the Heart.........................318
Asthma Warning..318
Lead Alert..319
Lead Poisoning Alert...319
Toxic Chemicals Self-Defense.................................319
Who Should Be Vaccinated for Hepatitis B?.............319
Weight-Lifting Danger..319
Drowning Fact..320
Plastic vs. Wood Cutting Boards.............................320
To Beat the Heat..320
Milk and Diabetes Connection................................320
Have a Foot Problem?...320
Who's Reading Your Medical Records?.....................321
Fibromyalgia...New Strategies for Controlling
    Mysterious Pain and Fatigue.............................322
Aneurysm Alert...323
Avoiding Drug Errors...323
Gas Fumes Danger..324
Checking Up on Your Thyroid Could Save Your Life......324
Daytime Sleepiness and Narcolepsy........................326

17 • WEIGHT SUCCESS

The 10 Secrets of Successful Weight Loss.............................327
Beer Drinkers Really Do Have Bigger Bellies.......................329
Why Diets Fail...329
Wonderful Ways to Keep Weight
    Off Once You've Lost It...330
Maximize Your Gardening "Workout" 331
Metabolism Slows with Age..332
Dieting for People Who Have Trouble Dieting.....................332
Surprising Calorie-Burner...333
The Fat Bank...333
Simple Secrets of Permanent Weight Loss............................334
Free Yourself from Food Cravings..335
Body Shape and Health Risk 336
A Diet for Life...336
Vegetarian Diets: Results Last Longer...................................336
Do Your Feet Hurt?..336
Lose Weight—Even While You're Sleeping..........................336
Diet Doctors' Weight-Loss Secrets…
    And How They Keep Weight Off..337
Calorie Buster..338
The Real Reason It's So Hard to Lose Weight.......................339
Proven Ways to Lose Weight Wisely 340
More on How to Control Food Cravings................................341
Scent Therapy Can Help You Lose Weight...........................341
How the Weight-Loss Scientists Lost Their Weight...............342
Another Benefit of Losing Weight 344
How to Tell How Many Calories to Eat Each Day.................344

18 • HEALTHY ATTITUDES FOR YOUR WORK AND HOME ENVIRONMENT

Carpal Tunnel Syndrome: New Preventive Steps...................345
Stand Up Straight...346
Healthier Computer Use I...347
Healthier Computer Use II..347
What HMOs Won't Tell You...347
Are You Taking Advantage of the
    Family and Medical Leave Act?...349
Everyone Has Anxiety—More…or Less 349
Workaholism Self-Defense...350
Hostility, Stress and Disease 352
Simple Stress-Reducing Office Routine 352
How to Reduce Job Stress..353
Indoor Pollutants…Easy Avoidance Strategies 354
Environmental Control of Allergies 356

19 • TAKING CARE OF YOUR EYES, EARS AND TEETH

The Simple Secrets of Avoiding Serious Eye Troubles...........357
A Sign of Diabetes?..359
Solutions for Bloodshot Eyes..359
Cataract Self-Defense…Sunglasses…
    Supplements…Surgery...360
Obesity and Cataracts..361
Protect Your Eyes with Good Nutrition 361
Asthma Danger...362
Glaucoma Busters 362
Glaucoma Treatment Without Side Effects............................362
Better Glaucoma Testing..362
Eye Exam Timetable...362
Eye Exercise 363
Itchy Eyes?...363
"Red Eye" Danger...363
Does My 10-Year-Old Need Bifocals?...................................363

Eyedrop Danger I...363
Eyedrop Danger II 364
Sunglasses Update 364
Eye Injury Reduction...364
Wraparound Sunglasses Offer Best Protection 364
Food for Your Eyes...364
Better Hearing..365
Free Hearing Test...365
Exercise May Improve Hearing..365
How to Prevent Hearing Loss 365
Earlobes…What They Can Tell You.......................................367
No More Earaches When Flying 367
Getting Help for Ringing in the Ears from
    Tinnitus Sufferer Dr. Stephen Nagler..............................367
Help for Teeth and Gums...369
Cleaner Kids' Teeth..369
Best Dental Floss..369
Better Brushing..369
Vegetarians Are at Higher Risk for Periodontal Disease.......369
Brushing and Flossing Are Not Enough 370
For Sweeter Breath...372
Laser Whitening Procedure..372
What Causes a Burning, Itching Sensation
    Inside the Mouth?...372

20 • KEEPING FIT PAYS OFF

Jack LaLanne's Fitness Magic...373
The Dangers of Too Much Exercise 375
Walking Your Way to Better Health.......................................377
Inexpensive Ways to Shape Up..378
Health Clubs Can Be Unhealthy 378
Beware of Health Club Scams 378
Exercise Beats Dieting..378
The Right Time to Exercise..379
Smarter, More Effective Exercising.......................................379
Exercise and Longevity..379
Dr. Kenneth Cooper's Exercise Plan 379
Better Weight-Lifting Workouts...380
Short Exercise Sessions May Be Better..................................380
Do-It-Yourself Sports Drink...381
How to Fight Arthritis with Exercise.....................................381
Exercise Is Good for Asthmatics..381
How to Stick with Your Exercise Regimen 381
Better Stationary Biking...382
Exercise vs. Insomnia...382
Exercise Surprise..383
"Tubing" Your Way to Strong Muscles...................................383
How to Get the Most Out of Your Workouts.........................384
Overrated Exercise Machines...385
Dance for Health and Fun..385
Better Sleeping...385
Finding the Fountain of Youth 385
Sore Muscle Relief...386
Hot Weather Jogging..386
Best Swimming Exercise...386
Exercising to Lose Weight..386
Easy Rheumatoid Arthritis Relief..386
Walking with Weights Works!..387
How to Develop the Exercise Habit.......................................387
Exercise vs. the Blues...388

21 • THE WHOLE YOU— THE MIND/BODY CONNECTION

Deepak Chopra's Secrets of Having Boundless Energy.........389
Mind/Body Techniques for Enhanced Wellness 391

20 Minutes a Day to a Much Happier,
   Much Healthier Life...392
How to Use Guided Imagery for Wellness...........................394
How to Use Your Mind to Improve Your Health.................395
Your Mind and Your Health..397
How to Make Your Mind Very Sharp.................................399
How to Stimulate Your Cerebellum 400
Mind/Body Made Easy...401
Empower Yourself..401
The Healing Power of Friendship......................................401
How the Great Self-Help Experts Help Themselves.............403
Exceptional Cancer Patients Live Longer and Happier........405
Intentional Healing: The Do-It-Yourself
   Way to Perfect Health 406
For Deep Relaxation: Yoga Made Very Simple....................408
Midlife Wisdom...409
Four-Step Plan for Beating Obsessions
   And Compulsions...411

22 • NATURAL WAYS AND HERBAL SOLUTIONS

Herbal Teas…How to Grow Them and Brew Them, Too.....413
Spices and Self-Healing...414
Ginger for Upset Stomach…and More...............................415
Medicinal Herbs: Growing Your Own to Improve
   Physical and Emotional Health........................416
Flower Remedies...417
When to Consider Alternative Therapies............................417
Treat Stress and Depression the Natural Way....................418
Effective Remedies from Your Kitchen Cabinet..................420
All About Herbal Remedies..420
Fight Allergies with Stinging Nettle 422
Alternative Remedies for Hay Fever..................................422
Healing Secrets from a Mayan Medicine Man 422
Safe, Simple Fix for Minor Injuries...................................423
Two Herbs that Calm the Colon.......................................424
Food and Healing..424
Fast Headache Relief Without Drugs.................................426
Natural Remedies for Fatigue...426
Natural Alternatives to Common Medications....................427
Natural Ways to Lower Your Blood Pressure......................429
Meditation Lowers Blood Pressure....................................430
Meditation and Pain Control..430
The Benefits of Massage 430
Secrets of Self-Healing from Chinese Medicine..................431
Ancient Chinese Secret for Relaxation and Better Health......432
Some Medicinal Oils Are Very Good for You 433
Eat Away Arthritis...434
Natural Remedies for Impotence.......................................435
Natural Year-Round Allergy Remedies...............................436
Natural Remedies for Pain Relief......................................437
Good Things About Ginkgo Biloba....................................438
Ginkgo Biloba Trap...438
Lavender and Insomnia..438

23 • HEALTH CARE SMARTS

Why Personal Medical Research Is So Important.................439
Making Sense of Medical News...441
The Terrible Truth About Medical Misinformation.............441
How Does Your HMO Stack Up?.......................................443
Picking an HMO...443
The Value of Lab Tests..444
Avoiding Anxiety During an MRI......................................444
Ulcer Testing 444
Genetic Testing Can Save Your Life…or Ruin It.................444
Easily Overlooked Medical Deductions 446
Refund Break for the Ill 446
Health Benefits Alert...446
Prostate Cancer Fact...447
Cancer-Prevention Checklist...447
Cellular Phones and Cancer Risk......................................447
You Can Catch Up on Sleep...447
Best Ways to Protect Your Lower Back..............................448
Back Injury Study..448
The Benefits of Allergy Shots...448
How to Tell if You Are Allergic to Nickel...........................448
Lyme Disease Update...449
Lyme Disease Self-Defense...449
Illness Can Be Good for You..449
To Avoid Spreading Cold Sores….....................................449
Hooray!! Lower Cost Prescription Drugs............................449
Help for Ex-Ex-Smokers...450
Heavy Smokers and the Nicotine Patch 450

24 • EMOTIONAL HEALTH MEANS A HAPPIER YOU

How Your Emotions Affect Your Health…
   Proven Ways to Stay Well...............................451
The Truth…and Your Health 453
All About Moods 453
Secrets of Inner Strength...454
Letting Go..456
A Survivor's Journey..456
Acupuncture Can Help Depression....................................458
How to Put Much More Happiness in Our Lives.................458
Gambling a Problem?...459
The Smart Way to Handle Negative Emotions.....................459
Overcoming Fear of Failure..461
How to Overcome Emotions that Hold You Back................463
Extreme Shyness Is a Health Problem:
   How to Overcome It 465

25 • NEW WAYS FOR THE 21ST CENTURY

Alternative Medicine Moves Mainstream.............................467
How to Get Your HMO to Cover Alternative
   Medical Treatment...470
Magnets Stop Pain…Ease Arthritis…Help
   Heal Broken Bones and More.........................470
Chinese Medicine Works Well on Americans, Too 471
Placebo Power: How to Harness It....................................473
The Seven Simple Steps to a Century of Great Health.........474
All About Light Therapy..476
All About Prolotherapy..477
How to Harness the Amazing Power of
   Your Immune System.....................................478
More About You…Your Immune System
   And Much Better Health.................................480
Head Trauma Advance...482
Heart Failure and Biofeedback...482
Electrostatic Massage..482
Abdominal Aneurysm Treatment......................................483
"Super Glue" vs. Sutures...483
Multiple Sclerosis Breakthrough.......................................483
Nausea Relief 483
Hidden Drug Dangers..484

26 • STOP THE PRESSES

Nobel Prize Winner's Breakthrough—Prevent
  Heart Attack and Stroke with Nitric Oxide 485
How to Prevent a Heart Attack 487
Five Little-Known Ways to Lower Heart Attack Risk............487
How to Predict Heart Disease..488
Cheap, Safe and More Effective than Statins 489
The Supplement that Slashes Cholesterol
  54% Better than Statins...490
Breakthrough Therapies for Heart Disease,
  Cancer—and Varicose Veins 491
Surprising Stroke Risks Even Doctors Overlook 492
Latest Developments in Stroke Rehab....................................494
Cancer Vaccines Offer New Hope..496
Skin Cancer: Debunking the Myths..497
Prostate Cancer Fighter..499
Best Herb for Male Urinary Tract Problems...........................499
Longevity Boosters from the World's
  Longest-Lived People..499
Stop Memory Loss Before It's Too Late 501
Test Your Memory...502
You Can Prevent Alzheimer's Disease....................................503
The Truth About Brain Food...505
Common Drugs Fight Alzheimer's..507
Natural Healers...508
The Oxygen Cure...509
Vibrant Health via Nutraceuticals..511
Scents to Boost Energy, Mood, Memory and More...............512
Healing Herbs 513
Natural Sex Boosters...515
Alleviate Neck and Back Pain with Fish Oil...........................517
Drug-Free Ways to Treat Pain 517

Duct Tape Really Can Cure Warts 519
Mighty Matcha..520
Amazing! Salsa Stops Disease 520
Supercharge Your Immunity with Just a Few Herbs 520
Nature's Virus Killers for Colds and Flu.................................522
Shorter Flu Recovery..524
What You Need to Know to Protect Yourself
  from the Deadly Bird Flu 524
Are Antibacterial Soaps Making You Sick?............................526
Sinus Infection Relief..527
How to Eat Fruits and Vegetables Safely................................527
Better Weight Loss 528
The Calcium Diet 529
Weight-Loss Secret..530
The TV Workout 530
A Stronger Body in Only 30 Minutes a Week 530
Exercises that Help with Everything You Do.........................532
Vinegar May Help Fight Diabetes...533
Reduce Diabetic Nerve Pain 534
Are You Taking Too Many Medications? 534
How Safe Are Your Vitamins and Minerals?..........................536
Do Your Supplements Really Work? 537
Emergency Room Self-Defense...538
Important Medical Tests Doctors Don't Tell You About 538
Nobel Prize Winner Who Discovered Real Cause
  of Ulcers Tells All 540
You May Have this Stomach Bug and Not Even Know It.......542
Asthma Breakthrough..543
New Treatment for Incontinence...543
Can Earwax Removal Help Hearing Loss?..............................543

INDEX 545

1

Best of Bests

The Time/Health Connection

Stephan Rechtschaffen, MD
Omega Institute for Holistic Studies

Do you have enough time in your life? When I pose this question to people attending my wellness seminars, only one or two people say *yes*—out of 50 or more.

The others—like most of us—suffer from "time poverty." These individuals are so busy trying to go faster, do more and buy more that they never get a chance to just experience being alive.

Inevitably, time poverty leads to psychological stress...and to stress-related ailments like heart disease, diabetes, fatigue, insomnia and high blood pressure.

THE HISTORY OF TIME

Most of us are so used to living by the clock that we think we *must* live by the clock. But the modern clock wasn't invented until the 16th century. Even the hourglass didn't see wide use until the 13th century.

Without clocks to control them, our ancestors experienced time as a series of moments defined by *nature's* pace—not as an endless parade of deadlines.

We *can* return to this wonderful sense of timelessness. I've developed a technique called *timeshifting*. This technique helps demonstrate that your experience of time is under your control. It lets you transform time from your master into your servant.

People come to my seminars expecting tips on time management. What they don't realize is that "managing" time only turns up the speed on the treadmill of life.

What I teach is *time awareness*. It's not about being more efficient. It's about slowing down and focusing on one thing at a time. It's

Stephan Rechtschaffen, MD, cofounder and chairman, Omega Institute for Holistic Studies, 150 Lake Drive, Rhinebeck, NY 12572. He is author of *Timeshifting: Creating More Time to Enjoy Your Life*. Doubleday.

1

a process governed by a single rule—*live life in the now.*

FIND YOUR OWN RHYTHM

The rhythms that rule our lives are not fixed, though they may seem to be. It's just that our *internal* rhythms have fallen into sync with the rhythms of the world around us.

This process by which internal rhythms synchronize with external rhythms is called *entrainment.*

Timeshifting involves becoming aware of these external rhythms. Then you can *choose* to entrain with a slow, peaceful rhythm…or stay in sync with the rhythms of your environment, but in a more relaxed way.

FEEL YOUR EMOTIONS

Right now, put aside this article and spend a few minutes doing nothing—no TV, no books or magazines, no chitchat.

How did you feel? When I ask my seminar participants, the usual answers are "anxious," "guilty" or "sad." Sound familiar?

Good news: If you allow yourself to "stay with" your sorrow, rage, anxiety, etc., these negative emotions quickly lose their "charge." You'll feel free—and no longer compelled to replay old issues in your mind.

EXPAND THE MOMENT

I like to tell the story of the Zen monk and the tigers. To elude a hungry tiger, a monk climbed halfway down a cliff, until he was hanging by a branch above a ledge that held… a second tiger.

Beside the branch grew a strawberry bush. With his free hand, the monk picked a berry, popped it into his mouth and thought, "How delicious!"

Try to be like the monk. Consciously expand each moment of your life, free of regret about the past (tiger #1) or fear of the future (tiger #2). Remember—in the present there is no stress.

TIMESHIFTING EXERCISES

●**Develop rituals that help you stay "in the moment."** Let the ringing of a telephone signal you to pause and take a deep breath before answering…or gaze at a favorite photo when you feel anxious. One acquaintance of mine keeps a prism on her desk to look at when she feels worried. *Other rituals to cultivate…*

●**Do one thing at a time**, giving it your full attention. Pause for a few minutes after finishing one task before beginning another.

●**Take several three- to five-minute "mini breaks"** during the day to focus on your breathing. Slowly fill your lungs, then slowly release the air. Imagine watching your breath as it goes in and out.

Close your eyes and relax. Notice how your body feels. What does the room smell like? What sounds do you hear?

●**Get to meetings early** so you can compose yourself before others arrive.

●**Learn to timeshift in the midst of "busyness."** While waiting for a phone call or standing in line, shift into the present.

●**Create time boundaries.** Each day, set aside some time to devote entirely to yourself. During this period—ideally 15 minutes or so before work or after dinner—permit no meetings, no phone calls, no worries.

●**Honor the mundane.** We tend to focus on the day's highlights—a business luncheon, going to the movies, meeting someone for a date, etc. But to get the most out of life, we must learn to treasure mundane events, too.

If you're sweeping the floor, for example, bring full attention to the act. Notice the play of your muscles, the floor's appearance, the sound the broom bristles make, etc.

●**Create spontaneous time.** One of the happiest days of my life came during a forced layover in New Delhi, after my flight was postponed for 24 hours. I felt as if the day had been given to me, free of responsibilities or goals.

Nothing in particular happened that day, but the *spontaneity* of it all made it seem magical.

Paradoxically, I now *schedule* spontaneous time. You can, too. Open your date book to a day three weeks hence, and pencil in your own name. Set aside a few hours for an unplanned drive…or for just lying in bed.

●**Create time retreats.** Once a year, spend a week or more doing something extraordinary. I'm not talking about a jam-packed vacation, but a retreat into nature—anything that lets you shift to a slower rhythm.

Whatever your retreat involves, it should help you entrain to a slower, more peaceful pace.

How to Stop Worrying About Disease

Carla Cantor, coauthor, with Brian Fallon, MD, of *Phantom Illness: Shattering the Myth of Hypochondria.* Mariner.

Everyone worries about getting a serious illness *sometime*. But when occasional concern turns into a morbid obsession that interferes with daily life—it represents a more serious psychological problem.

Hypochondria is surprisingly common. One in 10 people who visit doctors' offices have the disorder to some degree…and three out of four patients have emotional problems that exacerbate their physical symptoms.

Unfortunately, few primary-care doctors take hypochondria seriously. Psychotherapists, too, have a poor track record. As a result, the majority of hypochondriacs suffer needlessly.

Good news: The outlook for hypochondriacs who get proper treatment is now excellent—thanks to psychoactive drugs, along with refinements in cognitive-behavioral and psychodynamic therapy.

WHAT CAUSES HYPOCHONDRIA

Hypochondriacs are *not* feigning illness. Their symptoms are *real*—but it's their interpretation of these symptoms that is unbalanced.

Everyday aches and pains are—to the hypochondriac—evidence of serious illness.

Hypochondria usually begins in the 20s or 30s—I was a college freshman when my hypochondria struck—although it can develop at any age. The condition is often portrayed as a woman's disorder, but it's just as common among men.

Single people seem to be especially susceptible. Psychologists theorize that's because they spend more time alone—and solitude encourages obsession about one's own health.

Some researchers believe that hypochondria has a biological basis—a pattern of neural "misfiring" in the brain that makes the individual unusually sensitive to physiological sensations.

Upbringing may also be a factor. Studies show that children of hypochondriac parents go to the emergency room more often—and show more disability and suicidal behavior—than children from normal families.

Presumably, the children are simply mimicking their parents' behavior.

It has also been theorized that parents who are overprotective unwittingly cause their children to grow up to be excessively vigilant about their health.

Others believe that hypochondria is simply a strategy for coping with emotional trauma—the death of a loved one, divorce, etc. The emotional pain caused by such trauma is so overwhelming that the person "buries" it under an obsession with disease.

EFFECTIVE MEDICATIONS

Though Prozac and related drugs have FDA approval for treating depression and obsessive-compulsive disorder (OCD), they are also effective against hypochondria.

In a study, 70% of hypochondriacs who took Prozac daily improved after 12 weeks.

Typical dosage: 60 to 80 milligrams (mg) a day. That's a bit higher than the 20 to 40 mg used to treat depression.

PSYCHOTHERAPY

Two forms of therapy are especially helpful…

•**Cognitive-behavioral therapy.** Patients learn to recognize the irrational statements they make to themselves…and learn new ways to interpret and respond to their symptoms.

With the therapist's help, patients confront the discomfort that arises in the absence of repeated trips to the doctor, endless discussions of symptoms and other rituals…and learn to replace them with alternative methods of relaxation—breathing techniques, relaxation exercises and cognitive strategies.

For referral to a cognitive-behavioral therapist in your area, contact the American Psychiatric Association (APA), 1000 Wilson Blvd., Suite 1825, Arlington, VA 22209 (888-357-7924). *www.psych.org.*

•**Psychodynamic therapy.** In this form of therapy—the traditional "talk cure"—patients explore how their fear of disease might serve an emotional function, such as avoiding other painful feelings and conflicts. They receive support in confronting these conflicts and finding constructive ways to deal with them.

For more information on psychodynamic therapy, contact the APA (see previous page).

WHO SHOULD SEEK HELP

Seek help if you answer "yes" to any of these four questions...

• **When you hear about an illness,** do you fear you have it?

• **Do you often ask family and friends** to reassure you that you're not ill?

• **Are you obsessed with one particular disease?**

• **Do you "doctor shop"**—go from doctor to doctor, rejecting one diagnosis after another?

If you suspect you may have hypochondria, consult a therapist with training and experience in treating the disease.

MORE HELPFUL RESOURCES

• **Obsessive-Compulsive Foundation**, 676 State St., New Haven, CT 06511 (203-401-2070, *www.ocfoundation.org*).

• **New York State Psychiatric Institute**, 1051 Riverside Dr., New York 10032 (212-543-5000, *www.nyspi.cpmc.columbia.edu*).

Creating Your Medical Family Tree To Save Your Life

The late Victor Herbert, MD, JD, chief, Mount Sinai Nutrition Center and Hematology and Nutrition Research Laboratory, Veterans' Affairs Medical Center, Bronx, NY. He is coauthor of *The Healing Diet: How to Reduce Your Risks and Live a Longer and Healthier Life if You Have a Family History of Cancer, Heart Disease, Hypertension, Diabetes, Alcoholism, Obesity, Food Allergies.* Macmillan.

If you have only a vague idea of your family's medical history, you may be setting yourself up for needless health problems.

All chronic diseases—including asthma, rheumatoid arthritis, multiple sclerosis, heart disease and cancer—have a hereditary component. Knowing that you carry the gene for a particular disease gives you a chance to prevent that disease...or to deal with it at its earliest stage, when it's more likely to be curable.

The key to gaining this invaluable knowledge is making a brief history of ailments that run in your biological family. A medical family tree is simple to create. More important, it pays off.

Example I: One of my patients, a 20-year-old man, discovered a family history of *hemochromatosis*, an often deadly disease in which the body absorbs too much iron. When a blood test showed that he suffered from a mild iron overload, he corrected the problem by donating blood on a monthly basis and giving up his daily iron supplement.

Example II: After her mother died of ovarian cancer, a 31-year-old woman put together a medical family tree. Using it, an oncologist determined that this woman and her sisters each had a 50% chance of developing ovarian cancer, too. So far, aggressive screenings and dietary strategies have kept the sisters cancer-free.

Example III: Another tree revealed a genetic link between five female relatives stricken with autoimmune disorders, including lupus, rheumatoid arthritis and a condition called Boeck's sarcoid. A dietician's question revealed that each woman had been taking alfalfa pills and vitamin E —both of which bring out latent genetic autoimmune disorders. When they stopped taking the supplements, symptoms gradually disappeared in four of the five women.

These are *not* isolated cases. In one study, 25,000 medical trees were responsible for identifying 43,000 individuals at high risk for hereditary ailments—and who were great candidates for preventive treatment.

It's easy to collect data on your immediate relatives, but don't stop there. Go back as many generations as possible—even if you must do some digging.

Don't worry if the information you unearth is inexact or incomplete. Anything that adds to the big health picture of your family could be helpful.

GATHERING INFORMATION

Make a list of all your living biological relatives...and any friends, neighbors, coworkers, etc., who can provide information on those who have died. If your family is small, interview relatives by phone.

Or, consider holding a family reunion—and add your tree-making project to the agenda.

Helpful resources: Medical records and death certificates can be obtained from doctors and hospitals, as well as from bureaus of vital statistics and state and county archives.

In addition, you can send a self-addressed, stamped, business-sized envelope to the National Genealogical Society (3108 Columbia Pike, Suite 300, Arlington, VA 22204) for more information. *www.ngsgenealogy.org.*

CREATING YOUR TREE

Get a piece of sturdy paper, measuring at least 36 inches wide and 30 inches long. Fold it into fourths, horizontally. Each section will represent a single generation.

If you plan to cover more than four generations, get bigger paper and fold it into more sections—or attach additional sheets.

Spread the paper flat on a table. In the bottom section, tape the health questionnaires on your children and/or those of your siblings.

In the section just above, tape your questionnaire and those of your spouse and spouse's siblings.

Above your own information, place your parents' and their siblings' information, and so on.

Position all the remaining questionnaires so that they branch outward and upward in the traditional family tree pattern.

Too much work? You can purchase a ready-made chart from the National Genealogical Society...or create your own using a computer program such as Windows *Family Tree Maker* (Genealogy.com, *www.genealogy.com*).

HOW TO USE YOUR TREE

Once your chart is complete, take it to your doctor. Ask him/her to study it for patterns of disease through the generations—and to identify family members who may be at risk.

Good news: Discovering that you are likely to carry the gene for a particular disease does not necessarily mean you will develop it. In many cases, a simple blood test will pinpoint your degree of risk.

Example: If breast cancer runs in your family...*and* your percentage of body fat is 20% or more above mean desirable body fat for your sex

and age...*and* your blood test shows elevated levels of estrogen, your doctor may order more rigorous tests and frequent checkups.

Almost certainly, the doctor will also recommend lifestyle modification. Whether a genetic predisposition leads to disease—or is suppressed—is at least partly determined by diet, exercise, smoking and other controllable factors.

Many genetic disorders, such as diabetes and some cancers, are triggered in part by obesity. Other conditions may be prevented by following a particular diet.

Example: If colon polyps run in your family, you should be examined regularly by a gastroenterologist...and eat a calcium-rich diet. Such a diet has been shown to help suppress polyps and colon cancer.

Once your family medical tree has alerted you and your doctor to a possible predisposition, controlling your lifestyle and getting regular checkups will give you the best chance of beating the genetic odds.

Secrets to Staying Healthy—and Happy— While Traveling

Karl Neumann, MD, clinical associate professor of pediatrics, Weill Medical College of Cornell University, New York City. He is also editor of Traveling Healthy Newsletter.

No matter what your destination or why you're traveling, fatigue, stress, an upset stomach or worse can spell disaster for your trip.

Fortunately, the wear and tear of travel can be kept to a minimum with simple advance planning.

Here are some easy ways to make your travel more comfortable—and healthful...

SELF-CARE CHECKLIST

Your chief consideration when packing for a trip is where you're going, how long you'll be away and what the climate is like at your destination. But no matter what sort of trip you're planning, bring along a well-stocked self-care kit. *It should be easily accessible in your carry-on luggage and should contain some or all of the following...*

●**Antacid.** Familiar store-bought remedies such as Maalox, Mylanta, Gelusil, Tums or Rolaids combat the stomach upset, heartburn and abdominal cramping sometimes caused by unfamiliar food or drink—or overindulgence in either.

●**Diarrhea remedy.** Over-the-counter preparations like Imodium A-D, Kaopectate or Pepto-Bismol are all effective at stopping diarrhea. Tablets are easier to take along on a trip, although the liquid forms of these medications usually offer faster relief.

●**Laxative.** On the road, constipation is often more of a problem than diarrhea.

Reason: Your diet while traveling is apt to lack high-fiber foods. Also, it may be difficult while you are traveling to maintain a regular exercise routine. Take along some Metamucil, FiberCon or Senokot just in case.

●**Antihistamine.** The over-the-counter medication Benadryl is effective against a host of potential allergens and irritants and is well-tolerated by most people. If you have to stay alert, ask your doctor about Claritin. It's now available without a prescription and it causes little or no drowsiness.

●**Antibiotic.** For tooth abscesses, severe bronchitis, festering skin wounds or other stubborn bacterial infections, ask your doctor to prescribe an antibiotic in advance.

Caution: Antibiotics should be used *only under a doctor's supervision.* Call your doctor at home for instructions if you need to use one.

●**Motion sickness remedy.** Dramamine or Bonine tablets are effective medicines.

Caution: Dramamine and Bonine can cause drowsiness. Avoid them if you have to stay alert.

●**Athlete's foot remedy.** Be sure to include antifungal foot powder or solutions like Lotrimin, Micatin or Tinactin in your travel kit, since showers in hotel rooms and fitness centers are not always fungus-free.

Also helpful: Rubber thongs for the shower.

●**Sunscreen, sunglasses and a wide-brimmed hat.** These are a must for travel to sunny places or if you intend to be outdoors for extended periods of time.

Important: Your sunscreen should have an SPF of at least 15 and should guard against both UVB and UVA rays.

●**Insect repellent.** For adults, look for one that contains 20% to 30% DEET.

●**Aspirin, acetaminophen or ibuprofen.**

●**A decongestant, as well as a supply of facial tissues.**

You might also want to bring along a basic first-aid kit containing an antibacterial cream or ointment, bandages, gauze, thermometer, scissors and tweezers.

If you wear corrective lenses, pack a spare pair of contacts or eyeglasses—plus your prescription.

If you intend to swim in unchlorinated water, take along a remedy for swimmer's ear, an infection marked by redness, itching and pain of the outer ear canal. I recommend an over-the-counter preparation called Vosol.

FIGHTING JET LAG

Anytime you fly across several time zones, you disrupt the body's circadian rhythms. The resulting jet lag should be thought of not as a special problem, but as another form of manageable stress. *Ways to control it...*

●**Avoid drinking alcohol during your flight.** Alcohol is a depressant, and can aggravate lethargy and fatigue, two classic symptoms of jet lag. It can also cause restlessness, which can disturb your sleep or keep you from sleeping altogether. And because it acts as a diuretic, alcohol can leave you feeling dehydrated.

●**Limit your consumption of caffeine.** Like alcohol, caffeine is a diuretic that can leave you feeling dehydrated and out of sorts. Too much caffeine can also cause nervousness, anxiety, tremors and insomnia.

●**Drink plenty of water.** Studies have shown that even slight dehydration can cause listlessness and fatigue and can even make you prone to mental errors—symptoms similar to those of jet lag.

Bear in mind that you may be dehydrated even *before* departure.

Reason: Your eating and drinking patterns may be erratic in the hours before your flight. Breathing dry cabin air only increases this dehydration and its enervating effects. To stay hydrated, drink plenty of water or other nonalcoholic beverages before and during your flight—one eight-ounce glass every two to three hours. Don't wait until you feel thirsty—by then you may already be dehydrated.

SAFE FOOD AND DRINK

Regions of the world fall into three "tiers"...

- **Europe, North America and Australia.**

- **Israel and the Caribbean.**

- **The rest of the Middle East, most of Africa, the Far East** and other developing regions.

Anytime you travel to the second or third tier, you must be especially vigilant about what you eat and drink. *Self-defense...*

- **Eat cooked food while it is still hot.** Make sure meats are well-done. Throughout developing countries, undercooked beef and pork are major sources of tapeworms and other parasites. Likewise, all poultry, seafood and vegetables should be fresh and thoroughly cooked.

- **Avoid peeled fruits** and those with broken skin. Watch out for raw vegetable salads, too. They can be contaminated with bacteria from the food preparer's hands or from the water used to rinse the vegetables.

- **Avoid custards, pastries and other baked desserts.** These foods are often contaminated with microbes that trigger gastric distress, especially if improperly refrigerated.

Exception: Served hot from the oven, these foods are generally safe. If you want dessert, stick to wrapped candy or fresh fruit that you peel yourself.

- **Stick to bottled or canned beverages.** Don't use ice cubes, which might be contaminated. Avoid milk, milk products and foods that are prepared with them unless you are positive that they have been properly pasteurized.

- **Avoid bread that has been left in open baskets**—it may have been exposed to flies and other disease-bearing insects. If you're not certain whether bread has been properly stored, remove the crust and eat only the *interior* of the loaf.

WATCHING OUT FOR INFECTIOUS DISEASES

If you are planning a trip to the tropics, get immunizations *at least one month before your departure.* Frantic, last-minute efforts to obtain shots only compound the ordinary stress occasioned by an overseas journey. And multiple immunizations require several shots over a period of days or weeks.

A 24-hour hotline run by the Centers for Disease Control and Prevention (CDC) (800-232-4636 or 877-394-8747, *www.cdc.gov*) provides recorded messages outlining immunization requirements and recommendations for international travel.

To avoid malaria, ask your doctor about taking prophylactic drugs. Some must be taken one week before you travel to ensure that adequate blood levels of the drug are reached before you arrive—and that any adverse reactions occur before you leave for your trip.

How to Read Your Body's Messages

Martin Rush, MD, a psychiatrist in private practice for more than 30 years who lives in Middletown, OH. He is author of *Decoding the Secret Language of Your Body.* Fireside.

Many physical problems, from mere discomfort to chronic pain to serious illness, have psychological as well as physical roots.

Of course, viruses, bacteria, muscle strain and other physical factors play a large role in making us feel awful. However, these troublemakers are more likely to do damage if we are also troubled by distressing emotions—such as fear, anger, guilt or sadness.

The problem isn't the negative *emotions* themselves—everyone feels them at one time or another. It's *repressing* these emotions that gets our bodies into the act. When we stuff our feelings inside instead of expressing them, the body's response is to send a physical signal—which can't be ignored so easily.

In my 30-plus years as a family physician and then as a psychiatrist, I've noticed that when people identify the stressful situation that preceded a physical symptom—and then talk about the feelings associated with that situation—the physical problem often goes away and their emotional burden lightens as well.

I do not mean to trivialize illness, nor do I claim that talking about your feelings is a substitute for good medical treatment. Physical problems are very real and may well require physical intervention. But if the emotional roots of a problem are neglected, the issue will keep showing up in the body—in one way or another—until it's resolved.

DECODING YOUR BODY'S LANGUAGE

How do you uncover the hidden emotions that are behind a physical problem? Try thinking back on the stresses that were present in your life just before the illness occurred...or simply review recent events that might have upset you.

Since you might not recognize certain situations as upsetting, it's a good idea to have a friend (or therapist) help you with this step. Others may spot connections you missed.

Once identified, get those painful feelings off your mind (and body) by talking to someone about them.

If you have trouble identifying the source, pick up clues from the physical location of the problem. Although each person's situation is unique, I have observed a number of common themes in my patients (and myself).

COLD HANDS AND FEET

When hands and feet get cold or numb, it's usually because the nervous system has signaled the arteries to contract, reducing blood supply to the extremities. What causes this to occur? I've noticed that the phenomenon often seems to strike people who are reluctant to

"reach out" for their desires—they're afraid of getting the very thing they want.

Example I: The old cliché about brides or grooms getting "cold feet" isn't just an expression—it's a genuine physical phenomenon that expresses the conflict between the longing for connection and the fear of responsibility.

Example II: When I took up skiing in my 50s, my feet and hands got so icy cold—no matter how many layers of socks and mittens I wore—that I couldn't enjoy myself. As I thought about the issue, I remembered that although I had always longed to learn to ski, this pastime had been beyond my family's means. I realized that I was terrified of enjoying the kind of carefree pleasure that was denied my parents.

As I faced this conflict, I became more relaxed...and now I'm quite comfortable on the slopes!

SORE THROAT

For many people, the throat is where they store tension when they have been slighted, insulted or otherwise rejected. These wounds to the spirit create an urgent need for reassurance, comfort and love.

On a primitive level, we associate those yearnings with food—and especially the security we felt as nursing infants.

Years later, when we feel rejected, the throat contracts instinctively, as though to re-create that old feeling of comfort. But when comfort isn't forthcoming, the protective mucus that lines the back of the throat dries up, leaving the area vulnerable to incoming germs.

When your feelings are hurt, say so—to yourself, to the person who hurt you (if appropriate)...and to other people, if the insult was serious. Be sure the people you tell about the incident can be depended upon to respond with the kindness and reassurance you crave.

BOWEL TROUBLE

Constipation, irritable bowel syndrome (IBS) and other problems related to elimination tend to be associated with holding in "nasty" feelings—anger, spitefulness, jealousy, disappointment—because we're afraid people won't like the "real" us.

Hemorrhoids are another expression of this conflict.

Example: A woman in one of my psychotherapy groups was plagued with constipation. No one in the group had ever heard her raise her voice. Encouraged to talk about her childhood, she described growing up as the middle sibling and learning to keep her feelings to herself in order to avoid confrontation. As an adult, she continued to squelch her own needs in favor of tending to the demands of her husband and children. As she became more comfortable discussing her feelings freely with the group, she gradually learned to stand up for herself, and constipation ceased to be a problem for her.

LOWER BACK PAIN

Carrying too much weight can cause the muscles supporting the back to go into spasm, leading to acute or chronic pain. The excess weight can be physical or emotional—when we feel overburdened and want someone to take care of us for a change.

Example: A middle-aged man developed back trouble after his aging mother came to live with him and his wife. He loved his mother and wanted to help her, but having her join the household and arranging for her care put him under a great deal of stress. He didn't want to hurt her feelings by airing his complaints—and he also felt selfish and guilty about resenting her.

When he was finally able to talk to his wife about his feelings, he no longer felt as though he were carrying the burden alone. Once his back didn't need to speak for him, the pain lessened dramatically.

HOW TO DEAL WITH HIDDEN FEELINGS

Though many people do find therapy valuable, you don't necessarily have to talk to a therapist to discharge these emotions. A friend, relative, colleague or member of the clergy can be just as helpful—if that person can be counted on to be supportive.

You may not even need a long, drawn-out ranting session. Often it's enough simply to acknowledge the previously buried feeling ("That made me really mad") and have someone affirm your reaction ("I can see why you felt that way").

If you're concerned about wearing out your friends or being viewed as a complainer, spread the burden around. Mention the issue briefly to a few different people. You'll feel better each time you talk about it.

Dr. Joyce Brothers's Secrets of Winning The Ever-Changing Game of Life

Joyce Brothers, PhD, the nationally renowned psychologist. She is author of numerous books, including How to Get Whatever You Want Out of Life. *Ballantine.*

I don't believe in luck. I believe that good fortune comes through hard work and preparation, so that you are able to take advantage of life's big opportunities when they present themselves to you.

However, there are steps you can take to ensure that your efforts are well placed and you can recognize opportunities when they appear.

CLARIFY YOUR ASPIRATIONS

The first and most important step is to discover what you really want out of life. Before dreams can come true, you have to identify them.

This, of course, is one of the most difficult discussions you'll ever have with yourself. Most of us find identifying our goals and aspirations too broad to ponder and too difficult to answer.

In fact, most people know what they want out of life—*on a subconscious level.* The goal is to bring the knowledge up to our conscious levels, where it can be articulated and achieved.

Helpful: Quick—ask yourself right now what you want most in the world and, without stopping to think, write down the first three things that come into your head. Read your list, and put it away.

Repeat the process weekly for six weeks. At the end of six weeks, take out all the lists and study your answers. You will find a pattern—the responses that repeat themselves are your dreams.

If that doesn't show you what you want most in the world, you will at least have a much clearer idea.

MASTER THE ART OF POWER READING

Almost every goal we set involves improving ourselves through studying material with which we are unfamiliar. The ability to read and retain what you need to know in a hurry is the basic tool for getting what you want.

The problem is that few people have efficient techniques for absorbing written materials, so progress is slow. *Here is my five-step strategy—it works no matter what you want to study...*

●**Get an overview.** Whether it's one document or a stack of books, rapidly skim the material. If you don't need to absorb the material overnight, decide how many days you can devote to it. Then divide the text into even amounts.

●**Divide each day's material into three equal parts.** Plan to spend the most time on the second part. Since our brains learn most easily at the beginning and end of a study session, the middle section will give you the most trouble.

●**Internal command.** As you read the first part, tell yourself that when you're done, you're going to close the book and recite what you've read. This internal command sets your mind so you can concentrate better.

●**Turn over the material when you've finished the first part.** The goal is to recite aloud the essence of what you've read. I suggest turning over the material because we tend to be unconscious cheaters.

●**Recite aloud the major points of what you just learned.** Even better, write them down while you're reciting. There's a direct relationship between senses and memory. The more ways your brain senses something, the better you remember it. When you finish, check your work against the material to be sure you are right—or to see what needs more work.

Important: When reciting material, pause for a few seconds between sections. Otherwise, new information won't be retained.

Repeat steps three, four and five with the remaining sections.

CREATE A POSITIVE "HALO EFFECT"

What psychologists call the *halo effect* has nothing to do with goodness or godliness. It has to do with your aura and how it affects other people's first impressions of you.

The impression you leave with others who could be helpful to you will create a halo effect that radiates out to color their opinion of everything you do in the future.

Five rules for creating a great impression with other people...

●**Appear knowledgeable and smart.** Before meeting new people, determine what subjects are likely to come up in conversation and learn as much as you can about those subjects. The goal isn't to appear as a know-it-all but as someone who is informed and well-read.

●**Avoid smoking**, excessive drinking and other bad habits. All create a negative impression and shift the focus away from you and to your habit.

●**Be on time.** Not only is lateness discourteous, it makes people think you don't value their time. Lateness is a sure way to create a negative halo effect.

●**Get the person's name right**, and use it a few times while speaking.

●**Don't talk too much**—or interrupt the person speaking. There is a great deal of power in silence, especially if you are attentive to the person speaking.

LEARN THE SUBTLE ART OF FLATTERY

No matter how successful people become, nearly everyone has an inferiority complex. So when you tell people they are talented, marvelous or brilliant, they will appreciate the compliment and be much more likely to do things for you.

The most effective flattery always comes from the heart. The best compliments come from people who truly believe what they are saying and recognize areas of real interest to the person being flattered.

Learn to appreciate aspects of other people's personalities or work. Be confident enough in yourself to recognize *their* strengths.

Secondhand flattery is also tremendously effective.

Example: "Greg told me that everyone over in your office is excited about the new project you started. Congratulations."

STRIVE TO BECOME ENGROSSED IN YOUR WORK

In every endeavor, there are moments of magic experienced by people who are acting with total involvement. This peak experience —similar to the high long-distance runners experience—is what psychologists call *flow*.

To achieve this state, avoid doing what is easy. Instead, focus on challenging yourself, and work at it as intensely as you can.

But don't pick an overwhelming challenge that exceeds your limits. Choose the kind that stretches you and pushes your limits.

You must also set aside a significant span of uninterrupted time. It is virtually impossible to switch into a flow state in less than half an hour. It is *absolutely* impossible to do so if you are bedeviled by interruptions.

Use It...or Lose It Physically...Mentally

Martin Groder, MD, a Chapel Hill, NC, psychiatrist and business consultant. He is coauthor of *Business Games: How to Recognize the Players and Deal with Them*. Bottom Line Books.

The longer you neglect your talents and special skills that were developed over the years, the harder it is to restore them and the less likely you'll be able to bring them back to their old levels of excellence. Once you've reached the point of no return, you probably won't even make the effort.

The deterioration of our abilities occurs due to disuse, and this law applies equally to both your mental and physical abilities—to chess as well as to tennis.

WHY WE LOSE IT

Much of the decline in strength and stamina that we blame on age is actually due to the disuse cycle. Slow down, and it gets harder to pick up the pace again—so the natural tendency is to slow down even more.

Activities as diverse as shooting pool, playing the piano, speaking a foreign language or responding sexually are coordinated by complex interactions of nerve cells in the brain.

When you practice, these neurons actually grow microscopic filaments to connect to one another. It's a process known as *arborization*. When you stop practicing, these connections wither away.

Every time you learn new skills or master fresh areas of knowledge, neurons secrete growth hormones that foster arborization, thus stimulating their own growth and the growth of their neighbors.

BRAIN DRAIN

Part of the brain is devoted to learning, striving to meet challenges and dealing with frustration, while another part takes care of establishing habits and routines. Let one part atrophy, and its functions are taken over by the areas that are used more.

When you stop challenging yourself and expanding your skills, that part of your brain goes quiet and brain activity shifts to its humdrum mode. The more you let yourself become stodgy and fail to challenge yourself, the harder it is to reactivate that part of your brain.

Motivation is often a major victim of this process. Once you let your skills decay, it's harder to feel excited.

Example: Playing piano poorly...or not seeing results from exercising...isn't very rewarding, so you're tempted to let the activity slide altogether rather than make the effort to correct the situation or merely stay at a level that matches your abilities.

A LITTLE PRACTICE

Finding the time to maintain skills in the midst of our busy lives may seem an elusive goal. But it's important to remember that in midlife or beyond, you get the most benefit from the first small effort. By practicing your skills, even just a little each week, you will be able to exercise the capacities that are important to you.

Practicing many of your skills just a little bit is more important than concentrating on just one or two.

How much practice is enough? There's no universal rule, but when it comes to physical exercise, a workout every other day for 20 to

40 minutes appears to be enough to keep you in shape…and healthy.

In music, too, it appears that a half-hour to one hour of practice every other day will maintain a significant level of skill.

So—using what you don't want to lose at least two to three times every week for a half-hour to an hour is a good minimum for which to strive.

MAKE PRACTICE COUNT

To ensure the time you devote to maintaining your skills is well spent, take yourself, your talents and your strengths seriously enough to optimize the conditions for fruitful practice. *Here's how to do it…*

● **Use the right equipment.** If you're walking to maintain fitness, get good walking shoes. Want to hone your piano-playing skills? Get the piano tuned. It will make the experience more rewarding and increase the odds you'll keep doing it.

● **Make practice enjoyable.** Some people like to walk, run or bike alone…while others need to feel the support of fellow strivers in a gym or health club. Ask yourself what works best for you.

Example: Will sharing your essays with others motivate you to keep writing? Join a workshop or organize a writers' group on your own.

● **Find your level of practice and stick with it.** Some people want to keep their skills sharp in a relaxed way, without strain, as an enjoyable leisure pursuit. Others prize the exhilaration of feeling themselves tested and stretched.

Let your personal preference guide you in choosing whether you practice your skills for fun or find challenging opponents who will force you to stretch.

● **Know your limits.** A big mistake many people make when practicing is falling into the "pro" trap. They don't bother practicing their skills because they know they won't ever become the champions they so admire.

Admire those who have achieved excellence, but don't model yourself after them. Realize your limitations, and remind yourself that the goal is to keep your abilities alive, not to conquer the world.

BE KIND TO YOURSELF

Attitude plays a big role in how well you perform and whether you stick to your practice regimen. A positive outlook fuels your determination to keep your capacities sharp, while negativity kills motivation. *Helpful…*

● **Be generous and accepting toward yourself**, particularly if you're trying to retain or regain competence in an area where you were once highly skilled.

● **Accept the role of a student**, even if your endeavor is something at which you once excelled.

● **Don't match your performance against memories** of a younger self at the peak of your powers…at a time when lots of practice had honed your skills.

● **Be a kindly, patient teacher or coach to yourself**, the kind who throws the ball to a kid a thousand times before the child learns to catch it properly. Summon up thoughts of past mentors. Enlist patient, supportive companions who will encourage you.

Important: Keep bad coaches and negative role models out of the picture. Listen for that nasty self-critical inner voice—we all have one—and silence it. Avoid "friends" who will sap your confidence.

PRACTICE PEOPLE SKILLS

The abilities you need to get along with others—communicating, working as part of a team, compromising, making helpful judgments instead of destructive criticisms—also need practice to stay sharp.

If you work at home, as increasing numbers of people do today, you may lack the day-to-day interaction that maintains these parts of your personality.

Solitude is important as well. People who are constantly surrounded by others—mothers who have young children…anyone who works in a busy office and comes home to a lively house—can lose the capacity for quiet and reflection.

12 Quick and Easy Things You Can Do to Improve Your Health

Harold H. Bloomfield, MD, a leading psychological educator for 25 years. A best-selling author, he is coauthor of *The Power of 5*. Rodale Press.

No more excuses. Here are some ways to boost your health and happiness—*in five minutes or less.*

1. Inhale an energizing scent. Research suggests that lemon and peppermint scents are energizing. To exploit this finding, have an occasional cup of lemon or peppermint tea...or chew peppermint gum. Keep a bottle of peppermint and/or lemon extract to sniff...add a couple of drops to a small scent dispenser...or experiment with potpourri containing other energizing scents such as pine, jasmine, lavender or orange.

2. Sip ice water. It keeps your cells hydrated *and* helps you burn calories. *Reason:* Whenever you drink something cold, your body raises your metabolism to keep your body temperature from falling. That process burns calories—eight 16-ounce glasses of ice water will burn an extra 200 calories per day.

Strategy: Start the day with eight to 16 ounces of ice water. Sip a 16-ounce glass every hour or two, keeping one next to you at work and at home. All told, you should drink eight glasses a day. Finish up by 7 p.m.—to avoid having to use the bathroom after you go to bed.

3. Practice "one-breath" meditation. You don't have to spend years mastering meditation. This one-breath method is a powerful, straightforward relaxation technique that can be practiced anytime, anywhere. Try it whenever you feel fatigued or out of sorts.

What to do: Sit in a comfortable chair. Straighten your back, relax your shoulders and take a deep breath. Let the air "open" your chest. Imagine it filling every cell in your body. Hold the breath for a moment, then exhale, releasing every bit of tension.

Also helpful: One-touch relaxation. Place your fingertips just in front of your ears. Inhale

and clench your teeth. Hold for five seconds. Exhale, and let your jaw muscles go loose.

Repeat this exercise three more times, using half the original tension, then one-fourth, then one-eighth. Then take a deep breath, press your fingertips against your jaw, let it go slack and say, *Ah-b-b-b.* Imagine you are breathing out tightness.

4. Minimize noise at home and at work. Loud or irritating sound creates severe emotional and physical tension. Fortunately, many aggravating noises can be silenced.

Strategy I: Place foam pads under blenders and other kitchen appliances...and under printers, typewriters and other office machines.

Strategy II: Before buying an air conditioner or another potentially noisy appliance, compare noise levels of different brands. Use noise-absorbing insulation around dishwashers.

5. Bask in bright light. Most people get a powerful surge of energy from sunlight or bright indoor light. Try moving your desk chair closer to a window...or, better yet, take a five-minute outdoor walk every few hours.

Also helpful: Each day, get five minutes of nonpeak sun (before 10 a.m. or after 3 p.m.) without sunscreen or sunglasses to enjoy the full mood-lifting effects of sunlight.

Indoors, replace incandescent or fluorescent bulbs with full-spectrum "daylight" bulbs from a lighting or health-food store. *Cost:* $9 and up for bulbs, $16 and up for tubes.

6. Do abdominal exercise. Use this technique while sitting at your desk or while stuck in traffic. Sit up straight. Place hands on hips with thumbs pointing toward your back. Exhale slowly and completely, pushing the last air out forcefully with your lower abdominals.

Repeat up to 10 times a day. You might try one or two stomach-flattening sessions just before meals, at stoplights on your commute or each time you sit down at your desk. These exercises are great muscle toners for the lower abdomen.

7. Perform mental "cross-training." Cross-training is the process by which you "stretch" your mind in as many different directions as possible by engaging in a variety of mental and physical activities. Word puzzles and other games are an easy way to perform this cross-training. Pick a random sentence from the newspaper, then rearrange the words to make a new sentence…play Scrabble or do crossword puzzles…challenge a friend to chess or checkers.

8. Cook with "nutriceuticals." These are vegetables, herbs and spices that have specific healing properties…

●**Garlic and onions** boost the immune system, helping prevent colds.

●**Basil, cumin and turmeric** help prevent cancer of the bladder and prostate.

●**Black pepper, jalapeños, hot red peppers and mustard** all boost your metabolism for several hours. That helps burn fat.

●**Cinnamon** helps metabolize sugar, keeping your blood sugar levels steady.

9. Check your reading posture. Poor posture—leaning over a desk, for instance—can cause tension headaches, vision problems and pain in the jaw and/or neck.

Self-defense: Bring reading material up to your field of vision or use a book stand to hold a book at the proper angle. If you spend a lot of time on the telephone, get a headset. Don't cradle the phone between ear and shoulder.

10. Do trigger-point therapy. Wherever you feel tense, feel for a tight band of muscle tissue—a trigger point. Press or squeeze it with light to moderate pressure. Continue pressing for five to 10 seconds, then release.

11. Curb indoor pollution. Whenever possible, keep your windows open. All gas appliances should be checked annually and properly vented to the outside to limit their output of carbon monoxide. Use exhaust fans in the bathroom, kitchen and garage whenever you use these rooms. Make your home and office smoke-free.

12. Do absolutely nothing. "Lyming" is the Caribbean art of doing nothing—without feeling guilty about it. Try lyming frequently to give your brain time to process all the information it receives over the course of a day.

Helpful: Take a five-minute "mental vacation" every few hours. Picture your favorite beach or other getaway place. The idea is to escape the rat race briefly—but completely.

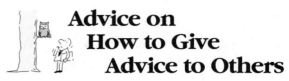

Advice on How to Give Advice to Others

Jeswald W. Salacuse, Henry J. Braker Professor of Commercial Law, Fletcher School of Law and Diplomacy at Tufts University in Medford, MA. He is author of *The Art of Advice: How to Give It and How to Take It.* Crown.

There is an art to giving advice. When you have mastered the art, people will listen to what you say…and come back for more. Both you and those who consult you will benefit from the relationship.

BENEFITS OF ADVISING OTHERS

Professionals are paid very well for their expert advice. But there are other reasons for giving advice.

●**Parents advise their children** out of love and concern for their welfare.

●**Senior managers counsel junior executives** because of idealism, friendship and good sound business. Just knowing that other people want your advice boosts your own self-esteem.

ADVISING IS AN ART

To be a good adviser it is not enough to provide information, no matter how accurate. You must be able to form relationships with others that can help them find the best solutions to their specific problems.

Example: A good parent knows what his/her children should do—and must be able to talk to them in a way that shows he understands their concerns.

HOW TO GIVE ADVICE

Good advice is the product of a three-step process…

●**Understand the other person's particular problem and objectives.** Your goal is not to demonstrate your own superior wisdom, but to help someone else solve his problem. To do that, always listen closely to what the other person says. Try to discover how he got into the current situation…exactly what problem he wants you to help him solve…how he hopes to benefit from your advice.

To help another person open up to you: Break the ice by starting off with something relevant about yourself...encourage him to discuss the problem in his own way...don't interrupt...don't anticipate...never suggest a solution before you understand the problem.

Example: An unhappy wife tells you about her husband's inattention and prolonged absences from home and asks your advice. Don't immediately tell her to change all the house locks, empty out the joint checking account and call a divorce lawyer. If you draw her out some more, you may find that she really wants to rebuild her relationship with her husband, whose troubled business is threatened with bankruptcy.

Important: Understand your precise role. Before you start dispensing advice, make sure the other person really wants it. He may just be looking for a sympathetic listener.

If the other person wants your advice, determine whether you are qualified to give it.

Ask yourself: Do I have the knowledge, skills and time I need to help this person?

Example: Martha often helps other people fill in standard tax returns. While helping a recently widowed friend, she discovers a tax problem outside her experience. Martha should not just go ahead and guess what her friend should do. She should tell her to get professional assistance. If the friend has never dealt with financial matters, Martha could help her find the right adviser.

●**Identify and evaluate the options and explain them as clearly as possible.** Don't try to be a solo performer—and don't always apply your favorite solution to a particular problem. You may know more about the technical details of the problems other people face...but they know better than you how well any proposed solution will fit them.

Example: If a couple about to retire asks your advice, don't automatically tell them to sell their big house, invest the profits and move to a small condo. They may prefer, for instance, to keep the house so they can put up many relatives and friends who come to visit.

●**Let the other person make the decision.** After you give your best advice to the person who consulted you, remember that he—not you—will have to live with the consequences.

That does not mean you wash your hands of any responsibility. In most cases, you should leave the decision entirely up to the

person who asked your advice. But it is appropriate for you to intervene in the decision if he asks explicitly what you would do...or wants to do something immoral or very risky ...or does not understand the likely outcome of a particular choice.

ETHICAL RULES OF ADVISING

Do no harm. The person who has chosen you as an adviser thinks you will be able to help him.

Make sure before you give any advice that following it will not cause him harm. Give pure advice. Your job is to help someone else make the right decision, not to benefit yourself.

A good adviser is loyal to his client and committed to giving the best advice. He shows respect to the person who consulted him, is careful to use his full attention and skill to find the best solution and is reliable in keeping his promises.

Important: As an adviser, you need your own adviser—someone trustworthy to give you counsel on difficult problems.

KNOW WHEN TO STOP

When you have given the advice the other person needs to solve his problem, step aside. *Reasons to quit...*

●**The individual who approached you has reached the goal he originally sought.** Make sure you understand the goal clearly from the very beginning of the task.

Example: If your children ask your opinion about a house they are thinking about buying, do not assume that if they purchase it they will want your unsolicited advice on how to furnish it.

●**You are in over your head.** If this happens to you, explain the problem frankly—like Martha in the earlier example, who agreed to help her friend with her taxes but then found that the job exceeded her knowledge and her capabilities.

●**Your situation changes.** You may want to retire from the role of advice-giver or just don't have the time or energy needed to keep advising someone.

If he is continuously relying on your advice, give him adequate notice that you are no longer available and—if he really needs good advice

—try to steer him to someone who can take your place.

BOTTOM LINE

People who ask for your advice are really paying you a compliment. They are showing very high regard for your expertise and judgment. Make sure you repay it by giving the best advice possible.

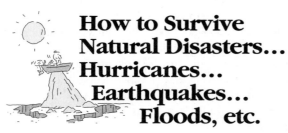

How to Survive Natural Disasters... Hurricanes... Earthquakes... Floods, etc.

Betsy Shand and Janice McCann, coauthors of Surviving Natural Disasters. *DIMI.*

If you think that you'll never be hit by a natural disaster, you're not alone. That's what people in New Orleans thought before Hurricane Katrina.

Reality: There's hardly a home in the country that is truly safe from some type of disaster, ranging from major catastrophes, such as a major flood, to relatively minor emergencies, such as electrical blackouts and freak snow storms.

Good news: Commonsense precautions go a long way in avoiding loss of property and life.

Though the list of precautions might seem long, they can be taken over a period of weeks or months. And once you have the measures in place, there's little left to do except cope with the next disaster with greater peace of mind.

EMERGENCY PROVISIONS

Think of weathering a disaster as a little like camping out in your own home, where electricity and water have been cut off. *Store in a closet or other convenient location...*

●**Food that can be eaten with little or no preparation**, such as peanut butter, whole-grain crackers, baby food, powdered milk and cold cereal.

●**Several gallons of water**, which you can buy in bottles at the supermarket.

●**Food and water** for a pet if you have one.

●**A first-aid kit** that contains not just the standard items such as bandages and iodine— but also scissors, needles and thread and several days' supply of whatever medication you're currently taking. Kits can be bought from the Red Cross, camping-supply shops and most drugstores.

●**Flashlights with batteries stored separately** so they'll stay fresh.

●**Cash.** If electricity goes out, banks and Automatic Teller Machines will not be working.

●**An extra pair of eyeglasses** or contact lenses.

●**A ladder and basic tools**, including a crowbar, screwdriver, saw and hammer.

Keep a full or nearly full tank of gas in your car. The last experience you want is seeing an empty gas gauge while you're racing to escape rising flood waters. (Don't store gasoline outside your car's tank.)

DOCUMENT DEFENSE

Since disasters often destroy homes and their contents, store copies of important documents and vital information with a trusted friend. *Examples...*

●**A copy of your insurance policy** and the phone number of your agent.

●**Your attorney's name and number.**

●**A list of health problems**, medication and your doctor's number.

●**The location of your safe-deposit box** and an extra key.

●**Banking information**, such as Certificates of Deposit and checking account numbers.

As a rule, choose an out-of-town friend to hold these items since a neighbor's house may be just as vulnerable as yours.

DISASTER TRAINING

First-aid training does more than let you help the injured. It also builds up a sense of confidence that can be vital in getting you through a disaster. The Red Cross, YMCAs, YWCAs, community centers and many hospitals offer courses in first aid. Courses in preventing and surviving fires are offered by most fire departments. But even if you don't take a course, make your own plan to evacuate in case of fire. *Key elements of the plan...*

●**Install smoke alarms and/or sprinklers.** (Insurance companies often lower their rates on homes with sprinklers.)

●**Store towels, water and a rope ladder** under your bed. In case of fire, you can often buy lots of escape time by soaking towels in water and stuffing them under doors to block incoming smoke.

●**Keep fire extinguishers in appropriate places around the house.**

●**Sleep with the doors closed.**

●**Plan an evacuation procedure**, and practice it periodically, just as you'd go through a fire drill.

Beware of items that can become hazardous in a disaster...

●**Difficult-to-see power lines** that have fallen or are dangling.

●**Water pipes, electricity lines and gas mains** in your home. Ask utility companies to show you how to shut them off. That's what to do if water is leaking, if you smell gas or if you suspect an electrical problem after a disaster.

NEIGHBORHOOD TEAMS

Organize a neighborhood disaster committee whose members can come to each other's aid in the event of an emergency. Working as a team, neighbors can often save a home if, for example, the owners are away and a gas main has ruptured.

Many residents have skills or equipment that can be invaluable in a disaster.

Examples: Doctors, carpenters, plumbers or neighbors with generators or cellular phones.

Key: A system that lets homeowners signal their postdisaster status to the rest of the neighborhood. Pin large white, yellow or red ribbons to your door or other conspicuous location.

White means all is okay. Yellow indicates residents are fine but need some assistance. Red signals an emergency and the immediate need for help.

THE RIGHT INSURANCE

Few events are more disheartening than surviving a disaster only to discover that insurance won't cover your property loss. *To avoid the problem...*

●**Buy a homeowner's policy** that covers the *replacement* of your home and contents. Many policies cover only the current value. That means if a Regency chair is destroyed in a fire, insurance pays only the *current* value of a chair, not the replacement value of the antique.

●**Choose an insurance policy that pays your living expenses** for an adequate period of time for putting your house back in living condition.

●**To document the value of your home and its contents**, keep all receipts for items you buy. Then photograph or videotape your possessions, or consider hiring a professional appraiser to put a price on items for which you don't have receipts.

How to Avoid the All-Too-Common Common Cold

David A.J. Tyrrell, MD, retired director of the Common Cold Unit of the British Medical Research Council in Salisbury, England.

We hear reports of all kinds of remedies for the common cold, from sucking on zinc lozenges to rubbing garlic on your clothes. To find out what medical science has to say about such remedies, we talked to Dr. David A.J. Tyrrell, one of the world's foremost experts on the common cold.

●**What causes colds?** Colds are caused by any of several hundred different viruses specially adapted to grow in the nose (*rhinoviruses* and *coronaviruses*). That's why it has proven impossible—so far—to make a reliable vaccine. We simply haven't been able to come up with one that's effective against all the viruses.

Smokers are particularly vulnerable to colds. Tobacco smoke dries out the mucus membranes lining the mouth and nose, impairing their ability to fend off viruses. Moderate drinkers (those who have the equivalent of one glass of wine a day) seem to be less susceptible.

One thing that does not affect your risk of catching a cold is being cold. Over the years, there have been various studies in which volunteers got soaked in cold baths or stood out in the rain. These people did not catch colds at a higher rate than people who stayed warm and dry.

This doesn't mean it's a good idea to go out in wintry weather without warm clothing. Being cold can precipitate bacterial pneumonia and other serious ailments.

●**How do colds spread?** Scientists disagree on this. Many think the virus spreads when a person inhales tiny virus-laden droplets of mucus and saliva liberated by the sneeze of an infected person. Some evidence suggests that it's possible to catch a cold simply by being close (within a yard or so) to an infected person.

Other scientists think the virus spreads via hand-to-hand contact...or by touching an object recently touched by an infected person, then touching the germ-laden hand to the face.

●**What can I do to avoid colds?** Since we can't count on others to stay at home when they're ill, it pays to avoid sitting or standing near anyone you suspect has a cold...and to watch where you put your hands and wash them often.

●**Does vitamin C prevent colds?** Despite its popularity, vitamin C has never been proven either to prevent or cure colds. Study after study has found no real difference in the incidence, duration or severity of colds between people who took vitamin C (up to 3,000 milligrams a day) and those who did not take C.

●**What about flu shots?** They prevent certain types of influenza but won't keep you from catching a cold.

●**Does psychological stress increase my vulnerability to colds?** Absolutely. Several years ago, I did a series of studies in collaboration with Sheldon Cohen, PhD, a Carnegie Mellon University psychologist.

We found that people who had recently been through a stressful experience—job loss, the death of a close relative or even desirable forms of stress like getting married—were more prone to colds than other individuals.

We found an almost twofold difference in infection rates among the most- and least-stressed individuals.

●**What's the best way to treat a cold?** While there's no way to cure the common cold, there are ways to make the symptoms more bearable...

●**Drink liquids** to keep mucus membranes moist.

●**Soothe a sore throat with warm, sweet drinks,** such as tea with honey. Or gargle with salt water.

●**Inhale water vapor** from a steam kettle or a hot bath or shower to help clear nasal passages. A hot bath is relaxing as well.

●**Keep the air moist** by using a humidifier or a kettle.

●**What about over-the-counter medications?** Take aspirin, acetaminophen or ibuprofen to reduce pain and fever.

Aspirin should not be given to children under 12 (some sources say 19) because of the risk of Reye's syndrome. Aspirin can cause stomach upset, and acetaminophen occasionally causes liver damage. Ibuprofen has a good safety record, although it, too, can cause stomach upset.

A decongestant containing *ephedrine* constricts dilated blood vessels, reducing swelling and secretion of mucus. It's best to take this drug in nose drops or nasal spray, because the effect will be localized.

Taking any drug orally exposes the entire body to its effects. Never use a nasal decongestant spray or drops for more than a week. If you do, you risk a "rebound" reaction, in which congestion worsens and the body becomes dependent on the drug.

●**Should I see a doctor if I have a cold?** In most cases, that's unnecessary. But if symptoms persist for more than a week, or you have high fever or a pus-like nasal secretion, you may have developed a bacterial infection on top of your cold. In such cases, see a doctor immediately. Ask if you need antibiotics—which, by the way, are *ineffective* against colds.

Children under age three, elderly people and those with lung or heart trouble are at greater risk of potentially deadly complications. They should notify a doctor at the first sign of anything more than a very mild cold.

The doctor should also determine whether you have a cold or the flu. A mild case of flu is often indistinguishable from a cold...and a severe cold may resemble the flu. Although both are characterized by sore throat, runny nose and cough, influenza usually involves muscle aches, headache and high fever.

The antiviral drugs *rimantidine* (Flumadine) and *amantadine* (Symmetrel) and the newer drugs *oseltamivir* (Tamiflu) and *zanamivir* (Relenza), an inhaled medication, can hasten recovery from influenza. However, they're effective only if taken soon after the onset of symptoms.

●**Is it okay to exercise with a cold?** There's no evidence that exercise prolongs or exacerbates a cold. Indeed, some people say they feel better afterward. But don't push yourself if you feel terrible.

●**Are any popular home remedies helpful?** Many old-fashioned remedies do seem to reduce discomfort, even if they don't actually get rid of the cold. For example, warm liquids like chicken soup soothe the throat, while the rising steam loosens up mucus. And tea made with ginger or another fragrant herb helps settle an upset stomach.

Menthol—mixed with hot water to make steam or rubbed in gel form on the upper lip —seems to clear clogged nasal passages.

Zinc lozenges, the herb *echinacea* and homeopathic products are said to be helpful in treating colds. But at this point, their effectiveness has not been proven.

How to Stop Sinusitis

Juan C. Guarderas, MD, division of allergy at the Mayo Clinic in Jacksonville, FL.

If you have a stuffy nose for more than a week or two, you may not be suffering from a cold—but from sinusitis. That's an inflammation or infection of the sinuses, the hollow spaces in the bones near the nose.

Among other functions, the four groups of sinuses warm and humidify air on its way from the nostrils to the lungs. A lining of mucus keeps the sinuses moist.

When everything's working right, tiny hairs called *cilia* sweep mucus from the sinuses down into the nose. But when the passages connecting the nose and the sinuses are congested—such as during a cold or allergy attack—the sinuses may fail to drain. Bacteria and/or fungi multiply in the trapped mucus, causing infection.

Sinusitis can lead to persistent cough or bronchitis—and can exacerbate existing cases of asthma. In rare cases, it can result in a life-threatening infection of the eyes or brain.

SYMPTOMS AND CAUSES

Sinusitis is usually marked by severe congestion...headache...mild fever...pain in the face or teeth...and a thick yellowish-green nasal discharge that continues all day and night. Some sinusitis sufferers are sensitive to shifts in barometric pressure—for example, on plane flights or during changes in the weather.

The common cold, in contrast, is characterized by watery white or yellow mucus that clears up as the day goes on. Allergies are often accompanied by itching and watering eyes.

Most cases of sinusitis occur during or shortly after a cold. Other cases are caused by allergies...tobacco smoke or other respiratory irritants...mouth infections...or anatomical problems, such as nasal polyps or a deviated septum, that obstruct sinus drainage.

Forty percent of cold-related sinus attacks get better without treatment as sinuses begin to drain again. But sinusitis often becomes chronic, creating long-term changes in the delicate lining of the sinus (the *mucosa*).

Chronic sinusitis may damage the cilia or acidify the mucus, leading to further irritation and inflammation. Over time, repeated bouts of sinusitis can permanently narrow the opening of the sinuses into the nose.

TREATING ACUTE SINUSITIS

The standard treatment for acute sinusitis is a course of antibiotics lasting 10 to 14 days...plus oral decongestants and nasal spray.* Antihistamines are not recommended because they can be too drying.

Caution: Using over-the-counter decongestant nasal sprays for more than five days can produce a "rebound" effect, in which the sprays themselves cause the nose to clog up.

With antibiotics, it's important to take the full course—even *after* you start feeling better. Otherwise, you create prime breeding conditions for drug-resistant bacteria.

Another good treatment for acute sinusitis is *saline irrigation.* When done under a doctor's supervision, it can be highly effective at reducing nasal and sinus congestion.

What to do: Each morning, fill a clean, narrow-tipped plastic squeeze bottle with a mixture comprised of one teaspoon salt to one pint lukewarm water. As you lean over a sink, squirt the solution into your nose until it's all gone. The solution will drain out. Be sure to clean the container and tip after each use.

TREATING CHRONIC SINUSITIS

Chronic sinusitis is harder to treat. In addition to decongestant sprays and pills, a three-week course of antibiotics is often helpful. If there's still no improvement at that point, see an allergist or otolaryngologist.

To pinpoint the source of your sinus trouble, this doctor may recommend an X ray or CT scan...or perform endoscopy.

Via this simple procedure—done in the doctor's office—the doctor can determine whether you have nasal polyps or another anatomical obstruction. If so, surgery to remove polyps or to widen the sinus opening slightly may be helpful.

*Most doctors recommend over-the-counter decongestant sprays like Afrin or Neo-Synephrine...saline sprays like Ocean...or prescription steroid sprays like *beclomethasone* (Beconase).

If your sinusitis is diagnosed as allergy-related, it may be necessary to avoid dust, animal dander and other allergens.

Nasal medications such as steroid inhalers may also provide some relief.

If you've had sinus trouble in the past and want to avoid recurrence, take precautions whenever you have a cold—to keep it from turning into a sinus attack.

Use decongestants and nasal irrigation...and avoid flying, scuba diving and other activities that involve rapid changes in air pressure.

Indigestion...How to Be Rid of It Forever!

Henry D. Janowitz, MD, former head, division of gastroenterology, and professor of medicine emeritus, Mount Sinai School of Medicine in New York City. He is author of *Good Food for Bad Stomachs.* Oxford University Press.

Indigestion affects millions of Americans each year. This catch-all term encompasses a wide array of complaints—from "acid stomach," belching, nausea, bloating and distention...to much more serious problems, such as peptic esophagitis, gallstones and stomach cancer.

The leading source of gastrointestinal distress is heartburn, technically known as gastroesophageal reflux disease (GERD). At one time or another, nearly all of us have experienced this burning sensation behind the breastbone. Often it's accompanied by a rush of highly acidic fluid into the back of the throat, leaving an unpleasant burning sensation there as well. Reflux occurs when the movement of food and digestive juices in the digestive tract causes stomach acid to back up into the esophagus.

Reflux may also arise from defects in the esophageal sphincter—the muscular "gateway" between the esophagus and the stomach.

This problem may be caused by a hiatal hernia—a weakness in the diaphragm, the muscular wall that separates the abdominal cavity from the lungs. *Other possible reflux triggers...*

●**Caffeine and cigarettes.** Both cause excessive secretion of stomach acid.

●**Fatty foods.** Fats are hard to digest, so fatty foods stay in the stomach longer than carbohydrates or proteins.

●**Alcohol.** While it doesn't induce reflux directly, it can cause erosion, swelling and inflammation of the stomach lining.

●**Ulcers.** Scar tissue from previous duodenal or peptic ulcers sometimes blocks the passage of food through the stomach.

●**Diabetes and viral infections.** They interfere with stomach motility by several mechanisms, including direct injury to nerves leading to the stomach or encouragement of overgrowth of intestinal bacteria.

Untreated reflux can cause chronic inflammation of the esophagus (esophagitis), a serious disorder marked by hoarseness, bleeding, pain, scarring, difficult swallowing, nausea and frequent awakening at night.

ANOTHER COMMON COMPLAINT

Nonulcer dyspepsia (NUD) is another common stomach complaint.

Symptoms: Gnawing stomach pain, nausea and vague acidity. These symptoms often mimic those of a peptic ulcer, although the stomach is otherwise normal.

Sometimes NUD is marked more by a feeling that the stomach is not emptying quickly enough. Food seems to linger too long, leading to fullness, swelling and gassiness. These symptoms can begin well before a meal is over...or up to two hours later.

No one knows exactly what causes NUD, but studies point to disturbances in the muscular action of the stomach, duodenum or esophagus.

RX FOR TROUBLED STOMACHS

While Maalox, Mylanta, Tums, Rolaids and other over-the-counter antacids are often helpful, it's better to *prevent* indigestion in the first place. *Prevention strategies...*

●**Eat three square meals a day.** Or, if you prefer, eat several small, light meals. Never skip breakfast or lunch with the intention of "making up for it" at the end of the day. Stuffing yourself at one sitting only increases pressure inside the stomach—and with it, the possibility of reflux.

●**Don't lie down too soon after eating.** Reflux is more likely to occur when you're lying down. So avoid late-night snacks and "siestas" during the day.

If you must sleep immediately after eating, be sure to keep your chest elevated. Put several pillows under your head, insert a foam wedge under your mattress or put the head of the bed on blocks.

If you crave a late-night snack, try drinking a cup of herbal or decaffeinated tea—fluids leave the stomach faster than solids.

●**Take steps to avoid constipation.** It raises abdominal pressure, making reflux more likely. Eat fiber-rich foods...drink plenty of fluids...exercise regularly...avoid tight belts or girdles...and keep excess weight off.

●**Avoid greasy or highly seasoned foods.** *Examples:* Curries, Szechuan dishes and dishes made with chili powder. If you've experienced indigestion after eating such foods in the past, be especially careful to avoid them.

BEYOND SELF-HELP

If your discomfort persists, seek professional help. To help the doctor make an accurate diagnosis, prepare a detailed account of symptoms—how long you have had them and under what circumstances.

Example: A gnawing or burning pain above the navel within one to three hours after eating can signal an ulcer. A thorough checkup should consist of a general physical exam, a blood and stool test and an upper GI series with barium in the stomach and esophagus.

In order to clearly see the esophageal lining, the doctor may perform an upper GI *endoscopy*, in which he will use a viewing probe called an *endoscope.*

Some prescription remedies are designed to reduce the irritating effects of reflux by suppressing stomach acidity or neutralizing the acid already secreted. Others clear the esophagus, strengthen its sphincter muscle and help empty the stomach—in the proper direction.

A class of drugs called *histamine 2 blockers,* along with medications such as Prilosec, stop production of hydrochloric acid in the stomach—especially overnight when it is most likely to accumulate and back up. The histamine 2 blockers Pepcid, Tagamet and Zantac are available over-the-counter, and help the pain of heartburn.

If tests confirm full-blown esophagitis, caffeine, tobacco and alcohol must be strictly forbidden, along with aspirin and other nonsteroidal anti-inflammatory drugs (NSAIDs).

The suggestions on diet and sleep must also be followed rigorously, and prescription medications must be continued for months even after all symptoms have disappeared.

The most striking new information about stomach ulcers is the discovery that the bacterium *H. pylori,* if present, must be eliminated by antibiotics to ensure that there will be lasting healing of the problem.

THE BRAIN–GUT CONNECTION

The brain is intimately linked to the stomach, esophagus and small bowel through a direct "rapid transit" system of nerve pathways —as well as through the slower, more indirect route of chemical "messengers," or hormones.

Such internal connections help explain why stress and emotional upset affect our digestive health so dramatically. Emotional disturbances of this kind change the brain's chemical activity, which in turn sends distress signals back to the gastrointestinal tract.

Your ability to tolerate stomach problems depends in large measure upon your disposition. For reasons unknown, some people have an unusually low tolerance for disturbances of the GI tract, whether these disturbances are caused by reactions to food, psychological stress or illness.

In such cases, stress management, relaxation, guided imagery and various other types of behavior-modification techniques are often helpful. Thus, a consultation with a psychologist, therapist or other mental health professional is often a vital part of any "cure" for a troubled stomach.

Cosmetic Surgery... The Best Solutions

Kimberly A. Henry, MD, a plastic and reconstructive surgeon in private practice in Greenbrae, CA. She is coauthor of *The Plastic Surgery Sourcebook.* McGraw-Hill.

Cosmetic surgery means more than nose jobs and breast implants. There are now hundreds of different procedures designed to take care of everything from wrinkles and scars to sagging skin and loose jowls.

FURROWED BROW

Deep vertical lines between the eyebrows can usually be eliminated with *Botox,* a toxin derived from the same microbe that causes the deadly ailment botulism.

Injected between the brows, Botox paralyzes the facial muscle causing the wrinkles. The procedure takes about 10 minutes. Results last for three to six months. *Cost:* $200–$400 per injection.

TIRED-LOOKING FACE

Although collagen injections work well for isolated facial wrinkles, they are not very effective for a face that is "tired-looking" all over. The best remedy for such a face is usually laser therapy.

Laser light causes collagen in the skin to shrink, eliminating wrinkles for about nine years. That's how long it takes facial wrinkles to form.

Several different kinds of lasers are now in use. For mild wrinkling, the best bet is the newly approved *erbium* laser. It combines good results with a brief recovery period.

The skin is red for three or four days. You can go back to work within a week. *Cost:* $100 to $3,000.

Avoid: Dermabrasion and chemical peels. These once-popular treatments for removing facial wrinkles yield unpredictable results. They can also cause scarring or lightening of the skin.

DEEP WRINKLES OR SCARRING

For acne scars or *deep* wrinkles caused by years of smoking and/or sun exposure, the best approach is once again laser therapy. But instead of the erbium laser, it's better to use the more powerful *carbon dioxide* laser.

Carbon dioxide laser therapy takes only 90 minutes, but the recovery period often lasts up to 10 days.

During the first week of this postoperative period, it's a bit like having a bad sunburn. The skin peels and crusts over. Pain medication is often needed. After seven to 10 days, the crust falls off, leaving behind new, pink skin. *Cost:* $2,000 to $6,000.

SAGGING JOWLS OR NECK WATTLES

For loose skin on the face or neck, the best treatment is a face-lift or neck-lift. In this four-hour operation, the surgeon makes an incision in front of and behind the ears.

Then he/she lifts the skin off the underlying muscles and fat of the face and tugs it back till it's snug.

Face-lifts are done on an outpatient basis. The recovery period lasts seven to 10 days. At that point, the stitches are removed, and you can return to normal activity. *Cost:* $7,500 to $30,000.

Good news: A new variant of the traditional face-lift procedure reduces the slight risk of nerve damage associated with the older procedure. *Supra-platysmal* face-lift involves repositioning only the superficial layers of skin.

The surgeon repositions the cheek fat and removes some fat around the jaw. *Cost:* $3,300.

Since neither type of face-lift can completely eliminate wrinkles, many patients opt to have laser therapy approximately six weeks after the face-lift.

FLABBY HIPS, THIGHS AND ARMS

With America's obesity problem continuing unabated, liposuction has become the most popular cosmetic surgery procedure.

In conventional liposuction, the surgeon sucks out fat using a thin tube (*cannula*) inserted through the skin. Most surgeons now use *tumescent liposuction*, in which fluids containing essential salts and sugars along with a local anesthetic and *epinephrine* to control bleeding are injected into the area being suctioned.

Unlike conventional liposuction, tumescent liposuction allows safe removal of *lots* of fat—up to 22 pounds at a time. *Cost:* $2,500 per site.

Some surgeons are starting to use *ultrasonic* liposuction instead. It involves use of a special probe that "melts" fat before it's sucked out of the body.

ENLARGED BREASTS IN MEN

The standard approach to this problem is to make an incision around the outside of the nipple and then cut away the excess fat.

This method generally yields good results, especially when used in combination with liposuction. *Cost:* $2,500 to $3,000.

FINDING A GOOD COSMETIC SURGEON

Picking a surgeon certified by the American Board of Plastic Surgery is not enough. *You must also look for a surgeon who has...*

• **Treated someone you know,** with good results and

• **Performed the procedure several times.**

Best strategy: Consult two or three cosmetic surgeons. Listen to their recommendations, and see how your personalities mesh.

For a list of board-certified plastic surgeons in your area, contact the national referral service of the American Society of Plastic Surgeons at 888-4-PLASTIC. *www.plasticsurgery.org.*

All About Dizziness

Brian W. Blakley, MD, PhD, professor and chairman, department of otolaryngology, University of Manitoba, Winnipeg, Canada. He is coauthor of *Feeling Dizzy: Understanding and Treating Dizziness, Vertigo and Other Balance Disorders.* Wiley.

In the absence of other symptoms, occasional mild dizziness is nothing to worry about. *But see a doctor right away if dizzy spells recur...if they're severe enough to force you to lie down...or if they're accompanied by...*

• **Double vision.**

• **Incontinence.**

• **Arm and/or leg weakness.**

• **Difficulty speaking or swallowing.**

●**Severe headache.**

These symptoms are suggestive of stroke, brain tumor, aneurysm or another potentially life-threatening problem.

COMMON TYPES OF DIZZINESS

●**A mild turning sensation.** This can be caused by almost any systemic ailment, including transient ischemic attacks, multiple sclerosis...even AIDS.

Some women have mild turning during menstruation—or as a side effect of hormone replacement therapy or menopause.

●**Imbalance.** This swaying or wobbling feeling can be caused by flu, infection, arthritis, compression of the spinal cord, diabetes or another metabolic disorder.

Imbalance can also be caused by alcohol abuse, depression or anxiety (rapid breathing reduces the flow of oxygen to the brain)...or by certain medications, including cough medicines and blood pressure drugs.

●**Vertigo.** This sensation of spinning often accompanies migraine headaches as well as many diseases.

●**Feeling of faintness.** This is often a result of *postural hypotension,* the brief period of reduced blood pressure that occurs when someone abruptly stands or sits up.

Several medications can contribute to postural hypotension, including antihypertensives, antihistamines, sedatives and antipsychotics.

With proper treatment, most cases of dizziness disappear. However, some cases resist treatment—including those that are caused by multiple sclerosis, AIDS and menstruation. In these cases, the patient simply has to learn to live with the problem.

EAR AND BRAIN DISORDERS

Persistent dizziness not linked to an underlying illness usually involves brain or inner ear trouble.

●**Benign paroxysmal positional vertigo** (BPPV) occurs when a person moves his head in a certain position—typically when he lies on his back, then rolls quickly to one side.

BPPV itself isn't life-threatening, but it can be deadly if it occurs while driving an automobile or standing up.

BPPV in people under 50 is often caused by head trauma. Even a light bump can be enough. In people over 50, BPPV can occur after illness, or be caused by degeneration of the nerves in the middle ear. In some cases, BPPV appears for no apparent reason.

●**Vestibular neuronitis** is sudden vertigo that occurs a few days or weeks after recovery from a viral infection. Often it's accompanied by nausea and/or vomiting. *Likely cause:* Inflammation of the vestibular nerve, which connects the brain and inner ear.

●**Ataxia** is a loss of coordination. It's usually caused by the death of brain cells, although it can also be caused by vitamin deficiencies or heavy drinking. Most common among elderly people, it often comes on gradually, and is generally irreversible.

●**Ménière's disease** is a set of related symptoms, including vertigo attacks...roaring, ringing or hearing loss in one ear...a feeling of fullness in the ear. Most cases are caused by fluid buildup in the inner ear. Ménière's usually strikes between the ages of 30 and 50. Symptoms tend to recur, lasting an hour or more at a time. They range from mild to debilitating.

●**Ear infection** that causes fluid to accumulate in the middle ear can cause everything from mild imbalance to severe vertigo.

GETTING GOOD TREATMENT

There's no easy way to test the balance mechanisms in the ear and the brain, so your doctor may have trouble pinpointing the cause of your dizziness. If he/she fails to take a complete medical history...or does not take your dizziness seriously...or has little experience with dizziness, find another doctor.

Best: An otolaryngologist or neurologist working in a dizziness clinic. For the name of one near you, contact the American Academy of Otolaryngology–Head and Neck Surgery. One Prince St., Alexandria, VA 22314. 703-836-4444, *www.entnet.org.*

Doctors use several tests to check for inner ear damage. The tests I use most often are the hearing test (audiogram) and two more specialized tests, *electronystagmography* (ENG) and the *rotary chair exam.*

ENG looks at eye movements caused by electrical stimulation of the vestibular system. The rotary chair exam measures eye movements as the patient sits in a computer-controlled rotating chair.

The best antidote for inner ear ailments is *time*. Inner ear damage usually heals within a few weeks or months. Fluid buildup from ear infection also tends to disappear in a few weeks.

Even persistent nerve damage usually stops causing dizziness after several months. The brain simply learns to re-sort incoming information (much as it adjusts to the rocking of a ship).

Vestibular neuronitis often persists until the underlying inflammation clears up. That can take years—though medicine, bed rest and rehabilitation exercises are helpful.

Dizziness may be *permanent* in those suffering from ataxia, multiple sclerosis or other central nervous system disorders.

Treatment for Ménière's disease may involve surgery to relieve accumulation of fluid, but diuretics and/or steroids can provide significant relief.

If you do have surgery, make sure the surgeon is certified in otolaryngology. *To check credentials:* Contact the American Board of Medical Specialties, 866-ASK-ABMS, *www.abms.org.* Dizziness usually subsides within eight weeks of surgery.

In some cases of dizziness, the mild sedative *meclizine* (Antivert) brings short-term relief. *Scopolamine* is even more effective…but also causes more side effects, including drowsiness and dry mouth. *Caution:* These drugs should be used for no more than a week or two, during severe episodes.

REHABILITATION EXERCISES

Many people with dizziness benefit from rehabilitation exercises. These speed the brain's adaptation process by enhancing neural connections in the inner ear. In fact, rehabilitation exercises are helpful for most balance problems, with or without a doctor's supervision. *Two helpful exercises…*

Horizontal head rotations: Sit down. Face forward. Turn your head to the right, then the left, going back and forth. Start slowly and

increase the speed of rotation of your head as much as you can in 20 seconds. Repeat, starting on the other side.

Vertical head rotations: Sit down. Face forward. *Position I:* Turn your head 45 degrees to the right. *Position II:* Move the top of your head from its vertical position so that your left ear moves toward your left knee and your head is horizontal. Alternate between positions 1 and 2 as fast as you can for 20 seconds. Repeat for the other side.

These exercises should be repeated two to three times in each session. Three sessions per day should be performed.

How to Win the Chronic-Pain War

Norman Marcus, MD, medical director of the Norman Marcus Pain Institute, New York City. He is coauthor of *Freedom from Pain.* Fireside.

If you suffer from headaches, back pain, neck pain or joint pain that persists for more than six to eight weeks, you may be experiencing chronic pain.

The good news is that now you can do more than just put up with it.

ORIGINS OF CHRONIC PAIN

The body requires about six weeks to heal following major injuries—broken bones, surgical incisions, etc. The pain associated with those injuries, however, can be felt long after the body has healed.

The acute or short-term pain that immediately follows an injury is directly related to how much damage the body has sustained. But pain that persists longer than might be expected following such conditions is chronic pain—and it is *not* related to the amount of damage that was sustained.

For years, chronic pain has been thought of as a disease itself and, therefore, the favored approach was managing the pain rather than looking for a cause of the pain.

CAUSES OF CHRONIC PAIN

Muscles are the major cause of chronic pain. They produce pain in four ways.

Emotional stress is the chief culprit that makes us tense our muscles without even being aware of it. Not surprisingly, all the day-to-day stress we experience affects the body. You tense your muscles, and you feel pain. And that pain may travel to different parts of the body.

Most chronic pain should not be seen as evidence of disease. It may, however, serve as your barometer of tension. The other causes for muscle pain are weaknesses and stiffness, spasm and trigger points.

HOW TO REDUCE CHRONIC PAIN

•**Tune in to what your body is telling you.** If you are experiencing persistent pain, you have a problem and should get help. Unfortunately, many doctors may not be able to help with your back or neck pains.

Reason: Although about 80% of the human body is made of muscle, most doctors are not taught a "hands-on" approach to examining muscles or evaluating the possible effects of muscle tension, weakness or spasm. As a result, muscle-related pain may not be recognized by your doctor or managed appropriately.

If previous pain-management strategies have not worked for you, look for a doctor who has expertise in muscle-related pain. Screen potential doctors to see if they incorporate evaluation and treatment of muscles in their pain-management regimens.

•**Stop thinking of the pain as a disease.** It will be more difficult to get rid of your pain if you make it the focus of a lot of worry and concern.

Try to carry on with as many normal daily activities as you can. Don't be afraid of movement, even if it's a little uncomfortable. Movement is necessary for chronic pain sufferers because muscle inactivity worsens the pain.

•**Begin a moderate exercise program.** This does not mean taking strenuous aerobics classes…or jogging five miles a day. In fact, both types of exercise should be avoided.

Better: Start a walking or swimming program, beginning with a modest distance and grad-ually increasing your goal as you feel more comfortable. Work with your doctor to develop the appropriate regimen for you. Work up to 30 to 40 minutes of exercise, three or four times a week.

Always remember that a proper exercise program starts with relaxation techniques such as meditation…then limbering and stretching prior to the initial exercise…followed by a cool-down period, which ends with relaxation again.

In addition to helping you stretch and strengthen, the process will help your mind release tension and stress, the major causes of chronic muscle-related pain.

If your pain is associated with danger signs —fever, chills, night sweats, headaches and malaise—it could indicate an underlying disease or potentially serious problem. You should consult your doctor.

IDEAL EXERCISE

•**Walk outdoors.** When you walk, you go a little faster, a little slower, take a bigger step, then a smaller step. That's natural for the body and a great way to exercise to eliminate chronic pain. Don't worry about the speed at first. Increase your distance by about 20% every few days. Aim to walk two to three miles each day.

•**Use a stationary bike** with the seat adjusted so you can extend your legs a little less than full extension. A stationary bike offers a good aerobic workout—if it is done with minimal tension at first and slowly built up in difficulty. If your back hurts on an upright bike, try a recumbent one.

•**Cross-country ski machines** offer a great workout if you are fit enough.

•**Swimming is terrific.** But if you have back pain, doing multiple laps with a crawl may result in overarching your back, causing more pain. If you have back pain, the back stroke and the side stroke are safer.

EXERCISES TO AVOID

•**Do not use any type of exercise machine that forces your body** into awkward positions to which you are not accustomed.

•**Do not overdo any muscle-strengthening exercise.** Three to four repetitions of any movement is sufficient. Then you should move on to the next exercise. You may return to any of the completed exercises for another set but only if you are completely free of pain.

●**Avoid stair-step exercises.** They can produce pain and soreness from the repetition of one movement. These leg exercises involve only ascending—not descending—motion for an aerobic workout. It's better and cheaper to simply walk up and down a staircase.

●**Avoid exercising on treadmills,** since they also force you to repeat the same motion at the exact same pace over and over again. The body is not made to handle that type of repetitive motion.

Beating Arthritis Pain

Jason Theodosakis, MD, MS, MPH, assistant clinical professor of medicine and former director of the preventive medicine residency training program at the University of Arizona College of Medicine in Tucson. He is coauthor of *The Arthritis Cure: The Medical Miracle that Can Halt, Reverse and May Even Cure Osteoarthritis.* St. Martin's.

The 16 million Americans who suffer from osteoarthritis* tend to rely on aspirin, ibuprofen and other nonsteroidal anti-inflammatory drugs (NSAIDs) to control their pain.

But NSAIDs do nothing to treat the underlying condition. Consequently, arthritis pain tends to worsen with time. In addition, NSAIDs can trigger a host of troublesome side effects, including digestive problems and high blood pressure.

Worst of all, new evidence suggests that NSAIDs can *aggravate* arthritis by blocking synthesis of *proteoglycans*, key molecules that help draw much-needed water into dry, damaged joints.

Breakthrough: The daily use of two nutritional supplements—*glucosamine* and *chondroitin*—controls pain, boosts joint mobility and helps undo the cartilage damage that is the hallmark of osteoarthritis.

*Osteoarthritis is one of 100 different kinds of arthritis. It is caused by the degeneration of the cartilage lining the joints.

Glucosamine and chondroitin work together to block the action of cartilage-destroying enzymes...promote the flow of water and nutrients into cartilage...and boost the activity of cartilage-producing cells called *chondrocytes. The supplements have been proven effective in studies around the world...*

●**In a double-blind study conducted in Portugal**, 40 arthritis patients were given either 1.5 grams (g) of glucosamine or 1.2 g of ibuprofen a day. Ibuprofen's pain-reducing effect faded after two weeks. Glucosamine relieved pain for the study's full eight-week duration.

●**A double-blind study of 80 arthritis patients in Milan, Italy**, found that 1.5 g a day of glucosamine reduced symptoms by 73% after 30 days. Patients who were given a placebo experienced only a 41% reduction in symptoms.

●**In a French study**, 120 people with knee or hip arthritis were given chondroitin or a placebo. After three months, the chondroitin group reported significantly less pain than the placebo group.

I can personally vouch for the effectiveness of glucosamine and chondroitin. Five years ago, my osteoarthritis—the result of chronic sports injuries—became so bad that I was forced to use crutches and a wheelchair.

After a search of the medical literature on arthritis uncovered several references to glucosamine and chondroitin, I began taking both supplements. My symptoms diminished within two weeks...and disappeared within four weeks. Several months later, a medical exam revealed that the cartilage in my joints had actually repaired itself.

USING THE SUPPLEMENTS

Glucosamine and chondroitin are available at drugstores and health-food stores. They're available without a prescription, but it's best to use them under the supervision of a sports medicine specialist, a rheumatologist or an orthopedic surgeon.

How much of each supplement should you take every day? That depends upon your body weight. *I use these guidelines...*

Less than 120 pounds: 1,000 milligrams (mg) glucosamine…800 mg chondroitin.

Between 120 and 200 pounds: 1,500 mg glucosamine…1,200 mg chondroitin.

More than 200 pounds: 2,000 mg glucosamine…1,600 mg chondroitin.

I tell my patients to divide each dose into halves, taking the first half in the morning, the second half in the evening—preferably with food.

As their arthritis pain subsides, I have them reduce the dosage. Symptoms generally begin to diminish within six weeks.

Important: Potent as these supplements are, they are only part of an effective arthritis treatment regimen. Here are the other key components.

ANTIOXIDANTS

Since the cartilage damage associated with arthritis is caused in part by cell-damaging *free radicals*, I urge my patients to take daily antioxidants. *The "ACES" antioxidants are particularly effective at controlling free radicals…*

●**Vitamin A**…5,000 international units (IU) a day.

●**Vitamin C**…4,000 mg a day.

●**Vitamin E**…400 IU a day.*

●**Selenium**…200 micrograms (mcg) a day.

It's also a good idea to eat foods rich in *bioflavonoids*. These compounds make *collagen*—the tough protein that is a primary constituent of cartilage—stronger and less prone to inflammation.

Bioflavonoid sources: Green tea, berries, onions, citrus fruits and pitted fruits, such as cherries and plums.

REGULAR EXERCISE

Walking, swimming and other forms of exercise are key elements of any arthritis regimen.

Exercise boosts production of synovial fluid, the nutrient-rich "broth" that lubricates the joints. It also strengthens the muscles, tendons and ligaments that support the joints…extends your range of motion…and boosts your flexibility.

Challenge: Finding an exercise that won't trigger additional pain. I often refer my arthritis

*Due to the possible interactions between vitamin E and various drugs and supplements, as well as other safety considerations, consult your doctor before starting a vitamin E regimen.

patients to a physical therapist. He/she can tailor a fitness regimen to suit your specific needs—and limitations.

To find a physical therapist in your area, contact the American Physical Therapy Association at 800-999-2782 or online at *www.apta.org*.

Caution: People who bill themselves only as "personal trainers" often lack the training required to work safely and effectively with arthritis patients.

BODY MECHANICS

Some cases of arthritis are caused by misaligned joints or other "body mechanics" problems. Such problems place undue stress on the joints, causing cartilage to break down.

To identify body mechanics problems, I often ask my arthritis patients to have a biomechanical analysis, which looks at how they walk, work and move about.

A typical analysis involves videotaping your movements and/or using electronic "force plates" to measure forces on the soles of your feet as you walk. Once problem areas are pinpointed, you'll be shown how modifying your movements can reduce the mechanical stresses on your joints.

Example: A woman with severe arthritis pain in her ankle was told by three different doctors that she had to give up tennis. She was also informed that she needed surgery to stabilize the joint. Her gait *appeared* normal, but a biomechanical analysis showed that it was putting unusual stress on her right knee, ankle and foot. She spent a few hours learning how to walk correctly and bought a different pair of shoes. Within two weeks, her pain was gone.

Biomechanical analysis is available from sports medicine doctors and practitioners who have completed a fellowship in sports medicine. It costs $100 to $1,000, depending on the equipment used.

WEIGHT LOSS

Each step you take subjects your knee and hip joints to forces that are 2.5 to 10 times your body weight. That's why it's essential to stay slim if you want to control arthritis pain.

Example: The knees of a 200-pound man must bear up to one ton of weight whenever he squats or walks downstairs.

If you're overweight, take steps to lose the excess weight. If your weight is normal, make sure it stays that way.

Beating Joint Pain

David S. Pisetsky, MD, PhD, chief, division of rheumatology at Duke University Medical Center in Durham, NC. He is author of *The Duke University Medical Center Book of Arthritis*. Fawcett.

A sudden twinge in an elbow, shoulder, knee or another joint is probably *not* arthritis. Most forms of arthritis develop slowly, striking first in the hands.

Instead, you've probably irritated the soft tissue around the joint. This ailment—really a family of ailments including bursitis, tendinitis and carpal tunnel syndrome—calls for a slightly different approach to treatment than arthritis.

Soft-tissue inflammation is not a natural consequence of aging. Most cases can be traced to excessive exercise...or to a job-related activity involving repetitive motion. The pain is usually apparent within 24 hours of overuse. It can range from a dull ache to shooting pain.

COMMON SOFT-TISSUE INJURIES

•**Rotator cuff tendinitis** affects the tendons that hold the shoulder joint in place. Common among swimmers and other athletes, this ailment can make it hard to get dressed or lie down.

•**Shoulder bursitis**—very common among gardeners and house painters—is caused by repeated pressure on shoulder *bursae*, fluid-filled "cushions" that protect the joints. It becomes painful to move the arm away from the body.

•**Tennis elbow** strikes carpenters, gardeners, mechanics, dentists...and tennis players who use poor form or a tightly strung racket. The pain makes it hard to shake hands or lift a briefcase.

•**Carpal tunnel syndrome** is an inflammation of tissue surrounding the median nerve of the hand. Symptoms include weakness, pain, burning or aching in the wrist and/or hand. Usually caused by repeated hand motions, like those used by checkout clerks, seamstresses and computer operators.

•**Prepatellar bursitis** involves inflammation of the bursa in front of the kneecap (patella). It is common in people who must stand or kneel for extended periods. The pain is rarely severe.

•**Shin splints** involve pain in the front of the lower leg. Most cases are caused by repetitive exercise—especially running on hard surfaces. This can injure muscle and tendon tissue.

•**Achilles tendinitis**—inflammation of the Achilles tendon—is common among basketball and squash players and runners (especially those who run on concrete or in flimsy shoes). Symptoms include pain, swelling and tenderness in the heel.

•**Plantar fasciitis** involves a tear in the ligament connecting the arch to the heel. It causes a burning pain on the sole of the foot and the heel, making it painful to walk or stand on your toes. Common among runners.

•**Trochanteric bursitis** is inflammation of the bursa near the hip. Symptoms include pain in the hip and thigh, especially when you walk, rise from a chair or lie on the affected side.

FINDING OUT WHAT AILS YOU

If you experience sudden pain, tenderness or swelling in a joint, consult a doctor at once. *His/her initial examination of you should include...*

•**Complete medical history.** Tell the doctor what preceded the injury, including whether the problem is chronic or an isolated case.

•**Physical exam of the joint.** The doctor should manipulate your limb to see if and how your range of motion is limited.

•**Review of systems.** Asking about symptoms in different systems of the body, such as fever or weight loss, is the only way to be sure there is no underlying illness, such as gout or joint infection.

The doctor may x-ray the joint—to check for swelling and anatomical abnormalities, such as worn cartilage. If a more detailed picture is needed, he/she may order an MRI scan.

Most cases of soft-tissue inflammation can be treated by a primary-care physician.

Caution: With doctors under increasing pressure from insurers, soft-tissue injuries often get superficial treatment—a recommendation of rest and a prescription for anti-inflammatory drugs. This works in some cases, but it's also how short-term problems can turn into chronic joint ailments.

If your pain doesn't respond to treatment within a few weeks, consult an orthopedist or rheumatologist.

FIRST-LINE TREATMENT

First, it's essential to stop whatever activity caused the injury in the first place, at least until the inflammation has healed.

Your doctor may choose to put the joint in a sling for a few days. Immobilization should be done only when absolutely necessary, however…and then only for a few days. *Reason:* It can cause muscle weakness.

An ice pack often helps during the first 24 to 48 hours after the onset of pain. Once the pain subsides, you can use a hot water bottle, heating pad or hot bath to improve joint mobility.

For pain and swelling, doctors often recommend aspirin or another nonsteroidal anti-inflammatory drug (NSAID)—typically *ibuprofen* (Motrin), *naproxen* (Aleve) or *indomethacin* (Indocin). Indomethacin is especially popular because of its effectiveness and rapid action.

Acetaminophen (Tylenol) is not a NSAID. It works on pain—but not inflammation. It may not be effective for overuse injury.

For maximum effectiveness, NSAIDs must be taken in high doses. Since these doses can cause stomach upset, bleeding and other side effects, NSAID therapy requires close supervision by a doctor.

CORTICOSTEROIDS AND PHYSICAL THERAPY

If NSAIDs fail to reduce the inflammation, your doctor may inject the affected bursa with cortisone or another corticosteroid. Although they may be effective, corticosteroids can cause increased vulnerability to infection as well as other side effects.

Some doctors give steroids right away. I prefer to wait at least 10 days to see what effects rest and NSAIDs have.

Physical therapy is also very helpful. I start my patients on gentle "range-of-motion" exercises as soon as possible. Your doctor can show you one or more that are appropriate for your injury.

Some soft-tissue injuries stem from improper joint movements, which are often caused by muscle weakness. In such cases, I recommend strength training.

If you're new to strength training, consider hiring a physical therapist for a few sessions—to be sure you're using proper form. Do *not* begin strength training without a doctor's supervision.

To find an accredited therapist in your area, contact the American Physical Therapy Association at 800-999-2782, *www.apta.org.*

SURGERY

For chronic or severe joint pain—especially in older people—orthopedic surgery may be the only option. Several procedures are used, from minimally invasive arthroscopic surgery to full-blown joint reconstruction. *Cost:* Several thousand dollars.

PREVENTING RECURRENCES

If exercise caused your injury, you may be able to return to your former level of intensity —but only gradually, over several months… and only after carefully analyzing the mechanical problems that caused the injury in the first place.

If the inflammation stemmed from an anatomical problem, consider replacing the offending activity with one your body can better handle. Switch from running to cycling, for example, or replace tennis with swimming.

For job-related tendinitis or bursitis, ask your doctor to refer you to an occupational therapist. He will carefully analyze your work movements and find ways to reduce stress on your joints.

A switch in equipment often helps. *Examples:* Wearing shoes with good cushioning and firm heel support…playing with a lightweight, shock-absorbent tennis racket…using a cushioned pad when kneeling…and using a raised, padded bar to support your wrists when typing.

Beating Migraines

Fred Sheftell, MD, president of the American Council for Headache Education, and director and founder of the New England Center for Headache, Stamford, CT. He is coauthor of Headache Relief for Women. *Little, Brown and Co.*

Migraine isn't just any headache. It's a severe, throbbing pain that can keep you home from work, disrupt your family life…and leave you with significant disability.

Migraines are *very* common. In fact, they affect 18% of women and 6% of men in the US. Without treatment, they can recur year after year.

A typical migraine…

- **Occurs on one side of the head.**

- **Is of moderate to severe intensity.**

- **Interferes with daily activity.**

- **Is exacerbated by physical activity** like coughing, walking or climbing stairs.

- **Is accompanied by nausea,** vomiting or sensitivity to light and sound.

Most migraine sufferers (migraineurs) can recognize what's called a *prodrome* in the 24 hours leading up to a migraine—sudden depression or exhilaration, increased or decreased appetite, disruptions in sleep, etc.

About 15% of migraine sufferers "see" flashing lights or strange shapes just before the headache hits. Such hallucinations are known collectively as an *aura.*

There's no easy way to tame migraines. But when migraineurs get good medical care and take an active role in their treatment, nine out of 10 can reduce a once debilitating problem to a minor inconvenience.

WHAT TRIGGERS MIGRAINES

A migraine starts with abnormal electrical activity in the cerebral cortex, the thinking part of the brain. It spreads quickly to the hypothalamus and the midbrain.

Levels of the brain chemical *serotonin* rise and then drop sharply, making blood vessels swollen and inflamed.

Though the migraine predisposition is inherited, most *individual* attacks are triggered by either dietary or environmental factors…

- **Alcohol** (especially beer and red wine).

- **Erratic meal and/or sleep schedules.**

- **The artificial sweetener *aspartame*** (NutraSweet).

- **The flavor enhancer *monosodium glutamate*** (MSG).

- **Processed meats** and other foods containing the preservatives nitrates or nitrites.

- **Aged cheeses,** freshly baked bread, chopped liver and other foods that contain the amino acid *tyramine*…and chocolate, which contains *phenylethylamine.*

- **Perfume or cigarette smoke.**

- **Caffeine withdrawal.** To avoid trouble, it's best to have no more than one five-ounce cup of coffee a day.

- **Psychological stress.** Most migraines occur when the period of stress is *over.* That's why migraines are common *after* exams or holidays.

HOW TO PREVENT ATTACKS

The first step in controlling migraines is to keep a "headache diary." Record the frequency and severity of your attacks…as well as the foods you consumed during the 24 hours prior to each attack. *Other key strategies…*

- **Maintain a regular schedule.** Eat at the same times each day. Keep consistent sleep hours seven days a week. Don't "sleep in" on weekends.

- **Take vitamin supplements**—vitamin E, consult your doctor for appropriate dosage… vitamin B-2, 400 milligrams (mg) a day…vitamin B-6, 50 mg a day. Vitamin supplements help stabilize levels of estrogen and serotonin.

• **Schedule "nurturing" time** during which you listen to music, read, play with your dog or cat, etc.—anything you find enjoyable and relaxing.

• **Practice a relaxation technique** like yoga, meditation, deep breathing or biofeedback once or twice a day for 15 minutes.

Deep breathing: Loosen your clothing and sit in a quiet place. Breathe in as you count to five, then out to the count of five. Silently repeat to yourself, "Breath in relaxation, breath out tension."

Biofeedback: With this high-tech relaxation aid, you're hooked up to a mechanical unit that measures skin temperature or muscular tension. With practice, you will learn how to raise the temperature or loosen the muscle. Either way, your body relaxes.

When traveling: Give yourself plenty of time to pack. Don't carry heavy bags using a neck or shoulder strap. Avoid alcohol during airplane flights.

• **Exercise regularly.** Physical activity relieves stress and boosts levels of *endorphins*, the body's pain-relieving chemicals. At least three times a week, have a moderate, *noncompetitive* workout. Competitive exercise boosts your stress level.

MOST EFFECTIVE MEDICATION

If migraines persist despite these lifestyle changes, taking *daily* medication may prove to be helpful.

Over-the-counter (OTC) painkillers like acetaminophen, aspirin, ibuprofen and naproxen are often effective in *treating* an attack.

If you do not respond to one of these medications, "combination" analgesics like Excedrin or Anacin may help. These products combine aspirin or acetaminophen with caffeine, which constricts swollen blood vessels and enhances pain relief.

If OTC remedies don't work, ask your doctor about Tylenol with codeine...Fiorinal (aspirin plus a mild sedative)...and Midrin (acetaminophen plus a muscle relaxant and a drug to shrink swollen blood vessels).

For *preventing* attacks, daily use of the beta-blockers *propranolol* (Inderal) and *nadolol* (Corgard) is often effective.

The calcium channel blocker *verapamil* (Calan, Verelan) and antidepressants such as *amitriptyline* (Elavil), *nortriptyline* (Pamelor) and *fluoxetine* (Prozac) are also effective.

Although *methysergide* (Sansert) is often effective, it can scar the lungs, kidneys and heart. If it must be used for more than five months, periodic chest X rays, MRI scans of the kidneys and other tests should be performed to make sure no harm is taking place.

What about alternative remedies? Some migraineurs get relief from a daily dose of the anti-inflammatory herb *feverfew*, which is available at health-food stores. Others get relief from fish oil supplements.

TO THE RESCUE

• **Acupressure** may offer relief to some migraineurs. At the first sign of a headache, press the web between your thumb and index finger, on the same side as your headache, for five minutes.

• **Sumatriptan** (Imitrex) is the biggest advance in migraine care in more than a century. One self-injection relieves most migraines within 60 minutes. The pill form is also effective, but it takes longer.

Beware: Don't use sumatriptan if you have heart disease—it narrows blood vessels. If you're at risk for heart disease (men over 40, family history of heart attack, smoking, blood pressure over 140/90, cholesterol over 220), the doctor may want to administer the first dose in the office, and check your electrocardiogram.

A sensation of pressure in the chest after a dose of sumatriptan is common. But if the drug causes chest *pain*, discontinue it.

• **Dihydroergotamine** (Migranal) is as effective as sumatriptan but takes longer to work. Inhaled and injectable versions of dihydroergotamine (DHE) and sumatriptan are very helpful when vomiting makes it impossible to keep pills down.

Best Ways to Prevent Colon Cancer

Samuel Meyers, MD, clinical professor of medicine at Mount Sinai School of Medicine, New York City. He is coauthor of the medical textbook *Bockus Gastroenterology*. W.B. Saunders.

If someone told you that a 20-minute medical test literally could save your life, wouldn't it be foolish to refuse it? Unfortunately, millions of Americans are doing just that when they fail to get periodic colon cancer screening.

Result: Each year, up to 57,000 Americans die unnecessarily from the disease.

Here's what you must know to protect yourself against colon cancer...

SCREENING WORKS

Almost all malignancies of the large intestine and rectum start out as *premalignant polyps*, flat or mushroom-shaped growths that are harmless but may become cancerous. If a polyp is detected and removed, cancer will *not* develop. That's why screening—regular exams to detect polyps or cancer in its earliest stages—is crucial.

The most recent screening guidelines, published by the US Multisociety Task Force on Colorectal Cancer in February 2003, recommend screening for *all* men and women beginning at age 50. If you have already had surgery for polyps or colon cancer—or if you have inflammatory bowel disease, such as ulcerative colitis or Crohn's disease—your risk for colon cancer is increased and you should have colonoscopy on a schedule determined by your doctor.*

Screening options...

• **Colonoscopy every 10 years**. This screening test is the most accurate and has been shown to prevent 85% to 90% of colon malignancies.

*People with a close relative (parent, sibling or child) who has had colon cancer or polyps should start regular screening with colonoscopy at age 40 (or five years earlier than the youngest diagnosis in the family). If you have two close relatives with the disease, have a colonoscopy every five years. If three relatives, you should have genetic counseling and possibly start colonoscopy screening at age 25 or younger.

Many health insurance plans now pay for screening colonoscopy, as does Medicare. Without health insurance, the procedure costs about $3,000.

Unfortunately, colonoscopy has a reputation for being embarrassing and painful. Both criticisms are overblown. Most patients say colonoscopy is not nearly as bad as they had expected.

What's involved: While you are sedated, a flexible, one-half-inch diameter tube that employs digital video optics is threaded through the anus and passed through the large intestine, enabling the doctor to see your entire colon lining on a video monitor. The procedure itself usually takes no more than 20 minutes.

Many people find the preparation, which involves laxatives to empty the bowel, much more unpleasant than the colonoscopy itself.

Until recently, the standard bowel preparation method involved drinking four liters of a bad-tasting colon-cleansing solution, such as *GoLYTELY*, the night before. Newer products now make the process less unpleasant...

• *Phospho-soda* also tastes bad, but you only take several tablespoons dissolved in liquid the night before and the morning of the procedure.

Helpful: While you can mix it with any clear liquid, most patients prefer to mix it in ginger ale to make it more palatable.

• *Visicol* contains the same ingredient but is in tablet form. Instead of downing a liquid solution, you swallow a total of 40 tablets in multiple doses.

Helpful: Whatever bowel prep method you use, consume at least three eight-ounce glasses of fluid the night before to prevent dehydration. You can drink any liquid, but a sports drink that contains electrolytes is preferred.

• **Sigmoidoscopy every five years.** This test is less invasive than colonoscopy and requires less preparation (an enema the night before and the morning of the procedure) and no sedation. Because the procedure is less thorough than colonoscopy, it identifies only 50% of colon malignancies.

What's involved: A flexible tube, like that used in a colonoscopy, is passed through the lowest third of the large intestine (sigmoid colon), where half of all tumors occur.

Sigmoidoscopy appeals to people who don't want to be sedated. The procedure, which costs about $400, is also less expensive than colonoscopy.

Important: On a subsequent day, you should return to take a barium enema, followed by an X-ray, to view the remaining two-thirds of the colon. A barium X-ray costs about $500.

Although sigmoidoscopy combined with a barium X-ray screens the entire colon, it is still less accurate than colonoscopy.

• **Fecal occult blood test once a year.** People who don't want to undergo colonoscopy or sigmoidoscopy can opt for this test. It is the least accurate screening option and only reduces colon cancer rates by one-third.

Typical cost: $5.

What's involved: A chemical applied to stool samples detects traces of blood, which would suggest the presence of polyps or tumors. No preparation is required, but you must avoid certain foods (such as red meats and broccoli) for three days and medications (such as aspirin) for a week before to ensure accuracy. Since the test detects blood, taking aspirin, which can cause internal bleeding, could trigger a false positive.

Some people find the procedure unpleasant because it involves using a small wooden stick to smear small bits of your own stool on specially treated cardboard. If blood is detected, you'll need to have a colonoscopy.

NEW TEST

Virtual colonoscopy uses computed tomography (CT) to provide detailed radiographic pictures of the colon. It is relatively noninvasive, requires no sedation and can be done at your radiologist's office. It does require the same kind of preparation as colonoscopy.

This test is less accurate than conventional colonoscopy—it detects 75% to 80% of polyps larger than one centimeter, but just 40% to 50% of smaller ones. Health insurers will *not* pay for it.

Typical cost: $900.

It may be a good option for people with heart or lung disease, for whom sedation can be risky.

Aspirin Therapy Reduces Colon Cancer Risk

John A. Baron, MD, professor of medicine, Dartmouth Medical School, Hanover, NH, and leader of a study of 1,121 people who had polyps removed during routine cancer screening, presented at a meeting of the American Association for Cancer Research.

In a recent study, daily use of baby-strength aspirin—81 milligrams—reduced the recurrence of colon polyps by 19% in people who had polyps removed previously. Polyps can become cancerous.

If you have a family history of colon cancer: Ask your doctor whether you should take a daily low-dose aspirin.

Caution: Don't start aspirin therapy if you are allergic to aspirin or have bleeding problems.

 # Prostate Cancer: What Every Man Must Know Now

E. Roy Berger, MD, a medical oncologist and prostate cancer specialist affiliated with North Shore Hematology-Oncology Associates, East Setauket, NY. He is coauthor of *Updated Guidelines for Surviving Prostate Cancer.* 1st Books Library.

For such a small gland, the prostate causes big trouble. This year alone, 200,000 men will be diagnosed with prostate cancer.

The disease kills almost as many men as breast cancer kills women.

SCREENING IS ESSENTIAL

Little is known about what *causes* prostate cancer, although men who eat a high-fat diet seem to be at greatest risk. That's why *screening* is essential.

Caught in its early stages, prostate cancer can usually be cured with surgery or radiation, and possibly helped by drug therapy. Key, of course, is catching the tumor *before* it spreads.

Self-defense: Once a year, starting at age 50,* all men should undergo…

- **Digital rectal examination** (DRE). The doctor inserts a finger into the rectum to feel the prostate gland for nodules or firmness suggestive of cancer.

- **Prostate-specific antigen test.** This blood test measures levels of prostate-specific antigen (PSA), a protein secreted by the prostate. Elevated PSA levels suggest the need for further evaluation.

It's important to realize that PSA levels increase with age. A level that's normal for a man of 80, for instance, may suggest prostate cancer in a man of 45.

For men 51 or older, a level above 3.5 suggests the need for further tests. Above age 70, the cutoff is 6.5.

GETTING A PROPER BIOPSY

If your PSA is high, or if the digital exam reveals a suspicious lump, it's prudent to have the prostate biopsied.

Problem: Some doctors take just one or two tissue samples. To be sure to find any tumor (and to estimate its size), however, the doctor must take at least six tissue samples.

OTHER IMPORTANT TESTS

Some prostate tumors grow fast, others slowly. A slow-growing tumor might cause no trouble for years—without any treatment. A virulent tumor calls for immediate, aggressive intervention.

Science has yet to find a foolproof method for telling one type of tumor from the other. However, a tumor's *Gleason score* can help you pick appropriate treatment. The Gleason score is an indication of how "aggressive" the cancer cells are.

Two other tests are often helpful when making the treatment decision…

- **Ploidy analysis**—how much DNA the tumor contains. A tumor that has either more or less DNA than normal is likely to spread.

- **Polymerase chain reaction (PCR) test.** This test can show whether the tumor has spread long before other tests.

*Start screenings at age 40 if your father or brother had prostate cancer or if you are African-American. Risk is significantly higher among these men.

WATCHFUL WAITING

If tests indicate that the tumor is small and slow-growing, treatment may be unnecessary.

As long as PSA levels stay low and the tumor grows slowly, "watchful waiting" may be appropriate. All you have to do is have a checkup every two months, including a DRE and PSA test.

Watchful waiting is generally more reasonable for a man of 70—who is likely to die of other causes before a sluggish tumor causes any trouble—than a 50-year-old.

THE CASE FOR SURGERY

If the cancer is confined to the prostate, surgical removal of the gland—a procedure called *radical prostatectomy*—is sometimes curative. Following surgery, up to 70% of men become impotent. Up to 5% become incontinent.

Innovation: *Nerve-sparing prostatectomy.* In this procedure, the surgeon is careful not to sever the delicate nerve bundles next to the prostate that control erection. Nerve-sparing prostatectomy is a trade-off. You're less likely to become impotent, but there's more risk that some cancerous tissue will remain.

WHAT RADIATION HAS TO OFFER

In traditional radiation therapy, a machine zaps the prostate with high-intensity X-rays.

For cancer limited to the prostate, this *external beam radiation* (EBR) may be as effective as surgery. Unlike prostatectomy, it doesn't involve weeks of recovery.

Up to 50% of men who undergo radiation therapy become impotent. Incontinence is generally not a problem.

Brachytherapy is a form of radiation that is sometimes performed on an outpatient basis. In this procedure, tiny "seeds" of radioactive iodine or palladium are implanted within the prostate.

Since brachytherapy causes less damage to surrounding tissues, the impotence rate is only about 15%, the incontinence rate close to 0%. Brachytherapy delivers more radiation to the tumor.

Seed radiation seems to be just as effective as prostatectomy at curing the disease.

HORMONE THERAPY

For prostate cancer that has spread to other tissues, prostate surgery and radiation are unlikely to extend life.

In such cases, the best strategy is to block action of *testosterone* and *dihydrotestosterone*. Secreted primarily by the testicles and adrenal glands, these male hormones spur growth of prostate cancer cells—wherever they appear in the body.

Doctors can "shut down" the testicles by administering drugs called *LHRH agonists*...or by surgically removing them in a procedure called *orchiectomy*.

Doctors also prescribe the drugs *flutamide* (Eulexin) or *bicalutamide* (Casodex), which block hormonal action at the cellular level. This combined hormone therapy is the treatment of choice for metastatic prostate cancer.

In a study of men with metastatic cancer, those who got combined therapy lived 1½ years longer than those who got single hormone therapy. Combined therapy is also used —with surgery or radiation—to treat cancer limited to the prostate.

EXPERIMENTAL APPROACHES

In *cryotherapy*, the prostate is destroyed by freezing. Even with a highly skilled surgeon, this experimental therapy often causes impotence. Since it's never been widely used, there are no long-term survival statistics.

Research suggests that *modified citrus pectin*, a powder derived from citrus fruit, helps stop prostate cancer from spreading. But this potential lifesaver won't be ready for several years.

SUPPORT GROUPS

Any man with prostate cancer should find out about support groups in his community. To find a support group or cancer specialist in your area, contact Patient Advocates for Advanced Cancer Treatments (PAACT) at 616-453-1477, *www.paactusa.org*.

With all the treatment options, any man with prostate cancer should consult *three* doctors—a urologic surgeon, a medical oncologist and a radiation specialist familiar with brachytherapy.

Colon Cancer Self-Defense Essentials

Peter R. McNally, DO, professor, division of gastroenterology, University of Colorado Health Sciences Center and director of clinical gastroenterology and endoscopy, Denver Health Medical Center. He is author of the medical textbook *GI/Liver Secrets*. Mosby.

Colon cancer kills more people than any other malignancy except lung cancer. One American in 20 will develop colon cancer in his/her lifetime—usually after age 50.

Tragically, 90% of colorectal cancers could be avoided through early detection.

DETECTION MEANS PREVENTION

Colon cancer doesn't just come out of nowhere. Most cases develop from a polyp, a premalignant growth on the lining of the colon.

Periodic screening offers a way to spot tumors early...and to find and remove polyps while they're still benign. It takes five to 10 years for a polyp to turn cancerous. *Here's what to do...*

● **Age 40 to age 50.** Have an annual *digital rectal exam* (DRE). The doctor inserts a gloved finger into the rectum and feels for suspicious growths.

● **After age 50.** Each year, have a DRE and a *fecal occult blood test*. In this test, you'll be asked to put a smear of stool on a specially treated card on three successive days, while following a special diet.

If the test shows blood—or if you're at high risk for colon cancer—the doctor will examine the full length of your colon with a long, flexible viewing scope (colonoscope). Any polyp that is found is removed during the procedure.

Because *colonoscopy* can cause discomfort, you will probably be given an intravenous sedative like Demerol or Valium.

Undergo *flexible sigmoidoscopy* every three years unless you've had a recent colonoscopy. Using a short, flexible tube inserted into the rectum, the doctor inspects the lower one-fourth of the colon. That's where most tumors develop.

The procedure causes only mild discomfort, so it's usually done without sedation.

WHO IS AT HIGH RISK

Colon cancer runs in families. Your risk is above average if one or more of your first-degree relatives (parents or siblings) has had the disease.

In such cases, it's prudent to have a flexible sigmoidoscopy every three to five years, starting at age 35.

A rare hereditary condition known as *familial adenomatous polyposis* dramatically raises your risk of colon cancer. If genetic tests reveal that you have this condition—in which hundreds of polyps form in the colon—screening should begin in adolescence.

If you've had one polyp removed, you're likely to develop more. Have a colonoscopy every three years.

Ulcerative colitis and Crohn's disease are also associated with an elevated risk. Anyone who has either condition for 10 years or more should have an annual colonoscopy.

REDUCING RISK WITH DIET

Colon cancer is rare in regions where vegetables and grains make up the bulk of the diet. It's common in the US and other Western nations where the diet is largely based on meat.

Implication: A diet rich in fruits, vegetables, beans and whole grains prevents colon cancer. The American Cancer Society recommends at least five servings of these foods each day.

While it's hard to determine exactly which components of this healthy diet are protective, research has zeroed in on several candidates...

●**Low fat.** There is a clear link between dietary fat and colon cancer. Fats boost the body's production of bile acids, which promote rapid cell growth.

●**High fiber.** The indigestible part of plant-based foods, fiber moves food through the bowel quickly—reducing its contact with carcinogens and bile acids.

Wheat bran is more protective than fruit and vegetable fiber. Oat bran has little impact on colon cancer risk, though it does reduce cholesterol levels.

Get at least 25 grams (g) of dietary fiber per day—from whole grain cereals and breads and vegetables, fruits and beans.

●**Calcium.** Some studies suggest that calcium protects the colon by neutralizing bile acids and fatty acids.

Consume at least 1,000 milligrams (mg) of calcium each day—ideally through diet, not supplements.

●**Antioxidants.** Low blood levels of vitamins C and E and beta-carotene seem to confer an increased risk of colon cancer.

Eat lots of citrus fruits and dark-green and yellow vegetables—these are the best sources of antioxidants.

WHAT ELSE MAY HELP

●**Exercise.** A sedentary lifestyle increases the risk of colon cancer. Like fiber, physical activity reduces the risk by hastening the passage of waste through the body. It also stimulates blood flow to the colon.

Walk briskly or do some other exercise at least 30 minutes, three days a week.

●**Nonsteroidal anti-inflammatory drugs** (NSAIDs). As several studies have shown, individuals who have taken aspirin or ibuprofen regularly for years face a reduced risk of colon cancer.

Unfortunately, there is not enough evidence to justify taking aspirin or NSAIDs strictly for cancer prevention.

●**Estrogen.** There are studies that suggest that postmenopausal women who take estrogen are less likely to develop colon cancer than similar women who don't take estrogen, though the risks of heart attack, stroke and breast cancer and blood clots may outweigh this benefit.

WATCH OUT FOR SYMPTOMS

See a doctor at once if you experience changes in bowel habits...blood in the stool...rectal pain...and/or recurrent abdominal cramps.

The earlier cancer is detected, the better the chance for cure.

Often-Overlooked Causes of Chronic Fatigue

Ronald L. Hoffman, MD, medical director of the Hoffman Center in New York City. He is author of *Tired All the Time: How to Regain Your Lost Energy.* Poseidon.

If you feel tired all the time, you have lots of company. Each year, Americans make 500 million visits to the doctor seeking treatment for fatigue.

Many people who frequently feel tired fear they have the debilitating condition *chronic fatigue and immune dysfunction syndrome* (CFIDS).

If your fatigue has persisted for more than six months or is accompanied by sleep disturbances, joint pain, headaches, inability to concentrate or short-term memory loss, you may indeed have CFIDS.

In such cases, it's best to seek treatment from a CFIDS specialist. For a list of specialists in your area, contact the CFIDS Association of America, Box 220398, Charlotte, NC 28222. 704-365-2343, *www.cfids.org.*

Good news: Only about 10% of my patients with fatigue actually have CFIDS. Most of the rest are suffering from "garden variety" fatigue, caused by too little sleep or exercise, poor dietary habits or other easily correctable problems.

THYROID PROBLEMS

Many cases of chronic fatigue are caused by over- or underproduction of thyroxine. That's the thyroid hormone responsible for regulating how energy is consumed by the body's cells.

Overactive thyroid: Symptoms of hyperthyroidism include fatigue, anxiety, insomnia, heart palpitations and bulging eyes. This condition is treated with thyroxine-blocking drugs... or with surgery or radioactive iodine to destroy the thyroid gland.

Underactive thyroid: Suspect hypothyroidism if you feel depressed or lethargic, chill easily, are gaining weight or suffer from premenstrual syndrome (PMS), muscle aches, dry skin, eczema, hair loss, low libido, a hoarse throat or frequent colds or flu.

If you're experiencing any of these symptoms, it's a good idea to check your basal body temperature. Insert a thermometer under your armpit as soon as you awaken, before getting out of bed. Record results for three consecutive mornings.

A basal temperature of 97.4 degrees or lower suggests hypothyroidism. Your doctor can give you a blood test to confirm your suspicions.

Most doctors treat hypothyroidism with synthetic levothyroxine (*Synthroid*). However, some patients show more improvement when they take *natural* thyroid hormone (derived from beef or pork).

If Synthroid doesn't relieve your symptoms, ask your doctor to consider that alternative.

ADRENAL INSUFFICIENCY

Anyone whose fatigue is accompanied by malaise, frequent illness, allergies or low blood pressure or sugar may be making too little of the adrenal hormone *dehydroepiandrosterone* (DHEA).

Adrenal insufficiency is usually caused by autoimmune disease...or by adrenal gland damage stemming from long-term use of cortisone.

If a blood test reveals low levels of DHEA, you might need to take it in pill form.

In Europe, DHEA has long been used to boost immune function and combat fatigue—though few American doctors have much experience with the drug.

To find an endocrinologist familiar with DHEA, call the American College for Advancement in Medicine, 888-439-6891, *www.acam.org.*

DIABETES

Adult-onset diabetes is an often-overlooked source of persistent fatigue. To rule out this condition, ask your doctor for a *fasting blood glucose test.*

The normal range of insulin is 80 to 100 mg per deciliter of blood. If you fall above that range, eating a special diet and getting regular exercise can help lower blood sugar levels. That should boost your energy.

HORMONAL PROBLEMS

In men, chronic fatigue may be caused by abnormally low levels of testosterone. Men suffering from this problem (which can be spotted with a simple blood test) can boost their energy levels by taking testosterone supplements.

Hormone problems can cause fatigue in women, too. But tests for hormone imbalances in women are often inaccurate.

Instead of relying on a blood test, women should suspect hormone problems if…

• **Their fatigue is cyclical,** getting worse prior to menstruation and improving afterward.

• **They experience weight gain** of more than five pounds prior to each period.

• **They perpetually crave sugar,** spicy foods or chocolate.

• **They experience migraines** or breast tenderness when taking birth-control pills.

To treat hormone-related fatigue, women should reduce their consumption of alcohol, meat and dairy products…eat more dietary fiber and less sugar and refined foods…take supplements of *gamma linolenic acid* (GLA).

GLA is found in primrose oil, borage oil and black currant seed oil, available at health-food stores.

Women with extreme PMS-related fatigue should ask their doctor about having a *Meyer's cocktail* once a month. That's an intravenous drip of calcium, magnesium, and vitamins B and C.

FOOD ALLERGIES

Chronic, mild food allergies can cause fatigue. Suspect allergies if you have dark circles under your eyes…are frequently irritable…feel foggy or depressed…or have frequent infections or dry skin.

Cravings for particular foods or cycles of energy and fatigue also suggest food allergies —especially to wheat and dairy products. These foods can cause the body to produce an energy-sapping morphine-like substance.

Consider a medically supervised fast of one to four days, to see if your energy increases.

Add foods back to your diet only with the doctor's permission.

ENVIRONMENTAL TOXINS

If you can't find another source of fatigue, you may be suffering from exposure to indoor pollutants. *Usual culprits…*

• **Benzene.** In linoleum and degreasers.

• **Formaldehyde.** In new carpets and new drapes.

• **Lead.** In tap water and house paint.

• **Mercury.** In dental fillings and in some house paints.

• **Nitrogen dioxide.** Released by kerosene heaters, gas stoves and furnaces.

• **Trichloroethylene.** Used in dry cleaning.

Have your home tested for environmental toxins. For companies that test air and water, look under "Laboratories–Testing"—in the *Yellow Pages.*

One reputable firm is RCI Environmental, 17754 Preston Rd., Suite 101, Dallas 75252. 972-250-6608.

If toxins *are* a problem, install carbon-based water and air filters. Make sure your home is well-ventilated so that fumes can escape.

Another option is to fill your home with house plants to help filter the air.

Your doctor should test your blood for chemical markers of contaminants…and your hair for lead, mercury and other toxic metals. If traces of toxins are found, ask him/her about adding selenium, vitamin E, beta-carotene, garlic and sodium alginate to your diet. They help rid the body of toxic metals.

THE ROLE OF SUGAR

In many cases, fatigue is the result of eating too much sugar. Sugar and refined carbohydrates make your blood sugar rise. This signals the pancreas to produce insulin. Too much insulin leads to *hypoglycemia* (low blood sugar), which causes extreme fatigue.

If you suspect hypoglycemia, ask your doctor for an oral *glucose-tolerance test.* If, during the test, you experience heart palpitations, mental confusion or extreme fatigue, or feel dizzy or shaky, suspect a sugar problem—even if your doctor says your blood sugar levels are normal.

Treatment is simple—stop eating sugar. *Also helpful:* Eating six small meals instead of the usual three big meals. Small, frequent meals help stabilize blood sugar levels.

Finally, ask your doctor about taking ergogenic (energy-generating) dietary supplements, including vitamin B-15...L-carnitine...octacosanol, a wheat germ extract...ginseng.

High Blood Pressure... The Silent Killer

Vincent Friedewald, MD, clinical professor of medicine at the University of Texas Medical Branch, Galveston. He is author of Ask the Doctor: Hypertension. *Andrews McMeel.*

High blood pressure is the most overlooked health problem in the US. Only 14 million of the estimated 70 million Americans who have it are getting adequate treatment.

The rest may *feel* fine, but they're at increased risk for stroke, heart attack, kidney failure and other ailments.

To find out more about detecting and treating this "silent killer," we spoke with prominent cardiologist Dr. Vincent Friedewald...

●**When is blood pressure considered high?** Any pressure above 120/80 is potentially problematic. We used to think that only the second (diastolic) number mattered. Now we know that the first (systolic) reading is important, too.

Hypertension is ranked in stages...

	Systolic	*Diastolic*
Prehypertension	120 to 139	80 to 89
Stage 1	140 to 159	90 to 99
Stage 2	greater than 160	greater than 100

●**My blood pressure is only slightly elevated. Is that cause for concern?** Even Stage 1 hypertension can cause serious health problems. Everyone should try aiming for an optimal blood pressure reading of 115/75.

●**What causes high blood pressure?** We don't know the full story. However, blood pressure is a reflection of how hard your heart is pumping...and of the size of your *arterioles*, special blood vessels that act as gatekeepers

between the arteries and the capillaries, the tiniest blood vessels.

Arterioles dilate or narrow according to nerve signals from the brain, which bases its "decisions" on feedback from nerve endings near the heart. These nerve endings constantly monitor your blood pressure.

This feedback loop boosts your pressure when you exercise or undergo psychological stress and lowers it when you're asleep or relaxed.

In hypertension, blood pressure is *consistently* higher than it should be—whether you are stressed or relaxed.

Ninety percent of people with high blood pressure have *primary* (essential) hypertension. This condition seems to be largely hereditary, although excess weight, lack of exercise, high salt intake, alcohol consumption and age can also play a role.

●**What about the other 10% of cases?** They're the result of other ailments—typically kidney disease, thyroid or adrenal gland problems or sleep apnea. Once the underlying disease is diagnosed, blood pressure can usually be controlled.

●**How do I know if I have high blood pressure?** Have a doctor measure it...or buy and use your own blood-pressure monitor. *Cost:* $35 to more than $100. Ask your doctor to make sure it's properly calibrated.

A *single high* reading—especially a diastolic reading *above* 90 or a systolic reading *above* 140 —may be cause for concern. However, it does *not* necessarily mean you have hypertension.

A single measurement may not be representative of your blood pressure throughout the day. And about one in five people who visit the doctor exhibit high blood pressure *simply because they're nervous.*

Your doctor must be careful to distinguish real hypertension from this "white-coat" variety. Aggressive treatment of white-coat hypertension can be dangerous.

To tell if your blood pressure is *consistently* high, you must take several readings—preferably over a period of days or weeks.

If you are diagnosed with hypertension, your doctor should follow up with a thorough physical exam. *This exam should include an electrocardiogram, a urinalysis and blood tests for...*

- Blood lipids
- Calcium
- Complete blood count
- Creatinine
- Glucose
- Potassium
- Uric acid

•What can I do to lower my blood pressure? If it's just a bit high, you can probably nudge it down into the safe range by making a few lifestyle changes...

•Cut back on alcohol. Alcohol in any form raises blood pressure. Have no more than one ounce a day—the amount in two beers, a glass of wine or a jigger of whiskey.

•Exercise more. Get 30 to 60 minutes every day of moderate activity—walking, jogging, bicycling, etc. Becoming fit can lower your blood pressure by six to seven points.

•Lose weight. Overweight people who reduce their body weight by 5% to 10% often experience a significant drop in blood pressure.

•Quit smoking.

•Reduce sodium intake. Some people are salt-sensitive, others aren't. My advice is to stop using a salt shaker...and to avoid processed foods, which account for two-thirds of daily salt intake.

•Is there any special diet that can help? In addition to restricting your salt intake, try to eat calcium- and potassium-rich foods (especially fruits, grains and vegetables). These minerals promote excretion of sodium.

Being a vegetarian also seems to lower blood pressure. Vegetarians not only eat more fruits and veggies than their meat-eating peers, but are also thinner. Some people swear by magnesium supplements, fish oil, garlic and other purported pressure-lowering remedies. But there's no hard evidence that these products have any beneficial effect.

•When is it appropriate to treat hypertension with drugs? If you're more than a few points above normal, your doctor will probably prescribe antihypertensive medication *in addition to* lifestyle changes.

There is now a wide variety of very effective antihypertensives...

•Diuretics remove sodium and water from the bloodstream, shrinking blood volume and dilating arteries. Diuretics are especially effective in African-American and elderly individuals... and in individuals whose blood pressure is salt-sensitive. Diuretics can deplete potassium levels, so any patient taking them should have his/her potassium levels carefully monitored.

•Beta-blockers reduce the force of each heartbeat and block the release of hormones that boost blood pressure. Beta-blockers can cause fatigue, insomnia and sexual problems. They should be avoided by those with asthma or heart failure.

•ACE inhibitors slow key chemical interactions in the bloodstream that lead to hypertension. Relatively free of side effects, they can cause coughing and—rarely—swelling of the face and limbs.

•Calcium channel blockers (the *short-acting* form of *nifedipine*, such as Procardia, Adalat) have been linked to heart attack. Some doctors are questioning using calcium channel blockers as a first-line treatment for hypertension because they do not appear to provide the protective benefits of diuretics, beta-blockers and ACE inhibitors.

•Can hypertension be cured? Once you have essential hypertension, it never goes away. You'll have to monitor your blood pressure on a regular basis for the rest of your life. However, with a combination of lifestyle changes and well-tailored medication, most people can bring their pressure down to safe levels.

Lifesaving Breakthroughs In Stroke Treatment

Thomas Brott, MD, professor of neurology, Mayo Clinic, Jacksonville FL. He helped develop one of the most successful citywide emergency stroke treatment programs in the US.

Not long ago, stroke was considered untreatable. There was little doctors could do for the half-million Americans each year who suffer this devastating neurological problem.

Now: Armed with a "clot-busting" medication, doctors can prevent much of the brain damage caused by the most common form of stroke.

We spoke recently with Thomas Brott, MD, about the new developments in stroke care…

●**What are the new drug treatments we've been hearing about?** The first approach is to use a genetically engineered anticoagulant called *tissue-plasminogen activator* (TPA) to dissolve stroke-related blood clots. This brings oxygen to brain cells whose oxygen supply has been cut off by clots.

In the second approach, doctors treat brain cells with *neuroprotectors*. These experimental drugs prevent the "cascade" of chemical reactions that kill brain cells subjected to brief periods of oxygen starvation.

●**How effective are these treatments?** The jury is still out on neuroprotectors, but studies suggest that TPA increases the chance for total or near-total recovery from a stroke by 35% to 55%.

The hitch is that TPA works well only if it's given within three hours of the onset of the stroke. Since there was little they could do anyway, doctors used to take a "wait-and-see" approach to stroke. Now that effective treatments are available, doctors and patients alike should treat stroke as a medical emergency—just like heart attack.

●**How can I be sure to get prompt, effective treatment, should I suffer a stroke?** Know the telltale symptoms of stroke—and make sure anyone you live with knows them, too.

Typical symptoms include a loss of balance or coordination…a sudden inability to walk… numbness or weakness, particularly on one side of the body…and blurred or decreased vision, particularly in one eye or on one side of the visual field of each eye.

If the language area of the brain is affected, there may be an inability to speak, slurred speech or difficulty understanding what's being said.

If even *one* of these symptoms is present, call 911 immediately.

●**Is there any special procedure that should be followed?** To determine what type of stroke the patient has suffered, doctors should order a *computed tomography* (CT) scan of the head within one hour.

Five out of every six stroke patients have what is known as an *ischemic* stroke. It's caused by a blood clot that blocks the flow of blood to the brain.

The other likely possibility is *hemorrhagic* stroke. It's caused by the rupture of a blood vessel in the brain.

If the CT scan and other tests indicate that the patient has had an ischemic stroke, doctors should administer TPA right away.

●**Is TPA widely available?** Virtually every hospital pharmacy in the US now has TPA. But not every emergency room is staffed with doctors skilled at administering the drug.

TPA is *very* tricky to use. About 6% of people who get it experience bleeding in the brain. And—TPA is off-limits to many patients with high blood pressure…those taking *warfarin* (Coumadin) or another blood thinner…and those who have problems with their platelet count or blood sugar levels.

●**When will neuroprotective drugs be available?** Several neuroprotective drugs are now in Phase III clinical trials (the last hurdle before FDA approval).

Other promising neuroprotective agents—including *aptiganel, nalmefene, citicoline* and *anti-ICAMA-1 antibodies*—may still be years off.

●**Are any other promising treatments on the way?** Other stroke drugs currently in Phase III trials include the clot-dissolving drug *prourokinase* and *ancrod,* a blood thinner derived from pit viper venom.

Another promising treatment involves temporarily reversing the direction of blood flow in the large veins of the body. Researchers hope that this "retrograde" blood flow therapy will be even more effective than TPA at dislodging clots from blood vessels within the brain.

●**Who is at greatest risk for stroke?** Risk for stroke goes up with age—doubling each decade after age 55. You can't do anything about your age, of course, but if you have any of the risk factors for stroke, ask your doctor about treating the underlying disorder.

You should also ask your doctor about taking aspirin or another blood thinner.

Evidence suggests that aspirin therapy reduces the risk for stroke—especially in those who have the heartbeat abnormality known as *atrial fibrillation.*

●**What are the risk factors for stroke?** High blood pressure...elevated cholesterol ...atrial fibrillation...diabetes...previous heart attack...and cholesterol deposits in the carotid arteries in the neck. A doctor can check for such blockages using ultrasound.

For Serious Medical Emergencies

Stephan Lynn, MD, director of the department of emergency medicine at St. Luke's-Roosevelt Hospital Center in New York City. Dr. Lynn is also author of *Medical Emergency!* Diane Books.

When a serious health emergency strikes, our first instinct is to panic. That's because most of us don't know what to do in such a situation. *Here are the most serious medical conditions—and what to do until help arrives...*

HEART ATTACK

Chest pain is the most common symptom of a heart attack, which occurs when an artery is blocked by a blood clot. This stops blood flow to the heart and damages the cardiac muscle.

Symptoms: Crushing pain in the middle of the chest, which may radiate to the jaw, neck, shoulders, back or arms...shortness of breath ...sweating...nausea and/or vomiting.

How to help yourself or someone else: If the symptoms last longer than three to five minutes and are particularly severe or aren't relieved by antacids...

●**Call an ambulance.** Never drive yourself to the hospital since there is a strong possibility that you may pass out. Paramedics can provide early medical care—ambulances carry defibrillators, the machines that can restore a normal heart rhythm and prevent death.

●**Take an aspirin.** It's been shown to limit damage from a heart attack.

●**Lie down, breathe slowly and keep calm.** Anxiety and activity can increase heart damage.

STROKE

As the name implies, a stroke hits suddenly —when a blood clot or hemorrhage affects the brain, preventing blood and oxygen from circulating.

Symptoms: Unexpected numbness and weakness that usually affects one side of the body...vision disturbances...an inability to speak.

How to help yourself or someone else: Have the person sit down immediately so he/ she doesn't fall...call an ambulance...make sure the airway is open by tilting the head back and the chin up.

SHORTNESS OF BREATH

Many conditions can cause severe shortness of breath—pneumonia...asthma...inhalation of toxic fumes or smoke...bronchitis...an airway obstruction...a blood clot in the lungs...or a heart attack.

Symptoms: Nostrils that open wide...an Adam's apple that moves up when you inhale... the need to use neck muscles to breathe...discomfort when you inhale...gasping...dizziness and/or fainting.

How to help yourself or someone else: Call an ambulance, which will supply you with oxygen while taking you to the hospital...sit with your head elevated...breathe slowly and deeply...remain calm.

ALLERGIC REACTION

A serious allergic reaction can occur after eating certain foods, receiving an injection, taking a drug or getting an insect bite or sting. Many times the cause is unknown.

Symptoms: Severe or sudden hives, itching or a rash...flushed skin...swollen tissues around the mouth and in the airway...breathing difficulties such as wheezing…physical weakness…nausea…dizziness and/or collapse.

How to help yourself or someone else: Call an ambulance. If you have a known allergy and carry an *epinephrine* injection, immediately give yourself a shot or have someone else do it.

If you don't have *epinephrine*, take an antihistamine. *Diphenhydramine* (Benadryl) can be bought without a prescription. Apply ice to the affected area to reduce the swelling and itching. Lie down.

FRACTURE

It can be difficult to distinguish a mere sprain from a more serious fracture without an X-ray.

Symptoms: Fractures are signaled by intense pain or swelling, an inability to use a body part—hip, wrist, arm, shoulder, ankle, leg—or an obviously misshapen or broken extremity or body part.

How to help yourself: When in doubt go to a hospital emergency room. *While you're in transit, follow the RICE procedure if you can…*

Rest…

Ice the injury to reduce swelling…

Compression. Wear an elastic bandage around the extremity to provide support…

Elevate the body part so blood and other fluids won't pool there.

Important: If you're not in severe pain or don't obviously have a break, you can do the RICE procedure for 24 to 48 hours and see if the injury improves. If you do not notice any improvement, see a doctor.

How to help someone else: Don't move or bear weight on the injured part. You may make a splint out of a rolled-up magazine. If there is severe pain, multiple injuries or bleeding, call an ambulance.

AT THE EMERGENCY ROOM

Gaining appropriate attention and priority in the emergency department depends upon "planning for your emergency" and carefully communicating with personnel once you are there.

●**Create a list that you can always carry with you.** Include your medical problems, your medications and your allergies, as well as your name, address and phone number and your insurance information.

●**Know how to call an ambulance in your community** and which emergency rooms are best for your special needs.

●**Communicate effectively by speaking slowly**…telling the doctor or nurse exactly what happened to you. Don't expect that medical personnel will already know what's wrong or why.

●**Understand that a triage nurse** will determine the order in which you will be seen based upon his/her assessment of your medical needs compared with those of others who are waiting.

Easy Ways to Save Big Money on Prescription Drugs

Donald L. Sullivan, RPh, PhD, associate professor of pharmacy practice, Ohio Northern University, Ada, and author of *The Consumer's Guide to Generic Drugs: The Complete Reference Book for Anyone Using Prescription Drugs.* Penguin.

No doubt you already know that you can often save on costly medications by asking your doctor for a prescription for generic equivalents. *Here are five more cost-cutting tricks…*

●**Ask for free samples.** Doctors are deluged with drug samples from manufacturers—but they don't always distribute these samples to their patients.

Ask, and you may get a week or more of a pricey drug for free.

Caution: Check expiration dates. Forgo samples that have been sitting around the doctor's office for too long.

●**Use mail order or the Internet—**but only when appropriate. Buying prescriptions by mail or on the Internet can be an economical, convenient way to purchase drugs. However, many mail-order pharmacies use nonpharmacists to fill prescriptions.

While a pharmacist does do a final check, the volume of drugs being processed is very high—and mistakes are possible.

Going the mail-order or Internet route also means you lose the benefit of a face-to-face meeting with your pharmacist—who can warn you about drug interactions or answer your questions on the spot.

Bottom line: If you want to use mail order or the Internet, do so only with drugs you're familiar with—ideally, drugs you must take on a long-term basis. That way, you reduce your risk of taking the wrong drug or falling victim to unforeseen drug interactions.

●**Don't let your insurance company impose limits** on prescription length. If your doctor writes a prescription for a 90-day supply of pills, your insurer may approve only a 30-day supply.

Limiting your prescription in this manner helps the insurer cut costs...but costs you money and extra trips to the drugstore.

Loophole: If you need 90 days of pills but your insurer covers only 30 days, ask your doctor to substitute "take as directed" instead of "take once a day" on the prescription form.

That makes it hard for the insurance company to calculate how many pills comprise a 30-day supply. You'll be able to get the full 90-day supply filled.

Caution: Find out how often the drug should be taken, and write it yourself on the bottle.

●**Avoid time-release formulations.** Many prescription drugs are available in both time-release and non-time-release forms. Time-release pills are much more convenient because they don't have to be taken as often as their "plain" counterparts. But they're also more costly.

●**Look into patient-assistance programs.** Under such programs—offered by most pharmaceutical makers but rarely publicized—individuals short on cash because of job loss or another financial setback may qualify for free prescription medication.

In most cases, all that's required is your doctor's certification that you're unable to afford a costly but necessary medication.

Call the manufacturer directly to find out if a particular drug is available through such a program—and what the terms are.

The Importance of Support Groups for Chronic Illness

David Spiegel, MD, associate chair of psychiatry and behavioral sciences at Stanford University School of Medicine in Stanford, CA. He is author of *Living Beyond Limits: New Hope and Help for Facing Life-Threatening Illness.* Ballantine.

If you're suffering from arthritis, diabetes, cancer or another serious or chronic illness, participating in a support group can boost your emotional and even your physical well-being.

Unfortunately, few people who could benefit from participating in a group do so.

Some of us shy away from support groups because we fear we'll be too embarrassed to discuss our problems with strangers. Of course, members of a support group don't remain strangers for long.

Others view support groups as a source of emotional "hand-holding" for people who are weak or insecure.

In fact, group participants spend little time feeling sorry for each other. They help one another face their problems head-on—*and it really pays off*.

WHAT THE RESEARCH SHOWS

●**Breast cancer.** In a study at Stanford University, 86 women with advanced (metastatic) breast cancer were randomly assigned to one of two groups.

One group received standard medical care. The other group got identical care *plus* weekly sessions with a support group. At the end of the first year, women who had participated in the support group felt less anxious and depressed than the women who had not participated in the group. They also reported half as much physical pain as the other women.

Long-term follow-up showed something that was even more remarkable—that the support group participants lived an average of 18 months longer.

●**Malignant melanoma.** University of California at Los Angeles researchers conducted a randomized trial of 80 melanoma patients.

The 40 patients assigned to the control group received standard medical care. The other 40 patients in the experimental group got standard medical care—and they participated in weekly support group sessions.

When tested six weeks later, the experimental group reported less anxiety and depression than the control group. Six years later, 10 members of the control group had died. Only three of the experimental group had died.

●**Diabetes.** A University of Chicago study found that male diabetics who participated in support groups were less depressed than similar men who did not participate in support groups.

HEIGHTENED IMMUNITY

What accounts for these dramatic findings? One theory is that the social support created by a group boosts the immune system by reducing the psychological stress associated with serious illness, and is known to interfere with immunity.

This theory is supported by the UCLA study, which found unusually high levels of immune system cells called *natural-killer cells* in patients who participated in support groups.

MUTUAL ENCOURAGEMENT

Support group members also encourage each other to take better care of themselves physically. Some act as advocates for one another, making sure they get access to information and proper treatment.

Groups fight isolation by giving members a chance to talk to people who understand what they're going through—this at a time when family and friends may not know what to say.

Finally, support groups help people find meaning in their suffering. Because the group gives them an opportunity to use their own experiences to help others, many patients feel that some good has come from a bad situation.

FINDING THE RIGHT GROUP

If your doctor or a hospital social worker is unable to steer you to a group, visit the American Self-Help Clearinghouse Web site at *www.selfhelpgroups.org*.

The group's facilitator should be knowledgeable about group dynamics as well as about your specific illness and its treatment.

Look for a group headed by a doctor, psychologist, nurse or social worker. Fees should be reasonable—no more than $40 per person per session.

If you can't find a group near you, start your own. Post a notice at a hospital, clinic or church, seeking members who are dealing with the same illness. At the same time, start your search for a facilitator.

Many successful groups are run by their members (and have no leader). However, a professional facilitator is best equipped to handle members who get upset, try to dominate the discussion or keep avoiding important issues.

FOR MAXIMUM BENEFIT

You'll get the most out of your group by making a point to attend every session. It's much easier to establish a trusting environment if all of the participants commit themselves to showing up for the sessions.

Do not feel obliged to speak up. Realize, however, that you will get more from a group the more you talk about what you are going through...and the better you are at listening to other members.

2

Everyday Remedies

The Ultimate Guide to Infectious Disease

Winkler G. Weinberg, MD
Southeast Permanente Medical Group

Many of the diseases that seem to strike out of the blue actually have their origins in our personal habits. *Here's how to protect yourself and your family from infectious illnesses…*

WASH YOUR HANDS

Colds and flu are contracted not by being *near* a coughing, sneezing person, but by *touch*.

Self-defense: Wash your hands as soon as possible after touching someone who's ill… after touching something an ill person has touched…and just periodically when you're living or working with an infected individual.

Until you wash up, don't touch your eyes or nose. Those are the main entry points for cold viruses. For times when no sink is handy, carry a supply of alcohol-based wipes.

PREPARE FOOD CAREFULLY

Much of the meat and eggs in the supermarket are tainted with *salmonella*.

Escherichia coli (E. coli) is present in up to 4% of ground beef, pork, poultry and lamb. It's also found in unpasteurized milk and juice and other beverages.

To prevent food poisoning…

●**Refrigerate food immediately after preparing or serving it.** If it's been sitting out for more than an hour, throw it away.

●**Avoid steak tartare and raw or undercooked eggs.** Steer clear of Caesar salad and homemade eggnog and mayonnaise. If *any*

Winkler G. Weinberg, MD, chief of infectious diseases for Atlanta-based Southeast Permanente Medical Group. He is author of *No Germs Allowed: How to Avoid Infectious Diseases at Home and on the Road.* Rutgers University Press.

yolk from a contaminated egg remains liquid, salmonella can survive.

● **Wash utensils or surfaces that have been in contact with raw meat or eggs** before using them again.

● **Drink only *pasteurized* milk and juice.**

● **Avoid bottom-feeding fish.** Grouper, red snapper, amberjack and barracuda can harbor *ciguatera*, a disease-causing toxin.

● **Steam shellfish for at least 15 minutes.** Thorough steaming takes care of E. coli and other infectious agents that are commonly found in clams, oysters and mussels.

GUARD AGAINST TICK BITES

Most tick bites are benign. But since Lyme disease and other tick-borne illnesses can be hard to detect and treat, it's best to avoid getting bitten in the first place.

During tick season (April through the first frost), take these precautions...

● **When walking in wooded or grassy areas,** wear long-sleeved shirts and long, loose-fitting pants tucked into socks.

● **Use insect repellent containing DEET.** A 30% concentration is best. Put it on your clothing *and* any exposed skin.

● **If you have outdoor pets, use tick-killing powder or spray.** Your veterinarian can recommend a good brand.

● **Check yourself for ticks daily.** Have a family member check your scalp and other hard-to-see areas. Look closely—some ticks are the size of a pinhead.

If you find a tick, do *not* remove it with alcohol, petroleum jelly or a lighted match. These methods can cause the tick to regurgitate under your skin, raising your chance of illness.

Better: Using tweezers, gently grasp the tick and pull steadily *outward* at the same angle the tick is facing.

Keep the tick in a jar of alcohol, so it can be identified later if you develop a bull's-eye rash or other suspicious symptoms.

PREVENT URINARY INFECTIONS

Women who are prone to urinary tract infections (UTIs) may want to consider using a birth control method other than the diaphragm.

Spermicidal jellies and foams used with a diaphragm create an environment hospitable to bacteria.

Women should also urinate after intercourse to flush out infection-causing bacteria. UTIs are rare among men.

AVOID PARASITES IN WATER

In most areas, tap water is chlorinated to kill bacteria. But chlorination does not kill *Cryptosporidium* and other parasites.

Self-defense: If you have poor immunity, boil water for one minute or install a reverse-osmosis water purifier under your sink.

BE CAREFUL WHILE TRAVELING

Check with a doctor well in advance of your trip and get any recommended vaccinations.

In the US, Canada, Western Europe, Australia, New Zealand and Japan, food and water are usually safe. In other regions, eat only fully cooked or freshly peeled foods. Bring your own water...or drink carbonated beverages or wine.

Watch out for ice cubes and the mixers in mixed drinks.

To purify water: Boil it for at least one minute. Or—add 2% tincture of iodine (five drops per quart of water), and let it sit for at least an hour. This method is good for suspect tap water and water from a stream or lake.

If you visit an area where malaria and/or other insect-borne diseases are endemic, wear light, loose-fitting clothing and mosquito netting...use DEET spray...and stay indoors as much as possible.

LEGIONNAIRE'S DISEASE

Smokers, elderly people and individuals taking immunosuppressant drugs are at risk for Legionnaire's disease.

The bacteria that cause Legionnaire's are often found in shower heads, air conditioning systems and cooling towers—in the US and abroad.

Self-defense: Stay as far away as possible from cooling towers. And—before using an unfamiliar shower, sterilize the shower head by running the water at its hottest setting for five minutes.

Everything You Need to Know About Bacteria!

Linda R. Gooding, PhD, professor of microbiology and immunology at Emory University School of Medicine, Atlanta.

Though bacteria are often viewed as agents of disease, many of the billions of microorganisms dwelling inside our bodies are essential for good health.

"Friendly" bacteria—such as the lactobacillus and bifida cultures in yogurt—inhibit growth of yeast and other disease-causing organisms. There's even evidence that friendly bacteria help lower cholesterol levels.

Problem: Each time you take an antibiotic, you kill bacteria in your body—friendly and unfriendly alike. That raises your risk of diarrhea, yeast infection and food sensitivity.

Bacteria are also killed by cortisone, prednisone, birth-control pills, antacids—even stress.

To the rescue: A family of supplements known as *probiotics*. These blends of bacteria and rice or milk powder repopulate the bowel with friendly bacteria.

In a study at Long Island Jewish Medical Center, women who ate a daily cup of yogurt had fewer vaginal infections than women who didn't eat yogurt. The effect might have been even *more* significant had the women taken probiotics.

To keep your intestinal flora healthy, I recommend eating yogurt regularly. Most brands contain active cultures. Be sure to check labels if you're unsure.

Take probiotics in *addition* to yogurt if you have high cholesterol or chronic yeast infections…while traveling…or while taking antibiotics, steroids, birth-control pills or antacids.

Probiotics are available at health-food stores. Pick a brand that contains at least one billion live organisms per gram. Be sure to check the package's expiration date.

How to Stay Healthy on Your Next Airplane Flight

Adriane Fugh-Berman, MD, associate professor, department of physiology and biophysics, Georgetown University School of Medicine. She is author of *Alternative Medicine: What Works*. Lippincott, Williams & Wilkens.

Any long trip is tiring. But air travel can also cause health problems—colds and other respiratory infections, aches and pains, jet lag and even a potentially fatal condition known as *pulmonary embolism*. Fortunately, there are easy ways to prevent each of these problems.

COLDS

It's easy to catch cold while traveling by air. That's because the air inside most jets is recirculated. And so are the airborne germs.

Sitting far away from someone with a cough doesn't help. Since you're in a confined space, you're almost equally likely to be exposed to germs whether the source of the germs is 20 rows away or right next to you.

Making matters worse, the humidity inside a modern jetliner is usually 10% or lower. That's less humid than desert air. By drying the mucous membranes lining your nose, mouth and respiratory tract, low humidity makes it easy for viruses and bacteria to get a foothold.

To fend off "airliner germs," some people have resorted to wearing surgical masks during flights. I don't recommend that. But I do recommend boosting your immune system. The day before, the day of and the day after your departure, swallow one-half dropperful of *echinacea* tincture…along with 2,000 milligrams (mg) of vitamin C (divided into two 1,000 mg doses).

Drink 16 ounces of water or juice just before boarding the plane…and 12 ounces *each hour* while you're in the air. You might want to bring your own water bottle, in case the flight attendants are too busy to serve you.

BACKACHE AND NECK PAIN

Support your lumbar spine by placing a rolled blanket behind your back. If you plan to doze, a U-shaped neck pillow makes a big difference. I prefer *inflatable* pillows, since they take up less space in your carry-on bag. They cost about $10 and are available at luggage stores.

Two exercises are also helpful…

•**Shoulder circles.** Shrug your shoulders up and down, then roll them forward and back.

•**Head circles.** Tilt your head to the side, ear toward shoulder. Hold briefly, then raise your head back to center. Tilt to the other side, then return to center. Drop your chin to your chest, hold briefly, then return your head to its normal position. Tilt your head back, hold, then return to center.

JET LAG

The best way I've found to fight jet lag is to reset your biological clock with melatonin after your arrival. Two hours before your new bedtime, take 1 to 3 mg. Take it the next two days, too, if you have trouble adjusting to your new schedule. Exposure to natural daylight after your arrival will also help you adjust.

PULMONARY EMBOLISM

Hours of sitting almost motionless slows your circulation, raising your risk for pulmonary embolism. In this potentially deadly condition, a blood clot forms in the leg, then breaks away and travels to the lung—where it can interfere with the body's oxygen supply.

To keep blood from pooling in your lower extremities, take periodic walks during the flight. As you walk about the cabin, occasionally stand on your toes, then rock back on your heels.

If the seat belt sign is on, do the following exercises in your seat…

•**Heel rocks.** Sit with your back straight and feet flat on the floor. Lift your heels, then rock back on them. Then alternately flex and point your toes.

•**Leg lifts.** Press down on your left thigh with your left hand, and lift your thigh against this resistance. Repeat 20 times. Switch sides and repeat.

Water Therapy for Common Ailments

The late Dian Dincin Buchman, PhD, a New York City–based lecturer on water therapy and other alternative therapies, and author of several books, including *The Complete Book of Water Healing*. McGraw-Hill.

Ice packs, hot and cold compresses, medicated baths and other forms of water therapy were mainstays of folk medicine for centuries.

Today, high-tech medicine has eclipsed water-based treatments. Yet these treatments—safe, inexpensive and easy to use—remain valuable tools for easing discomfort caused by common ailments.

MEDICATED BATHS

We all know how relaxing a warm bath can be. But not everyone realizes that even *greater* benefits can be reaped by adding natural ingredients to the water.

•**Apple cider vinegar.** Add a cup to bathwater, and splash a handful over your shoulders, back and chest. That will invigorate you when you're fatigued.

This technique also helps restore the skin's germ-killing natural acidity, which is continually washed away by bathing.

To soothe poison ivy or sunburn, add *two* cups of vinegar.

•**Bran.** A bran bath eases itching, soothes dermatitis or other skin irritations and eliminates scaly patches.

Sew several handfuls of wheat or oat bran into a cheesecloth pouch. Soak the pouch in hot water for several minutes, then place in a tub filled with tepid water. Squeeze the pouch until the water turns milky.

•**Pine extract.** One capful in a warm bath helps open clogged pores, speeds healing of rashes and relieves muscle fatigue.

Pine extract is available at drugstores and health-food stores. Do not confuse it with pine *cleanser*, which will irritate the skin.

SALT MASSAGE

This energizing technique tones tissues, relieves stress and fatigue…and can help you ward off a cold.

Sit on the edge of a tub filled with warm water. Pour salt into a cupped hand. Slowly add water to the salt until you make a thick paste.

Using firm, circular motions, rub the paste over your body. Then rinse off the paste with a brief soak in the tub...or sponge it off with cold water. Be careful not to rub salt onto sores, cuts, etc.

HAND BATH

To ease writer's cramp, soak hands in hot water. To warm cold hands, soak them alternately in hot water (three minutes) and cold water (30 seconds). Repeat several times, ending with cold water.

Caution: Don't leave hands in cold water for more than a few minutes at a time.

COLD-WATER TREADING

Fill the tub ankle-deep with cold water. Holding onto a firmly anchored rail, march in place for a few seconds or minutes (as long as you can comfortably tolerate). Then rub your feet briskly with a towel.

Done twice daily, this technique creates a remarkable sense of well-being...and is great for relieving exercise-related leg cramps. Some believe that it builds resistance to disease as well.

Done at night, cold-water treading promotes sound sleep—yet it has an eye-opening effect when done in the morning.

COMPRESSES

To prevent or relieve headache pain, fold a washcloth in half, dip it in ice water and wring it out. Place it on your head or neck. Rewet it every few minutes to keep it cold.

To relieve a sore throat or laryngitis, fold a cotton cloth in thirds, wet it with cold water and wring it out. Wind it once around the neck and fasten with a safety pin. Over the cloth, wrap a wool scarf.

Leave this wrap in place as long as you like. With the cold trapped against the skin by the wool, the body continues to divert more warming blood to the area—helping break up congestion.

How to Feel and Look Younger

David Ryback, PhD, an antiaging/stress reduction consultant in Atlanta. He is author of *Look 10 Years Younger, Live 10 Years Longer,* which is available in editions for men and for women. Prentice Hall.

Practice stretching each morning. Regular stretching helps you feel more flexible and, as a result, you will feel and look younger. By stretching, you relax your muscles, and movements become more graceful and youthful.

• **Stand up straight.** By maintaining good posture, you'll look 10 pounds thinner. Practice in front of the mirror, and you'll notice that your stomach looks flatter, your torso appears longer and thinner—and you don't have that old, tired, hunched look.

• **Exercise at least 15 minutes a day.** Physical activity alleviates depression and improves your mood. It also sends more blood to the skin, giving your complexion a healthy, rosy, youthful glow.

• **Eat more fruits and vegetables.** A vegetarian or even a semivegetarian diet that includes lots of fruits, vegetables and grains will help you maintain a stable energy level. By eating sensibly, you can quickly increase your energy level and feel younger.

• **Reduce stress.** If left unchecked, stress puts unnecessary wear and tear on your body's internal organs and causes you to look tired and years older.

How to Break Bad Habits

William J. Knaus, EdD, author of *Change Your Life Now: Powerful Techniques for Positive Change.* Wiley.

To break a problem habit, you need to create a *will to change*—not an attempt to restrain yourself. Self-restraint against bad habits rarely works.

51

Example: Dieters usually gain back the weight they have lost. But a *will to change* is a command effort that allows experimenting with change, accepting its difficulty and moving ahead again even after inevitable backsliding.

Helpful: Deflect your attention from the habit to something else.

Example: Keep a pitcher of water in the refrigerator. Whenever you have a habit urge—of any kind—pour and slowly sip two glasses of ice water. This will often allow time for the urge to pass.

Simple Solutions For Incontinence

Kristene E. Whitmore, MD, chief of urology and female pelvic medicine, Drexel University College of Medicine, Philadelphia. She is coauthor of *Overcoming Bladder Disorders*. Perennial.

More than 13 million Americans have trouble controlling their bladders. Urinary incontinence is *not* a disease. It's a symptom of an underlying problem—diabetes, stroke, multiple sclerosis (MS), Parkinson's disease or even chronic bladder infection.

Obese people face heightened risk for incontinence. So do smokers and women—especially those who have recently had a baby. Passage of the baby through the birth canal often damages the abdominal muscles responsible for holding and releasing urine.

In men, incontinence is usually a result of nerve damage caused by surgery to treat prostate enlargement or cancer.

Good news: Incontinence can often be prevented—or controlled. If you're incontinent—or worried that you might become incontinent—avoid caffeine, alcohol, spicy foods, chocolate, artificial sweeteners and other bladder irritants...urinate before and after intercourse to expel infection-causing bacteria...and drink lots of water.

Do *not* drink large quantities of water at one time, however. Doing so causes the bladder to fill too rapidly. Have one sip every five to 10 minutes throughout the day.

Women: To keep pelvic floor muscles strong, do Kegel exercises.

Women with recurrent bladder infections should take a cranberry pill with each meal. The pills contain compounds that keep infection-causing bacteria from sticking to bladder walls.

Cranberries and cranberry juice also contain these compounds—but at lower levels.

Men: Ask your doctor about taking a zinc supplement and saw palmetto extract. Both have been shown to prevent or relieve prostate enlargement.

TYPES OF INCONTINENCE

Four out of five cases of incontinence can now either be cured or made better. *The first step is to identify which of the four types is involved...*

- **Stress incontinence** is associated with a weakness of the urinary sphincter, the circular valve-like muscle around the bladder neck and urethra that controls the flow of urine.

Coughing, laughing, etc., exert more pressure on the bladder than the sphincter can contain, and urine spills out.

Usual causes: Abdominal or pelvic surgery, childbirth, estrogen deficiency. Certain drugs, including alpha blockers and diuretics, make matters worse.

- **Urge incontinence** occurs when "overexcited" nerves cause involuntary contraction of bladder muscles. You have a sudden urge to urinate—but can't reach a toilet in time.

Usual causes: Parkinson's disease, multiple sclerosis, bladder infection, the bladder disorder *interstitial cystitis*, spinal cord problems, chemotherapy.

- **Overflow incontinence** occurs when weak bladder muscles or a urinary obstruction makes it hard to empty the bladder. Urine eventually overflows, like water over a dam.

Usual causes: Diabetes, enlarged prostate in men, prolapsed (dropped) bladder or uterus in women. The problem can also be caused by over-the-counter cold and allergy medications...or by the decongestant *pseudoephedrine*.

- **Functional incontinence** is a transient problem associated with stool impaction, restricted mobility, vaginal irritation and other conditions.

BLADDER TRAINING

The aim of bladder training is to empty the bladder *on schedule*—so that urine won't build up to the point where an accident occurs.

At first, urinate every 90 minutes. Gradually lengthen the interval between trips to the bathroom—up to three hours—until you find a schedule that's safe and convenient.

Helpful: A "voiding diary." For two to three days in a row, record how often you urinate—and when leakage occurs. Review the diary with your doctor.

KEGEL EXERCISES

Most people with stress or urge incontinence get partial relief if they strengthen the urinary sphincter. *To do Kegel exercises...*

- **Identify the muscle you want to train.** It's the same muscle used to control a bowel movement. If you have trouble identifying it, place a finger in your vagina (if you're a woman) or anus (if you're a man). Practice squeezing only the muscle around your finger.

- **For the first three to six days,** squeeze the muscle for three seconds at a time.

- **Over the next few weeks,** gradually build up till you can tighten the sphincter for 10 seconds at a time. Relax the muscle for 10 seconds after each contraction. Do 50 every day.

BIOFEEDBACK AND WEIGHTS

Biofeedback uses a special tampon, inserted in the vagina or rectum, to help you identify the muscles that need to be strengthened. The tampons are available by prescription.

Women whose incontinence is caused by weak abdominal muscles often benefit from vaginal "weight training." Cone-shaped weights are held in the vagina for 15 minutes, twice a day, as you go about your daily activities.*

HELPFUL MEDICATIONS

Drug therapy brings faster relief than do the nondrug approaches outlined above—but it often causes side effects.

Best approach: Start taking the medication when you begin bladder training, diet and

*To find out where you can purchase these and other incontinence products, call the National Association for Continence at 800-252-3337.

Kegel exercises. Gradually wean yourself off the drugs as the non-drug methods start to work.

- **Oxybutinin** (Ditropan), *propantheline* (Norpanth), tricyclic antidepressants like *imipramine* (Tofranil) are good for stress and urge incontinence. Side effects include dry mouth, constipation and dry skin.

- **Diet pills** containing *pseudoephedrine* are good for stress incontinence. Side effects include anxiety, insomnia, sweating. Do not use if you have high blood pressure.

THE SURGICAL OPTION

When other treatments fail to provide relief from incontinence, surgery may be the answer.

Several different forms of surgery are available, depending upon the exact nature of the problem and its severity.

Hemorrhoid Self-Defense

Mayo Clinic Health Letter, 200 First St. SW, Rochester, MN 55905.

Eat high-fiber foods—fresh fruits, vegetables and whole grains...drink plenty of water—at least six cups a day...stay active, which reduces pressure in anal and rectal veins that results from being in one position too long. Regular exercise also helps prevent constipation.

Prevention and Treatment of Common Foot Problems

Suzanne M. Levine, DPM, a podiatrist in private practice in New York City. She is author of *My Feet Are Killing Me!* (Fawcett), *Your Feet Don't Have to Hurt* (St. Martin's) and *50 Ways to Ease Foot Pain* (Consumer Guide).

Eighty-seven percent of Americans have foot trouble—bunions, corns, calluses, foot odor, etc. Despite their prevalence, however, such problems are *not* inevitable. *Most can be prevented via a simple five-step foot-pampering regimen...*

● **Soak your feet at the end of each day.** Use lukewarm water along with Dr. Scholl's Soap 'n Soak Instant Foot Bath or another product containing *sodium bicarbonate*. This compound lowers the skin's acidity, rendering it less susceptible to fungus and calluses.

After soaking, dry your feet thoroughly—especially between your toes.

● **Massage moisturizer into your heels after each soak.** Moisturizer will help prevent skin fissures and calluses. These problems are common in summer—especially if you wear open-heeled shoes.

● **Use foot powder twice a day.** After soaking at night and then again in the morning, dust your feet with Quinsana Plus Anti-Fungal Foot Powder or another product containing the perspiration-fighting agent *benzethonium chloride*.

Foot powder is especially beneficial during summer months, when foot perspiration is a big problem.

● **Inspect your toenails once a week.** If they need trimming, cut them straight across using a long-handled nail clipper. Each time you trim your nails, scrub your toes and the soles of your feet to remove calluses.

For dry skin, use Kerasal or another foot mask containing *salicylic acid* or another "keratolytic agent." This rids the feet of excess keratin, a moisture-repelling protein found in skin.

● **Do nightly foot exercises.** Before going to bed, spend a few minutes picking up a pencil with your toes...pressing on an imaginary accelerator pedal with each foot...and using your toes to trace the outlines of letters of the alphabet on the floor.

Nightly foot exercises help minimize the foot swelling that inevitably occurs during the day.

BUNIONS

These bony protuberances on the sides of the feet are caused by ill-fitting shoes and/or hereditary factors. They can lead to painful calluses, osteoarthritis and/or hammertoes.

Self-defense: Wear loose-fitting shoes. New shoes should be purchased at midday, when the feet are slightly swollen. Make sure there's a thumb's-width space between the front of the shoe and your longest toe.

To reduce redness and swelling: Use ice around the bunion.

Finger test: If a whitish area appears when you press down on a bump, you may not be suffering from a bunion but from bursitis, a condition that requires medical attention.

CORNS

These areas of yellowish, thickened skin atop or between the toes can be quite painful. They're usually caused by friction and pressure on the foot.

Self-defense: Soak your feet in water containing Epsom salts. Afterward, apply moisturizer and cover the area with plastic wrap. After 15 minutes, remove the plastic and use a pumice stone to smooth out the corn.

Also helpful: Orthotics or foam insoles. Orthotics, which are custom-made, cost $350 or more—but are usually covered by insurance. Insoles are available at drugstores for less than $15.

HAMMERTOES

This problem—twisted or misshapen toes that may overlap each other—is common among people who have high arches.

Self-defense: Relieve pressure on the toes by wearing shoes with wide toes...and by covering corns with corn pads, lamb's wool or bandages. In severe cases, outpatient surgery may be necessary.

HEEL SPURS

These bony growths protruding downward from the heel bones are typically caused by rapid weight gain...or from playing tennis or another sport that places pressure on the heels.

Heel spurs are often confused with *plantar fasciitis.* This condition is usually caused by excessive stress or pressure on the plantar fascia, the protective tissue under the soles of the feet.

Self-defense: Put foam or felt pads in the heels of your shoes...or purchase insoles to help raise the arches of the feet.

Each time pain strikes, elevate your foot and apply an ice pack to the heel for 20 minutes.

Over-the-counter painkillers are effective against both heel spurs and plantar fasciitis.

Also helpful: Exercises that stretch the Achilles tendons. Once a day, try picking up marbles with your toes…or lifting your toes while the soles of your feet are planted firmly on the ground.

COLD FEET

This condition usually stems from foods, drugs and/or behaviors that cause impaired circulation—caffeinated foods and beverages …appetite suppressants…and smoking.

Self-defense: Stop smoking. Cut down on caffeinated foods and beverages. Switch shoes at least once a day, wearing shoes of different heel heights. Shift your weight back and forth while standing. Each night, take a bath in lukewarm water.

Once a day, do these three circulation-boosting exercises…

Exercise #1: Cross your legs at your ankles, then try to pull them apart as you simultaneously resist. Hold for one minute. Switch sides, and hold again.

Exercise #2: Place the balls of your feet on a telephone book, with your heels resting on the floor. Push up and down. This exercise may be done sitting or standing for one minute.

Exercise #3: Lie on the floor with your feet pressed flat against the wall. For about one minute, "climb the walls" using your feet.

TOENAIL FUNGUS

This condition (*onychomycosis*) can lead to warped and discolored toenails.

Self-defense: Make a paste with lukewarm water and baking soda. Rub it on the affected area daily. Rinse and dry.

Also helpful: Wear cotton socks…change shoes twice a day…and use antibacterial drying powder and foot deodorant. Avoid garlic and other spicy foods if they cause your feet to perspire.

Do *not* use opaque nail polish. It darkens the nail bed, making it vulnerable to fungal growth.

If symptoms persist, ask your doctor for the oral medication *itraconazole* (Sporanox).

ATHLETE'S FOOT

Most cases are caused by *Candida*, the same yeast that causes vaginal infections, and/or by *T. rubrum*, another type of fungus.

Self-defense: Keep your feet dry. Change socks at least once a day. Avoid colored socks—some are made with dyes that promote the growth of fungus.

Use Tinactin, Halotex or another antifungal ointment or spray containing a broad-spectrum antifungal agent of the *azole* family.

FOOT ODOR

This condition is caused by bacteria that thrive on moist, sweaty skin. It can also be caused by eating spices, which can cause sweat glands to become overactive.

Self-defense: Cut back on spicy foods, and keep feet dry. Change shoes at least once a day. Air them out after each wearing.

Also helpful: Dr. Scholl's Odor Destroyers Medicated Powder and Johnson & Johnson's Odor-Eaters.

Heel Pain Relief

Carol Frey, MD, associate clinical professor of orthopedic surgery at the University of Southern California School of Medicine in Los Angeles.

Store-bought pads relieve heel pain more effectively than custom-made inserts. Researchers gave foot stretching exercises to 200 people suffering from a heel condition called *isolated proximal plantar fasciitis.*

In addition, the researchers provided the subjects with several different cushioning devices—ranging from off-the-shelf rubber and silicon cushions and insoles costing between $9 and $40, to custom-made orthotic arch inserts costing between $300 and $500.

Stretching plus the store-bought devices helped 81% to 95% of the sufferers. But when combined with orthotics, stretching relieved less than 70%.

Medicine Cabinet Must-Haves

Timothy McCall, MD, an internist, medical editor of *Yoga Journal* and author of *Examining Your Doctor: A Patient's Guide to Avoiding Harmful Medical Care.* Carol. *www.drmccall.com.*

Every medicine cabinet should have the following basics...

- **Acetaminophen** or aspirin for pain and fever.

- **An antihistamine** for hives or other allergic reactions.

- **Triple-antibiotic ointment,** adhesive bandages, gauze, tape for minor wounds.

- **Ipecac syrup** to induce vomiting in certain types of poisoning. (Call Poison Control before giving.)

- **Ace bandages** for strains and sprains.

- **Thermometer.**

- **Pointed tweezers** for splinters.

Extend the Life of Athletic Shoes

Carol Frey, MD, associate clinical professor of orthopedic surgery at the University of Southern California School of Medicine in Los Angeles.

Air shoes out for 24 hours after each use... pull out the insoles and stuff them with newspapers or paper towels and place in a well-ventilated area...never leave shoes in the sun or a hot car...never toss them into a washing machine.

Also: Don't try to resuscitate worn-out shoes by adding new insoles. Most shoe breakdowns occur in the midsole—the wedge of cushioning between the outsole and the upper. Insoles are designed to provide support, not replace the midsole.

Emergency Ice Packs

Peter Bruno, MD, associate professor of medicine at New York University in New York City and internist for the New York Knicks basketball team.

If ice cubes aren't available, use a bag of frozen peas. It will hug body contours, easing pain and helping to heal.

Important: Wrap the bag in a cloth to prevent ice burn...apply for 10 minutes at a time.

CPR to the Rescue

Richard O. Cummins, MD, professor of medicine, division of emergency medicine, University of Washington Medical Center, Seattle.

Rescuers should start CPR before calling 911 when trying to resuscitate a child or a young adult. Clear the airway, do one minute of chest compressions, *then* call 911. With individuals over age 30, call 911 first.

Reason: An older person whose heart stops is probably experiencing ventricular fibrillation. This heart condition requires prompt treatment by emergency personnel. But a young person whose heart stops usually has only an obstructed airway—which can be cleared by anyone with minimal training. If you lack CPR training, call 911 first, then return to the victim and try to help.

Music Fights Insomnia

Gail C. Mornhinweg, PhD, ARNP, professor of nursing, University of Louisville, KY. Her six-month study of 25 adults with insomnia was published in *Journal of Holistic Nursing,* 2455 Teller Rd., Thousand Oaks, CA 91320.

Patients who had trouble sleeping were given two cassette tapes—one of Baroque music, the other of New Age music. After listening to the tapes at bedtime, all but one of the patients said they fell asleep faster and slept longer than usual.

Also: Sleeplessness returned on nights when the patients did not listen to music.

How to Reduce Your Risk of Cancer

David Alberts, MD, director of Cancer Prevention and Control at the Arizona Cancer Center in Tucson.

Reduce your risk of colorectal cancer by eating a diet high in fiber and calcium. Ninety people at risk for colorectal cancer were given varying doses of calcium and wheat bran fiber supplements.

Result: The high-fiber group (13.5 grams [g] per day) produced 52% less bile acid than did the low-fiber group. Those who consumed the most calcium (15,000 milligrams [mg]) had a 35% reduction in bile acid production.

Theory: Fiber and calcium soak up these cancer-promoting acids. One ounce of Kellogg's All-Bran contains nearly 10 g of fiber...and one cup of milk contains 300 mg of calcium.

 # Can't Sleep?

Mark R. Pressman, PhD, director, Sleep Medicine Services, The Lankenau Hospital and Medical Research Center, Wynnewood, PA. His study of 80 patients was published in *Archives of Internal Medicine*, 515 N. State St., Chicago 60610.

Sleep disorders often go undiagnosed. If you awaken repeatedly at night to use the bathroom, see a doctor to rule out the possibility that you're waking because of a sleep disorder. In a study, 79% of patients who *thought* they were getting up to urinate were actually being awakened by sleep apnea, snoring or leg movements.

Good news: Most sleep disorders can be successfully treated.

Help for People Who Can't Fall Asleep

Rituals of Healing: Using Imagery for Health and Wellness by Jeanne Achterberg, PhD, psychologist and body-mind researcher, Big Sur, CA. Bantam Books.

Simply telling your body to sleep probably will not work. Instead, try *active imaging*, where you use images to bring you to sleep.

Examples: Imagine a calming, repetitive scene, like waves at the seashore. Or let your mind drift into the memory of what it feels like to go to sleep.

Remember your usual sleeping position, and allow yourself to feel your body floating or moving downward into a comfortable, restful state.

Elevation and Breathing

Norman H. Edelman, MD, executive vice president and chief medical officer, American Lung Association, 61 Broadway, New York City 10006.

People with breathing disorders feel better if they move to a lower elevation. The lower the elevation, the more oxygen is in the air and the easier oxygen is transferred to blood. Some people who live at high elevations will benefit from moving to sea level.

Control Pet Allergies

Martha V. White, MD, research director, Institute for Asthma & Allergy, Washington Hospital Center, 106 Irving St. NW, Washington, DC 20010.

Keep the pet outside, off the furniture and out of your bedroom. In most cases, it is the saliva and dander—the dead skin that flakes off and travels through the air—not the pet hair that causes the allergy problem. Also consider washing your dog or cat daily with water. Avoid frequent shampooing—it can release dander more quickly.

Feeling Forgetful?

Barry Gordon, MD, PhD, professor of neurology and cognitive science and founder of the Memory Clinic at Johns Hopkins University, Baltimore, and author of *Memory: Remembering and Forgetting in Everyday Life.* MasterMedia.

Boost your memory by deciding what you need to remember most and focusing on it ...paying close attention to anything you want to memorize...learning to remember in little bits over time, not trying to remember a large amount of information at once.

Also helpful: Designate a *memory spot* in your home where you leave things, so you don't have to bother remembering where you put the car keys...or use a pocket notebook or file cards to help jog your memory.

Does Drinking Coffee Help Control Hay Fever?

Vincent Tubiolo, MD, allergy, asthma and immunology specialist, Santa Barbara, CA.

In a study, hay fever sufferers given 400 milligrams of caffeine (equal to 18 ounces of coffee) reported a 51% reduction in symptoms, compared with a 19% reduction in those given a placebo. Caffeine blocks nasal inflammation caused by hay fever.

Trap: Caffeine can raise blood pressure and heart rate. This study is *not* an excuse for hay fever sufferers to drink more coffee.

All About Home Testing

Rosemary Soave, MD, infectious disease specialist and associate professor of medicine at New York Hospital–Cornell Medical Center, New York City.

Home diagnostic tests are reasonably accurate. Be sure to follow directions carefully.

To protect yourself: If you do not understand something, call the toll-free number on the package, or ask your pharmacist or doctor before using the test...always read the directions carefully before starting a test...check the packaging to make sure the test has not passed its expiration date...store temperature-sensitive test kits in a dark area away from heat and sunlight. *Also:* When doing a timed test, use a watch that clearly shows seconds.

Bee Sting First Aid

Recommendations from the American Academy of Allergy, Asthma & Immunology, 555 E. Wells, Suite 1100, Milwaukee 53202.

Remove the stinger if it is visible by scraping gently with a butter knife or credit card. Do not squeeze the area and pull with tweezers or fingers—that can release more venom.

After removing the stinger, wash the area with soap and water and apply a cold pack to reduce pain and swelling.

Though rare, serious allergic reactions to bee stings occur within minutes. If the person who has been stung collapses, develops hives or swollen lips or eyes or has trouble breathing, call 911 immediately.

A Shot to Relieve Constipation

Guiseppe Brisinda, MD, senior investigator, University Hospital Agostino Gemelli, Rome, Italy, and leader of a study of Botox use in people with constipation, published in *American Journal of Gastroenterology.*

Botox shots may relieve constipation if the condition is caused by inappropriate contraction or inability to relax pelvic-floor muscles. Ask your doctor about local injections of Botox if traditional approaches, such as eating fiber and taking laxatives, are not effective.

Drink Up!

Food and You by the editors of *Prevention* magazine Health Books. Berkley.

To drink your recommended 64 ounces of water each day…

●**Drink a glass as soon as you wake up**—to replenish fluids lost during sleep.

●**Have a glass of water before any meal or snack** to help control your appetite.

●**Buy a 64-ounce container and fill it every day**—then keep it near you, on your desk at work or the kitchen table at home, so you can see how much you are drinking.

●**To have chilled water all day**—freeze a partially filled plastic bottle overnight, then top it off with more water in the morning.

Three Quick Massages

Donna DeFalco, massage therapist, writing in *American Health*, 28 W. 23 St., New York City 10010.

Anchor your thumbs behind your ears and make circles on your scalp with your fingers.

Knead the palms of your hands with the opposite thumbs, starting where the hand joins the wrist and working toward the spaces between the bones of the fingers.

Close your eyes and place your ring fingers just below your eyebrows, near the bridge of the nose. Press gently, slowly increasing the pressure for five seconds, release, and repeat twice more.

Headache Prevention

Robert G. Ford, MD, director, Ford Headache Clinic, Birmingham, AL.

Taking five minutes to relax at the very first sign of trouble can help stop a headache.

Examples: If you're stopped at a red light, progressively relax your left leg, from toes to buttock, while your right foot stays on the brake pedal. *At the office:* Close your eyes for one minute every hour and take long, deep breaths.

At the first sign of a headache: Rub your hands together to create heat, then gently press the heels of your hands onto your eyelids. Close your eyes and give your face, scalp and neck a brief massage. Look away at a distant point—or stare at your hands for a minute.

Avoiding Headache Triggers

Bob Niklewicz, PT, MA, a physical therapist in private practice in Rohnert Park, CA.

A headache can be triggered by holding the neck in one position for a prolonged period—such as when working on a computer, driving or even bird-watching.

Self-defense: If you're prone to headaches, ask your doctor to help you pinpoint neck strain or other headache triggers.

Also helpful: Learn deep breathing and other relaxation techniques. Use good posture when standing or sitting.

Headache Relief

John G. Arena, PhD, professor of psychiatry and health behavior, Medical College of Georgia, Augusta.

Relaxation of the neck and shoulder muscles is the best way to relieve tension headaches. A study found that people who learned to relax their trapezius muscles reduced the intensity and duration of headaches by at least half. Relaxing these muscles proved far more effective than relaxing the forehead or using relaxation methods to relax all the other muscles of the body.

The headache sufferers taught themselves how to relax the neck and shoulder muscles by mental means until they discovered what worked best for them.

Beat Heartburn Without Drugs

Marvin Lipman, MD, chief medical adviser, Consumers Union, writing in *Consumer Reports on Health*, 101 Truman Ave., Yonkers, NY 10703.

Avoid foods that can trigger it—alcohol, chocolate, peppermint, spearmint and fat. Avoid caffeine in foods and over-the-counter pain medications. Avoid carbonated drinks. *Also:* If you are overweight, lose weight…if you smoke, quit.

For nighttime heartburn: Raise the head of your bed on four- to six-inch blocks, or use a wedge-shaped support to elevate the upper half of your body. Do not lie down with a full stomach.

For Better Driving With Arthritis…

Tammi Shlotzhauer, MD, assistant medical director, Rochester Clinical Research, Rochester, NY, and coauthor of *Living with Rheumatoid Arthritis.* Johns Hopkins University Press.

Stop frequently to get out and stretch in order to prevent stiffness and soreness.

Consider having lever aids installed on door and ignition keys, to make them easier to turn …and adding grab handles on the ridge of the roof inside the car to make entry and exit easier.

Keep medicines in the glove compartment, not the trunk, to avoid exposure to extreme temperatures…and carry snacks and a beverage so you can take the medicines on schedule. In cold weather, have someone warm up the car before you get into it.

Arthritis in the Kitchen

Arthritis: Stop Suffering, Start Moving by Darlene Cohen, certified movement therapist, San Francisco. Walker & Co.

If your fingers and wrists are stiff, it is tempting to do kitchen tasks with your upper arms, shoulders and upper back. But this can cause neck and shoulder aches.

Better: Look at kitchen chores as a way to exercise those joints and improve their mobility. But find ways to do the chores that do not strain painful areas too much.

Example: Use an extra-heavy, high-quality, sharp knife for chopping and cutting. Its weight can make it easier to cut without using a painful amount of wrist pressure.

Homemade Heating Pad

Allison P. Scheetz, MD, and David E. Mathis, MD, instructors of medicine, Mercer University School of Medicine, Macon, GA.

Fill a tube sock with uncooked rice, knot the top, then microwave on high for three minutes.

This creates a pad that will mold easily around any painful joint and hold its heat for about one hour—without risk of burns.

To Stop a Nosebleed…

Earl Schwartz, MD, spokesperson, American College of Emergency Physicians, Dallas.

Pinch nostrils and hold them together for five minutes. Tilt the head back only a little…not enough for blood to run down the throat. If the bleeding does not stop in five minutes, continue pinching nostrils for another seven minutes. If bleeding still continues, call your doctor.

Better Dandruff Shampoo Use

Richard Berger, MD, clinical professor of dermatology, University of Medicine and Dentistry of New Jersey, Robert Wood Johnson Medical School, New Brunswick, NJ.

Apply shampoo twice. Leave the first application on your hair for one to two minutes, then rinse and relather. Leave the second application on your hair for three to five minutes. That is how long the medication needs to work.

For serious dandruff problems: Ask your doctor about Nizoral, a potent antidandruff shampoo available over-the-counter.

Tongue Scraping

Ray Wunderlich, MD, a physician in private practice in St. Petersburg, FL. A specialist in preventive and nutritional medicine, he is author of *Natural Alternatives to Antibiotics*. Keats.

Cleaning the top of your tongue twice a day with a scraping device is a simple, inexpensive way to control even the most stubborn cases of bad breath...and to prevent infections in and around your mouth.

Every day, infectious bacteria, viruses, fungi and yeast—along with food particles and cellular debris—collect on the rough surface on the back of the tongue.

From this "staging area," these microorganisms launch infections that cause tooth decay, gum disease, sore throats and colds, as well as bad breath.

Why not simply clean the tongue with a toothbrush? That's far less effective at removing microorganisms, and it can cause gagging.

For best results, use a plastic tongue scraper, such as the one manufactured by Oolitt. Bend it in a U-shape, with the open end of the U pointing away from you and the serrated edge against your tongue.

Starting at the back of your tongue on the right side, sweep the serrated edge forward until it reaches the tip. Rinse any debris off the scraper, and sweep repeatedly until no more "gunk" is being collected. Then switch to the left side and repeat.

Do this twice a day, after breakfast and at bedtime, just before brushing your teeth. Rinse the tongue scraper after each use with 3% hydrogen peroxide.

If your dentist or local drugstore doesn't sell one, you can purchase a variety of easy-to-use Oolitts for all ages from Oolitt Advantage, Inc., P.O. Box 273653, Tampa, FL 33688. 877-332-7500, *www.oolitt.com. Cost:* $12 for an 18-month supply (six scrapers), plus shipping and handling ($3.50).

Better Toothbrushing

Michael W. Davis, DDS, a dentist in private practice in Brunswick, ME.

Slip the plastic spool from a roll of adding machine paper over the toothbrush handle. This enlarges the gripping surface, making brushing easier.

Avoid Bad Breath

Jon L. Richter, DMD, PhD, director, The Richter Center for Treatment of Breath Disorders, Philadelphia.

Clean your tongue with a tongue scraper or plastic teaspoon with the bowl pointing down...eat fibrous foods like apples...use breath mints or chewing gum to promote saliva flow.

Common causes of bad breath: Postnasal drip from a cold or allergy...mouth dryness—a side effect of many antihistamines and other medications...dieting, since less frequent eating slows saliva flow...sulfur-containing foods, such as garlic, onions, broccoli and cabbage...heredity—some people simply have more mouth odor than others...and hormonal changes, especially just before a menstrual period.

Jaw Pain Relief

Irwin D. Mandel, DDS, professor emeritus, Columbia University School of Dental and Oral Surgery, New York City.

Relieve jaw pain caused by *temporomandibular (TMJ) disorder* by giving your jaw a rest during painful episodes. Eat soft foods, and avoid extreme jaw movements like those involved in gum chewing, wide yawning, eating thick sandwiches and singing loudly. Apply moist heat or ice packs—whichever feels better—to the chewing muscles along the sides of the face. Keep a detailed pain diary to help you identify triggers and avoid them. It can help, when your mouth is closed, to keep your lips together and teeth apart.

Bike Helmet Fact

Diane Thompson, epidemiologist, Harborview Injury Prevention & Research Center, Seattle, who led a study of more than 3,000 cyclists treated for injuries at seven hospitals.

Bike helmets prevent injuries even in big collisions.

Study: Wearing a helmet reduces the risk of head injury by 69%...the risk of severe brain injury by 74%...and the risk of eye, ear, nose and forehead injuries by 65%. Helmets are important for all age groups.

 ## Quick Cures

Tim Clark, executive editor of *The Old Farmer's Almanac* for more than 20 years. The *Almanac* is published each September in three editions.

For hiccups: Briefly apply ice to the side of the neck—to interrupt the reflex that causes hiccups.

When craving sweets: Rinse your mouth with one teaspoon of baking soda dissolved in a glass of warm water. Do not swallow. Craving should disappear immediately.

Painless Adhesive Bandage Removal

Kathryn Marion, author, *Success in the Real World.* Virtualbookworm.com.

Soak a cotton ball in baby oil and wipe it around the sides of the bandage. In about 10 minutes, the adhesive will be softened—making bandage removal easy and painless.

Neck Pain Relief

Robert A. Lavin, MD, assistant professor of neurology, University of Maryland, Baltimore, whose study was published in *Archives of Physical Medicine and Rehabilitation*, 330 N. Wabash Ave., Suite 2510, Chicago 60611.

To ease neck pain, sleep on a water pillow. Volunteers who slept on pillows with adjustable water-filled pouches for two weeks reported better sleep and less pain when they awoke than those who slept on down-filled, foam or roll pillows. Water pillows are available from select home/health care stores. *Cost:* About $45.

Natural Air Filters

Bonnie Wodin, owner of Golden Yarrow Landscape Design, a garden consulting firm, Heath, MA.

Houseplants can serve as natural air filters. They can remove indoor air pollutants such as carbon monoxide and formaldehyde.

Best: Aloe vera, Chinese evergreen, elephant-ear philodendron, English ivy, ficus, golden pothos, corn plant, peace lily and spider plant.

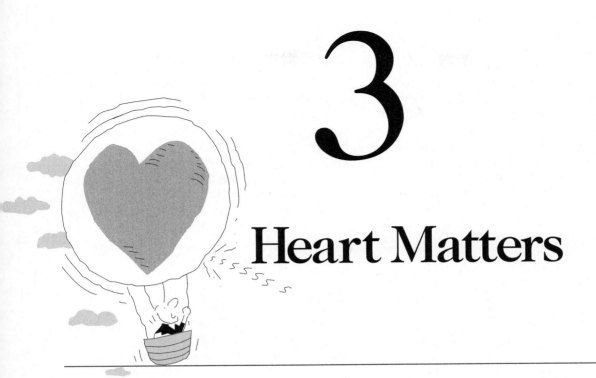

3

Heart Matters

It's Never Too Late to Start Taking Care of Your Heart

Harvey B. Simon, MD
Harvard Medical School
Massachusetts General Hospital

Some people mistakenly believe that if they've had bad health habits all their lives, it won't help to change now. But you can prevent—and in some cases even reverse—damage to your heart…no matter how old you are. And since heart disease is the number-one killer in America, it makes sense to do what you can to prevent it.

FOUR MAJOR LIFESTYLE CHANGES

The changes that can make an enormous difference in preventing heart disease…

•**Stop smoking.** Smoking is the greatest risk factor for coronary artery disease. It increases the chance of heart attack by 250%.

Even if you've smoked for years, stopping will improve your health. Heart rate and blood pressure will return to normal, and the risk of heart attack will fall until it matches that of people who never smoked.

•**Reduce blood cholesterol.** The most effective way to do this is by watching your diet. It isn't just cholesterol in food that raises levels in blood, it's the saturated fat—which stimulates the body to produce its *own* harmful cholesterol. The average American gets 37% of daily calories from fat. A much healthier level would be 30% or 15%.

Helpful: New food labeling regulations make it easier to estimate the fat content of the foods you eat.

Cholesterol reduction diet: Cut back on desserts and animal products—eggs, meat,

Harvey B. Simon, MD, associate professor of medicine, department of internal medicine and preventive cardiology at Massachusetts General Hospital in Boston. He is on the faculties of Harvard Medical School and the Massachusetts Institute of Technology and is a founding member of the Harvard Cardiovascular Health Center.

cheese and other whole dairy products. Increase your intake of vegetables, dried beans and whole grains. Switch from using butter or margarine in cooking to small amounts of olive oil, which appears to reduce "bad" LDL cholesterol but not "good" HDL cholesterol.

●**Exercise.** Exercise benefits the cardiovascular system by strengthening the heart muscle, improving circulation, raising HDL and lowering LDL cholesterol, reducing stress on arteries and fighting the formation of blood clots.

The best kind of exercise for the heart is aerobic—the kind that uses the large muscle groups for prolonged periods of time.

Examples: Biking, swimming, fast walking, running, stair climbing, rowing, racquet sports.

You're exerting yourself at the right level if you work up a sweat but don't feel out of breath. Any amount of exercise is helpful— even an hour a week. But you'll reap greater benefits if you work up to a total of at least three to four hours a week.

●**Lower your blood pressure.** One-fourth of American adults—and half of those over age 60—have high blood pressure, also known as hypertension. High blood pressure strains the heart muscle and damages the arterial wall, making people with hypertension more than twice as likely as others to have heart attacks.

The best way to lower blood pressure is to get the correct amount of minerals in your diet…

●**Reduce sodium.** Aim for less than 1,500 milligrams of sodium per day. Check food labels for sodium content. Sodium comes in many guises—the familiar table salt, as well as baking powder, baking soda, monosodium glutamate and soy sauce. Snack foods and processed foods tend to be especially high in sodium.

●**Increase potassium and calcium.** Many fresh fruits and vegetables are rich in potassium, including bananas, dates, oranges, cantaloupe, apples, raisins, potatoes, winter squash, lima beans, beets and broccoli. Healthful calcium-rich foods include skim milk, broccoli, spinach, fish and soybean products—particularly tofu.

OTHER WAYS TO HELP YOUR HEART

In addition to these four basic lifestyle changes for heart health, research suggests several other behaviors that may help to prevent heart disease…

●**Take aspirin.** Aspirin reduces blood clotting and has been shown to lower risk of a second heart attack. It's possible that aspirin may help to prevent a first heart attack as well.

Recommended dose: One baby aspirin a day, or one adult aspirin tablet every other day.

Caution: Check with your doctor before taking aspirin regularly. People who have ulcers, excessive bleeding or who are on other medications may need to avoid aspirin.

●**Eat fiber.** Numerous studies suggest that water-soluble fiber—the kind found in oat bran and also barley, prunes, beans and other legumes—reduces LDL cholesterol in the blood.

●**Eat fish.** Two to three servings of fish per week can reduce heart disease risk by about 40%.

Fish contains omega-3 fatty acids, which lower LDL and raise HDL, and may also reduce blood clotting and inflammation in the arterial walls.

●**Avoid secondhand cigarette smoke.** "Passive" smoking is thought to cause up to 35,000 deaths from heart attack in the US each year. At highest risk are people who live with someone who smokes or who work in smoke-filled environments. Try to reduce exposure as much as possible—ask smokers to consider your safety…or even leave the room when someone is smoking, if you must.

●**Take antioxidant vitamins.** There's some evidence that vitamins C, E and beta-carotene —which seem to fight the dangerous effects of unstable molecules in the body called free radicals—lower the risk of heart disease.

If you take supplements, stick to moderate doses—1,000 milligrams of vitamin C, 400 international units of vitamin E* and 10,000 international units of beta-carotene.

Caution: One study found that smokers who took beta-carotene supplements had a higher rate of death from lung cancer—so until further research is done, smokers should probably avoid these supplements.

●**Learn to cope with stress.** The link between emotional strain and heart disease is

*Due to the possible interactions between vitamin E and various drugs and supplements as well as other safety considerations, be sure to consult your doctor before starting a vitamin E regimen.

difficult to prove. However, if you're prone to anxiety or depression, learn more about stress-fighters—yoga, meditation, deep breathing or psychotherapy. You will be helping your heart —and you'll certainly enjoy life more.

Preventing Heart Disease

Harvey B. Simon, MD, associate professor of medicine, department of internal medicine and preventive cardiology at Massachusetts General Hospital in Boston. He is on the faculties of Harvard Medical School and the Massachusetts Institute of Technology and is a founding member of the Harvard Cardiovascular Health Center.

How can you minimize your risk of heart disease? *Most Americans are already familiar with the basics...*

• **Don't smoke.** Heart damage from tobacco causes 150,000 fatal heart attacks a year.

• **Eat less fat** (especially saturated fat). Less fat means lower cholesterol levels and reduced risk of obesity.

• **Watch your blood pressure.** A reading of 135/85 elevates the risk for heart attack and stroke. One in the normal range (below 120/80) is better.

• **Get regular exercise.**

If you're already making these efforts, terrific. But there's much *more* you can do to protect yourself.

WHAT CAUSES HEART DISEASE

Heart disease occurs via a three-step process:

Step 1: **Levels of LDL (bad) cholesterol get too high**...and/or levels of HDL (good) cholesterol fall too low.

Ideally, your total cholesterol should be under 200. Your level of HDL should be at least 35. Your ratio of total cholesterol to HDL cholesterol should be 4.5 to 1 or lower.

Step 2: **The arterial lining is injured**—usually via smoking or by having high blood pressure or blood sugar levels. This injury facilitates the entry of cholesterol from the blood into the artery wall.

Step 3: **A blood clot forms.** The growing cholesterol deposit disrupts the flow of blood. That causes blood clots to form. Eventually, a clot blocks the artery, causing a heart attack.

Lesson: A comprehensive heart disease prevention program must take aim at each step.

EAT LESS SALT

If you have hypertension, the less salt you eat, the lower your blood pressure is likely to be. And the lower your blood pressure, the smaller your risk of heart disease.

Tossing the salt shaker is a good start. But 75% of the sodium in a typical diet comes from salt that is hidden in processed foods.

Self-defense: Read labels. A bowl of canned soup can have up to 1,200 milligrams (mg) of sodium. That's half the 2,400-mg-per-day level recommended by health experts.

MORE POTASSIUM AND CALCIUM

Potassium has just the opposite effect of sodium—more means reduced blood pressure. But there's no evidence to suggest that blood pressure can be lowered by taking potassium supplements.

Better: Increase your intake of potassium-rich foods, such as bananas, oranges, dates, lima beans and potatoes.

Calcium also seems to play a key role in lowering blood pressure. For instance, blood pressure levels tend to be unusually low among people who live in areas with hard (calcium-rich) water and among those who eat lots of dairy products.

Lesson: If you are concerned about your blood pressure, eat more nonfat dairy products, dark green vegetables and tofu (bean curd). *Also:* Ask your doctor about taking Tums or another calcium supplement.

GET MORE DIETARY FIBER

Dietary fiber helps prevent heart disease by lowering cholesterol, blood pressure and blood sugar.

Sadly, most Americans get only one-third of the recommended 30 daily grams (g) of fiber.

Sources of dietary fiber: Beans, beets, prunes, citrus fruits and grains. It's a good idea to start your day with a breakfast cereal containing at least 10 g of fiber per serving.

EAT FISH TWICE A WEEK

Heart disease is quite uncommon among people who eat lots of fish. Certain unsaturated fatty acids unique to fish are thought to be responsible for this protective effect.

I urge my patients to eat at least four ounces of fish a week. *Best:* Rich, oily species like bluefish, mackerel, tuna and salmon.

What about fish-oil supplements? There's little evidence that they're beneficial.

ALCOHOL AND ASPIRIN

Study after study has proven that an *occasional* drink raises levels of HDL cholesterol. Men whose HDL is below 30 should consider having one or two drinks daily (one if you're a woman). One drink equals a glass of wine, a shot of distilled spirits or 12 ounces of beer.

Low-dose aspirin therapy—one-half tablet a day—is proven to prevent heart attacks in those who have heart disease.

Aspirin may also be beneficial for individuals *at risk* for heart disease. That includes men over 50 and postmenopausal women. There's no evidence that preventive aspirin therapy is beneficial to people with healthy hearts.

Caution: If you're allergic to aspirin, have ulcers or are prone to digestive bleeding, aspirin therapy is *not* for you.

CONSIDER TAKING ANTIOXIDANTS

Cholesterol damages arteries when it has been oxidized, via a chemical reaction analogous to rusting.

Fortunately, the body has enzymes that prevent oxidation by "mopping up" the unstable molecules (free radicals) that cause oxidation. Three antioxidant nutrients—vitamins C and E and beta-carotene—give this natural defense system a big boost, especially when taken in *combination.*

Sufficient levels of beta-carotene can easily be obtained by eating green and yellow vegetables, and vitamin C is abundant in citrus fruits. But it's hard to get much vitamin E from dietary sources, so I recommend taking a daily supplement.

WHAT ABOUT OTHER SUPPLEMENTS?

There's been much less research on chromium than on the "big three" antioxidants. But in one study, volunteers took 200 micrograms of the mineral three times a day.

Result: Levels of protective HDL cholesterol rose by 16%. That translates into a 20% reduction in the risk of heart disease.

If your HDL level is below 30, and it cannot be raised via weight loss, exercise or moderate alcohol consumption, ask your doctor about taking chromium supplements.

Important: Glucose tolerance factor (GTF) seems to be safer than the more popular supplement, *chromium picolinate.*

In another study involving more than 15,000 physicians, researchers found that those whose blood contained high levels of the amino acid *homocysteine* were more likely to have a heart attack. Homocysteine seems to damage artery walls and promote clotting.

To keep homocysteine levels down: Take a daily supplement containing vitamins B-6 and B-12 and folic acid.

MEDICAL TESTS

Your blood pressure, cholesterol and blood sugar should be checked each time you have a physical exam. That's once every year for people 50 or older and once every two to three years for people 35 to 49 years of age.

I'd also suggest an electrocardiogram with each checkup. Stress tests aren't necessary unless you're having chest pains or other heart disease symptoms.

Eating Right for a Healthy Heart and Long Life

Joe D. Goldstrich, MD, former medical director of the Pritikin Longevity Center in Santa Monica, CA, and author of *Healthy Heart, Longer Life.* Ultimate Health Publishing.

Researchers have identified three mechanisms by which to lower the risk of developing heart disease...

●**Lower the amount of LDL (bad) cholesterol in the blood.** An LDL level in excess of 100 confers an increased risk for heart disease.

●**Block *oxidation* of LDL cholesterol.** LDL cholesterol is benign until it has been oxidized. Only then can it be incorporated into obstructions along the walls of the coronary arteries. These obstructions are called *plaques.*

●**Control blood clotting.** Heart attacks occur when a plaque fissures or cracks, triggering formation of clots that block the flow of blood to the heart.

How do you set these mechanisms into motion? Regular exercise, avoiding smoking and keeping your blood pressure and weight under control are essential. But that's only the beginning...

HEART-PROTECTIVE FOODS

A diet low in saturated fat reduces levels of LDL cholesterol. *In addition, certain foods have extra power to protect the heart...*

●**Olive oil.** While it's a good idea to reduce consumption of *all* kinds of dietary fat (including oils), substituting olive oil for other oils helps keep your heart healthy.

The monounsaturated fats in olive oil reduce levels of LDL cholesterol while raising levels of HDL (good) cholesterol.

What makes monounsaturated fats superior to the polyunsaturated fats found in most other vegetable oils? They don't facilitate the conversion of cholesterol into its oxidized form.

●**Nuts.** Almonds and pistachios contain the same kind of monounsaturated fats found in olive oil. While nuts are too fatty to eat all the time, an occasional snack of almonds or pistachios could be beneficial to your heart.

●**Garlic.** In addition to reducing LDL and raising HDL, garlic helps prevent blood clotting.

If you don't like the taste of garlic—or worry about bad breath—take garlic capsules.

●**Fish.** Numerous studies have shown that the omega-3 oils in certain kinds of fatty fish (salmon, cod, sea bass, tuna, etc.) inhibit blood clotting and lower the risk for sudden cardiac death.

Try to eat fish at least once a week. Fish oil capsules can be rancid, and rancid oil *boosts* the oxidation of cholesterol.

●**Soy foods.** Tofu, miso soup, textured vegetable protein (TVP) and other soy products lower levels of LDL cholesterol. Researchers suspect that a compound in soy called *beta-sitosterol* is responsible for soy's cholesterol-lowering effect.

●**Red wine.** Any form of alcohol raises HDL cholesterol and reduces clotting. Red wine has additional benefits—if consumed in moderation (no more than two glasses a day). It contains clot-inhibiting *bioflavonoids* and *resveratrol,* a powerful antioxidant that guards cholesterol from oxidation.

VITAMIN SUPPLEMENTS

●**Vitamin E.** A potent antioxidant, vitamin E keeps LDL cholesterol from turning into its toxic form. Ask your doctor about an appropriate dose for you.

Of the many forms of vitamin E now available, capsules containing *d-alpha tocopherol succinate* are best. These capsules don't go rancid. Oil-filled vitamin E capsules sometimes do.

●**Vitamin C.** This antioxidant vitamin protects the smooth tissue that lines the coronary arteries against microscopic injuries caused by high blood pressure, smoking and high cholesterol. It's these injuries that are thought to provide a beachhead for plaques.

Studies suggest that a daily dose of at least 500 milligrams (mg) of vitamin C is best.

Since the usual form of vitamin C (ascorbic acid) can cause stomach irritation, it's better to get your C in the form of *calcium ascorbate* or *magnesium ascorbate.*

●**B Vitamins.** B-6, B-12 and folic acid all reduce blood levels of *homocysteine.* High levels of this clot-promoting amino acid are linked to heart disease.

It's best simply to take daily doses of the B vitamins. I usually recommend 100 mg of B-6 ...500 micrograms (mcg) of B-12...and 800 mcg of folic acid.

●**Carotenoids.** Beta-carotene is the best-known member of this family of antioxidants.

Studies suggest that another carotenoid called *lycopene* also offers protection against heart disease. Tomatoes are an excellent source of lycopene.

It's best to get your carotenoids in their natural form—red, yellow or leafy green vegetables. If you'd like to take carotenoids in supplement form, pick a supplement containing "natural mixed carotenoids."

MINERAL SUPPLEMENTS

●**Selenium.** This mineral is the raw material used by the body to make the antioxidant enzyme *glutathione*. People who take selenium supplements face a reduced risk for both heart disease and cancer. The usual dose is 200 mcg a day.

●**Chromium.** It helps keep levels of blood sugar in balance. Elevated blood sugar spurs the body to secrete insulin, and chronically high insulin levels can lead to obesity, high blood pressure and high triglycerides. All boost heart disease risk.

I advise my patients to take 200 mcg of *chromium picolinate* or *chromium polynicotinate*. These natural forms of chromium are safe and readily absorbed.

●**Magnesium and potassium.** Magnesium helps lower blood pressure by relaxing the tiny muscles that line blood vessel walls. Potassium lowers blood pressure by replacing sodium, a known provoker of high blood pressure.

The best way to get these minerals is from fruits and vegetables. Bananas and citrus fruits are especially good sources.

Heart Disease and Weight

Leslie Katzel, MD, PhD, associate professor of medicine at the University of Maryland School of Medicine, Baltimore.

If you are overweight, a key to reducing heart disease is losing weight. A study of men found that when they lost an average of 18 pounds over nine months, their risk of heart disease fell by 40%. Researchers found that this benefit did not automatically follow from simply changing the composition of the diet. It was necessary to lose weight by eating less, changing to fat-free and low-fat foods and/or exercising.

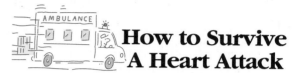

How to Survive A Heart Attack

William J. Cole, MD, director of the Coronary Care Unit at New York Downtown Hospital, and clinical assistant professor of medicine at New York University Medical Center, both in New York City.

Heart attack kills 600,000 Americans each year, making it the number one cause of death. But for every fatal heart attack, many more heart attacks do not prove fatal.

Why do some people succumb while others survive? To find out, we spoke with Dr. William Cole, a cardiologist who directs one of the busiest coronary care units in the US.

We can learn important lessons from heart attack survivors, according to Dr. Cole...

DON'T IGNORE SYMPTOMS

When lay people envision a heart attack (*myocardial infarction*), they tend to picture someone clutching at the chest, falling to the floor and losing consciousness. This scenario actually describes *cardiac arrest*, when the heart stops beating. The typical heart attack is far less dramatic.

Problem: Heart attack sufferers are often stoic. When they have chest pain or other symptoms suggestive of heart trouble, they think, *It must be something I ate.*

Many securities traders have sought treatment at my hospital only after being carried off the floor of the stock exchange. Many had endured chest pain for hours.

Why the delay in seeking treatment? In most cases, the individual was too frightened even to consider the *possibility* of a heart attack…or reluctant to risk embarrassment by calling an ambulance only to find out the problem was heartburn.

These individuals wait until they're in agony before seeking help. By the time they reach the emergency room, irreversible damage has often been done.

The most common symptom of heart attack is pain in the chest. But in some cases there is no pain—just a sensation that has been described as "someone sitting on the chest." The pain may radiate up the neck and down the arms.

Other symptoms: Sudden sweating, shortness of breath, tightness in the jaw or nausea.

In some cases, these signs occur several days before an attack. Because the sensations wax and wane, patients are tempted to ignore them. That's a *big* mistake.

Those at obvious risk for heart disease—smokers, overweight people and individuals with high blood pressure or elevated cholesterol—should be especially alert to these signals.

But heart attacks also strike—and kill—people with *no* known risk factors. If you or someone you know notices even mild symptoms, call a *doctor at once.*

GET TO THE HOSPITAL QUICKLY

If treatment is initiated during the first "golden" hour following a heart attack, mortality is only 1% to 5%. After four to five hours of delay, the mortality rate climbs to 12%.

Just 10 to 15 years ago, the death rate associated with heart attack victims who reached the hospital alive was 15% to 20%. Doctors could do little more than administer oxygen and morphine—to make the patient more comfortable.

Now: The death rate for these patients is 5% to 7%. Doctors have "clot-busting" drugs that actually restore blood flow to the heart. But the patient must still reach the hospital right away.

Helpful: Call 911 first. Then have someone call your doctor so he can alert the hospital that you're on your way. If the cardiac care team is expecting you, you'll be treated without delay.

GET AGGRESSIVE TREATMENT

Since the early 1980s, heart attack patients have received *thrombolytic therapy*—intravenous drugs that dissolve blood clots. The most effective clot-buster is *tissue plasminogen activator* (tPA).

In addition, nearly all heart attack patients receive aspirin (to thin the blood) and *heparin* (to prevent arteries from re-closing).

While thrombolytic treatment has brought about a significant decline in heart attack mortality, we can do *much* better. Studies suggest that a surgical procedure known as *acute angioplasty* is even more effective than clot-busting drugs.

In this procedure, an X-ray called an *angiogram* is used to pinpoint the blocked coronary artery. Then a small balloon is inserted into the artery through a catheter. The balloon is inflated, pushing aside the blockage and restoring blood flow to the heart.

Problem: Not all hospitals are equipped to perform angioplasty. If you must choose between two hospitals a similar distance away, ask to be taken to the one that is better equipped to do acute angioplasty. If this choice would prolong your trip by 15 minutes or more, it's probably better to go to the closer hospital.

PREPARE FOR EMERGENCIES

If a patient is at high risk of cardiac arrest, it's a good idea for his family members and coworkers to know cardiopulmonary resuscitation (CPR). In fact, *everyone* should learn CPR.

High-risk patients include people who have had prior episodes of cardiac arrest…have a weak heart muscle as a result of a prior heart attack or bypass surgery…or have a history of life-threatening irregularities in the heartbeat (arrhythmias).

These patients might also want to consider asking their doctor about purchasing their own defibrillator. That's the twin-paddled device doctors use to shock the heart into a normal rhythm.

Paramedics usually carry defibrillators, and many sports arenas have begun keeping their own units on the premises.

New, "smart" models are simple enough to be used by almost anyone—even without training. When placed on the victim's chest, these devices automatically monitor arrhythmias and—if necessary—administer a shock.

Unfortunately, the expense puts personal defibrillators out of the reach of many patients.

Some high-risk patients have been fitted with *implantable* defibrillators. *Cost:* About $20,000.

A Benefit of Having Friends

Blair Justice, PhD, professor of psychology, University of Texas School of Public Health at Houston and author of *Who Gets Sick.* Peak Press.

People who live isolated lives—without hugs, handshakes or other physical contact—are as likely to develop heart disease as those who smoke, eat high-fat diets and don't exercise.

Theory: Close connections with other people relieve stress and boost immunity. And—sharing one's troubles is a healthier coping mechanism than overeating, drinking or smoking.

Helpful: Regularly discuss what's going on in your life openly with your spouse...a friend ...or a family member.

Heart Trouble Predictor

James A. Blumenthal, PhD, professor of clinical psychology at Duke University Medical School, Durham, NC.

Mental stress tests help predict who is likely to have heart trouble, over and above physical stress tests. Researchers measured the blood flow in the hearts of 126 people undergoing mental stress tests such as solving difficult math problems rapidly. They found that

27% of those who showed an abnormal response to mental stress suffered a cardiac event within the next five years—more than twice the rate of those who showed a normal response.

Longer Life

Data from the *American Journal of Epidemiology,* 111 Market Pl., Ste. 840, Baltimore 21202.

The approximate number of years you can add to your life by adopting good habits that reduce the risk factors that lead to coronary heart disease...

- **Avoid diabetes** ....8 years
- **Exercise regularly** ....5.5 years
- **Avoid hypertension** ....5 years
- **Don't smoke** ....3 years
- **Maintain healthy weight** .....2 years

Symptoms of Angina Pectoris

Richard H. Helfant, MD, clinical professor of medicine, division of cardiology, University of California at Irvine, CA. He is author of *Women, Take Heart.* Penguin.

Tightness, pressure, heaviness or constriction in the center of the chest are symptoms of angina pectoris. Discomfort may start in the shoulders—more often on the left—or spread to shoulders from the center of the chest...then move down the arms or into the neck or jaw. Chest discomfort is likely to be caused by angina pectoris when symptoms are caused by physical activity, and usually disappear within minutes after activity stops.

Warning: Angina pectoris is the most common initial symptom of heart disease in women. If you have symptoms, see your doctor immediately.

Hypertension... What You Need To Know

Marvin Moser, MD, clinical professor of medicine at Yale University School of Medicine in New Haven, CT, and president of the Hypertension Education Foundation, Inc. He is author of *Clinical Management of Hypertension*. Professional Communications.

Some doctors have begun to rethink long-held views about the link between diet and blood pressure, thanks to two studies...

•A study conducted by Michael H. Alderman, MD, at Albert Einstein College of Medicine in the Bronx, New York, suggested that sodium restriction may not be beneficial—and could even be harmful—to people with high blood pressure.

•A study sponsored by the National Institutes of Health (NIH) showed that a low-fat diet rich in fruits and vegetables could lower even moderately high blood pressure without the need for medication.

To sort through these and other findings in the field, we sat down with one of the country's leading hypertension specialists, Dr. Marvin Moser...

•Are the new studies valid? Dr. Alderman's study did find that heart attacks were more common among hypertensives who ate very little sodium than among those who ate lots of sodium.

But the vast majority of the study's 2,900 participants consumed moderate levels of sodium...and showed no increased incidence of heart attack at all.

There are other potential problems with the study, including a lack of data on the specific treatments used.

Given these facts, I don't think Dr. Alderman's study should be considered in treatment decisions.

•If the study was flawed, why did it receive so much publicity? Because the Salt Institute—the leading lobby for the salt industry—is trying to use the study in an attempt to persuade the National Heart, Lung and Blood Institute (NHLBI) to change its long-standing recommendations regarding sodium consumption.

NHLBI guidelines call for consuming no more than 2.4 grams (g) of sodium per day. That's the amount contained in about 6 g of table salt (about 1¼ teaspoons).

The average American eats 10 g to 15 g of salt each day—the equivalent of two to three teaspoons.

•Then what is the bottom line regarding salt and high blood pressure? For someone with normal blood pressure, a low-sodium diet may not lower blood pressure by more than one to two points. This is a small number for an individual, but it could have a big impact on public health.

If everyone followed the NHLBI guidelines, the incidence of stroke would drop by approximately 7%.

•Isn't it hard to stick to a low-sodium diet? Not at all.

I tell my patients that they can help keep their pressure in check by going easy on the salt they use in cooking and at the table...and by minimizing their consumption of chips, canned soups, corned beef, hot dogs and other salty foods.

•What about salt substitutes? These products—which substitute potassium for sodium—are a great way to limit sodium consumption. But potassium tastes bitter.

Fortunately, a salt substitute called Cardia Salt Alternative tastes like ordinary salt. Ounce for ounce, it contains half the sodium, along with extra potassium and magnesium, which are believed to have a small but possibly beneficial effect on blood pressure.

•What about the NIH study? I believe the study is valid. It found that people who stick to a low-fat diet and consume lots of fruits and vegetables generally experience a seven- to 10-point drop in blood pressure.

•What explains the effectiveness of such a diet? Fruits and vegetables contain lots of potassium. Many doctors now believe that it's not sodium alone, but the ratio of potassium to sodium in the diet that affects blood pressure.

Ideally, we should all be consuming potassium and sodium in a one-to-one ratio.

The best way to do this is to avoid salty foods, as I mentioned, and to eat as many high-potassium vegetables and fruits as possible.

The best sources of potassium are baked potatoes and fruit—especially oranges and orange juice, cantaloupe and bananas.

You could take potassium supplements, but this would be rather expensive, since you would need several pills a day.

● **Does the NIH study suggest that lifestyle modification alone is enough to control high blood pressure?** For most cases, the answer is no.

If you follow a healthy diet, get regular exercise, reduce your alcohol intake and avoid smoking, you'll cut your risk for heart disease and reduce the likelihood that you'll *develop* high blood pressure.

But when it comes to reducing *existing* high blood pressure, these strategies alone generally aren't enough. Three out of four people with hypertension (defined as having a blood pressure of 140/90 or higher) must take anti-hypertensive medication.

For patients with mildly elevated blood pressure, I usually give lifestyle changes a couple of months to work before turning to medication. In severe cases, I generally prescribe medication right away.

● **Which blood pressure medication is most effective?** Two classes of drugs have been tested and proven to reduce long-term complications and mortality in people who have high blood pressure—they are diuretics and beta-blockers.

Diuretics, in particular, are underprescribed. Most antihypertensive drugs work better when used in combination with diuretics.

The long-term data on a third class of antihypertensive medication, ACE inhibitors, aren't in yet. My guess is that they'll demonstrate reduced mortality as well.

This may or may not be true for the fourth group of blood pressure drugs—calcium channel blockers. In fact, short-acting channel blockers such as *nifedipine* (Procardia) seem to make matters worse.

Surprisingly, doctors prescribe calcium channel blockers more than any other blood pressure–lowering drug. Perhaps that's because calcium channel blockers are heavily promoted by the drug companies that make them.

High Blood Pressure Mistakes Can Easily Be Avoided

Thomas Pickering, MD, director of the behavioral cardiovascular health and hypertension program at Columbia Presbyterian Medical Center in New York City. He is author of *Good News About High Blood Pressure*. Simon & Schuster.

Elevated blood pressure is a major risk factor for heart attack and stroke, along with smoking and high cholesterol.

With proper treatment, high blood pressure (hypertension) can be controlled.

Sadly, doctors and patients alike often err in their efforts to do so…

Mistake: **Ignoring systolic pressure.** Blood pressure is expressed as two numbers. The first represents *systolic* pressure—arterial pressure when the heart contracts. The second represents *diastolic* pressure—arterial pressure between beats. Hypertension is defined as a blood pressure of 140/90 or above.

Because the first studies linking heart disease with hypertension focused on diastolic pressure, doctors long assumed that just the second number was important.

Now we know that systolic pressure is an even bigger factor in heart disease than diastolic pressure.

Mistake: **Treating strictly by the numbers.** At what level does hypertension become so dangerous that treatment is required? Some doctors insist on treating any pressure of 140/90 or higher. Others wait until pressure rises above 160/95.

But no magic number applies to everyone. When deciding whether treatment is needed, your *overall* risk of heart disease and stroke is what's important.

A 65-year-old diabetic with high cholesterol might need antihypertensive medication for a pressure of 140/90. A healthy 35-year-old with a pressure of 150/95 may be able to lower those numbers with lifestyle modifications.

Mistake: **Relying on pressure readings taken in the doctor's office.** Blood pressure fluctuates throughout the day.

One in five patients labeled hypertensive actually has "white-coat" hypertension. Because of anxiety, their pressure reads high at the doctor's office—but is normal under other conditions.

White-coat hypertension usually requires no treatment, although it should be followed up.

To avoid needless treatment, I recommend *home monitoring*. This involves taking your own pressure two to three times a day to get a more complete picture of your blood pressure.

Home blood pressure readings are usually about five points lower than clinic readings.

When home monitoring gives equivocal results, I suggest *24-hour monitoring*. A Walkman-like device worn on the waist and attached to a blood pressure cuff on the arm automatically records blood pressure at 30-minute intervals.

Mistake: **Using an unreliable blood pressure monitor.** Many monitors designed for home use are unreliable.*

Before using your monitor, have your doctor calibrate it. Have your doctor check your technique, too.

Mistake: **Failing to rule out secondary hypertension.** Most high blood pressure is *primary* hypertension—there's no single underlying cause. In roughly 5% of all cases, however, high blood pressure is *secondary* to kidney disease, an adrenal gland tumor or another ailment. In such cases, it's essential to treat this underlying cause.

Your doctor should examine you carefully and do key diagnostic tests. *Two tests are especially important...*

•**Echocardiogram**, a noninvasive ultrasound exam, shows if hypertension has caused

*If you have access to the Internet, read more about home blood pressure monitors at *www.bloodpressure.com.*

the heart to become enlarged. If it has, medication is usually required.

•**The ankle-arm index test** is simple—but often neglected. Blood pressure should be roughly the same whether measured at the arm or the ankle. A lower reading at the ankle suggests a blocked artery in the leg. Such a blockage calls for aggressive treatment to lower pressure.

The ankle-arm test is especially important for people over 65.

Mistake: **Being too quick to begin drug therapy.** When pressure is only modestly elevated and there is no sign of kidney damage or heart enlargement, I generally recommend six months of lifestyle modification—weight loss, proper diet, exercise. Only if these *non-drug* strategies fail to lower the pressure do I prescribe antihypertensive medication.

Weight loss is the most important lifestyle change. If you are overweight, your pressure should drop five points for every 10 pounds you lose.

Mistake: **Drinking alcoholic beverages.** The finding that moderate drinking cuts the risk of heart disease has led many to act as if there were no downside to drinking. *There is.*

Alcohol can raise blood pressure significantly. Five or more drinks a day boosts systolic pressure by about five points...diastolic by about three. I urge my patients to have no more than two drinks a day—preferably of wine.

Mistake: **Not exercising properly.** After vigorous exercise, blood pressure stays low for hours. And getting into shape will *permanently* reduce your blood pressure and your risk of heart disease.

I recommend at least 20 minutes of running, biking, walking, etc., at least four days a week.

For strength training, weight machines are safer than free weights—because muscular contractions, which raise blood pressure, are not sustained as long with the machines. Push-ups and other calisthenics are OK.

Mistake: **Thinking that cutting back on salt will do the trick.** Only about half of all hypertensives are salt-sensitive. Their pressure drops if they cut back on salt and other sources of sodium. For the other 50%, avoiding salt makes no difference.

To find out if your blood pressure is affected by salt, avoid salt altogether for four weeks. See if there's any change.

Mistake: **Ignoring potassium.** There's now solid evidence that dietary potassium lowers blood pressure. Potassium-rich foods include bananas, oranges, beans, squash and sunflower seeds.

Watch out for potassium *supplements.* They can raise blood levels of potassium so high that dangerous disturbances in heart rhythm can result.

Mistake: **Ignoring the effects of other drugs.** Blood pressure can be raised by many prescription and over-the-counter drugs.

Examples: Pseudoephedrine, a decongestant found in many cold and allergy pills...and nonsteroidal anti-inflammatory drugs (NSAIDs) like *ibuprofen* (Advil).

If you take high doses of NSAIDs, ask your doctor about taking aspirin or acetaminophen instead. To set up an effective antihypertensive regimen, your doctor must know *all* the drugs you're taking.

Mistake: **Staying on medication indefinitely.** Most individuals who need pressure-lowering drugs must take them for life. *But not everyone.* Once a patient's blood pressure is under control, I try withdrawing medication. In many cases, the pressure stays down.

Alter your blood pressure medication regimen only under medical supervision—and with careful home monitoring. If pressure rises again, resume treatment.

Borderline Blood Pressure Risk

Christopher J. O'Donnell, MD, MPH, associate director, Framingham Heart Study, Framingham, MA. His analysis of health data on 18,682 men 40 to 84 years of age was published in *Circulation*, 560 Harrison Ave., Ste. 502, Boston 02118.

Even mildly elevated systolic blood pressure raises the risk for stroke and heart attack. Patients with elevations of systolic pressure (the "upper" number) between 140 and 159 and diastolic pressure (the "lower" number) 90 or below—had a 42% higher risk of stroke, 56% higher risk of dying from heart disease and a 26% greater chance of having a heart attack.

Systolic pressure represents blood pressure during contractions of the heart. Diastolic pressure is that between beats.

Best Place to Take Your Blood Pressure

Clarence E. Grim, MD, professor of clinical medicine, Medical College of Wisconsin, and director of the high blood pressure diagnosis and treatment center, St. Michael Hospital, both in Milwaukee.

Blood pressure readings taken at home are more accurate than readings taken in a doctor's office. The stress of being in a doctor's office (white-coat syndrome) can send blood pressure soaring—by as much as 23%.

Helpful: A home blood pressure monitor is available in most drugstores. Take readings three times a day (morning, afternoon, evening) for one week. Average your readings before your next doctor appointment.

Angioplasty Trap

James G. Jollis, MD, associate professor of medicine, Duke University Medical Center, Durham, NC. His review of 97,000 Medicare patient records was presented at a meeting of the American Heart Association.

Many cardiologists perform too few angioplasties to meet national standards.

Trap: Up to 6.8% of patients treated by inexperienced doctors suffer complications—including fatal ones. Only 4.6% of patients whose angioplasties are done by experienced surgeons develop such complications. To meet standards set up by the American College of Cardiology, a cardiologist must perform at least 75 angioplasties a year. Half of all cardiologists perform 40 or fewer a year.

Lesson: If you're scheduled for angioplasty, ask your cardiologist about his/her level of experience.

How Effective Are Implantable Defibrillators?

Eleanor Schron, RN, project director, National Heart, Lung and Blood Institute, Bethesda, MD. Her study of 1,016 patients suffering from severe heartbeat abnormalities was presented at a meeting of the North American Society for Pacing and Electrophysiology.

Implantable defibrillators are very effective. In a study, patients with an irregular heartbeat who were implanted with one of the cassette-tape-sized devices were 38% less likely to die than similar patients who relied solely on drug therapy. The defibrillator—which shocks the heart back to life after cardiac arrest—proved so superior to drugs that the study was stopped early. Up to 1,500 lives could be saved a year if patients who chose drug treatment instead received a defibrillator.

Beating Heart Disease: When Surgery Is Necessary...and When It's Not

Steven F. Horowitz, MD, chief of cardiology at Beth Israel Medical Center, New York City.

When fatty deposits narrow the arteries in your heart, the consequences can be deadly.

Reduced blood flow starves the heart of oxygen, causing an often severe form of chest pain called *angina*. You tire easily and may be unable to exercise. And your risk of heart attack is dramatically increased.

A technique known as *coronary artery bypass graft* (CABG) surgery has proven very effective at creating a detour around these potentially deadly blockages. But any form of surgery—especially open-heart procedures like CABG—is risky. In fact, 1% to 2% of individuals who undergo bypass surgery die in the hospital.

The risk is especially great for diabetics and hypertensives...and those who have already sustained a heart attack or have had previous bypass surgery.

Good news: Blocked coronary arteries can often be opened up via drug therapy...or less invasive surgical procedures—even lifestyle changes.

EVALUATING THE BLOCKAGE

If you develop chest pain or excessive shortness of breath upon exertion, or if you have other symptoms of coronary artery disease, your doctor will probably schedule some noninvasive diagnostic tests...

•**Stress electrocardiogram** (cardiac stress test) monitors the heart's electrical activity during strenuous exercise.

•**Thallium scans and positron emission tomography** (PET) check to see if certain areas of the heart are deprived of oxygen-rich blood.

If tests suggest significant blockage, your doctor will probably recommend angiography.

In this low-risk procedure, a narrow tube (catheter) is inserted through an incision in the groin and threaded up to the coronary arteries. Special dye injected through the catheter renders coronary arteries visible on X-ray equipment.

DRUG THERAPY

If the blockage is severe, your doctor may recommend immediate surgery. *In most cases, however, the first treatment is medication...*

•**Nitroglycerin** (Monoket, Imdur). Tiny pills containing this time-tested drug can be placed under the tongue at the first sign of angina...or supplied all day long via a skin patch or pills. It relaxes veins, diminishing the amount of blood returned to the heart. This allows the heart to work less. It also relaxes coronary arteries.

●**Beta-blockers** (Lopressor, Tenormin, Inderal). These oral drugs limit the heart's response to adrenaline in the bloodstream. Since the heart pumps more slowly, it needs less oxygen.

●**Calcium channel blockers** (Calan, Procardia, Cardizem). This family of oral medications relaxes arteries and lowers blood pressure. Some of these medications should not be used by those with heart failure. Short-acting *nifedipine* (Procardia) probably shouldn't be used at all with coronary disease.

Three other groups of medications may also be helpful...

●**Aspirin** may reduce the risk of heart attack by preventing platelets from sticking together and forming clots.

●**ACE inhibitors** (Capoten, Vasotec, Prinivil) are especially valuable in treating or preventing heart failure after a heart attack.

●**Cholesterol-lowering drugs** (Mevacor, Zocor, Pravachol, Questran and niacin) work primarily by lowering "bad" LDL cholesterol and, in some cases, raising "good" HDL cholesterol.

If your angina worsens despite drug therapy, your doctor will probably recommend bypass surgery or angioplasty.

ANGIOPLASTY

In this procedure, a catheter is used to introduce a tiny balloon into the coronary arteries. The balloon expands to squash the fatty deposits blocking the arteries.

If blockages aren't too numerous or severe enough to necessitate bypass, and drugs really aren't doing the trick, then angioplasty may be appropriate.

Angioplasty involves less pain and risk than bypass surgery. You may be out of the hospital in a few hours—at most a couple of days...and back to full activity shortly thereafter.

Drawback: In up to 50% of cases, the artery closes again—often within six months—and the procedure must be repeated.

In recent years, a variation on angioplasty has become popular. After the blocked artery is opened, a mesh reinforcing tube called a stent is inserted. With a stent, the chance of the artery closing again is cut by 50%.

CORONARY BYPASS

In bypass surgery, the chest is opened, the ribs are spread and the heart is cooled to a standstill while a heart-lung machine takes over. Blood vessels "harvested" from the leg or chest are grafted onto the coronary arteries in such a way that they carry blood around the blockage.

Bypass surgery is the only reasonable option if tests reveal obstruction of the left main coronary artery. Bypass is also the best bet if three or more coronary arteries are blocked and function of the left ventricle is diminished.

Bypass surgery requires at least four days of hospitalization, and several weeks of recuperation at home. It may take two to four months before you can resume a full, active life. The grafts generally stay open for five to 15 years but may close earlier.

LIFESTYLE MODIFICATION

We all know that a low-fat diet, exercise and stress reduction can help prevent heart disease. These strategies can also relieve angina —even reverse coronary artery disease.

You may have heard of the program developed by Dr. Dean Ornish, of the Preventive Medicine Research Institute in Sausalito, CA. His program is *not* a substitute for bypass or angioplasty if you have life-threatening artery blockage...or if you have unstable angina that does not respond to medication.

But for patients in the "gray zone" where neither Coronary Artery Bypass Graft (CABG) nor angioplasty offers any clear advantages, lifestyle intervention may be the best option.

The program involves...

●**A very low-fat vegetarian diet.** To reduce total fat to 10% of calories, participants learn to cook without oil or other forms of fat. The American Heart Association recommends that 30% of calories come from fat—but that's too high.

●**Aerobic exercise.** Brisk walking, jogging, stair-climbing or biking, at least three hours a week.

●**Yoga, stretching and meditation**—for an hour a day. Facilitates deep relaxation.

●**Group therapy.** To teach people ways to express their emotions and improve their relationships.

For the first three months, program participants come in three times a week for exercise, diet counseling, stress reduction and group therapy. For the next nine months, they come once a week.

By then, they have incorporated the diet, exercise and stress-reduction into their lives.

What to Do When The Doctor Says Bypass Surgery

Fredric J. Pashkow, MD, medical director of the Queens Medical Center Heart Institute in Honolulu. He is coauthor of *50 Essential Things to Do When the Doctor Says It's Heart Disease* (Plume) and *The Women's Heart Book* (Plume).

Since its introduction in 1967, coronary artery bypass graft (CABG) surgery has enabled thousands of people to survive severe coronary artery disease.

Coronary artery disease (atherosclerosis) occurs when fatty deposits form in the coronary arteries, restricting flow of oxygen-rich blood to the heart. Over time, atherosclerosis may lead to a form of chest pain called *angina* ...or to heart attack.

In bypass surgery, doctors reroute blood flow around arterial blockages, using blood vessels grafted from another part of the body, usually a leg.

The procedure has become so common that people tend to forget just how serious it is.

One surgeon slices open the chest, cracking the breastbone (sternum) to reach the heart, while another "harvests" the arteries or veins to be grafted. The heart is stopped for several hours as doctors attach the grafts.

Bypass surgery generally requires a hospital stay of four or more days, plus a one-month convalescence.

Bypass surgery is often the best therapy for heart disease, but it is not the *only* approach. *Other options to consider...*

LIFESTYLE MODIFICATION

As Dr. Dean Ornish and other researchers have shown, a low-fat diet (10% of calories from fat) can slow the progress of atherosclerosis—and in some cases reverse it. This approach is very effective when combined with cholesterol-lowering drugs called *statins.*

Drawback: The low-fat diet doesn't always work. And such a diet is hard to follow. Only about 15% of patients are motivated enough to stick with it.

ANGIOPLASTY

This procedure costs less and is less invasive than open-heart surgery. Often, the patient can go home the same day.

The surgeon inserts a catheter into a tiny incision in the leg and threads it into the coronary artery. A balloon on the tip is then inflated to flatten the plaque against the artery wall, widening the artery and easing the flow of blood.

Drawback: About 25% of the time, angioplasty has to be repeated to eliminate plaques that recur—sometimes within six months of the original operation.

To prevent recurrence, some cardiologists now use *stents*—tiny metallic tubes inserted into the artery to keep it open.

KEYHOLE SURGERY

This experimental procedure is a less invasive variant of conventional bypass surgery. Instead of cracking the chest, the surgeon makes a small incision between the ribs. Using an endoscope, he/she removes the *internal thoracic artery* from the chest and grafts it onto the coronary artery.

For *accessible* blockages, keyhole surgery should prove just as effective as CABG. But it's still too early to know its exact success rate.

WHICH APPROACH IS BEST?

Can you get by using one of these less invasive approaches? *The answer depends on several factors...*

●**Condition of the heart.** If the heart can pump enough blood despite the blockages, bypass surgery can probably be avoided.

Bypass surgery is preferable if the heart has been weakened by heart attack.

•**Location and number of blockages.** The more severe and numerous the blockages, the greater the need for bypass surgery.

Bypass is preferable to angioplasty if blockages are "upstream" (close to the point where the arteries branch off of the aorta)…if the patient has one or more blockages of the *left main coronary artery*…and/or if two or all three coronary vessels are blocked.

•**Level of chest pain.** If angina isn't relieved by medication, bypass is probably the best option.

Angioplasty may be more appropriate if the patient has had just one tiny heart attack, with minimal damage to the heart…has just started to experience angina…or is highly motivated to follow a low-fat diet and regular exercise regimen.

If your doctor recommends bypass, consult a bypass surgeon *and* a cardiologist who specializes in angioplasty.

WHAT TO DO *BEFORE* SURGERY

Anyone who decides to have bypass surgery can increase the chance of a successful operation by doing the following…

•**Find a good surgeon.** He should be board-certified in cardiothoracic surgery. In addition, he should perform at least 150 bypass operations each year. Fewer than that, and he may lack the necessary expertise.

Some patients are uncomfortable asking a surgeon about these details. But good surgeons are happy to share this information— and you want only the best. If the surgeon seems defensive, find another one.

•**Check out the hospital.** It should perform at least 200 bypass operations a year, with a death rate of less than 1.5%.

The hospital should be accredited by the Joint Commission. To inquire about a hospital's status, contact them at 630-792-5800, *www.jointcommission.org.*

•**Stop smoking.** Smoking in the 10 days before surgery increases the risk of pneumonia and other surgical complications.

•**Avoid aspirin.** If you take aspirin on a regular basis (to prevent heart attack, for instance), ask your cardiologist about stopping temporarily. Doing so will reduce the risk of excessive bleeding during and after surgery.

•**Rethink diet and exercise habits.** Doctors once thought that bypass surgery would allow patients to carry on their high-fat, low-exercise lives as before. That's simply untrue. To keep your newly grafted vessels healthy, you must keep fat intake low and get regular exercise.

If you have diabetes: Ask your doctor about "tight control" of your blood sugar before surgery. The better you manage your diabetes, the lower your risk of postoperative infection.

It's essential to continue to monitor your cholesterol level after surgery—and take steps to control it with diet, exercise, stress management and—if necessary—cholesterol-lowering medication.

Better Bypass Surgery

Frederick St. Goar, MD, director of interventional cardiology and clinical research, Cardiovascular Institute, 2660 Grant Rd., Mountain View, CA 94040.

Recovery is faster with a procedure called "port access" coronary artery bypass graft surgery than with ordinary bypass surgery. In conventional surgery, the surgeon must make a 12-inch incision in the chest. Port access surgery requires only one three-inch and two one-inch incisions.

New Surgical Procedure For Heart Failure Sufferers

Anthony P. Furnary, MD, associate director, Starr–Wood Cardiac Group, Portland, OR. His 12-month study of cardiomyoplasty in 68 heart failure patients was published in the *Journal of the American College of Cardiology*, 3655 Nobel Dr., Ste. 630, San Diego, CA 92122.

Cardiomyoplasty involves transplanting muscle tissue from the patient's own back to the ventricles of the failing heart. A pacemaker-like device implanted at the same time stimulates the transplanted tissue to contract, assisting the heart as it pumps. Cardiomyoplasty is especially promising for older patients who fail to respond to less drastic treatments, yet who have other medical problems that disqualify them for a heart transplant.

Open-Heart Surgery Breakthrough

Karl Krieger, MD, the Philip Geier Professor of cardiothoracic surgery, New York Presbyterian—Weill Cornell Medical Center, New York City.

Open-heart surgery can now be performed without multiple transfusions. The drug *erythropoetin* boosts red cell count prior to surgery, while *aprotinin* helps stop postoperative bleeding.

More: The surgeon uses a machine to collect blood lost during surgery, then transfuses it back into the patient. Ordinarily, open-heart surgery requires up to four units of blood—and each carries a chance of being tainted with a disease-causing virus. If you're scheduled for surgery, ask your doctor about these strategies.

Saving Your Heart Without Bypass Surgery ...Without Angioplasty

John A. McDougall, MD, medical director of the McDougall Program for controlling heart disease. He is author of *The McDougall Program for a Healthy Heart.* Penguin.

For anyone with heart disease—even for anyone at *risk* for heart disease—it may seem as if time is running out.

But having treated thousands of heart patients in my clinic over the past 10 years, I know that there is time to recover cardiovascular health in nine out of 10 cases. This can usually be accomplished *without* angioplasty or bypass surgery.

Anyone eager to prevent or cure heart disease must learn to avoid fatty foods and other dietary "poisons."

I'm often asked, "How often can I eat steak and eggs without hurting my heart?" I reply, "How often can you smoke without any ill effects on your body?" The only honest answer to both questions is *never.*

DRAMATIC CHANGES ARE POSSIBLE

Most of the people who participate in my two-week program are seriously ill. Many have already had a heart attack. Others take medication for chest pain (angina) or high blood pressure.

By the time they leave our clinic, most have significantly lowered their cholesterol and blood pressure...and stopped taking medicine. The vast majority go on to live full lives.

This remarkable transformation involves three simple steps...

• **Eliminate *all* excess fat from your diet.** That means substituting fruits, vegetables and grains for red meat, chicken, dairy products, eggs, oils, cakes and candies and refined and processed foods.

• **Get daily aerobic exercise.** Patients in my program are required to walk for at least 30 minutes a day.

• **Learn to manage psychological stress** — without resorting to overeating or other self-destructive behavior. Massage, meditation and group discussion are all effective ways to do this.

THE SKINNY ON FAT

The typical American gets a whopping 40% of his daily calories in the form of fat. It's this fat that clogs the coronary arteries with the fatty streaks (plaques) that cause heart attack.

Dietary fat endangers your heart by...

• **Causing red blood cells to clump.** That slows circulation, reduces oxygen in the blood and raises blood pressure.

• **Creating new plaques** and making them prone to rupture.

• **Causing existing plaques to grow.**

• **Causing abnormally rapid clotting of the blood.** That can lead to arterial occlusion if a new plaque bursts.

●**Causing release of hormone-like compounds.** Called *prostaglandins,* these compounds boost the clumping effect.

To keep plaques from forming, the American Heart Association (AHA) suggests limiting daily fat intake to 35% of calories. Yet studies show that even at this level of fat intake, new plaques *continue* to form. Amazingly, the AHA stands by its misguided recommendation.

HOW HEART ATTACKS OCCUR

Many people think that a heart attack occurs when an *old* plaque grows so big that it occludes a coronary artery.

Actually, most heart attacks occur following the rupture of a *newly formed* plaque—which contains liquid fat and cholesterol.

This rupture leaves a wound on the artery wall—which is quickly capped with a blood clot. This clot can grow quickly, becoming so large that it occludes the artery and stops blood flow to the heart.

The implication? Heart attacks can occur even when the coronary arteries are relatively plaque-free. As I tell my patients, you play Russian roulette *each time you eat a fatty meal.*

THE MCDOUGALL PROGRAM

My diet separates foods into three categories...

●**Eat all you want.**

●**Brown rice**, wheat, corn, oatmeal and other whole grains.

●**Whole-grain products**, including noodles, breads, pancakes and waffles. Make sure they contain no fats or oils.

●**Potatoes and yams.**

●**Squash.**

●**Peas**, lentils, lima beans and string beans.

●**Green and yellow vegetables.**

●**Cucumbers**, onions, peppers and tomatoes.

●**Beets**, carrots, turnips and other root vegetables.

●**Mild spices and herbs.**

●**Eat in moderation.**

●**Fruit**, fruit juice and dried fruit (up to three servings a day).

●**Sugar** and artificial sweeteners.

●**Salt.**

●**Alcohol.**

●**Fatty plant foods**, including nuts, peanut butter and tofu.

●**Avoid.**

●**Red meat**, poultry, fish, seafood, eggs, milk and milk products like butter, cheese, yogurt and sour cream. Even *nonfat* dairy products should be avoided. They contain proteins that can trigger an artery-damaging immune response.

I allow fatty foods *only* on special occasions—eggs on Easter...turkey on Thanksgiving ...cake on your birthday.

●**Cooking oil.** Instead, use a nonstick pan or wok. Sauté with water, soy sauce, wine, tomato juice, lemon or lime juice or Worcestershire sauce.

When baking, replace the oil in the recipe with half the amount of applesauce, mashed bananas or soy yogurt.

●**Sulfites.** These preservatives, used in wines and in salad bars, can cause an allergic reaction.

When buying packaged food, read labels carefully. Avoid products containing fats and oils, including monoglycerides, diglycerides and/or hydrogenated or partially hydrogenated fats or oils. Before making long-term dietary changes, discuss your nutritional needs with a doctor or dietician.

ONE MAN'S STORY

Charles Schaefer of Santa Rosa, CA, suffered his heart attack at age 46.

After undergoing balloon angioplasty, he was told he would probably need bypass surgery. At the time, his cholesterol was 220—average for Americans. His weight and blood pressure were normal, too.

After leaving the hospital, he went on my diet. His cholesterol immediately fell to 180. He then visited my office, and I put him on a cholesterol-lowering drug that brought his level down to 150. He also began walking or bicycling several times a week.

Four years later, treadmill stress tests show that his coronary arteries are wide open. His heart is healthy, and he feels in better shape than ever.

"If I had stayed on the same rich American diet that I had been on," says Mr. Schaefer, "I would not be alive today."

Bypass Surgery Dangers Are Real

Dennis T. Mangano, MD, PhD, professor of anesthesiology, University of California, San Francisco, and founder and director of the Ischemia Research and Education Foundation.

Heart bypass surgery leads to stroke and other brain damage more often than people realize—one out of 15 patients who undergo surgery and one out of six patients over age 75 will suffer serious damage.

Greatest risk: Older patients...women... prior stroke sufferers...people with diabetes or hypertension.

Prior to surgery: Make sure your surgeon uses techniques designed to reduce stroke risk —echocardiography (to locate the safest place for instrumenting the main artery) and drugs to prevent blood pressure drops—and pays attention to the temperature of fluids used to rewarm the heart and brain. Your surgeon should check for evidence of stroke within 90 minutes of the operation...and consider aggressive treatment for complications.

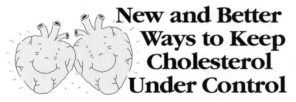

New and Better Ways to Keep Cholesterol Under Control

Daniel Rader, MD, director of preventive cardiology at the University of Pennsylvania Health System in Philadelphia.

For decades now, cardiologists have been warning us that a high level of *low-density lipoprotein* (LDL, or "bad") cholesterol means an increased risk of heart attack.

In the United States, the average total cholesterol level is 210...the average LDL cholesterol level about 140.

But a growing consensus of doctors now believe that these average levels may be *too high* to ensure a healthy heart.

Each year, more than 800,000 Americans suffer their first heart attack. And—many of these people have average cholesterol readings.

Doctors now think that your level of LDL cholesterol should ideally be no higher than 130. At that level, the fatty arterial deposits (plaques) that cause heart attacks are less likely to form.

LOWERING ELEVATED LEVELS

If your LDL cholesterol is 130 or higher...

•**Switch to a diet low in fat.** The average American gets 37% of his/her calories from fat. To lower the amount of fat in your diet, eat less meat and more fruits and vegetables...substitute nonfat milk for whole milk...and eat more oat bran and other forms of soluble fiber. *Also:* Ask your doctor about taking *psyllium* (Metamucil).

Saturated fat should account for no more than 10% of your daily caloric intake.

The body uses dietary fat to make cholesterol. Few people realize it, but eating too much fat is worse for your heart than eating too much cholesterol. It's okay to eat eggs once or twice a week.

•**Get more exercise.** Aerobic exercise—at least 20 minutes, three or four times a week— brings moderate reductions in LDL cholesterol.

Exercise also increases levels of *high-density lipoprotein* (HDL) cholesterol. That's the "good" form associated with reduced heart attack risk.

DO YOU NEED DRUG THERAPY?

What if your LDL cholesterol level is 160 or above despite a good diet and exercise regimen? Cholesterol-lowering medication may be appropriate—if you smoke, have high blood pressure or diabetes and/or have a family history of heart attack. Even in the absence of these risk factors, drug therapy may be appropriate.

Three tests can give you information about your risk...

•**Lipoprotein (a) test.** High levels of this blood component—often represented as Lp(a) —have been linked to heart attack. Normal Lp(a) levels are 20 or lower.

•**Homocysteine test.** Individuals with high levels of this amino acid in their blood are prone to heart attack. Your homocysteine level should be 10 or lower. Folic acid supplements help reduce levels of homocysteine.

•**Ultrafast computed tomography (CT) scan.** This 20-minute noninvasive test can check your coronary arteries for calcium. Calcified plaques are a sure sign of heart disease—and may predict future risk of heart attack.

If these tests suggest an elevated risk, your doctor may recommend cholesterol-lowering medication.

WHICH DRUG IS BEST?

The most widely used cholesterol-lowering drugs are the "statins." Your doctor may recommend a statin, such as *pravastatin* (Pravachol) or *simvastatin* (Zocor). These two have been shown in large-scale studies to reduce heart attack rates.

Your doctor may also recommend high doses of the vitamin *nicotinic acid* (niacin). Although it is quite effective at lowering cholesterol, niacin can cause facial flushing and elevated blood sugar or uric acid. People taking it must be closely monitored by a doctor.

HDL AND TRIGLYCERIDES

Low levels of HDL cholesterol are associated with increased risk for heart attack. If your HDL level is less than 35, ask your doctor what you can do to raise it.

Studies suggest that HDL can be raised by niacin therapy…moderate alcohol consumption (one or two drinks a day)…and vigorous exercise.

A triglyceride level of 250 or higher is associated with increased heart attack risk, although high triglycerides pose less of a threat than high cholesterol.

Triglyceride levels can usually be lowered via weight loss, exercise and a diet low in fat and—especially important—sugar.

If you have high triglycerides, ask your doctor about substituting fresh fruit for fruit juices, which are extremely high in sugar.

ALTERNATIVE APPROACHES

People who eat lots of fish have a lower risk of heart disease. But there's no evidence that fish oil capsules have the same effect. In some people, they actually *raise* LDL.

Fish oil capsules can help reduce extremely high triglycerides (over 1,000). If you have high triglycerides, ask your doctor if fish oil capsules are appropriate. Heavy consumption of garlic has been shown to bring modest reductions in cholesterol. But garlic *pills* have not been shown to work. There's no harm in taking them, but don't substitute them for proven cholesterol-lowering medication.

ALREADY HAD A HEART ATTACK?

If you have had a heart attack or have heart disease, your LDL cholesterol should be less than 100. There is a good chance you may need medication to reach this goal.

Doctors are beginning to think that medication may be appropriate for virtually all heart attack survivors. A study published in *The New England Journal of Medicine* suggests that they are right. In this study, more than 4,000 heart attack survivors with average LDL cholesterol levels were given *pravastatin* or a placebo. Over the next five years, those who received pravastatin suffered 24% fewer heart attacks than those who got the placebo.

Lesson: If you've had one heart attack, reducing your cholesterol can reduce your risk of another—even if your cholesterol level is not elevated. Your new target for LDL cholesterol should be 100 or lower. Currently, only one in four heart patients achieves this level.

Bottom line: Reducing cholesterol levels prevents heart attacks. If diet and exercise don't do the job, medications are effective and very safe.

For a Better Echocardiogram

Nelson B. Schiller, MD, professor of medicine, anesthesiology and radiology at the University of California, San Francisco.

For a better ultrasound exam of the heart (echocardiogram), ask the doctor about squeezing a tennis ball during the procedure. Doing so boosts blood pressure and heart rate, making it easier for the doctor to spot heart and circulatory system problems. Doctors commonly use echocardiograms to gauge damage to the heart following a heart attack.

Aspirin and Anger

Murray A. Mittleman, MD, DrPH, associate professor in the department of epidemiology, Harvard School of Public Health, Boston.

Aspirin may reduce the risk of heart attacks for angry people. A study of 1,623 people found that angry people were more than twice as likely to suffer a heart attack within two hours after feeling angry than they were at other times.

The connection between anger and heart attacks was not found, however, in members of the group who took aspirin regularly.

It has long been recommended that people take one aspirin tablet (or half a tablet daily) to reduce heart attack risk. Aspirin makes heart attacks less likely by minimizing the chance of formation of potentially dangerous blood clots.

Researchers think that the same works to counteract the effects of adrenaline and other anger-generated stress hormones that make clots more likely to form.

Better than Aspirin

Michael Gent, DSc, department of clinical epidemiology and biostatistics, McMaster University, Hamilton, Ontario, Canada. His study of 19,185 volunteers who had suffered heart attack, stroke or clogged arteries in their legs was published in *The Lancet*.

The blood thinner *clopidogrel* is better than aspirin at warding off heart attack and stroke. Clopidogrel cuts the risk of new heart attacks and strokes by one-third, compared with one-fourth for aspirin.

More: Volunteers who took this drug were less likely to suffer gastrointestinal bleeding than those who took aspirin. The drug may be appropriate for patients with heart disease and/or peripheral arterial disease.

Heart Health Trap

Bruce Yaffe, MD, an internist in private practice, Yaffe, Ruden and Associates, 201 E. 65 St., New York City 10021.

If your doctor has prescribed Procardia or Adalac for you, make sure it is the long-acting form.

The FDA now requires that older, short-acting forms of these calcium channel blockers for high blood pressure or angina carry a warning label because some studies have linked them to an increased risk of heart attack.

These studies have little relevance for people taking the newer, long-acting forms. The newer calcium channel blockers control hypertension by keeping a steady level of the drug in the body, rather than allowing the amount to fluctuate rapidly, which may be dangerous.

Work Hours May Be Hazardous

Ichiro Kawachi, MD, PhD, professor of social epidemiology and director, Harvard Center for Society and Health, Harvard School of Public Health, Boston.

In a study, risk of heart attack was 70% higher among nurses who worked rotating shifts than among coworkers who worked regular hours.

Likely culprit: Stress resulting from disruption of the body's daily biological clock. This causes release of stress hormones such as epinephrine, norepinephrine and cortisol. In turn, these hormones raise blood pressure, reduce glucose tolerance and increase wear and tear on the cardiovascular system.

Cholesterol Drug Benefits

James Shepherd, MD, professor of pathological biochemistry at the University of Glasgow Medical School, Scotland.

The cholesterol-reducing drug *pravastatin* may prevent heart attacks in men who have elevated cholesterol levels but no history of heart disease.

Researchers in Scotland studied more than 6,000 apparently healthy men between age 45 and age 64 with high cholesterol levels. Those who took the drug suffered 28% fewer deaths from heart disease, and 31% fewer nonfatal heart attacks, than a similar group that took a placebo.

Helping Blood Vessels Work Properly

David G. Harrison, MD, professor of medicine and director, division of cardiology, Emory University, Atlanta.

A study of people with high cholesterol found that their artery walls didn't expand when they were supposed to (e.g., after exercise). After researchers gave these patients cholesterol-lowering drugs, known as statins, for nine months, they found that the artery walls began to dilate properly and blood pressure had dropped. Arteries that don't open properly prevent blood from moving through the body quickly enough in times of stress, and are associated with heart attacks and other cardiovascular problems.

Best Heart Disease Treatment

Nanette Kass Wenger, MD, professor of medicine at Emory University School of Medicine, and chief of cardiology at Grady Memorial Hospital, both in Atlanta.

Individually prescribed programs of exercise and diet and other risk-reduction programs reduce mortality rates among heart disease victims by 25%—but fewer than one-third of patients who could benefit from such programs are enrolled in them.

Why: Many doctors fail to refer appropriate patients because they do not know of local programs, and many patients have inadequate insurance coverage. Exercise programs pose no health risk even for older patients.

Useful: A free booklet, *Recovering from Heart Problems Through Cardiac Rehabilitation*, #96-0674 is available by contacting the Agency for Healthcare Research and Quality at 800-358-9295, *www.ahrq.gov.*

Easy Disease Risk Reducer

The late Ralph S. Paffenbarger, Jr., MD, professor emeritus of epidemiology at Stanford University School of Medicine, Stanford, CA.

A follow-up of the famous 1978 study of 20,000 Harvard alumni confirmed its findings that middle-aged and older men who exercised moderately had half as many heart attacks as their contemporaries who did not exercise.

A Smoke-Free World

Alan Blum, MD, director, Center for the Study of Tobacco and Society, University of Alabama, Tuscaloosa. Dr. Blum is the founder of Doctors Ought to Care (DOC), an antismoking group long recognized for its service to public health.

More than 46 million people have successfully stopped smoking. Most people who succeed in giving up smoking do so only after making three to five attempts, so failing once or twice is no reason to give up. After stopping, health improves no matter how long you've smoked or how old you are. The extra risk of heart disease that results from smoking decreases by 50% within one year, then continues to drop to zero after 15 years. And after five years, the risk of stroke faced by former smokers drops to the level faced by persons who have never smoked.

Timing Is Critical

Charles Hennekens, MD, professor of medicine, Harvard Medical School, and chief of preventive medicine at Brigham and Women's Hospital, Boston.

Taking an aspirin during—or very soon after—a heart attack reduces the risk of death significantly. A study of more than 17,000 patients worldwide found that those who took aspirin within 24 hours of the first symptoms were 23% less likely to die from a heart attack than those who did not.

When aspirin was taken along with the clot-dissolving drug *streptokinase*, the death rate dropped by 42%. It is believed that aspirin prevents production of prostaglandins, substances that encourage blood to clot. Blood clots can block blood vessels that carry vital oxygen to the damaged heart.

Height and Heart Disease

Donna Parker, ScD, assistant professor (research), community health, Brown University, Providence, RI.

Men over five-feet, 10-inches have an 80% lower risk of heart disease than men under five-feet, five-inches.

Possible reasons: Poor childhood nutrition—or prenatal nutrition—may stunt growth and affect adult health. Also, arteries in the hearts of shorter people are narrower, possibly increasing blockage risk.

Self-defense: Short men should focus on controllable risks—smoking, blood pressure, exercise, diet, weight. Results were inconclusive for shorter women—but they should be similarly cautious.

Average height: Around five-feet, nine-inches for men...five-feet, four-inches for women.

Even a Little Is Too Much

James Shepherd, MD, professor of pathologic biochemistry, University of Glasgow Medical School, Scotland. His five-year study of 6,595 men 45 to 64 years of age with cholesterol levels of 250 to 300 was published in *The New England Journal of Medicine*, 10 Shattuck St., Boston 02115.

Until recently, most doctors agreed that cholesterol-lowering drugs should be reserved only for patients at highest risk for heart disease.

Finding: Otherwise healthy patients with mildly elevated cholesterol who took *pravastatin* (Pravachol) had 31% fewer heart attacks than those who got a placebo.

Test Results Can Vary

Glen Griffin, MD, former primary care physician who now lectures on following a low-fat diet and coauthor of *The New Good Fat, Bad Fat: Lower Your Cholesterol and Reduce Your Odds of a Heart Attack*. Fisher.

Cholesterol test results can vary. Factors affecting results include illness and pregnancy.

Helpful: Have your doctor perform two or more tests before you make any major lifestyle changes.

Important: Cholesterol testing should include a determination of your HDL ratio—the ratio of total cholesterol to HDL ("good") cholesterol. A healthy ratio is *under four.* This measure is a much better predictor of heart disease risk than overall cholesterol readings.

Exercise and Heart Attack

Wayne Chandler, MD, professor of laboratory medicine, University of Washington, Seattle, who led a study of 44 men and women around age 66.

Men and women who biked, walked or jogged three times a week over a period of six months were less likely to suffer blood clots—and potentially fatal heart attacks—than those who did only flexibility exercises.

Their blood was also less likely to clot in the morning, the time of day when heart attacks are most likely to occur. This study may be the first to finally explain exactly how exercise helps prevent heart attacks.

Also: Those whose fitness levels improved the most during the study were least likely to suffer blood clots, but benefits vanished once they stopped their regular exercise routine.

More Harm than Good?

William E. Boden, MD, professor of medicine at the University of Connecticut School of Medicine and director of cardiology at Hartford Hospital. His study of 920 heart attack survivors was presented at a meeting of the American College of Cardiology.

A common heart test does more harm than good for survivors of one type of heart attack. *Angiography*—an X-ray procedure in which a catheter is threaded into the heart—may be too invasive for survivors of non-Q-wave heart attacks.

Study: The death rate among non-Q-wave heart attack survivors who underwent angiography was 34% higher than the rate among those who received a noninvasive heart test instead. Physicians can distinguish a Q-wave heart attack from a non-Q-wave heart attack via a simple electrocardiogram (EKG).

Hooray! Heart Help!

Tomas A. Salerno, MD, professor of surgery at the University of Miami and chief of the division of cardiothoracic surgery at Jackson Memorial Medical Center, Miami.

One type of operation may allow many patients with failing hearts to avoid transplants and enjoy near-normal lives.

The operation, developed by Randas J.V. Batista, MD, a Brazilian surgeon working in a primitive rural hospital, involves removing a slice of muscle from the left ventricle of patients with severely enlarged hearts. This surgery enables the remaining part of the heart to pump more effectively. US physicians who have observed the procedure in Brazil are exploring how it can be improved via high-tech medical techniques.

 ## Hunting Danger

Susan Haapaniemi, MS, exercise physiologist, William Beaumont Hospital, Royal Oak, MI.

The excitement of spotting the prey can trigger a heart attack in hunters with clogged arteries. In a study of 25 hunters, spotting a deer caused the hunters' heart rates to soar. One hunter's heart rate shot up from 78 to 168 beats per minute—and he was seated.

Self-defense: Get in shape before hunting season begins…rest frequently while hunting…avoid tobacco, caffeine and alcohol…and hunt with a buddy. *Also:* Hunters and nonhunters alike should wear bright orange when venturing into the woods during deer season.

Personality Danger

Mark Goodman, PhD, behavioral medicine specialist, and George Moran, MD, chief of cardiology, Union Memorial Hospital, Baltimore. Their 18-month study of 41 angioplasty patients was published in *Mayo Clinic Proceedings*, 200 First St. SW, Rochester, MN 55905.

Heart patients with Type A (hostile) personalities are more likely to need repeat angioplasties.

Background: More than one-third of heart patients who undergo angioplasty to open a blocked coronary artery eventually need to have the procedure repeated—because the artery closes back up. This process is called *restenosis.*

Study: Type A patients were 2.5 times more likely to experience restenosis than their calmer counterparts. *Theory:* Type A people have high levels of adrenaline in their blood. Adrenaline causes arteries to constrict.

Needed: Further study to determine if Type A patients can use relaxation techniques to reduce their risk of restenosis.

Mother's Diet and Heart Disease Link

David J.P. Barker, MD, PhD, director, Medical Research Council Environmental Epidemiology Unit, University of Southampton, Southampton, England.

Your risk of heart disease and other illnesses is linked to your mother's diet during pregnancy. An undernourished mother is more likely to give birth to a small baby. Small birth size is linked to insulin resistance (a condition that can lead to diabetes)...high blood pressure...and two major risk factors for heart disease—elevated triglycerides and low levels of HDL (good) cholesterol.

Fish Oil and Heart Attacks

Christine M. Albert, MD, associate professor of medicine, Harvard Medical School, Boston.

Fish seems to fight heart attack. In a study, men who ate fish at least once a week were 50% less likely to die of coronary artery disease than men who ate fish less than once a month. The more fish they ate, the lower their risk.

Theory: Compounds in fish—probably omega-3 fatty acids—are beneficial to the heart. *However:* Fish oil capsules may not benefit the heart, since they don't contain all the compounds found in fish.

Cutting Heart Attack Death Risks

Arthur Moss, MD, professor of medicine, University of Rochester Medical Center in Rochester, NY, leader of the study of almost 200 heart attack survivors, published in *The New England Journal of Medicine,* 10 Shattuck St., Boston 02115.

Implanted heart defibrillators could cut the risk of death by 50% for people who survive a first heart attack and have erratic heartbeats. The battery-powered implants work like the external defibrillators routinely used by emergency personnel—they shock the heart back into normal rhythm during a cardiac arrest.

Beta-Blockers and Heart Attacks

Stephen Soumerai, ScD, professor of ambulatory care and prevention at Harvard Medical School, Boston. His study was published in *The Journal of the American Medical Association*, 515 N. State St., Chicago 60610.

Older heart attack patients who were given *beta-blockers* lived longer. A five-year study of 5,300 Medicare patients found that those who used beta-blockers after heart attacks were 43% less likely to die within two years than those who did not. Researchers believe that if physicians prescribed beta-blockers for all eligible patients, it would save about 7,000 lives per year. The heart-slowing beta-blockers cost only about $3 per month, compared with $30 to $50 per month for the more frequently prescribed—but less effective—calcium channel blockers.

Garlic and Cholesterol Link

Manfred Steiner, MD, PhD, professor of medicine, East Carolina University School of Medicine, whose study was published in *The American Journal of Clinical Nutrition*, Baylor College of Medicine, 1100 Bates St., Houston 77030.

When otherwise healthy men who had high cholesterol took garlic supplements for six months, their cholesterol levels dropped 5% or more. The supplements contained seven grams of aged garlic—equivalent to 10 to 15 grams of cooked garlic or two cloves of fresh garlic.

Possible explanation: Garlic reduces LDL ("bad") cholesterol, although it had no effect on HDL ("good") cholesterol.

Psychological Stress Danger

Debra K. Moser, DNSc, RN, professor of cardiovascular nursing, University of Kentucky, College of Nursing, Lexington. Her nine-month study of 86 heart attack survivors was published in *Psychosomatic Medicine*, Box 1550, Hagerstown, MD 21741.

Severe stress in the aftermath of a heart attack increases the chance of complications. All heart attack survivors experience some anxiety, but some are more anxious than others.

Study: Patients who felt more anxious following a heart attack were 4.9 times more likely to suffer angina, heart spasms, another heart attack or dangerous heart rhythms than their less anxious counterparts. Almost 20% in this high-anxiety category suffered complications, compared with 6% of low-anxiety patients.

Theory: Severe anxiety causes the body to produce *catecholamines* and other stress-related chemicals that thicken the blood.

Helpful: Unrestricted visiting with friends and family...and relaxation therapy.

Triglyceride Levels

Michael Miller, MD, director, Center for Preventive Cardiology, University of Maryland Medical Center, Baltimore. His study of triglyceride levels in 492 men and women was presented at a meeting of the American Heart Association.

Safe triglyceride levels may not be so safe after all. Current guidelines call for triglycerides to be no higher than 200. But a study found that people with levels between 100 and 200 had twice the risk of dying from a heart attack as those with levels below 100. They were also twice as likely to require bypass surgery or another procedure to clear blocked coronary arteries.

To keep triglyceride levels down: Get regular exercise...minimize consumption of sugar and saturated fat...and boost intake of omega-3 fatty acids. Sources of omega-3 fatty acids include sardines, mackerel, tuna, fish oil capsules and flaxseed oil.

Stroke Risk Reduction

Gregory W. Albers, MD, director, Stanford Stroke Center, Stanford University Medical Center, Palo Alto, CA. His study of atrial fibrillation in 309 elderly patients was published in *Archives of Internal Medicine*, 515 N. State St., Chicago 60610.

To cut their risk of stroke, individuals experiencing a type of irregular heartbeat known as atrial fibrillation should usually be treated with blood thinners like aspirin or *warfarin* (Coumadin). In a study, 82% of these patients were found to be at high risk for stroke, yet only 64% were being treated with either drug. Many doctors are hesitant to prescribe Coumadin because they are not prepared to do the necessary monitoring of patients and/or they fear bleeding complications.

Early Treatment Is Best

Eric J. Topol, MD, chief of genomic medicine and translational science, Scripps Health, San Diego, CA.

Starting treatment earlier could reduce heart attack deaths by 15%. On average, treatment now starts almost three hours after the onset of symptoms.

Self-defense: If you have symptoms of a heart attack, seek treatment immediately.

Danger symptoms: Pain or pressure in the chest that lasts more than a few minutes...pain radiating to shoulders, neck or arms...lightheadedness...nausea...shortness of breath.

4

Your Doctor and You

The Smart Way to Pick a Physician

Timothy McCall, MD

Finding a good primary-care physician has always been important. It's especially true today, with health maintenance organizations (HMOs) playing an ever-expanding role in the delivery of health care.

In most HMOs and other managed-care plans, your primary-care doctor acts as the "gatekeeper." He/she decides when you can see a specialist, get physical therapy, be hospitalized, etc.

Since HMO doctors may receive financial incentives to keep costs down, it's important to find someone who'll balance the insurance company's desire to maximize profits with your own health needs.

How do you find a good doctor? Whether you belong to an HMO or have traditional insurance coverage, much of the conventional wisdom is misguided.

Some experts say to choose a doctor on the strength of his/her credentials. It is sensible to find out where your doctor went to medical school and whether she's board-certified. But a doctor who went to a prestigious medical school like Johns Hopkins may have graduated last in his class. You might be better off with someone who excelled at the Medical College of Who-Knows-Where. Surprisingly, credentials can be misleading.

Other experts say it's best to ask friends and family members to recommend a doctor. That's not always a good idea.

Most people are pretty good at judging bedside manner, and that's important. But some doctors with a pleasant manner don't practice good medicine. Few people are actually equipped to judge a doctor's medical judgment and skills.

Timothy McCall, MD, an internist, medical editor of *Yoga Journal* and author of *Examining Your Doctor: A Patient's Guide to Avoiding Harmful Medical Care*. Carol. *www.drmccall.com.*

A more reliable way to find a good doctor is to get a recommendation from a medical insider. If you know someone who works in a hospital or clinic, that person probably knows the scuttlebutt about local doctors—which ones are good and, more important, which ones you should avoid.

Once you've found a few good prospects, how do you narrow the field?

Conventional wisdom says to interview each doctor until you find one you feel comfortable with. Many physicians will agree to a brief "get acquainted" session. It's not a bad idea. You may learn a bit about a doctor's bedside manner and maybe even his medical philosophy.

Ultimately, though, it's not the doctor's credentials or reputation or what he says that matters. What matters is how well he practices. Contrary to popular belief, just about anyone can judge that.

Start by reading up on any condition you're diagnosed with and any drug you're prescribed. The more you know, the better your ability to assess a doctor's knowledge and skills.

Probably the easiest thing to determine is whether the doctor is spending enough time with you.

A careful interview and a thorough physical exam are the foundation of good medical practice—and they take time. So do explaining things and answering questions.

Since clinics and HMOs are pressuring doctors to spend less time with their patients, I believe the amount of time a doctor spends with you is the best single indication of how concerned he is with your welfare. A doctor who's willing to buck the system to give you the time you need may also be more likely to go to bat for you if your insurer tries to deny you a needed service.

The process of evaluating a doctor should be ongoing. There's only so much you can find out about a doctor before your first appointment. Over time you'll learn much more.

It's like choosing a job or a college. You make your best guess, but you often don't know what you've got till you've had it for a while.

How to Get the Most from Your Doctor–Patient Relationship

Bernard Lown, MD, professor emeritus of cardiology at Harvard University School of Public Health in Boston. He is author of *The Lost Art of Healing*. Ballantine Books.

Does your doctor really care about you …or just treat you? As a doctor with more than 40 years of experience, I can attest to the fact that a good doctor–patient relationship greatly reduces the anxiety associated with being sick. It also improves the likelihood that you'll get good medical care.

Lesson: It pays to examine a doctor's demeanor at least as carefully as you examine the diplomas hanging in his/her office.

Here are seven signs that you've come to the right office…

● **You talk with the doctor** *before* **disrobing.** If upon arriving for your first appointment, you are led to an exam room and asked to take off your clothes, you're at a patient "mill"—not a doctor's office.

Your first meeting with the doctor should be in his private office—while you are fully clothed. His initial goal should be to put you at ease. The best way to do that is via a few minutes of conversation. Forcing you to shiver naked under a thin gown is not the way.

● **The doctor offers his hand to you.** Extending a hand in greeting is a small but significant sign of respect. I wouldn't condemn a doctor who didn't shake hands with his patients, but it counts as a strike against him.

Similarly, does the doctor assume that it's fine to call you by your first name? Doing so is a sign of disrespect. A good doctor asks his patients what they wish to be called—then respects their wishes.

● **The doctor is on time.** A doctor may want you to *think* he's late because he has given priority to patients sicker than you. That's rarely the case.

Consistent lateness is inevitably the result of poor management, overbooking and/or arrogance—an indifference to the time of others.

A good doctor shows respect for his patients by seeing them on time.

● **The doctor is not interrupted by phone calls.** Your doctor's concentration is broken every time he answers his secretary's buzz. I've forbidden my assistant to interrupt me except for a dire emergency. A good doctor responds to phone calls between patients.

● **The doctor is optimistic.** A doctor's mood influences not only a patient's emotional status, but also his/her medical outcome. Words can either heal or harm, and a good doctor knows this.

Your doctor should be upbeat no matter what your condition. There's always *something* that can be done to help—even if it's just to lessen your anxiety. I tell my patients that they no longer have to worry about their illness because I'll be the one taking over that duty from now on.

● **The doctor takes a careful history.** Seventy-five percent of the information needed to make an accurate diagnosis comes from taking a careful and detailed patient history.

This makes sense. While a doctor may know a great deal about a particular illness, he knows little about how that illness manifests itself in you. Only you can reveal that, and only if he pays attention to what you tell him.

Your doctor should question you closely not only about your medical condition, but also about your work, social relationships and any other aspects of your life that might be affecting your health. Taking a good medical history is the single most important sign of good doctoring.

● **You** *feel* **cared for.** Each time you leave your doctor's office, you should feel better emotionally, if not physically. You should feel that the doctor took your concerns seriously and answered all your questions.

The doctor should talk in terms you can understand, but you should never get the feeling you're being talked down to.

Mostly, you should have confidence in the doctor not just because of his expertise, but because he's another human being who has made a commitment to care for you.

HOW'S YOUR DOCTOR?

If you've broken your foot and the best orthopedist in town is gruff and rushed, so be it. Since you'll be under his care only for a limited period of time, his expertise is more important than his personality.

But I wouldn't be so quick to excuse a difficult demeanor in my primary care physician.

If your doctor doesn't meet all the criteria listed above, let him know. You might even give him a copy of this article—just to get the conversation going.

How to Get The Best Care From Your Doctor

Richard L. Sribnick, MD, an internist in private practice in Columbia, SC. He is coauthor of *Smart Patient, Good Medicine: Working with Your Doctor to Get the Best Medical Care.* Walker & Co.

Although conscientious doctors try to provide good care for all patients, they tend to do their best work for patients with whom they have good rapport.

The doctor-patient relationship, like any other, requires effort to make it work. *Here's how to improve yours...*

● **Speak clearly and concisely when describing your symptoms.** Though a physical exam and lab tests may follow, the first—and often critical—ingredient for an accurate diagnosis is how well you describe your symptoms.

A good description reduces the risk of misdiagnosis...and helps you avoid needless diagnostic tests and surgical procedures.

Helpful: Prepare your spiel ahead of time —in writing. If you wait until you're half-clothed in the office, you may have a hard time expressing your thoughts clearly. *Four key issues...*

● **When** did the problem first appear?

● **Where** is it located? Be specific. "Pain in the temples" is better than "a headache."

● **How** does it feel? Is it a stabbing pain? Throbbing? How often does it occur? How long does it last?

•**What** brings it on or makes it worse? What relieves it? What other symptoms occur at the same time?

If you have several problems, list all of them as soon as the doctor walks into the examination room. Let *him/her* decide which to pursue first.

Say you've been experiencing chest pain. How do you describe your symptoms to the doctor?

Wrong: "My chest feels funny sometimes at work. It's probably just stress."

A busy doctor may dismiss this problem as trivial, and not investigate further.

Right: "I feel like there's a fist tightening in the center of my chest. This chest pressure began several weeks ago and lasts for a couple of minutes each time. I first noticed it after walking up two flights of stairs at work. I felt better after I stopped to rest."

Such a description will alert the doctor to the possibility of heart disease, and the need for diagnostic tests like angiography.

•**Be calm—but not stoic.** If you don't look like you're in pain, the doctor may fail to appreciate just how much it hurts. If you make light of a symptom, he is likely to do so as well.

Important: Share your concerns. If you fear that your headaches are being caused by a brain tumor, for instance, say so. But do so *after* you've described your symptoms. That way, the doctor's thinking won't be biased.

Whatever you do, *don't* panic. If you do, the doctor may be tempted to order needless tests and procedures to comfort you.

•**Adopt a positive attitude.** Some patients exhibit a negative, almost accusatory attitude when talking to the doctor. It's an attitude exemplified by statements such as, "I want my money's worth here, and I don't want you to cut any corners."

Such an attitude puts the doctor on the defensive. That can lead to hostility, and it's hard for a doctor to provide good care when he's mad at you.

If you tend to leave your doctor's office feeling shortchanged of time or attention, you may need another doctor.

If you have this feeling with several different doctors, odds are you need a new *attitude*. Discuss the situation with a friend whose judgment you respect.

•**Don't put up with rudeness.** If you feel you've been treated poorly by the doctor or his staff, let him know. Just be sure to do so diplomatically. Make it clear that your purpose is problem-solving, so you can work better together.

Wrong: "Why do I always have to wait? Isn't my time important too?"

Right: "How can I minimize the time I have to wait?"

Always wait until the *end* of your visit to voice any complaints. That way, the doctor can turn his full attention to your medical problem—without being distracted by his own defensiveness.

•**Take steps to avoid frustration.** Minimize waiting for appointments by scheduling routine visits for the first slot after the doctor's lunch hour.

If that slot is unavailable, ask for the first appointment in the morning.

If the doctor agrees to "work you in" between appointments, ask in advance how long you'll have to wait. That will give you a sense of control—and reduce your frustration.

Phone strategy: Unless it is a true emergency, don't expect to speak with the doctor right away.

Tell the receptionist you would like the doctor to call you as soon as it's convenient.

In an emergency, of course, don't hesitate to ask the nurse to interrupt the doctor.

Prescription refills: Call during office hours, not on evenings or weekends. Call from home or work—not the pharmacy. Ask the doctor or nurse approximately when the prescription will be phoned in.

•**Show your appreciation.** Like everyone else, doctors want to feel good about their work…and they have affection for patients who express their appreciation for their efforts.

Don't be afraid to say "thank you" to your doctor. A simple note can really make a doctor's day—and improve the quality of your care.

How to Get the Most From Your HMO

Timothy McCall, MD, an internist, medical editor of *Yoga Journal* and author of *Examining Your Doctor: A Patient's Guide to Avoiding Harmful Medical Care.* Carol. *www.drmccall.com.*

If you're not already enrolled in a health maintenance organization (HMO) or other managed-care plan, you may be soon. More than 170 million Americans receive coverage through some form of managed-care (HMO, PPO, POS) plan.

The number in traditional fee-for-service insurance is decreasing every year, and even these plans increasingly incorporate managed-care features.

The rules are very different in this new system. To get good care, you must understand how managed care works and adjust your approach accordingly.

The first thing to understand is how the financial incentives for doctors have changed. Under the fee-for-service system, insurance companies paid doctors for every service rendered. Each time doctors stuck in a needle, ran a cardiogram or took out someone's tonsils, they were paid.

Unfortunately, doctors responded to this arrangement by doing millions of needless tonsillectomies and other procedures. As a result, medical costs skyrocketed, with health care consuming a larger and larger chunk of the GNP.

HMOs came along and changed the way doctors are paid. Although they use dozens of different systems, the bottom line in many plans is this—*the less the doctor does, the more money he or she makes.*

It's common for doctors to receive a flat monthly fee for every patient under their care. Under this arrangement, known as capitation, the cost of lab tests, procedures and other care comes out of the doctor's pocket. If the doctor orders an $80 X-ray, $80 is deducted from his paycheck.

Frequently, HMOs give bonuses and assess monetary penalties according to how much the doctor spends. For example, many HMOs reward doctors who limit the number of patients they hospitalize or who minimize referrals to expensive specialists. Using a technique known as "economic credentialing," managed-care plans terminate doctors who spend too much on patients.

To further limit costs, HMOs set up barriers to care. Under most managed-care plans, you can't see a specialist without being referred by your primary care doctor. Visits to the emergency room require pre-authorization. And it can take weeks—even months—to get an appointment.

Given these new realities, here's how to protect your interests. If you're thinking of joining an HMO or are already enrolled, learn as much as you can about the plan. Read the membership materials carefully. If possible, talk to current and former members about their experiences with the HMO in question.

Since your primary care doctor functions as the "gatekeeper"—blocking or granting access to specialists—choosing a good gatekeeper can be vital. You want someone who, if necessary, will appeal on your behalf if you need a special test or an extra day in the hospital.

It's often hard to tell much about a doctor from the brochures, so again, talk to other members, even people you bump into in the waiting room.

If you feel that you're being unjustly denied services you need, don't be afraid to really fight for them. If politely making your case to your doctor doesn't work, try appealing to an administrator. All HMOs have formal grievance procedures.

Finally, the more you can learn about any medical conditions you have, the better position you'll be in to assert yourself. HMO doctors have a difficult time saying no to reasonable, well-informed patients.

Don't forget, though, much of the medical care we've come to expect really isn't necessary. Sometimes you really don't need that $80 X-ray.

How to Get the Very Best Possible Medical Care

Peter H. Berczeller, MD, former professor of clinical medicine, New York University School of Medicine, New York City. A practicing internist from 1960 until his retirement in 1992, he is author of *Doctors and Patients: What We Feel About You.* Lisa Drew Books.

Visiting the doctor can be a stressful experience—whether the visit is for a routine checkup or to diagnose a troubling symptom. And with so much negative press about health care these days, anxiety among patients seems to be at an all-time high. Soaring costs, needless tests, faulty diagnoses and uncaring doctors are but a few of the chief complaints patients have today.

As a result, there's growing tension—even hostility—between doctors and patients.

In some cases, this tension is beneficial to patients—as when it motivates them to take a more active role in their treatment, for example. In other cases, doctor–patient tension leads patients to act in ways that are self-defeating and detrimental to their care.

Here's how to be a better patient—and how to bring out the very best in your physician…

●**Choose a doctor who is emotionally accessible.** Ideally, you want someone who conveys a sense of genuine concern, interest and involvement…and in whom you feel you can confide.

Do *not* select a doctor solely for his/her technical expertise. If I had a choice between a genius doctor and one who was merely competent but warm and humane, I'd pick the latter.

Reason: Easy, open communication between doctor and patient is essential both to the diagnosis and the healing process.

●**Tell your doctor all your concerns.** If it's your first visit, come prepared to give a complete medical history. If your records are on file with another doctor, make sure they've been transferred to the new doctor. On subsequent visits, report in detail any symptoms or changes you've experienced since your last visit. If you tend to be forgetful, bring a written list of all your concerns to your appointment.

●**Dress and behave appropriately.** Although the doctor is working for you, it's important to treat him with respect. Proper attire and courteous behavior not only are polite, but they can enhance your care. When I was seeing patients, I have to admit that I tended to listen just a little bit better when the patient was nicely dressed and well-spoken.

Proper attire and courteous behavior on the part of both the doctor and the patient help to dignify their interaction—entirely appropriate, given the serious nature of what patients and doctors talk about.

●**Tell the doctor if you're dissatisfied with your medical care.** Being honest and direct helps clear the air and puts your relationship on a better footing.

Some patients keep their negative thoughts to themselves, fearing that complaining will simply antagonize the doctor…and that he will retaliate by providing inferior care. Such thinking is misguided. In fact, because good communication is critical to receiving good health care, there's nothing most doctors like more than an open, honest patient.

Bonus: By revealing your inner feelings, you'll make it easier for your doctor to help you cope with the anxiety or helplessness that often accompanies illness. In other words, telling your doctor how you feel is a little like undergoing psychotherapy.

●**Don't expect your doctor to be perfect.** Doctors are human, and they make mistakes. While a big mistake is reason to find a new doctor, inconsequential ones are no cause for alarm.

Solution: You and your family must be assertive, vigilant and actively involved in your care. Politely question all medications given to you. Any allergies you have should be detailed in your medical record—but be sure to mention them to the doctor just in case.

If you're to be hospitalized, ask friends and relatives to watch out for you. Tell them to alert the doctor or nurse if they notice you don't look right.

●**Don't be put off if your doctor sometimes appears uncertain.** Far from being a liability, a doctor's uncertainty can be very helpful—it can even lead to better care. The best doctors don't try to project a sense of omniscience. Rather, they realize that there's always something else they can learn...and that there's always room for improvement in their performance.

•**Know when to get a second opinion.** An unusual physical finding, a lab test that doesn't make sense, an unexpected worsening of your condition—all suggest the need for a second opinion.

Problem: Some patients are too timid to seek one, fearing that doing so will offend their doctor. While some doctors are defensive about the prospect of an outside consultation, most are perfectly happy if the patient wants to seek another opinion.

Other patients are too *quick* to seek a second opinion—sometimes seeking one even before the first one has been rendered. I think it's best to wait until your doctor has had a chance to make a diagnosis and plan a treatment strategy.

Give your doctor a chance to set the scene properly—to find order in the random set of symptoms and findings and to give your condition a name.

To do this, a doctor must order appropriate diagnostic tests and observe you over a period of time. Hard as it is to believe, there's a logic and rhythm to each illness. Some take weeks or even months to identify—even if your doctor is first-rate.

There's simply no substitute for the imagination, enthusiasm and—most important—the concern that comes from a conscientious doctor who has been involved in your care from the outset. That's why the timing of other opinions is so critical.

•**Don't let family members become obstacles to your treatment.** Loved ones are invaluable as sources of emotional support. But too often they get in the way of your treatment—by interfering with the doctor's decisions...or by being hostile toward the doctor in a misguided attempt to show love for you.

A doctor who asks family members to leave a patient's room is not trying to demonstrate his power. Chances are, he simply wants an opportunity to form his own impression of the patient—without outside interference.

It's surprising just how much information can be obtained from a patient if there's nobody there to speak for him.

•**Develop a solid, caring relationship with one doctor.** While it's sometimes necessary to "fire" a doctor or to get a second opinion, some patients run from doctor to doctor haphazardly. *Skipping from doctor to doctor...*

•**Makes you easy prey for quacks** and other practitioners eager to exploit your obvious anxiety and subject you to needless tests and expensive treatments.

•**Delays your diagnosis.** The workup required for a diagnosis usually begins anew each time a new doctor is consulted.

•**Leads you to get the diagnosis you want to hear**—rather than the diagnosis that's most accurate.

For true healing to occur, a one-on-one, caring relationship with your doctor is essential. You should maintain this relationship with a primary doctor even if your condition necessitates consulting a specialist...or, getting a second opinion.

Doctors are not magicians. Leaving one—especially someone who has a good track record with you—and seeking out another is not usually the answer. The new "magician" will probably not cure you any more quickly, and switching mid-illness will probably cause even more delay in making you better.

Questions to Ask When Your Doctor Recommends a Specialist

Charles B. Inlander, a consumer advocate and health-care consultant based in Fogelsville, PA. He was founding president of the nonprofit People's Medical Society, a consumer health advocacy group in Allentown, PA. He is author of numerous books, including *Take This Book to the Hospital With You.* St. Martin's.

Finding the best medical specialist takes more than just getting a name and phone number from your doctor. *Steps to take...*

● **First ask your doctor why you are being referred to this particular specialist.**

Trap: Referrals are often professional courtesies. This may mean that a fellow colleague isn't likely to contradict your doctor's recommendations or that you may not be getting the name of the best person to confirm a diagnosis or treat your condition.

Important: Find out if your doctor knows the specialist's success rate in treating your problem. This is basic information that your doctor should know about the doctor to whom he is referring you.

● **Ask your doctor for a list of all the likely medical causes of your condition before you seek another opinion.** Similar symptoms can exist for different problems. Find out from your doctor the most likely causes of your problem...and the most remote causes. This information will help you when you seek another opinion.

Example: Hearing loss can indicate that you have damage to the eardrum—or a brain tumor. But the specialists who can diagnose and treat these conditions are in different fields. One is an ear, nose and throat specialist...and the other one is a neurologist or a neurosurgeon.

You can save yourself a lot of time and money by learning—and prioritizing—all your options before you shop around.

● **Once you have a diagnosis, find out how many times the specialist has treated your kind of problem within the last year.** Volume is critical, although the ideal volume depends on the problem being treated. For common problems, such as heart surgery, a specialist should treat hundreds of people a year. For rarer conditions, 10 to 20 cases is acceptable.

If the specialist's office is reluctant to share this information, consider seeking treatment elsewhere.

● **Get the name of a specialist who can give you a second opinion.** Up to 80% of second opinions on *treatments* don't agree with the first. Twenty percent of second opinions disagree with *diagnosis*. That's why it's important to seek several opinions.

If you have trouble finding someone, call the national headquarters of that specialty's association for a few names.

If you live in a rural or suburban area that doesn't have a concentration of specialists with the breadth of experience you need, it's worth it to get in the car or on the plane and go somewhere that does.

● **Find out if there are other treatment options.** Get a treatment plan from each doctor whom you see for an opinion. Then phone a prominent medical school in your state and ask to speak to the person who chairs the department under which your problem falls— for example, the orthopedic surgery department if surgery has been recommended for a knee injury. He/she may be willing to tell you about recent medical advances in the field. You can also do your own research through a local medical school library or an online medical database.

How to Find a Doctor of Alternative Medicine

For a free referral to an alternative doctor in your area, contact the American College for Advancement in Medicine, 24411 Ridge Rte., Ste. 115, Laguna Hills, CA 92653, 888-439-6891, *www.acam.org.*

Is Your Doctor Listening?

Robert A. Murden, MD, professor of clinical internal medicine and director, geriatric medicine, Ohio State University Medical Center, Columbus. His six-month study of 818 subjects was published in *Medical Care*, 8848 Winding Ridge Rd., Indianapolis 46217.

Doctors aren't good at listening to patients their own age. If your doctor seems to be a poor listener and he/she is roughly your age, consider looking for a new physician who is significantly younger or older.

Better Doctor–Patient Communications

Timothy McCall, MD, an internist, medical editor of *Yoga Journal* and author of *Examining Your Doctor: A Patient's Guide to Avoiding Harmful Medical Care*. Carol. *www.drmccall.com.*

Don't be intimidated by your doctor's manner. Decide what you want to talk about before your appointment—and make a list if necessary. Maintain eye contact with your doctor, both to show that you're participating in the process and to encourage the doctor to deal more directly with you. Don't let your doctor avoid answering your questions or make insensitive comments that go unchallenged. If your efforts to improve communications fail, consider finding another doctor.

The Right Way to Talk to Your Doctor

Timothy McCall, MD, an internist, medical editor of *Yoga Journal* and author of *Examining Your Doctor: A Patient's Guide to Avoiding Harmful Medical Care*. Carol. *www.drmccall.com.*

While most people know that it's important to talk to the doctor, what they really focus on are diagnostic tests like X-rays, blood analyses and electrocardiograms.

If a doctor fails to order tests, many people believe that he or she hasn't taken their complaints seriously.

But studies have shown that in three out of four cases good doctors arrive at an accurate diagnosis just by talking with their patients. The physical exam yields another 12% of diagnoses. Lab tests and X-rays account for only about 11%.

Even when tests do lead to a diagnosis, often it's information gleaned from the interview that enabled the doctor to decide which tests were necessary.

The beauty of the medical interview is that it's inexpensive and—unlike medical tests—it has no undesirable side effects. Time spent talking also builds rapport—and that in itself can be very therapeutic.

To get the most from the patient interview, the doctor must devote enough time to it. Unfortunately, physicians are under increasing pressure from insurance administrators and health maintenance organizations to cut down the length of office visits. As a result, many doctors have begun to skimp on the interview. But good doctors resist the pressure and spend the time to do the job right.

Doctors and patients alike have a role to play in making the most of their time together.

Doctors must use good interview techniques. The first rule is to allow the patient to talk without needless interruption. Sounds simple enough. But one study found that, on average, doctors listened to their patients for only 18 seconds before interrupting. Once interrupted, patients rarely return to what they had intended to say. As a result, important clues are lost.

It's also poor technique if the doctor attempts to control the conversation by barraging you with yes or no questions. This tactic results in less accurate information and missed diagnoses. Doctors should favor open-ended questions like, *What's bothering you?* or *Is there something you're worried this might be?*

Smart patients help their doctors get the most from the interview by preparing for their appointments. Before you go in to see your doctor, plan what you'd like to cover. Write down all your questions, but be realistic. It's impossible to cover a whole laundry list in a few minutes. Stick with those items of greatest importance to you. If you can't cover everything you need to, schedule a return visit.

If you're going in to have a specific symptom evaluated, ask yourself: When did it start? When does it happen? How long does it last? Is there anything that makes it better or worse? Have I ever had anything similar?

If the problem is pain, try to pinpoint its location in your body. Is the pain sharp? Crampy? Does it feel like pins and needles?

Honesty and openness are vital to a good medical interview. Unfortunately, doctors and patients tend to avoid embarrassing topics like sexuality and incontinence. Steering away from such areas can compromise your medical care.

Sexual difficulties, for example, can provide important clues to such problems as diabetes, thyroid disorders and medication side effects. And in this age of AIDS, knowledge of a patient's sexual habits can help the doctor recognize early symptoms and—more important —teach the patient how to avoid becoming infected in the first place.

Considering the importance of the medical interview, maybe it's time you had a little talk with your doctor.

Is There Something Your Doctor Isn't Telling You?

Timothy McCall, MD, an internist, medical editor of *Yoga Journal* and author of *Examining Your Doctor: A Patient's Guide to Avoiding Harmful Medical Care.* Carol. *www.drmccall.com.*

Doctors depend upon their patients to be open and honest in discussing their health concerns. But there are a few things that some doctors prefer their *patients* didn't know.

Here's what your doctor may not be revealing to you...

● **"I've been sued for malpractice."** Many doctors who have been sued—even repeatedly —continue to practice without their patients having any idea. Most malpractice settlements are shrouded in secrecy by agreements that prevent the information from ever becoming public. Since doctors may not want to reveal past disciplinary actions against them either, you may want to check out information collected by the Public Citizen health research group.

This consumer advocacy group publishes information on disciplinary actions against doctors. To obtain a report on actions taken against doctors in your state, contact the group at 202-588-1000 or online at *www.citizen.org.* The report costs $10.

● **"I'm years out of date."** Medical information is mushrooming so fast that no doctor can keep up completely. But some doctors do a better job than others.

To tell if your doctor is up-to-date, learn as much as possible about any condition you're diagnosed with. Start with consumer health guides, articles in magazines and newsletters or the Internet. For more information, spend time at your local library. You'll be able to spot doctors who are dangerously behind the times.

The federal government and hundreds of consumer organizations provide free or low-cost health information. And, for a fee, private health research firms will provide you with a detailed report on your ailment.

● **"The HMO pays me a bonus for not referring you to a specialist."** Most health maintenance organizations and other managed-care plans give doctors financial incentives for keeping costs down. Doctors get bonuses for such things as reducing the number of referrals to specialists, keeping patients out of the hospital and cutting down on MRI scans and other expensive services.

Since it's hard to learn this information from the plans themselves, I recommend discussing the matter with your employer's benefits manager.

If that doesn't work, ask your doctor directly. You might say, "It's not that I don't trust you, Dr. Smith, but I've been reading a lot about HMOs lately and would appreciate knowing if the doctors have any financial incentives to limit certain services." Some plans forbid doctors from revealing how they're paid. If your doctor says he or she cannot tell you, that's a bad sign.

● **"I'm not what I claim to be."** A study in *The New England Journal of Medicine* revealed that many doctors who call themselves specialists have never had the required training or passed the rigorous exam required for board certification. In teaching hospitals medical students sometimes fool patients by introducing themselves as "Dr. So and So."

To find out if a particular doctor is certified, call the American Board of Medical Specialties (866-ASK-ABMS). Better HMOs and hospitals generally check the credentials of their doctors—but it certainly doesn't hurt for you to check, too.

If you're hospitalized, insist that anyone rendering care tell you his name and training. This will help you spot poorly trained aides who—

in an attempt to cut costs—hospitals are now substituting for registered nurses.

What you don't know—and what your doctor may not be telling you—could indeed hurt you. Unless you do your homework.

Protect Yourself From Your Doctor's Financial Interests

Marc A. Rodwin, PhD, JD, professor of law and co-director of the health law concentration, Suffolk University Law School, Boston. He is author of *Medicine, Money and Morals: Physicians' Conflicts of Interest*. Oxford University Press.

We trust our doctors to make our health the highest priority—to "do the right thing" when ordering tests, prescribing drugs, etc. In taking the Hippocratic Oath, they swore to do just that.

Like the rest of us, however, doctors must earn a living. And sometimes the treatment a doctor prescribes—or withholds—has a direct bearing on his/her own financial well-being.

DOCTORS, HOSPITALS AND LABS

Some doctors have a financial stake in a diagnostic lab, hospital or another local health-care facility. Others don't have a direct stake—but have a close relative who does.

With such an arrangement, each referral the doctor makes is, effectively, a self-referral. Each time he orders a $1,000 MRI exam or puts you in the hospital, he turns a profit—or turns a profit for someone to whom he's closely tied.

Such an arrangement tempts doctors to order needless tests, recommend needless operations and hospitalizations, etc.

Or doctors may be tempted to send you to a hospital that handles their bills or provides them with other perks—even when another hospital is better equipped to treat your specific ailment. Doctors who have a financial stake in a health-care facility make referrals to it more often than doctors who lack such an interest, studies have shown.

Self-defense: Ask your doctor, "What financial ties or other arrangements do you have with the lab (or hospital) you're sending me to?" The fewer ties, the better.

In areas with few doctors, it may be impractical to reject a doctor simply because he owns a share of a local diagnostic lab. You may not have a choice. Or—your illness may require immediate attention, leaving you little time to consider other options.

But if you have a choice, a doctor's financial ties are a factor to consider—along with his training, reputation, etc.

NEEDLESS PROCEDURES

Doctors who work under the traditional "fee-for-service" system get paid for each service they render to patients. With such a setup, it's always in a doctor's financial interest to do more procedures—not fewer.

Most doctors manage to resist the obvious temptation to perform needless surgery, order superfluous diagnostic tests, etc. But the profit motive can—and sometimes does—cloud clinical judgment.

Self-defense: If your doctor recommends endoscopy, hysterectomy, catheterization or another invasive diagnostic test or elective (non-emergency) surgery, get a second opinion. Find a physician with no ties to your doctor—ideally someone who practices at another hospital.

DRUG COMPANY GIFTS

For almost any illness, a range of treatment options is available. But drugmakers spend millions of dollars on marketing campaigns designed to convince doctors that drug therapy is the best route.

And—each drugmaker spends millions on advertisements that are designed to convince doctors to use its drug. These efforts don't end at advertising.

Kickbacks are illegal. But drugmakers find other ways to ensure that doctors think of their products when they reach for a prescription pad.

Usual approach: Showering doctors with inexpensive gifts such as pens embossed with the name of the drug being promoted...or coffee and danish in the doctors' lounge.

In the past, drug companies have also been known to offer doctors...

99

●**All-expenses-paid weekends** at resorts hosting "educational seminars" on new drugs.

●**Super Bowl tickets.**

●**Cash payments** for participating in "market research."

Bottom line: The drug your doctor prescribes may be the one he's been persuaded to prescribe. That might not be the cheapest drug or the most effective one for your condition.

Self-defense: If you have a chronic condition such as arthritis or asthma, find out which drug (or nondrug therapy) is best for you. Explore all of the alternatives.

Conduct research at your local library or on the Internet...consult a drug reference book such as Dr. Sidney M. Wolfe's *Worst Pills Best Pills II* (Pantheon)...and/or contact the National Self-Help Clearinghouse (212-817-1822, *www.selfhelpweb.org*) to locate a support group in your local area.

Once your research is done, ask the doctor, "What makes the drug (or treatment) you've chosen a better choice than other drugs (or treatments) that are available?" Be sure to inquire about any possible side effects.

PERILS OF MANAGED CARE

Many health maintenance organizations (HMOs) pay doctors a monthly fee for each patient, rather than for each service. The doctor is paid the same sum whether he sees you once a year or 20 times. Performing procedures or scheduling follow-up visits means that he does more work without getting paid more.

This arrangement—called *capitation*—keeps costs down by encouraging doctors to provide *less care.* The risk, of course, is that a doctor might withhold care a patient needs.

HMOs also limit spending via *risk sharing.* Here, the doctor and the HMO share the financial risk for the cost of services. Risk sharing discourages doctors from making referrals, ordering tests, hospitalizing patients or recommending costly treatments.

Lawsuit: A woman claimed risk sharing discouraged her doctor from ordering a biopsy despite her symptoms of breast cancer. By the time her cancer was diagnosed, it had spread.

Self-defense: Ask your doctor, "What percentage of your income depends on risk sharing incentives and bonuses?" The larger the percentage, the more likely his judgment will be compromised.

To Take Charge of Your Medical Care...

Richard N. Podell, MD, clinical professor of family medicine, Robert Wood Johnson Medical School, New Brunswick, NJ. He is author of *When Your Doctor Doesn't Know Best.* Simon & Schuster.

Choose a doctor whose office hours fit your schedule—and who is available by phone. Research your symptoms before an appointment and prepare a list of questions. Take notes on the answers. Keep a journal with dates of shots, illnesses, aches and pains to help pinpoint problems more quickly. Ask to see your records and have them explained to you.

To Control Your Medical Costs...

Charles B. Inlander, a consumer advocate and health-care consultant based in Fogelsville, PA. He was founding president of the nonprofit People's Medical Society, a consumer health advocacy group in Allentown, PA. He is author of numerous books, including *Take This Book to the Hospital With You.* St. Martin's.

Negotiate with your doctor to keep charges in line. Find out what other doctors in your area charge for the same procedure. Make mention of your research to your doctor and ask him/her to accept the rate charged by his peers.

Also: Work out fees for regular treatments —for instance, a charge only for a shot when you need one regularly, instead of an extra charge for an office visit each time. And—try to get flat rates for some procedures, such as being charged one price for having several moles removed instead of a rate per mole.

GPs Often Err When Prescribing Psychiatric Drugs

Cecilia P. Kane, MD, department of psychiatry, Emory University School of Medicine, Atlanta.

General practitioners (GPs) may not keep up with the trends in prescribing psychiatric medications...or they may prescribe dosages that are too high or too low.

Shocking: Of 145 *diazepam* (Valium) prescriptions dispensed by general practitioners at one hospital, 43% were for patients over 65—even though the drug is not recommended for older patients.

To Prevent High Blood Pressure in The Doctor's Office

Claude Le Pailleur, MD, clinical cardiologist, Hôpital Necker, Paris. His study of 42 adults with high blood pressure was published in *Behavioral Medicine*, 1319 18 St. NW, Washington, DC 20036.

Limit conversation with your doctor before he/she takes your blood pressure.

Background: Many people whose blood pressure is normal at other times experience a sudden rise in pressure at the doctor's office. *Cause:* Anxiety associated with interacting with the doctor. This "white coat" effect—named for the doctor's garb—makes it hard to get an accurate reading.

Study: Hypertensive patients who talked with the doctor before having their blood pressure checked had a sudden rise in blood pressure. This effect was more drastic during discussions of stress and disease than during chitchat. During periods of silence, blood pressure rapidly fell.

Dirty Hands and Doctors

William R. Jarvis, MD, associate director for program development, Division of Healthcare Quality Promotion, National Center for Infectious Diseases, Atlanta.

Doctors wash their hands between patients only 50% of the time. Dirty hands spread everything from colds, flu and diarrhea to pneumonia and toxic shock syndrome.

Self-defense: Always make sure your doctor washes his/her hands before touching you.

Medical Hygiene

Jeffrey Jones, MD, associate professor of medicine, Michigan State University College of Human Medicine, East Lansing. His study and survey were published in the *Annals of Emergency Medicine*, Elsevier, 360 Park Ave. So., New York City 10010.

Dirty stethoscopes may be spreading illness. In a test of 150 stethoscopes, 133 were found to harbor staphylococcus bacteria. Asked how often they cleaned their stethoscopes, 48% of doctors said daily or weekly ...37% said monthly...and 14% said once a year or *never*. While there have been no reported cases of infection spreading via dirty stethoscopes, outbreaks of drug-resistant bacteria have been linked to germ-laden blood pressure cuffs...thermometers...latex gloves... even doctors' white coats.

At greatest risk: Patients with burns or open wounds. Always ask if the doctor has cleaned his/her stethoscope.

Is Your Doctor Up-to-Date?

Charles B. Inlander, a consumer advocate and health-care consultant based in Fogelsville, PA. He was founding president of the nonprofit People's Medical Society, a consumer health advocacy group in Allentown, PA. He is author of numerous books, including *Take This Book to the Hospital With You*. St. Martin's.

Find out if he/she has been certified or recertified by calling the American Board of Medical Specialties, 866-ASK-ABMS.

Ask the doctor how he completes the *continuing* medical education requirements imposed by all states. Find out if your doctor teaches or does research at a local medical school—which would make him more likely to have current knowledge.

MDs and Continuing Education

99 Questions You Should Ask Your Doctor and Why by Paul H. Keckley, PhD, associate professor of medical administration, Vanderbilt University School of Medicine, Nashville. Rutledge Hill Press.

Continuing medical education is crucial to a doctor's ability to maintain his/her skill and training in the latest medical research and procedures. Ask your doctor how many hours of continuing medical education credits he averages in a year. And do your own research in areas of particular concern to you—then bring the material to your doctor's attention in case he has not seen it.

Plan Ahead for Medical Emergencies

Managing Your Health Care: Making the Most of Your Medical Resources by the late Martin Gipson, PhD, professor of psychology at University of the Pacific, Stockton, CA. Pathfinder Publishing.

Ask your doctor where to call and where to go to in case of emergency. Anticipate medical care needs before the weekend—do not ignore symptoms during the week that might become emergencies on the weekend. If communicating with doctors by phone, describe symptoms yourself—not through someone else—if possible.

Prescription Danger

Daniel Albrant, PharmD, president, Pharmacy Dynamics, a health care consulting company in Arlington, VA.

When writing prescriptions, few doctors take into account the patient's weight.

Trap: Most of the standard dosages are calibrated for a 155-pound person.

Example: For some drugs, a 130-pound person needs 10% to 15% less medication. Taking too much can cause nausea, drowsiness—or worse.

Self-defense: If you weigh less—or more—than 155 pounds, talk to your doctor to make sure he/she is prescribing the proper dosage.

When to Look for A New Doctor

John J. Connolly, EdD, president and CEO, Castle Connolly Medical Ltd., New York City, and editor and publisher of *America's Top Doctors*. Castle Connolly.

If your doctor has a poor bedside manner…is vague or evasive with explanations…is never on schedule…can't make a diagnosis…orders too many tests…discourages you from seeking a second opinion…doesn't protect patients' privacy…has an unpleasant office staff.

Women and Their Doctors

Lila Wallis, MD, a clinical professor of medicine at Weill Cornell University Medical College and a former president of the American Medical Women's Association, Alexandria, VA.

Women must be more aggressive about their own health care. Studies show that some male doctors are not as attentive to the needs of their female patients as they are to the needs of their male patients. This does not mean that women should only see female doctors.

Vital for women: Come to your appointments prepared with questions…fill out the health questionnaire thoroughly…make notes of the doctor's answers to your questions as well as any advice…and be sure the doctor explores all the options for treating a particular problem.

Helpful: If a doctor has taken a course on *women's* health.

Easier Dental Visits

Thomas McGuire, DDS, dentist specializing in preventive care, founder of the Dental Wellness Institute, Sebastopol, CA, and author of *Tooth Fitness: Your Guide to Healthy Teeth.* Diane.

For less stressful dental visits, plan to go before noon, when you can expect to have more energy. Take an aspirin an hour before the appointment to head off minor pain. Bring a book to pass time in the waiting room, and keep your mind occupied. Work out a stop signal with the dentist and assistant so you can let them know if you're feeling pain. Divert your attention by raising your foot or arm a few inches from the chair and holding it there. Concentrating on that makes it hard to focus on the dental procedure.

How to Tell a Good Dentist from a Bad One

Marvin J. Schissel, DDS, vice president of the New York chapter of the National Council Against Health Fraud, 8639 Woodhaven Blvd., Woodhaven, NY 11421. He is coauthor of *The Whole Tooth: What You Must Know to Find a Good Dentist, Keep Healthy Teeth, and Avoid the Incompetents, Quacks, and Frauds.* St. Martin's Press.

How do you tell a good dentist from a bad one? Here's what to look for…and look *out* for.

THE TIME FACTOR

At each checkup, your dentist should spend about 30 minutes examining your teeth and removing the plaque and mineral deposits known as tartar.

Filling a cavity could take 15 to 60 minutes, depending on the extent and location of the decay.

Also: A good dentist does not shuttle back and forth between his/her patients.

This might enable him to squeeze in a few more patients, but can a dentist who flits about the office really focus on his work? Not very likely.

TREATING GUM DISEASE

Gum disease is caused by bacteria that breed in "pockets" between the gum and the root of each tooth. Your dentist should measure the depth of these pockets using a *periodontal probe.* If your dentist fails to do so, remind him.

The best way to prevent gum disease—and to treat mild cases—is via meticulous scaling (scraping) of tartar and plaque, which harbor the disease-causing organisms.

But some dentists save time by having their patients *self-treat* gum disease by gargling at home with hydrogen peroxide and baking soda.

Problem: There's no evidence that peroxide/baking soda is more effective than ordinary brushing. It will not remove tartar.

THE EQUIPMENT FACTOR

Just because a dentist has the latest equipment does *not* mean that he provides cutting-edge care. In fact, some impressive gadgets have little impact on the level of care.

Example I: Some dentists show their patients video close-ups of areas of decay using an *intraoral camera.* This system provides dramatic pictures. But too often unscrupulous dentists use the camera to persuade patients to have unnecessary work.

Example II: Some dentists use a *Cavitron* to dislodge tartar from under the gum line. This device, which blasts tartar with high-frequency vibrations, can save time when the buildup is heavy. But even if he uses a Cavitron, a good dentist always finishes tartar removal by hand.

THE TRUTH ABOUT FILLINGS

For years "holistic" dentists have urged patients to have their old silver fillings (which contain mercury amalgam) replaced with fillings made of plastic composite.

These practitioners maintain that mercury leaches out of silver fillings, poisoning the body and causing multiple sclerosis and other diseases.

Yet there is no solid evidence linking silver fillings to health problems. A very few people are allergic to mercury, but they rarely develop anything more than a rash.

If a filling cracks or falls out, of course, it must be replaced. But steer clear of any dentist who urges you to replace intact fillings for health reasons.

Composite fillings blend in with the tooth color, so they're good for teeth in the front of the mouth. But amalgam costs less and lasts longer than composite, so it's still the best choice for out-of-sight fillings.

NEEDLESS EXTRACTIONS

Even badly decayed teeth can usually be saved with fillings or crowns (perhaps in conjunction with a root canal procedure).

But these time-intensive procedures are often poorly reimbursed by dental insurance companies. Consequently, some unscrupulous dentists save time by simply pulling such teeth.

If your dentist recommends pulling a tooth, ask him why the tooth cannot be saved. If you're not convinced by the explanation, get a second opinion.

5

The Truth About Medicines

Where to Get Information On the Drugs You Take

Timothy McCall, MD

rug side effects represent more than just an annoyance. They're one of the most frequent causes of hospitalization in the US. Some of these side effects occur as a result of a mistake by a doctor or pharmacist. Others occur when patients take their medicines incorrectly. Either way, your best protection is to learn as much as possible about every drug you're prescribed.

Ideally, your doctor would give you all the drug information you need. But that doesn't always happen. Many patients leave the doctor's office without knowing even the most basic information—such as how many times a day to take the drug or whether it should be taken with food.

Under managed care, the drug information problem is only getting worse. The length of the average doctor's appointment continues to decrease, with many appointments now lasting less than 10 minutes. That means the doctor has less time to explain things.

Good doctors still make the effort. When you walk out of the office, you should know the generic *and* brand names of any drug you've been prescribed. You should also know the dosage, how to take it and what to do if you miss a dose.

The doctor should also explain common side effects, as well as the symptoms that suggest a serious problem—and what to do if they appear.

Many doctors and clinics now offer patient handouts that explain medications. They're a great idea as long as they're written in plain English—and if they aren't used as a substitute for the brief question-and-answer session that should be a part of every doctor's appointment.

Timothy McCall, MD, an internist, medical editor of *Yoga Journal* and author of *Examining Your Doctor: A Patient's Guide to Avoiding Harmful Medical Care.* Carol. *www.drmccall.com.*

Another good source of drug information is your pharmacist. He/she should be able to answer virtually all drug-related questions. Be sure to ask him for the "package insert" that comes with the drug.

Although the typical insert is written in nearly impenetrable "medicalese," look through it anyway. Keep it around, too, in case you develop a problem later on.

Be sure to list for your doctor and pharmacist *every* medicine you're taking. That goes for over-the-counter as well as herbal preparations, since these can interact—sometimes with serious, even fatal, results—with prescribed drugs. What *they* don't know could hurt you.

Have all your prescriptions filled at one pharmacy—ideally one with a computerized prescription system. That way, your entire medication history—including any drug allergies you might have—will be contained within a single file. This makes it easy for your pharmacist to spot any potential drug interaction or allergic reaction.

Managed care is affecting pharmacists as well as doctors. Independent drugstores, which often provide the most personalized attention, are being squeezed out by the big chains and mail-order houses, which offer HMOs deep discounts.

Chain stores and mail-order drugs may save you money. However, you probably won't get much drug information from them. That means you must do more homework and find resources. Fortunately, several good consumer guides to drugs are available.

Recommended: Dr. Sidney M. Wolfe's *Worst Pills, Best Pills* (Pocket Books), Dr. James Rybacki's *The Essential Guide to Prescription Drugs 2006* (HarperCollins) and Joe and Teresa Graedon's *The People's Pharmacy* (St. Martin's).

You can also get reliable drug information via the Internet. If you have access to a computer (at home or at your local library), here are two sites to try: RxList at *www.rxlist.com* and Aetna InteliHealth at *www.intelihealth.com*.

These Cholesterol Drugs Prevent Cancer, Alzheimer's and More...

Majid Fotuhi, MD, PhD, assistant professor of neurology, Johns Hopkins University School of Medicine, and director of the Memory Disorders Unit at Sinai Hospital of Baltimore. He is author of *The Memory Cure: How to Protect Your Brain Against Memory Loss and Alzheimer's Disease.* McGraw-Hill.

Sheldon Marks, MD, associate clinical professor of urology and clinical lecturer in radiation oncology at the University of Arizona College of Medicine, Tucson. He is author of *Prostate & Cancer* (Perseus) and directs the men's health message board at *WebMD.com.*

Boris Draznin, MD, PhD, professor of medicine at the University of Colorado School of Medicine, Denver, and associate chief of staff of research at Denver Veterans Affairs Medical Center. He is author of *The Draznin Plan: The Thinking Person's Guide to Diabetes.* Oxford.

The group of drugs called *statins* lowers LDL ("bad") cholesterol and reduces the risk of heart attack by as much as 50% and stroke by 25%—but that's not all. Recent research suggests that statins have other remarkable health benefits, too.

Statins, which include *atorvastatin* (Lipitor), *pravastatin* (Pravachol), *simvastatin* (Zocor) and others, limit the amount of cholesterol produced in the liver. They have powerful anti-inflammatory and antioxidant effects that prevent cell and tissue damage. The majority of patients who take them experience few or no side effects, though the drugs can be dangerous for some.

More studies are needed before doctors can recommend taking statins solely for Alzheimer's and cancer, but people with diabetes should ask about statin therapy.

ALZHEIMER'S DISEASE
Majid Fotuhi, MD, PhD

Large observational studies suggest that people who take statins may reduce their risk of getting Alzheimer's by 30% to 70%. Statins also may delay the onset of Alzheimer's symptoms.

How they work: Patients who have Alzheimer's disease accumulate higher-than-normal levels of amyloid proteins, which form gumlike insoluble plaque in the brain. The immune system detects this plaque and releases inflammatory molecules in an attempt to destroy it. Persistent inflammation damages surrounding brain cells without breaking down the plaque. Statins may reduce brain damage by controlling this inflammatory process.

CANCER
Sheldon Marks, MD

Statins may help prevent cancer. An Israeli study of 3,342 patients found that those taking statins were about 50% less likely to get colon cancer. Other studies indicate that statins can reduce the risk of prostate cancer by up to 56% and risk of breast cancer by 30%.

How they work: Statins may block the activation of an enzyme complex (*proteasome*) that breaks down proteins. Inhibiting this process may cause cancer cells to die rather than proliferate. It also is possible that statins block cell signals that can trigger cancerous cell division.

DIABETES
Boris Draznin, MD, PhD

Most diabetes patients should consider taking a statin drug, according to recent American Diabetes Association guidelines. The Heart Protection Study found that people with diabetes could reduce their risk of having a heart attack or stroke with statins, even if their cholesterol levels were normal. The guidelines recommend statins for diabetics over age 40 who have total cholesterol of 135 or higher.

Marijuana Can Be Effective Medicine

John P. Morgan, MD, professor of pharmacology at the City University of New York Medical School in New York City. He is coauthor of *Marijuana Myths, Marijuana Facts.* Lindesmith Center.

Marijuana is an effective treatment for several serious medical conditions. Thirteen states—Alaska, California, Colorado, Hawaii, Maine, Maryland, Montana, Nevada, New Mexico, Oregon, Rhode Island, Vermont and Washington—and the District of Columbia, have taken steps to legalize medical marijuana.

But federal laws still make it a crime to possess or use marijuana—whether it's for recreational or medical purposes.

Medical marijuana expert John P. Morgan, MD, explains the health benefits of marijuana…

•**For which ailments is marijuana effective?** Marijuana has been clinically proven to be excellent therapy for…

•**Nausea and vomiting.** People undergoing cancer treatment can get fast relief from these common side effects of chemotherapy.

•**Muscle spasms.** Marijuana can relieve spasms in multiple sclerosis patients and individuals with spinal cord injuries.

•**Glaucoma.** Marijuana reduces pressure within the eyes. It can help prevent eye damage as well as discomfort.

•**AIDS-related "wasting."** Marijuana is an excellent appetite stimulant. It can reverse malnutrition and the extreme weight loss (cachexia) associated with AIDS.

Anecdotal evidence suggests that marijuana helps with migraines, insomnia and chronic pain.

•**Given these benefits, why isn't medical marijuana widely used?** Along with heroin and LSD, marijuana is classified as a Schedule I substance. That means that it is considered dangerous and without medical value. Reclassifying it as a Schedule II drug would allow doctors to prescribe it under controlled conditions.

But until federal laws change, the average patient considers marijuana too risky…and the average doctor is unwilling to recommend it.

•**Do people get "high" when using marijuana as medicine?** Regular smokers of marijuana tend to develop a tolerance to the high.

•**Is marijuana addictive?** Few people who use medical marijuana develop a physical or psychological dependence on it.

In a recent study, researchers found marijuana no more addictive than caffeine.

Antibiotics: Too Much Of a Good Thing?

Timothy McCall, MD, an internist, medical editor of *Yoga Journal* and author of *Examining Your Doctor: A Patient's Guide to Avoiding Harmful Medical Care.* Carol. www.drmccall.com.

The development of antibiotics in the 1940s was one of the biggest breakthroughs in medical history. Many infections that had been deadly—pneumonia, meningitis, dirty wounds, tuberculosis—suddenly could be treated.

Unfortunately, antibiotics proved so effective in treating these *bacterial* infections that many doctors started to prescribe them for colds and other *viral* infections—for which antibiotics are completely ineffective.

Doctors should know better—but they are often only too willing to oblige their patients, who often request antibiotics.

One study found that doctors prescribed antibiotics for two out of three patients with colds. Some gave antibiotics to virtually every cold sufferer who walked in the door.

Needless antibiotics waste billions of dollars. And when you take an antibiotic you don't need, you risk side effects ranging from yeast infections to life-threatening allergic reactions. And as you may have heard, the rampant overuse of antibiotics is fueling the development of drug-resistant bacteria.

Many antibiotics that were once highly effective have now been rendered useless—and the problem is getting worse all the time. We risk returning to an age in which there is no effective treatment for certain infections.

The key, of course, is to use antibiotics only when you really need them. That way, they'll be more likely to work. *Here's what I recommend...*

• **Don't ask your doctor for antibiotics.** Given how often antibiotics are overprescribed, if your doctor says you don't need one, chances are you don't. If your condition worsens, you can always return.

• **If antibiotics are prescribed, take the full course of pills.** Many patients stop taking antibiotics when they feel better. That's a big mistake. If the infection is not quite eradicated, the bugs are likely to develop resistance.

• **If you find any leftover antibiotics in your medicine chest, throw them out.** Some people who fail to finish a course of antibiotics save their leftover pills, thinking they can use them later for another illness.

But taking antibiotics before you see the doctor thwarts his efforts to diagnose you. You probably won't have enough pills to treat an infection properly anyway.

• **Take antibiotics for a sore throat *only* if you get a clear diagnosis of strep.** If you have a sore throat, your doctor should order a throat culture—and prescribe antibiotics only if the culture indicates Group A streptococcus bacteria. In adults, fewer than 10% of sore throats are caused by strep.

• **If you're over age 65 or have a chronic illness, get a pneumococcal pneumonia vaccine.** The *Pneumovax* vaccine prevents the leading cause of bacterial pneumonia—which is one of the leading causes of death.

• **When you get sick, listen to your body.** Many of the requests I get for needless antibiotics come from people who refuse to slow down when they get sick. When you're ill, you need rest. If you go to work when you're not up to it, you risk infecting your coworkers and staying sick longer. You probably won't get much work done either.

• **Don't let a doctor prescribe antibiotics without examining you in person.** In these days of cost-cutting, HMOs and some doctors now try to cut costs by having you *not* come in for a visit. Instead, they'll offer you a prescription for an antibiotic—often one that isn't needed—over the phone. This strategy is convenient for doctors and patients—and good for business. In general, though, it's lousy medical care.

Medication Errors Can Be Avoided...Easily

Joe Graedon, one of the country's foremost experts on drug interactions. He has served as a consultant to the Federal Trade Commission on nonprescription drug advertising and as a member of the advisory board of the University of California (San Francisco) Drug Studies Unit. He is coauthor, with Teresa Graedon, PhD, of many books on health topics, including *Deadly Drug Interactions: The People's Pharmacy Guide* and *The People's Pharmacy: Completely Revised and Updated!* St. Martin's.

Each year, mistakes involving prescription and over-the-counter drugs cost the US economy $20 billion in hospitalization expenses...and kill 140,000 people.

Here's how to avoid "medication misadventures"—taking the wrong drug…overdosing…suffering a drug-induced allergic reaction, etc.

INTERACTING WITH YOUR DOCTOR

Before every doctor's appointment, jot down in order of importance all your medical concerns and/or symptoms. If you suspect that a rash or any other new symptom is drug-related, make that a priority. Such a problem could be life-threatening.

Most doctors have a limited amount of time to spend with their patients, so it is essential to start with the most urgent problem. If you ramble on about several other problems, the doctor may interrupt you—or you may get sidetracked—before you reach the important one.

Occasionally, psychological stress caused by seeing a doctor makes it hard to "take in" everything the doctor says. In such cases, take along a tape recorder. That way, you can record the doctor's comments and review them when you're more relaxed.

Important: Be as diplomatic as possible when making your recording. Let the doctor know that you simply want to avoid any confusion following his/her instructions.

Alternative: Ask a friend or family member to accompany you to your appointments. Have him/her take written notes regarding the doctor's instructions.

NEW PRESCRIPTIONS

Before accepting a new prescription, give your doctor the following information…

•**A complete list** of all prescription, over-the-counter (OTC) and recreational drugs you take, including vitamins, cold remedies, alcohol and tobacco.

•**Any allergy or sensitivity** you may have to any food or drug.

•**Any special diet** you may be following.

•**Any condition** for which you are already receiving a doctor's care.

Women: Let the doctor know if you are pregnant or attempting to become pregnant.

Ask the doctor for written information about the drug, its side effects and how to take it. Try to read this literature before you leave the office—but ask for a copy to take home with you.

Questions to ask: Are there any precautions or warnings of which you should be aware? Should you avoid certain foods, drugs or vitamin supplements while taking the medication?

Failure to get answers to these questions can cause serious problems—even death.

Example: A family of antidepressants called MAO inhibitors (Marplan, Nardil and Parnate) is extremely dangerous when taken in combination with certain other antidepressants…with cheese or soy sauce…or with certain OTC cold preparations.

Never take any medication without knowing its purpose. Is the drug intended to alleviate symptoms? If so, which symptoms? Is it intended to cure an ailment? Which ailment?

Get explicit instructions about how the medication is to be taken. A simple "three times a day" is inadequate. Find out the correct dosage and at what times of day the drug should be taken.

Ask if the medication should be taken with food or on an empty stomach.

What if you miss a dose? Should you take the dose as soon as you think of it? Or should you simply skip that dose and "double up" on the next one?

Your doctor should double-check for potential interactions between your new prescription and any medications you're already taking by consulting a reference text or a computer program. It is also a good idea for you to buy a reference book to double-check drug information.

If you experience any unexpected side effects once you begin taking a new medication, let your doctor know right away. Have your doctor tell you which side effects or symptoms require immediate attention.

Caution: Do not stop taking the medication without consulting your doctor. Abruptly stopping certain medications can trigger irregular heart rhythms, convulsions or even heart attack.

AVOIDING PHARMACY MISTAKES

Some patients routinely ask their doctor to "phone in" their prescriptions to a pharmacy. Doing so can be a big mistake—especially when a new prescription is involved.

Reason: Drug names often sound alike—especially when heard over the telephone in a noisy drugstore. The ulcer medication *Zantac*, for instance, can easily be confused with the antianxiety medication *Xanax*.

Your doctor should provide you with a written prescription form. This form should be printed clearly, in English, including the drug's brand and generic names, along with detailed instructions. Abbreviations should not be used.

Do not accept sloppy handwriting. In a survey, more than half of pharmacists acknowledged that a doctor's sloppy handwriting had caused them to make prescription errors.

Example: One patient who was supposed to get the anti-inflammatory drug *Tolectin* was instead given *Tolinase*, a diabetes drug. She developed pseudosulinoma, a serious condition that mimics excess insulin production.

Bottom line: If you can't read the prescription, odds are the pharmacist won't be able to either.

To further minimize errors, make sure your prescription is filled by the pharmacist. Because they have less training than pharmacists, pharmacy technicians are more prone to errors. If you're not sure who is filling your prescription, ask.

Finally, visit your pharmacy between the hours of noon and 3 p.m. In most drugstores, that's the slowest time of day. Avoid having a prescription filled immediately before or after work. That's the busiest time of day.

DRUG INTERACTION SELF-DEFENSE

Use one pharmacy for all your family's prescriptions. That way, you can be certain that the pharmacist is familiar with all your medications…and alert to potential interactions.

If possible, find a pharmacy that uses a computerized patient profile system to track the various medications family members are taking. Ask the pharmacist to check the computer for potential interactions. Be prepared to wait —or come back at another time—if the pharmacist needs to check your prescription with your doctor.

Your pharmacist should also check your new prescription for possible interactions with alcohol…or with OTC medications. *Such interactions can cause big problems…*

Example I: The antibiotic *tetracycline* can be rendered inactive by a single Tums tablet.

Example II: Even small quantities of alcohol can cause a serious reaction in someone taking an antihistamine, tranquilizer, sedative or pain reliever.

Like your doctor, your pharmacist should provide instructions on how to take the drug, potential side effects and any foods or drugs to avoid.

How to Measure Dosages

Michael Leff, editor, *Consumer Reports on Health*, 101 Truman Ave., Yonkers, NY 10703.

Use a real measuring spoon to portion out medicine—not a tableware spoon. Tableware spoons may hold from *half*…to twice as much as a measured spoon.

The Eight Most Common Medication Mistakes… And How to Avoid Them

Harold M. Silverman, PharmD, a pharmacist and health-care consultant in Washington, DC. He is author of *The Pill Book: The Illustrated Guide to the Most-Prescribed Drugs in the United States.* Bantam.

Many people unwittingly reduce the effectiveness of the drugs they take— or worse, cause themselves great harm —by mishandling their pills. *The most common drug traps and how to avoid them…*

Trap #1: **Failing to double-check your prescription.** Drug-dispensing mistakes are rare, but they do occur.

In his/her haste, a doctor may prescribe the wrong drug or dosage. The pharmacist may misread the doctor's handwriting…or reach for the wrong bottle of pills when filling your prescription.

Self-defense: Before handing the prescription form to the pharmacist, jot the drug name and dosage on a piece of paper.

When you pick up the bottle of pills, compare the label with your note. If you suspect a mistake, call your doctor.

Also, consider keeping a copy of *The Pill Book* (Bantam) or *Physicians' Desk Reference* (Thomson PDR) on hand. These books contain photos of pills.

Trap #2: **Being unaware of a drug's side effects.** Doctors are supposed to tell patients about a drug's possible side effects. But they don't always do so—because they don't want to "scare" their patients.

Prescription drugs can cause a variety of troublesome side effects, including sexual problems like diminished sex drive, impotence and retrograde ejaculation (in which semen is ejaculated "backward" into the bladder). If you are unaware that your medication is causing such a problem, you may worry yourself sick.

Self-defense: Before taking *any* newly prescribed drug, ask your doctor and pharmacist about side effects.

If you experience a problem, ask about taking a lower dose or switching to a substitute.

Trap #3: **Taking one drug that interacts with another.** Nine out of 10 pharmacies now have sophisticated drug-dispensing software that screens for drug interactions.

Each time you come in with a new prescription, the pharmacist runs a computer check. If the drug interacts with any other drug you're taking, the pharmacist alerts you.

But such systems work only if you have all your prescriptions filled at one pharmacy.

If you patronize different drugstores, you risk subjecting yourself to side effects and/or not receiving the drug's full benefits. You may even fail to discover that you have two prescriptions for the same drug from different doctors—and are double-dosing yourself.

Self-defense: Stick to one pharmacy. If you're taking several drugs and are uncertain about interactions, ask your pharmacist or doctor for a "brown bag" session. Put all the drugs you take in a bag, and bring it in. Review the name and dosage of each drug, and what each is for.

Be sure to schedule your brown bag session in advance. Otherwise, the pharmacist or doctor may be too busy to spend enough time with you.

Trap #4: **Combining certain prescription and nonprescription drugs.** In recent years, several drugs that used to be available only by prescription have gone on sale over-the-counter (OTC).

This cuts costs for consumers, but it makes it harder for doctors to monitor their patients for potentially dangerous drug combinations.

Example I: In rare cases, nonsteroidal anti-inflammatory drugs (NSAIDs) like *ibuprofen* (Motrin), *naproxen* (Aleve) and *ketoprofen* (Orudis) can cause kidney damage. If you have kidney disease, avoid large doses. Don't take them on a long-term basis.

Example II: The acid blocker *cimetidine* (Tagamet) interacts with the antidiabetes medication *sulfonylurea…benzodiazepine* tranquilizers like Valium…and calcium channel blockers like Adalat and Procardia.

Self-defense: If you're taking a medication on a long-term basis, ask your doctor if any OTC drugs interact with it.

Or—buy your OTC drugs where you have your prescriptions filled, and check with your pharmacist before taking the two together.

Trap #5: **Storing drugs incorrectly.** No doubt you have already heard that heat and humidity degrade drugs. Yet most of us continue to store our medications in the bathroom —the hottest, most humid room in the house.

Even if you cannot discern any degradation, your pills probably are becoming less potent.

Self-defense: Store all prescription and OTC drugs in a cool, dry spot—your bedroom closet, for example (or in the refrigerator, if the drug is supposed to be refrigerated).

If you have children in your house, make sure to keep the drugs out of their reach.

Trap #6: **Failing to have the dosage adjusted after a major change in body weight.** If you lose a lot of weight, a dose that was once correct may become a harmful overdose. Conversely, a significant weight gain may lead to under-dosing.

Self-defense: If you lose or gain more than 10% of your body weight, alert your doctor immediately so that he can adjust your dosage accordingly.

Trap #7: Using prescription drugs without medical supervision. Many people hang on to unused pills, thinking they will save a few bucks—and a trip to the pharmacy—if they get sick again.

Yet even if you get the same symptoms again, prescribing to yourself in this fashion is dangerous. Your new symptoms could stem from a different ailment—which calls for different treatment.

Self-defense: If you have pills left over after taking a course of medication, discard them. If you insist on hanging on to unused pills, at least call the doctor and get his approval before using them.

Trap #8: Disobeying the doctor's orders. When it comes to prescription medications, an amazing number of people simply don't follow their doctor's directions.

Some patients take more medication than was prescribed—on the erroneous "more-is-better" theory. Others take less than the doctor ordered—in a misguided effort to avoid side effects. Doctors call such behavior "patient noncompliance."

Self-defense: Take all medications according to your doctor's exact instructions. If you have trouble remembering to do so, devise a plan to jog your memory at the appropriate times.

For example, jot down your dosing schedule in your date book…carry your pill box in your pants pocket as a constant reminder…or pick up a combination pill box/alarm at your local pharmacy.

If you miss a scheduled dose, check with your doctor or pharmacist immediately about what to do. In some cases, it's best to continue with your regimen as if you hadn't missed a dose. In others, it's better to "double up" on a subsequent dose.

Dangerous Drug Interactions

Joe Graedon, one of the country's foremost experts on drug interactions. He has served as a consultant to the Federal Trade Commission on nonprescription drug advertising and as a member of the advisory board of the University of California (San Francisco) Drug Studies Unit. He is coauthor, with Teresa Graedon, PhD, of many books on health topics, including *Deadly Drug Interactions: The People's Pharmacy Guide* and *The People's Pharmacy: Completely Revised and Updated!* St. Martin's.

Every year, thousands of people combine drugs they are taking with other medications or foods that produce negative reactions. In most cases, they weren't aware there would be a problem, since the medications and foods seemed harmless.

Here are just some of the most common hazardous drug interactions—and what you can do to protect yourself and your family from harm.

DRUG/FOOD INTERACTIONS

No doubt your pharmacist has cautioned you to avoid taking certain antibiotics with dairy products. This combination can reduce the effectiveness of the medications.

But many pharmacists and doctors are unaware of some unusual drug/food interactions. *Foods that could cause problems with some medications…*

● **Grapefruit and grapefruit juice** contain compounds that can interact powerfully with medications—and cause devastating side effects.

Example: Blood pressure medications, such as Procardia and Adalat *(nifedipine)* and Plendil *(felodipine)*, are dangerous when combined with grapefruit, resulting in higher blood levels of blood pressure medications. Symptoms may include facial flushing, nausea, dizziness, confusion, palpitations or irregular heartbeat.

● **Green, leafy vegetables,** such as broccoli, brussels sprouts and cabbage reduce the effectiveness of the blood thinner Coumadin *(warfarin)*, a commonly prescribed blood thinner that prevents blood clots. These foods are rich in vitamin K, which helps the blood to clot. Coumadin, meanwhile, works by counteracting vitamin K's clotting action.

Consuming a small amount of vitamin K–rich foods daily probably won't pose a problem. But if you usually skip these vegetables and then overindulge, at a Chinese restaurant, for example, you reduce the drug's effectiveness and put yourself at risk for a blood clot or stroke.

●**Oatmeal and other high-fiber foods** may interfere with the absorption of Lanoxin (*digoxin*), a drug prescribed to control an irregular heart rhythm, which can lead to blood clots and stroke. Take Lanoxin two or three hours before or after eating high-fiber foods.

●**Salt substitutes** are used by people with high blood pressure. But they contain high amounts of potassium. If consumed with potassium-sparing diuretics such as Aldactone (*spironolactone*)—which are prescribed for high blood pressure or congestive heart failure—they can cause potassium levels to soar, increasing the risk of cardiac arrest.

●**Licorice and Lanoxin**—or a diuretic like Lasix (*furosemide*)—can lead to low levels of potassium, causing irregular heart rhythms and cardiac arrest. One piece of licorice probably won't hurt—but regular handfuls of licorice could be deadly.

PRESCRIPTION DRUG INTERACTIONS

●**Antibiotics vs. blood thinners.** Antibiotics like Flagyl and Protostat (*metronidazole*) can cause problems when taken with the blood thinner Coumadin. The antibiotics prevent the body from purging Coumadin, and if Coumadin levels get too high, life-threatening bleeding could occur.

If you are taking both metronidazole and Coumadin, you must be monitored carefully by your physician and have frequent blood tests.

Rx/OTC DRUG INTERACTIONS

Don't assume over-the-counter (OTC) medications are risk-free. Teamed with certain prescription drugs, some can cause complications. *Examples...*

●**Pain relievers.** Aspirin...Advil and Nuprin (*ibuprofen*)...Aleve (*naproxen*)...and Orudis KT (*ketoprofen*) can reduce the effectiveness of beta-blockers, such as Inderal (*propranolol*) and Lopressor (*metoprolol*), which are prescribed to treat high blood pressure.

If this happens, blood pressure can rise, increasing the risk of heart attack and stroke. If you are taking a beta-blocker, check with your doctor before adding a pain reliever. If your doctor prescribes a beta-blocker and aspirin, he/she should monitor your blood pressure.

●**Antacids** can inhibit the absorption of the heart and blood pressure medications Capoten (*captopril*) and Tenormin (*atenolol*), as well as Lanoxin.

And the activated charcoal added to counteract gas may reduce the effectiveness of a number of drugs, including tricyclic antidepressants such as Elavil (*amitriptyline*) and the diabetes medications Diabinese (*chlorpropamide*) and Tolinase (*tolazamide*).

●**Allergy and cough/cold remedies** that contain *pseudoephedrine, ephedrine* or *phenylephrine* should not be combined with a monoamine oxidase inhibitor antidepressant like Nardil (*phenelzine*) or Parnate (*tranylcypromine*). Your blood pressure could soar, leading to a hypertensive crisis and stroke.

GUARDING AGAINST INTERACTIONS

●**Make your doctors aware of the prescription and OTC drugs you are taking** and have your doctors check for interaction potential.

Ask them to consult drug reference books and/or computer reference programs before you leave the office.

●**Have all prescriptions filled at a single pharmacy,** preferably one that keeps computerized data on all your medications and can zero in on possible interactions. Tell your pharmacist about OTC drugs you are taking.

●**Make a list of key questions to ask.** When a new drug is prescribed, don't assume doctors and pharmacists are aware of every drug interaction—or if they are, that they will remember to alert you.

List the following questions and give copies to your doctor and pharmacist to fill out independently. If one contradicts the other, speak with both to get the correct answer.

- What is the medication's name?
- What is the dose?
- What time(s) should I take it?
- Should I take it with food? After eating? Before eating? How long?
- Should I avoid any foods?
- Are there vitamins or supplements I should avoid? Increase?
- Are there any precautions or warnings I should know about?
- Are there any contraindications that would make this drug inappropriate?
- What other prescription medicines should I avoid?
- Are there any OTC remedies I should avoid?
- What side effects are common with my medicine?
- Are there any side effects that are so serious you would want to know about them immediately?

If your doctor or pharmacist tells you that a drug won't interact adversely with another medication or food, don't assume that no interactions exist. Though rare, life-threatening interactions can go undetected by drug companies, the medical establishment and the Food and Drug Administration for months or even years after a drug hits the market.

So...if you experience any strange symptoms that cannot be easily explained, ask your doctor to contact the drug's manufacturer and file a report with the FDA.

Over-the-Counter vs. Prescription Drugs

Patricia Wilson, Associates & Wilson, a benefits consulting firm in Rosemont, PA.

While over-the-counter (OTC) drugs are generally less expensive than prescription drugs, insurance plans that cover all or part of the cost of prescription medications often make these drugs cheaper for plan participants than comparable uncovered OTC products.

Example: Two hundred milligrams a day of the heartburn medication *cimetidine* can cost as little as $60 per year for HMO members, while a year's worth of the over-the-counter drug Tagamet HB can cost $110 or more.

More than 50 prescription drugs have made the switch to drugstore shelves since 1972, and more are being considered for approval by the Food and Drug Administration every year.

Finish All Prescriptions

The late Ted Ferry, EdD, professor emeritus, Institute for Safety and Systems Management, University of Southern California, and author of *Home Safety Desk Reference.* Career Press.

Do not stop taking a medicine once you feel better—unless your doctor says it's okay. Prescription drugs often help you feel better before the underlying illness is cured. The end of symptoms does not necessarily mark the end of the disease.

Expiration Date Alert

Timothy McCall, MD, an internist, medical editor of *Yoga Journal* and author of *Examining Your Doctor: A Patient's Guide to Avoiding Harmful Medical Care.* Carol. *www.drmccall.com.*

Some medicines, like codeine, become more potent with age, while others lose effectiveness. Taking out-of-date medicine is an ineffective way to try to save money.

To make medicines last as long as possible: Do not store them in the bathroom. Bathroom heat and moisture can cause medicines to deteriorate prematurely.

Kids' Medication Overuse

James A. Taylor, MD, professor, department of pediatrics, University of Washington, Seattle.

More than half the three-year-olds in a major survey had taken at least one over-the-counter drug in the past 30 days.

Bottom line: Many children suffer side effects from the colorings, flavorings and alcohol in some kids' medicines. And—parents waste money on inappropriate drugs.

Prescription Drug Self-Defense I

Rosemary Soave, MD, infectious disease specialist and associate professor of medicine at New York Hospital–Cornell Medical Center, New York City.

To be sure your prescriptions are filled correctly, have your doctor note the purpose of the drug on the prescription, in addition to its name.

Reason: Many drugs have similar names, and some doctors' handwriting can be difficult to decipher.

Prescription Drug Self-Defense II

Charles B. Inlander, a consumer advocate and healthcare consultant based in Fogelsville, PA. He was founding president of the nonprofit People's Medical Society, a consumer health advocacy group in Allentown, PA. He is author of numerous books, including *Take This Book to the Hospital With You.* St. Martin's.

Mistakes on prescriptions are made *17 million* times a year. *To ensure that you don't take the wrong medication…*

When your doctor prescribes a drug, have him/her write down—on a separate piece of paper from the prescription—the exact name of the drug…dosage…number of times a day you should take it…and any side effects you should call to his attention. When you fill the prescription, compare the label with the doctor's note—and talk with your doctor about any discrepancies.

Caution: Mail-order or managed-care companies sometimes substitute drugs. Get your doctor's approval before you take a substitute.

Tell your doctor about all medications you use regularly—including over-the-counter drugs.

How to Save on Your Medicines

Rick Doble, editor and publisher, *Savvy-Discounts.com,* Box 96, Smyrna, NC 28579.

Buy double-strength pills (if your doctor will prescribe this way) and cut them in half with a pill cutter. Pill cutters cost $8 to $10.

●**Compare prices**—and include a discount mail-order pharmacy in comparison.

●**Always ask for generic medications.** When refilling a prescription, ask if a generic is now available. New ones come on the market regularly.

Aspirin? Tylenol? Advil? None of the Above?

Timothy McCall, MD, an internist, medical editor of *Yoga Journal* and author of *Examining Your Doctor: A Patient's Guide to Avoiding Harmful Medical Care.* Carol. *www.drmccall.com.*

Deciding on a pain reliever can be tough. Advertisements that tout one drug's advantages while slamming the competition are about as objective as political commercials.

For treating fever, headaches or routine aches and pains, different over-the-counter (OTC) painkillers are of similar effectiveness. But there are important differences.

●**Aspirin** is the least expensive OTC painkiller. But it's also the most likely to cause stomach upset. This can range from trivial indigestion to life-threatening hemorrhages.

No doubt you've heard that low doses of aspirin, taken regularly, help prevent heart attack and colon cancer. While aspirin does offer some protection against these ailments—other pain relievers don't—it also appears to raise the risk of bleeding into the brain (hemorrhagic stroke).

Aspirin therapy to prevent heart attacks is appropriate for people over age 50 with cardiac risk factors (high blood pressure, high cholesterol, etc.). I usually recommend a daily dose of 81 milligrams (one "baby" aspirin). Of course, you should check with your doctor.

•**Ibuprofen** (Advil, Motrin) and other newer nonsteroidal anti-inflammatory drugs (NSAIDs) are less likely than aspirin to upset the stomach. Ibuprofen is especially good for menstrual pain. But these drugs—including *naproxen* (Aleve) and *ketoprofen* (Orudis KT) —are by no means perfectly safe.

Each year, an estimated 10,000 Americans are hospitalized for intestinal bleeding caused by newer NSAIDs. One thousand die of such bleeding. These drugs can also cause kidney problems and reduce the effectiveness of some blood pressure medicines.

•**Acetaminophen** (Tylenol) is probably the safest OTC pain pill. But it's not entirely harmless. As Advil commercials correctly point out, drinking more than three alcoholic beverages a day while taking acetaminophen can cause liver damage. But if you drink that much alcohol and take ibuprofen or aspirin, your risk of a fatal intestinal hemorrhage also climbs.

For certain individuals, some drugs are better choices...

•**Anyone with a history of ulcers** should avoid aspirin and other anti-inflammatory drugs. Acetaminophen is usually a better choice.

•**Anyone with chronic hepatitis or another liver problem** should avoid acetaminophen. Aspirin or ibuprofen is better.

•**Heavy drinkers** should avoid regular use of all pain relievers. If one is needed, it should be taken at the lowest effective dose—and taken as infrequently as possible. Of course, the best bet is to cut back on drinking.

•**Elderly people** should generally stick to acetaminophen for treating minor aches and pains. Taking aspirin to prevent heart attack is a separate matter—one that should be discussed with a doctor.

•**For children,** acetaminophen and ibuprofen are safer than aspirin. When kids with influenza are given aspirin, they can develop a devastating illness called Reye's syndrome.

Whichever pain pill you choose, remember to use it sparingly. All drugs cause side effects.

If you do need a pain pill, forget all the marketing hype. Generic aspirin, acetaminophen and ibuprofen are every bit as effective as Bayer, Tylenol and Advil.

Painkiller Danger

William L. Henrich, MD, dean of the University of Texas Medical School and vice president for medical affairs at the Health Science Center, San Antonio, and chairman of the Consensus Conference on Analgesics, National Kidney Foundation.

Aspirin and acetaminophen, taken together over a long period of time, can cause kidney failure.

Self-defense: Avoid combination painkillers, such as Excedrin and Vanquish...and do not "mix and match" analgesic tablets. The National Kidney Foundation has called for a ban on over-the-counter cough, cold and headache remedies that contain both painkillers.

Insomnia and Painkillers

S. Lori Brown, PhD, MPH, research scientist officer, Food and Drug Administration, Rockville, MD. Her study was published in the *Journal of the American Geriatrics Society*, 11301 Wilshire Blvd., Ste. 309, Los Angeles 90073.

Insomnia can be caused by over-the-counter painkillers that contain caffeine. *Examples:* Aspirin-free Excedrin and Anacin. In a study of 2,885 patients, those who took caffeinated formulations of aspirin and acetaminophen were nearly twice as likely to report sleep problems as those taking similar noncaffeinated analgesics.

Tablets vs. Liquids

Malcolm Robinson, MD, clinical professor of medicine, University of Oklahoma College of Medicine, Oklahoma City. His study of 65 heartburn sufferers was published in *Gastroenterology*, American Gastroenterology Association, 4930 Del Ray Ave., Bethesda, MD 20814.

Researchers compared Tums E-X and Mylanta Double Strength tablets with the liquid antacids Mylanta II and Extra Strength Maalox. *Result:* The tablets were more effective at controlling heartburn and acid reflux.

Theory: When chewed, tablets mix with saliva to create a protective film that adheres to the esophagus longer than swallowed liquids do. *Also:* Chewing promotes production of saliva, which contains natural acid-fighting substances.

Economical Cholesterol Control

J. David Spence, MD, director, Stroke Prevention and Atherosclerosis Research Centre, University of Western Ontario, Canada.

The cholesterol-lowering drug *colestipol* (Colestid) can be used more economically *and* more effectively when mixed with the natural fiber supplement *psyllium*. Patients who took half (2.5 g) their usual dosage of colestipol, plus 2.5 g of psyllium, had greater declines in the all-important cholesterol-to-HDL ratio than when they took colestipol alone. Fewer side effects were reported with the mixture, too. Consult your doctor first.

Cholesterol Controversy

Bruce Yaffe, MD, internist, Yaffe Ruden and Associates, 201 E. 65 St., New York 10021.

The benefits of cholesterol-lowering drugs far exceed any cancer risk. Some research suggested that long-term use of two main classes of drugs, *fibrates* and *statins,* might lead to an increased risk of cancer. For people with greatly elevated cholesterol, that fear may be dwarfed compared to the immediate risk of a heart attack. Many years of experience show that the drugs cut heart attacks by 40%.

Aspirin Reduces Colon Cancer Risk

Edward Giovannucci, MD, professor of nutrition and epidemiology, Harvard School of Public Health, Boston. His review of health questionnaires completed by 121,701 women in 1976 was published in *The New England Journal of Medicine*, 10 Shattuck St., Boston 02115.

But the beneficial effects become apparent only after a decade or more of taking the drug. After 10 years, women who consistently took two or more aspirin tablets a week had a slightly lower risk of colon cancer than other women. After 20 years, the risk was nearly halved.

Important: Consult your physician before taking aspirin to reduce your risk of colorectal cancer.

Drug Scare Reality

Ralph E. Small, PharmD, professor emeritus of pharmacy and medicine, Medical College of Virginia Hospital, Box 980533 MCV, Richmond, VA 23298.

Prescription drug scare resulted from news reports that 25% of older Americans are taking drugs that could hurt rather than help them.

Reality: The risk is exaggerated—most problems with prescription drugs result from failing to follow doctor's instructions. In a small number of cases, drugs also may have adverse effects when taken in combination with over-the-counter remedies or other drugs that your doctor does not know you are taking.

Important: Always consult your doctor or pharmacist before combining any medicines.

Testosterone Patch Is Available

Adrian Dobs, MD, professor of medicine and oncology, Johns Hopkins Medical Institutions, Baltimore.

A testosterone patch can be used to treat men with *hypogonadism*—a condition in which the body produces too little testosterone, often leading to impotence and osteoporosis. Approved by the Food and Drug Administration, the patch is placed on the upper arm, abdomen, back or thigh—and releases the testosterone continuously. The patch is sold under the brand name *Androderm*—by prescription only. *More information:* See your doctor.

Daily Headache Syndrome

Robert D. Sheeler, MD, department of family medicine, Mayo Clinic, Rochester, MN.

D aily use of aspirin, acetaminophen, ibuprofen or other analgesics can create a rebound effect called daily headache syndrome.

Alternatives: Ice packs, heat, massage, relaxation therapy or other nondrug means. Use medications sparingly and only for more troublesome headaches.

All About Rebound Headaches

Joel Saper, MD, FACP, director, Michigan Head Pain & Neurological Institute in Ann Arbor.

R ebound headaches are becoming more common as people rely on over-the-counter (OTC) medications without consulting their doctors. OTC headache drugs can create headache rhythms that can only be controlled with ever-increasing doses.

Result: A form of addiction that requires detoxification. No other treatment will work until these medicines are eliminated.

Self-defense: Follow label directions carefully. Most specify not to use OTC medications for more than 10 days to relieve pain or more than three days to control fever—unless directed by a doctor...check ingredients carefully. Long-term use of these drugs for more than two days a week on a regular basis makes you vulnerable to the rebound potential.

Don't Self-Medicate

Stuart B. Levy, MD, president, Alliance for the Prudent Use of Antibiotics (APUA), Boston, and author of *The Antibiotic Paradox: How the Misuse of Antibiotics Destroys Their Curative Powers.* HarperCollins.

D on't take antibiotics prescribed for someone else—or even your own leftover pills.

Danger: Overuse of antibiotics has caused drug-resistant strains of bacteria—making antibiotics powerless against many infectious diseases.

Important: If you have an infection, ask your doctor to confirm that it is bacterial and that you need antibiotics.

Antidepressant Danger

Joe Graedon, coauthor of *Deadly Drug Interactions: The People's Pharmacy Guide* and *The People's Pharmacy: Completely Revised and Updated!* St. Martin's.

C ommon foods can cause headaches, fever, visual disturbances, confusion and a dangerous rise in blood pressure when eaten by individuals taking a prescribed antidepressant.

Self-defense: Avoid tyramine-containing foods while taking a monoamine oxidase (MAO) inhibitor—even for several weeks after you stop taking the drug. Tyramine-containing foods include avocados, bananas, bologna, broad beans, aged cheese, caviar, chicken liver (stored), miso soup, meat concentrate (in gravy), pepperoni, pickled herring, salami, summer sausage, soy sauce, wines (Chianti and vermouth) and yeast extract (marmite).

Attention Arthritis Sufferers

Guidelines from the American College of Rheumatology and the Arthritis Foundation, Atlanta.

The osteoarthritis drug of choice is *acetaminophen*, found in Tylenol. It has surpassed aspirin in popularity as an arthritis treatment because doctors say it is less likely to cause serious side effects.

Osteoarthritis treatment guidelines recommend first treating the disease with acetaminophen—then talking with your doctor about stronger drugs if the acetaminophen does not provide adequate pain relief.

Also helpful: Exercise to strengthen muscles...proper diet to maintain weight at a level that does not place extra stress on joints.

Break the Strep-Throat Cycle

Gary Ruoff, MD, family physician and researcher, Westside Family Medical Center, Kalamazoo, MI.

Take the *full course* of antibiotics prescribed by your doctor.

Most people use just enough antibiotics to relieve symptoms, then stop. This may result in symptomless infections that cause hidden damage (rheumatic fever)...a recurrence of the strep throat...or the transmission of strep throat to someone else.

Ulcerative Colitis and Nicotine Therapy

William J. Sandborn, MD, professor of medicine, division of gastroenterology, hepatology, internal medicine, Mayo Clinic, Rochester, MN. His four-week study of 64 nonsmoking colitis patients was published in *Annals of Internal Medicine*, 190 N. Independence Mall West, Philadelphia 19106.

Ulcerative colitis patients often benefit from nicotine therapy. Doctors have long observed that smokers rarely develop this chronic inflammation of the colon and rectum...and that nonsmokers with colitis often go into remission when they *start* smoking.

Study: Among patients who wore a nicotine patch, 39% showed improvement after four weeks, compared with 9% on a placebo patch. Many of the patients did not respond to *sulfasalazine* (Azulfidine), steroids and other conventional colitis drugs.

Lesson: If you have colitis, ask your doctor about using a nicotine patch.

Former Smokers and Nicotine Gum...

Harlan Krumholz, MD, professor of cardiology and epidemiology and public health at Yale University School of Medicine, New Haven, CT, and coauthor of *No If's, And's or Butts: The Smoker's Guide to Quitting.* Diane.

Nicorette gum should be used to help smokers quit. It should not be used to provide a long-term smoke-free source of nicotine—one of the most addictive drugs around. And don't expect that chewing this gum is enough to quit.

Most important: Making a commitment to quit...combined with as many other strategies as possible, including group therapy, visualization exercises and support of family, friends and doctors. *Note:* While there are some risks associated with nicotine gum, the risks from smoking are far greater.

Seizure Relief

Michael Privitera, MD, professor and vice-chair of neurology, University of Cincinnati College of Medicine.

The drug *topiramate* (Topamax) helps prevent seizures in the 30% of epilepsy patients who fail to respond to *phenytoin* (Dilantin) and other traditional antiseizure drugs. Topiramate reduces seizures by as much as 75% in some epilepsy patients. Side effects—including dizziness and coordination problems—largely disappear over time. About 30% of epilepsy patients—a total of 650,000 in the US—continue to suffer seizures despite the use of traditional antiseizure drugs.

Aspirin Therapy and Stomach Problems

Judith P. Kelly, MS, epidemiologist, Slone Epidemiology Center, Boston University School of Public Health, Boston.

Enteric-coated and buffered aspirin tablets are no easier on the stomach than plain aspirin. It's now popular to take an aspirin a day to help prevent heart attack. In a study, users of "aspirin therapy" were three times as likely to be hospitalized for stomach bleeding as those who didn't take aspirin regularly. They were equally likely to suffer bleeding no matter what kind of aspirin they took.

To avoid stomach trouble: Talk to your doctor about taking one-quarter tablet (or one baby aspirin)…and taking it with food.

Grapefruit Juice Danger

Paul B. Watkins, MD, director, General Clinical Research Center, University of North Carolina School of Medicine, Chapel Hill.

Grapefruit juice boosts the body's absorption of certain pills. The effect is especially pronounced with some sedatives and blood pressure drugs.

Self-defense: If you are already taking your medication with grapefruit juice—and are having no problems—you can continue to do so. But do not start drinking grapefruit juice with a sedative or a blood pressure medication without first talking with your doctor.

Channel Blockers and Cancer Link

Marco Pahor, MD, professor of medicine, Wake Forest University, Winston-Salem, NC. His study of calcium channel blocker use in 5,000 people over 71 years of age was published in *The Lancet*, 32 Jamestown Rd., London NW1 7BY.

Short-acting versions of this popular class of blood pressure drugs have been linked to cancer, as well as to stomach bleeding and heart attack. In one study, short-acting *nifedipine* (Procardia) raised cancer risk 72% in patients who took it.

Self-defense: If you're taking Procardia, ask your doctor about switching to a beta-blocker or a diuretic. Even if you're taking a longer-acting calcium channel blocker like long-acting nifedipine (Procardia XL) or *amlodipine* (Norvasc), it's a good idea to talk to your doctor.

Asthmatics and Inhalers

James G. Donahue, PhD, epidemiologist, Epidemiology Research Center, Marshfield Medical Research Foundation, Marshfield, WI, whose study of 16,941 health maintenance organization enrollees was published in *The Journal of the American Medical Association*, 515 N. State St., Chicago 60610.

Asthmatics who use inhaled steroids are *half* as likely to be hospitalized as those who use other—or no—medications. Inhaled steroids are most beneficial when used to treat persons with severe asthma.

Asthma Trap

Barbara P. Lukert, MD, director, Osteoporosis Clinic, University of Kansas Hospital, Kansas City.

Inhaled corticosteroids—often used to treat asthma—interfere with bone metabolism and may cause bone loss.

Self-defense: If you must take corticosteroids, ask your doctor about countering these side effects.

Possibilities: A daily diet containing at least 1,500 mg calcium…regular exercise…a low-salt diet. Evaluate estrogen levels for women and testosterone levels for men. *Also:* Ask your doctor about the antileukotriene asthma medications such as *zafirlukast* (Accolate). One glass of milk contains 300 mg calcium.

Shingles Treatment

Richard J. Whitley, MD, professor of pediatrics, microbiology and medicine, University of Alabama, Birmingham. His 21-day study of 208 volunteers 50 years of age or older was published in the *Annals of Internal Medicine*, 190 N. Independence Mall West, Sixth St. at Race, Philadelphia 19106.

Shingles respond well to the prescription drugs *acyclovir* (Zovirax) and *prednisone* (Deltasone). Blisters caused by this ailment (herpes zoster) healed faster in patients given the two-drug combination, compared with those given placebos.

Who Should Get the Hepatitis A Vaccine?

William S. Kammerer, MD, consultant, division of executive and international internal medicine, Mayo Clinic, Jacksonville, FL.

Travelers under 50 should get the vaccine (Havrix, VAQTA) if they expect to take two or more extended trips to Russia, Eastern Europe and/or tropical, developing countries within the next 10 years. If you'll be going only once, and plan to stay 10 days or fewer, *gamma globulin* injections represent a cheaper, though slightly less effective, alternative. Travelers 50 or older

should speak with their physician. The vaccine is given in two injections, six to 12 months apart. *Cost:* About $35 to $40 per dose.

Cut Your Risk of Getting an Ulcer

Robin I. Russell, MD, PhD, chief of gastroenterology, Glasgow Royal Infirmary, Glasgow, Scotland. His study of 285 arthritis patients was published in *The New England Journal of Medicine*, 10 Shattuck St., Boston 02115.

To avoid stomach trouble, arthritis patients who use aspirin for pain should ask their doctor about also taking prescription-strength *famotidine* (Pepcid).

Study: Ulcer risk fell by more than 50% when aspirin users also took Pepcid.

Caution: Over-the-counter famotidine (Pepcid AC) won't prevent ulcers…and might mask ulcer symptoms until they become severe.

Statins vs. Depression

Charles M. Blatt, MD, director of research, Lown Cardiovascular Foundation, Brookline, MA; assistant professor, Harvard Medical School, Boston; and leader of a study of 371 coronary artery disease patients, published in the *Journal of the American College of Cardiology*, 3655 Nobel Dr., Ste. 360, San Diego 92112.

Statins may lower depression risk when used continuously for years. This is in addition to lowering cholesterol, which usually is why they are prescribed. After average use of four years, patients on continuous statin therapy had a 30% to 40% reduced risk of depression and lower levels of anxiety and hostility. Each additional year of statin use lowered risks further.

Better Bowel Movements

Ervin Y. Eaker, MD, division of gastroenterology, University of Kansas Medical Center, Kansas City.

Severe constipation can sometimes be eased with the common gout drug *colchicine*. In a preliminary study, patients took oral colchicine for six weeks.

Result: The average number of bowel movements rose from two to six a week. Bloating, pain and nausea also dropped dramatically. If ongoing research corroborates these findings, colchicine could become the drug of choice for severe constipation.

Magnesium Poisoning

Bruce Yaffe, MD, an internist in private practice, Yaffe Ruden and Associates, 201 E. 65 St., New York City 10021.

Magnesium poisoning from antacids can occur in people who take large doses for a long time. Magnesium is also found in many laxatives and some pain relievers.

People most at risk: Those with improperly functioning kidneys...older people, since kidney function generally declines with age...people who have had intestinal surgery...those taking medicines that slow intestinal transit...anyone with longtime diabetes.

Self-defense: Use only the recommended amount of medicines that contain magnesium. If those doses do not help, do not increase them—see your doctor.

Medical History Danger

Thomas J. Romano, MD, PhD, rheumatologist in private practice in Wheeling, WV.

Don't forget about over-the-counter (OTC) medications if your doctor asks what drugs you take.

Common mistake: Thinking that OTC medications aren't "real" drugs. In fact, OTC drugs can affect the action of prescription drugs.

Example: One arthritis sufferer stopped responding to a prescription painkiller after she began taking a daily vitamin A pill. Two months after laying off the vitamin A, she once again got relief from the painkiller.

6

Health Secrets for Women

The Secrets of a Happy, Healthy Menopause

Wulf H. Utian, MD, PhD
Case Western Reserve University

Most women alive today will spend more than a third of their lives in their postmeno-pausal years. Menopause is often associated with uncomfortable symptoms like hot flashes, vaginal dryness and mood swings…and possibly a heightened risk of heart disease and osteoporosis.

Good news: There are now many ways to minimize the ill effects of menopause.

LIFESTYLE CHANGES

Without a doubt, the three most important ingredients for health before, during and after menopause are…

• **Proper diet.** Diet can do a great deal to prevent age-related ailments like heart disease, cancer and osteoporosis. By *proper*, I mean mostly fruits, vegetables and grains, and minimal fat, salt and sugar. If your eating habits aren't perfect, take a daily multivitamin.

To reduce your risk of osteoporosis, starting at menopause increase your consumption of calcium to 1,500 mg a day. And be sure to get at least 400 international units (IU) of vitamin D —from dairy products, vitamin supplements and/or sun exposure. (The skin makes vitamin D when exposed to the sun.)

Vitamin D boosts the body's absorption of calcium. One cup of milk contains about 300 mg of calcium and 100 IU of vitamin D.

• **Exercise.** Besides staving off heart disease and osteoporosis, regular workouts improve mood and overall well-being.

Best: "Weight-bearing" aerobic activities like walking, dancing, running and cross-country skiing…along with weight lifting. Try to fit in at least three 20-minute sessions a week.

Wulf H. Utian, MD, PhD, professor emeritus of reproductive biology at Case Western Reserve University School of Medicine in Cleveland.

•**Good habits.** Hot flashes can often be controlled by stopping smoking and limiting intake of alcohol, caffeine and spicy foods.

ALTERNATIVES TO HRT

If you choose not to go on hormone-replacement therapy (HRT), there are other options for relieving problems associated with menopause...

•**Alendronate** (Fosamax). When approved by the FDA, this drug was the first nonhormone remedy for osteoporosis.

In two large studies, alendronate was given in conjunction with daily calcium supplements. *Result:* Bone density increased by 8% at the hip and spine. The rate of fractures fell by 63%.

•**Calcitonin-salmon** (Miacalcin). This nasal spray is another option for osteoporosis. It's good for women who are more than five years past menopause and who have low bone mass. Two two-year studies have proven that the drug quickly increases bone mineral density in the spine, more slowly in the forearm or hip.

For maximum effectiveness, it must be taken with at least 1,000 mg of calcium and 400 IU of vitamin D a day.

•**Progestin.** If your only problem is hot flashes, oral progestin (without estrogen) may help. But it won't help other menopause symptoms...and it may boost your risk of heart disease.

•**Relaxation.** Biofeedback, deep breathing, yoga and meditation can all be used to reduce the intensity of hot flashes.

•**Vaginal lubricants.** If you experience vaginal discomfort during intercourse, Replens or K-Y Jelly can help. *Also helpful:* Having sex on a regular basis.

A PROMISING TREATMENT

The combination of a twice-daily slow-release fluoride tablet and 400 mg of calcium has been shown to reduce spinal fractures by 70% among women suffering from osteoporosis...and build bone mass in the hip and spine at the rate of 2% to 6% a year.

UNPROVEN REMEDIES

Some doctors believe that megadoses of vitamins E and C reduce menopause symptoms and cut the risk of heart disease and cancer. Vitamin E may also relieve hot flashes and vaginal dryness. However, their role in treating menopause symptoms remains unproven, especially when taken in supplement form. I don't recommend them.

Likewise, there's a lot of hype about herbal remedies like *dong quai, sarsaparilla, red clover* or *damiana*—but there's no evidence that any of these work.

The Great Hormone Debate

Christiane Northrup, MD, a physician in private practice in Yarmouth, ME, and former clinical assistant professor of obstetrics and gynecology at University of Vermont College of Medicine at Maine Medical Center, Portland. She is the author of *The Wisdom of Menopause*. Bantam.

Joyce Kakkis, MD, assistant professor of obstetrics and gynecology at the University of California-Irvine. She is in private practice in Long Beach, CA, specializing in HRT, and is the author of *Confessions of an Estrogen Evangelist*. KMG, Inc.

Recent media reports have stressed the dangers of hormone replacement therapy. But two eminent gynecologists, who have researched hormone therapy for themselves, say it's a bit more complicated.

Doctors have long recommended hormone replacement therapy (HRT) to not only prevent hot flashes and other menopausal symptoms, but also to curb the risk for heart disease and osteoporosis.

But when researchers recently halted a major study on the benefits of HRT, millions of women were forced to re-evaluate their options for controlling menopausal symptoms.

After five years of study, researchers at the Women's Health Initiative (WHI) found that women who took a daily tablet of equine estrogen (Premarin) and synthetic progesterone had a 26% higher rate of breast cancer, a 29% higher rate of heart attack and a 41%

higher rate of stroke than those taking a placebo. As a result of these findings, the 16,608 women being studied were instructed to stop taking the medications.

Is this the last word on HRT? For answers, we interviewed two leading experts in women's health—physicians who have addressed these questions for themselves and for their patients.

Christiane Northrup, MD, age 53, is menopausal (complete cessation of periods) and favors the use of natural treatments for menopausal symptoms.

Joyce Kakkis, MD, age 46, is perimenopausal (the years preceding menopause, when periods become irregular) and favors the use of HRT.

Here's what each doctor says about the current issues surrounding HRT...

DR. NORTHRUP

● **What is your opinion of the WHI study?** I felt that the study had major flaws from the outset. Women took a pill consisting of estrogen made from the urine of a pregnant mare, in combination with a chemically synthesized form of the hormone progesterone.

In all the years of human evolution, except for about the last 50, these chemicals have never been introduced into human bodies. And this so-called medicine—prescribed at the same dosage for millions of women, whether they weighed 110 or 210 pounds—was supposed to reduce the risk for heart disease, osteoporosis and other chronic degenerative diseases in the majority of women who took it. Given that the hormone dosages weren't individualized and didn't match those found in human females, I'm not surprised that there were adverse consequences.

● **Do you ever recommend HRT?** Yes. Some perimenopausal and menopausal women need hormones to control symptoms or feel their best. Working with her doctor, a woman should have her hormone levels checked and then decide what she needs. Some women's bodies, like mine, make adequate levels of hormones. Others don't. Some women feel best on HRT, while others don't. Women who have had their ovaries removed often need HRT for a few years.

If hormones are recommended, they should be *bio-identical*. This means they are chemically identical to the hormones manufactured in a woman's body, not patented animal versions or synthetic substitutes, which are so widely used today. And the doctor should check hormone levels every year, since a woman's body changes.

For myself, I wouldn't hesitate to use hormones if I needed them, but since my hormone levels are adequate and I don't have any health problems, I do not take them. Instead, I use natural alternatives to control my menopausal symptoms.

● **What do you use in place of HRT?** Soy does nearly everything HRT does without any of the side effects. I use soy to help control symptoms, such as hot flashes. Soy can also help control insomnia, dry skin and hair, depression and vaginal dryness, as well as strengthen the bones and heart.

The active ingredient in soy is *isoflavones,* a plant-derived "phytoestrogen" that acts like the estrogen found in the body. Do not take isolated soy isoflavones in pill form. Recent studies have shown that large amounts may increase breast cancer risk. Eat soy foods, including edamame (soybeans), soy milk, soy burgers and tofu.

● **How do you protect yourself against heart disease, bone loss and other age-related conditions?** In addition to eating soy, I follow some simple strategies. To build bones, I lift weights two to three times per week. Each day, I take 1,200 milligrams (mg) of calcium, 800 mg of magnesium and 400 mg to 800 mg of vitamin D—and get 15 minutes of sunlight without sunscreen in either the early morning or late afternoon. (I wear sunscreen the rest of the day.) To protect my heart, I take a brisk, 30-minute walk five times a week and eat a heart-healthy diet, including at least five daily servings of colorful fruits and vegetables.

DR. KAKKIS

● **What is your opinion of the WHI study?** I think the negative results of the WHI were overstated. By analyzing 10,000 of the study subjects on HRT, researchers found that eight additional women developed breast cancer, eight had a stroke and seven additional women developed heart disease each year, compared with those not taking HRT.

In light of these findings, should *everyone* stop HRT? I don't think so. Also, most experts think that women who get breast cancer within 10 years of starting HRT have a pre-existing condition that was simply accelerated by HRT. In other words, HRT is not the cause of their cancer.

The study also showed some benefits of HRT. Among the women analyzed, six fewer developed colorectal cancer and five fewer suffered hip fracture each year. Should women with a family history of colon cancer and osteoporosis stop HRT? I don't think so.

Finally, quality-of-life issues—hot flashes, insomnia, irritability and depression—were not addressed by this study. I do not intend to stop taking hormones on the basis of the WHI results, nor am I advising my patients to stop.

• **What's the best way to take HRT?** By using the lowest effective dose, which minimizes the risks. Typically, I start my patients at 25% to 50% of the standard dose of HRT. Then I monitor symptoms every six weeks and gradually increase the dosage only if the lower level is not working. The therapy is individually designed for each woman.

To get this type of treatment, a woman needs to work with a doctor who is familiar with the various options available for HRT. These include gels, creams, patches, pills and suppositories, as well as lower doses and "compounded" formulations, custom-blended by a compounding pharmacist.

If you don't find such a doctor, you're likely to be stuck with a standardized formulation that may not be right for you. The North American Menopause Society (NAMS) lists physicians who know about the latest in HRT. *To find a physician in your area:* Consult the NAMS Web site at *www.menopause.org.*

Once you've found the right doctor, you need to have blood tests to determine your hormone levels. Afterward, you should be re-evaluated by your doctor to see whether the therapy is working and to have it adjusted if it is not.

• **What do you take?** I take birth-control pills to control my perimenopausal symptoms. I'm still fertile, so the Pill acts as a contraceptive while providing the needed mix of hormones to prevent hormonal fluctuations for a perimenopausal woman my age. I intend to go from the Pill to low-dose HRT, and to take it for the rest of my life.

• **Do you use any natural remedies?** I eat edamame. It makes a delicious dish after 10 minutes of steaming. I have three, one-cup servings a week to control my perimenopausal symptoms.

I also take vitamin E to help control hot flashes and calcium to reduce muscle cramps, stabilize my mood and strengthen my bones.

Estrogen Trap

R. Graham Barr, MD, DrPH, assistant professor of medicine and epidemiology, Columbia University, New York City.

Estrogen replacement therapy (ERT) may contribute to asthma. *Recent finding:* Menopausal women on ERT have an 80% higher risk of developing asthma than women not taking hormones. *Theory:* Estrogen affects cells involved in the body's allergic or inflammatory response. *Important:* Women considering estrogen therapy should discuss these findings with their physicians. Asthma risk must be weighed against the potential benefits of ERT.

Wrinkle Remover

Stephen E. Chiarello, MD, a dermatologist in private practice in Port Charlotte, FL.

A "hand-sanding" technique lets doctors remove wrinkles without the high cost of the usual technique (laser resurfacing).

Called *manual dermasanding,* the technique involves injecting the wrinkled area with topical anesthetics. Wrinkles are then buffed away using a sandpaper-like material.

Strategies for Avoiding Troublesome Breast Cysts

Christiane Northrup, MD, a physician in private practice in Yarmouth, ME, and former clinical assistant professor of obstetrics and gynecology at University of Vermont College of Medicine at Maine Medical Center, Portland. She is the author of *The Wisdom of Menopause*. Bantam.

Breast cancer gets lots of media attention—and rightly so. But far more common is *fibrocystic breast disease*. At some point during their lives, 70% of women develop the fluid-filled, tender or painful breast lumps that characterize this condition.

We asked Christiane Northrup, MD, to answer the most common questions about breast cysts...

●**What causes breast cysts?** During ovulation and just prior to menstruation, fluctuating hormone levels can cause breast cells to retain fluid—resulting in cysts.

An estrogen/progesterone imbalance also appears to promote cyst development, but doctors don't know exactly how—or why.

In some cases, cysts are linked to abnormally high levels of estrogen. This is usually caused by eating too much fat.

Other women develop breast cysts despite having normal estrogen levels. *Good news:* The lumps usually disappear following menopause.

●**How can I tell a tumor from a cyst?** Cysts typically feel like a bunch of peas or grapes just under the skin. A painful lump is nearly always a cyst. Cancerous lumps are generally not tender.

●**Is breast cancer more common among women who get breast cysts?** In the 1970s, a few studies indicated that this might be the case. But subsequent research at the National Cancer Institute found that the vast majority of fibrocystic breast disease diagnoses did *not* involve an increased risk of cancer.

Exception: About 1% of women with fibrocystic breasts have *ductal atypia*. These abnormal breast cells sometimes turn cancerous.

●**If I discover a lump in my breast, what should I do?** Have your doctor examine it at once. He/she may want to obtain additional tests, such as a mammogram, sonogram or needle aspiration/biopsy.

If the lump contains fluid, odds are it's a cyst. It should disappear once the fluid is removed.

●**Are certain women more likely to get breast cysts?** Fibrocystic breasts are more common among women who are sensitive to caffeine...and those who have heavy periods, severe menstrual cramps and/or premenstrual syndrome.

●**The lumps in my breasts are very painful. What can I do for relief?** First, avoid all sources of caffeine. That goes for chocolate and caffeinated soft drinks, as well as coffee and tea. And don't overlook over-the-counter painkillers and diet aids. Many contain caffeine.

To keep your estrogen levels in check, adopt a low-fat, high-fiber diet. This diet should contain no dairy products...and should be high in whole grains, fruits, vegetables and beans. If dairy products are your primary source of calcium, be sure to take calcium supplements. After three months, add dairy foods back into your diet to see if they make a difference.

●**Are nutritional supplements helpful?** Many women get at least partial relief by taking a daily multivitamin or a daily pill containing vitamin E.

Also helpful: Selenium (24 to 32 micrograms [mcg] a day)...vitamin A (1,000 to 5,000 international units [IU] a day)...capsules of evening primrose oil, flaxseed oil or black currant seed oil (500 milligrams [mg] four times a day).

●**A friend of mine suggests that I try massage. Is that helpful?** Yes. Massage relieves discomfort by dispersing excess fluid to the lymph glands, where it's channeled out of the body.

What to do: Rub your hands together until they are warm, then massage each breast in concentric circles about 30 times. Use both hands, with your fingertips meeting in the middle. Move clockwise on the right breast, counterclockwise on the left breast.

For persistently painful breast cysts, I often recommend self-treatment with topical iodine. Iodine seems to affect estrogen's ability to bind to breast cells.

Apply iodine tincture in a three-inch-square patch to your upper thigh or lower abdomen. If the iodine stain fades within a few hours, apply it to another area of the upper thigh or lower abdomen.

Repeat these applications as long as they continue to fade within a few hours. When you can see a slight stain that persists for 24 hours, stop the treatment.

Easy Relief for Hot Flashes

Gregory L. Burke, MD, professor and chair, department of public health sciences, Bowman Gray School of Medicine, Wake Forest University, Winston–Salem, NC.

Try eating more soy. In a study, menopausal women who added 20 grams (g) of soy powder a day (about four tablespoons) to their diets reported reduced severity of hot flashes and night sweats.

Bonus: Their cholesterol levels also fell.

Theory: Soy contains *isoflavones*, compounds that mimic the beneficial effects of estrogen without its risks. Estrogen-replacement therapy raises the risk of breast and ovarian cancer. Soy powder, available at health food stores, can be added to juice, cereals and other foods.

Breast Cancer and Abortions

JoAnn Manson, MD, chief of preventive medicine, Brigham & Women's Hospital, Harvard Medical School, Boston.

The risk of breast cancer does *not* appear to be increased by abortion. This conclusion is based on a comprehensive study in which researchers studied the histories of 1.5 million Danish women born between 1935 and 1978. Because Danish law requires registration of all births, abortions and cancer cases, this study avoided reporting bias found in earlier studies in which some women who had undergone abortions may not have disclosed that fact to researchers. This bias may explain results in some earlier studies that suggested a link between abortion and breast cancer.

Evaluating Breast Lumps

Ellen Mendelson, MD, chief, section of breast imaging at Northwestern Memorial Hospital, and professor of radiology at Northwestern University Feinberg School of Medicine, both in Chicago.

A technique for evaluating breast lumps—*high-resolution ultrasound imaging*—can reduce the need for biopsies by 40%. This equipment is used in many breast imaging centers. Ultrasound can be used to distinguish lumps that are fluid-filled and not cancerous from those that are solid and require further evaluation. Solid masses with thin, sharp, smooth margins are often benign...those with jagged edges or irregular shapes may be malignant.

Breakthroughs In Breast Cancer Screening

Ellen Mendelson, MD, chief, section of breast imaging at Northwestern Memorial Hospital, and professor of radiology at Northwestern University Feinberg School of Medicine, both in Chicago.

One in eight—that's how many American women get breast cancer. But the diagnosis is not a death sentence. More than two million women in the US today have survived breast cancer. Many can thank screening techniques that detect the disease early—which often allows for additional treatment options and a better outcome.

MAMMOGRAPHY: A PROVEN TOOL

Women who get mammograms (X-rays of the breast) every one to two years have a lower risk of dying from breast cancer—about 20% lower for women in their 40s and about 25% lower for women in their 50s and 60s. Among breast cancer screening techniques, only mammography has been proven to reduce death rates from the disease.

Controversy: The American Cancer Society recommends that women age 40 and over have yearly mammograms. Yet in April 2007, the American College of Physicians advised against automatic yearly mammograms for women in their 40s, citing the physical discomfort of screening procedures & radiation exposure…and risk for false-positive results.

My view: Get annual mammograms beginning at age 40. *Reasons…*

•**The death rate reduction due to mammography,** though greater in older women, is still substantial in women ages 40 to 49.

•**Cancers in women under age 50 often grow faster and are deadlier** than those in older women.

•**The needle biopsy used to confirm or exclude a mammogram's findings usually is minimally invasive,** takes less than 30 minutes and leaves only a freckle-sized scar.

CAD MAMMOGRAPHY

With computer-aided detection (CAD) mammography, computer software analyzes a digital (rather than film) mammogram, marking suspicious areas. It now is offered by about 30% of mammography centers.

Controversy: A study in *The New England Journal of Medicine* found that CAD resulted in 31% more callbacks for additional tests and 20% more biopsies. Often, additional testing revealed no abnormalities.

My view: If a local facility offers it, it is preferable to use CAD (ask your doctor for a referral). *Reasons…*

•**CAD mammography increases detection of *ductal carcinoma in situ,*** perhaps cancer's earliest stage.

•**CAD mammography can spot various breast abnormalities.** Some may be cancer, some may not—but all merit subsequent testing.

ULTRASOUND: THE NEXT STEP

This noninvasive test is routinely performed after a suspicious area is found. It uses sound waves to create a picture (sonogram) that shows if the area is a harmless fluid-filled cyst —a harmless variation of normal tissue—or a solid mass that should be biopsied. Ultrasound is safe, painless, widely available, relatively inexpensive and usually covered by insurance.

The American College of Radiology Imaging Network will soon be presenting the results of a three-year study designed to show whether annual screening with mammography and ultrasound effectively detects cancer in women whose breasts are dense (have more glandular and connective tissue and less fatty tissue). If so, ultrasound may become a standard precancer screening technique for such women. Ultrasound may help distinguish between normal dense breast tissue and cancerous tissue, which also is dense.

MRI: THE NEW RECOMMENDATION

Magnetic resonance imaging (MRI) uses a magnetic field and radio waves to generate detailed pictures revealing cancers that mammograms may miss.

Note: Any woman recently diagnosed with breast cancer in one breast should have an MRI of the other breast.

The American Cancer Society recommends that women with the highest risk for breast cancer—20% or greater—receive a yearly mammogram and yearly MRI. *Any one of the following criteria places a woman in this group…*

•**Testing positive** on genetic tests for the BRCA1 or BRCA2 gene—linked to breast cancer.

•**Having a first-degree relative (mother, sister or daughter) who tested positive** for either gene.

•**Having two or more first-degree relatives with breast cancer.**

•**Having had chest radiation treatment for Hodgkin's disease** (a cancer of the lymphatic system).

MRI is very expensive, and insurance may not cover it. Women at moderately increased lifetime risk—a 15% to 20% risk—should talk to their doctors about the most appropriate screening method for them. *This group includes…*

•**Women with dense breasts.** Cancer is three to five times more likely to develop in dense breasts.

•**Women with fibrocystic (lumpy) breasts,** since such breasts often are dense.

• **Women who have had a biopsy that showed *lobular carcinoma in situ* (LCIS),** an irregular growth of noncancerous cells. LCIS increases breast cancer risk.

PROMISING TECHNOLOGIES

Several other breast cancer screening techniques show promise.

• **Gamma camera.** A woman is injected with a short-lived radioactive substance that gravitates to a diseased area, where it emits gamma waves recorded by the camera. Several companies recently have created gamma cameras specifically for breast imaging, and early test results are promising. Already some breast centers use gamma cameras as a next step after a suspicious mammogram—because the test is far less expensive than MRI.

• **Positron emission tomography (PET).** This technique scans the whole body to see if diagnosed breast cancer has spread. When radioactive glucose is injected into the body, cancerous tissues accumulate more of it...and emit more positrons (positively charged molecular particles), which appear as bright areas on the PET images.

Caution: A technique called *thermography* cannot accurately screen for breast cancer. Thermography detects tissues with higher temperatures—including inflamed or diseased tissues, not just cancer. Do not risk your health by putting your faith in it.

Milk and Breast Cancer Connection

Neal D. Barnard, MD, president of the Physicians Committee for Responsible Medicine, 5100 Wisconsin Ave., Washington, DC 20016. He is author of *Eat Right, Live Longer.* Three Rivers.

Milk has been connected to breast cancer through a growth hormone given to cows. The more milk you drink, the greater the risk.

Problems in children: Diabetes, anemia and colic.

Problems in adults: Arthritis, cataracts, anemia, infertility in women and ovarian cancer.

Best alternative sources of calcium: Dark green, leafy vegetables like broccoli, kale and collards (not spinach)...beans...calcium-fortified foods.

Avoid calcium wasters: Animal protein —including beef, poultry and fish...caffeine... salt...tobacco...a sedentary lifestyle.

Surprising High Heels Benefit

Suzanne Levine, DO, clinical podiatrist, New York Hospital–Cornell Medical Center, New York.

High heels can relieve heel and arch pain, often experienced by women after pregnancy or weight gain. They take pressure off those painful areas and move it to the ball of the foot.

Helpful: Wear heels of different heights at different times of the day to stretch muscles and tendons. The highest heel should be two-and-a-half inches tall. Also, avoid very thin heels.

A Bra/Breast Cancer Connection?

Adriane Fugh-Berman, MD, associate professor, complementary and alternative medicine, Georgetown University School of Medicine. She is author of *Alternative Medicine: What Works.* Lippincott, Williams & Wilkins.

Do brassieres cause breast cancer? Will switching to undershirts decrease your risk? Probably not. Although Sydney Ross Singer and Soma Grismaijer, the husband and wife coauthors of *Dressed to Kill: The Link Between Breast Cancer and Bras* (ISCD Press), maintain that the bra/breast cancer link is supported by scientific evidence, their "study" of this evidence is full of holes.

The bra/breast cancer theory was born several years ago in Fiji, when Grismaijer found a lump in her breast. Around the same time, her husband noticed the red marks on her body from her bra...and became convinced that the bra was to blame for her lump.

Grismaijer did not have the lump biopsied. Instead, she began a regimen of exercise, organic vegetarian food, purified water, herbs and vitamin supplements—and complete bralessness.

Guess what? The lump disappeared. But attributing its disappearance to not wearing a bra—as Grismaijer does—is ridiculous.

There's a good chance that the lump was benign. Grismaijer was pregnant when the lump was found, and hormonal changes during pregnancy are known to cause lumps.

After interviewing more than 4,000 women with and without breast cancer, the authors concluded that wearing a bra for more than 12 hours a day significantly increases the risk for breast cancer.

Unfortunately, this "finding" was unwarranted. Their study was conducted in a haphazard manner—without adherence to fundamental principles of scientific research. For example, no effort was made to ensure that the women in the two groups were similar in age, family history, medical history and other known risk factors for breast cancer.

The study was of such poor quality that it would have been disqualified from being published in a reputable medical journal. I'm afraid that's why it was packaged as a paperback book and directed at consumers instead of doctors.

The bottom line? There is simply no evidence that bras cause breast cancer. *Fortunately, there are other things women can do to reduce their risk...*

●**Eat more soy foods.** Tofu, tempeh, miso and soy milk all contain plant estrogens (phytoestrogens). These weak hormones inhibit the body's own production of estrogen, which may provide the "fuel" for breast cancer growth.

Neither soy oil nor soy sauce contain significant amounts of phytoestrogens.

●**Eat cruciferous vegetables.** Broccoli, cauliflower, brussels sprouts and kale affect estrogen metabolism in a beneficial way.

●**Think twice about estrogen-replacement therapy.** It's reasonable to use estrogen temporarily to treat hot flashes and vaginal dryness. But in general, long-term estrogen therapy is not a good idea. Estrogen can increase the risk of breast cancer.

●**Avoid pesticides.** Some pesticides contain estrogen-like compounds. Eat organic food whenever possible...and peel or wash all fruits and vegetables.

●**Eat a low-fat diet.** There is reason to believe that an extremely low-fat intake (less than 20% of calories from fat) is protective.

●**Exercise.** Women who exercise aerobically for more than three hours a week have a lower risk of developing breast cancer.

What about mammograms? They do not prevent breast cancer, but they reduce the risk of death from breast cancer by helping to find tumors in their early, treatable stages.

Smart Sports Bra Buying

James Dolan, MD, gynecological oncologist, Lutheran General Hospital, Park Ridge, IL.

Look for a bra made from soft fabric, especially in the nipple area...straps should be wide enough to support without digging into shoulders...avoid seams across the nipple area and bras with hook fasteners, which can chafe ...make sure that it won't ride up in the back or restrict arm movement. Be certain the chest band will stay in place and not roll up.

Most Breast Lumps Are Normal

Christiane Northrup, MD, a physician in private practice in Yarmouth, ME, and former clinical assistant professor of obstetrics and gynecology at University of Vermont College of Medicine at Maine Medical Center, Portland. She is the author of *The Wisdom of Menopause*. Bantam.

Human breast tissue is naturally very lumpy. But 20% of women who are between the ages of 25 and 50 have fibrocystic changes that produce unwanted, often painful lumps. These lumps are usually benign...but they can mask early detection of breast cancer.

Self-defense: Wear a supportive bra to minimize your discomfort...cut your salt intake to reduce swelling from water retention...perform breast self-examinations monthly...and see a doctor to make sure a lump is normal and not potentially troublesome.

Breast Implant Trap

Sherine E. Gabriel, MD, professor of medicine and epidemiology, Mayo Clinic, Rochester, MN. Her review of medical records of 749 breast implant recipients was published in *The New England Journal of Medicine*, 10 Shattuck St., Boston 02115.

One in four women who has breast implant surgery needs repeat surgery within eight years.

Usual reasons: Formation of hard tissue around the implant...ruptured implant...infection...chronic pain...nipple necrosis (tissue death).

Such complications are more common with implants put in following breast cancer (34% at five years) than with those put in for cosmetic reasons (12% at five years).

When to Schedule A Mammogram

Pamela A. Propeck, MD, radiologist, associate professor, department of radiology, University of Wisconsin, Madison.

Schedule mammogram appointments well in advance. It can take as long as eight weeks to get a routine mammogram screening. *Reasons:* Low reimbursement rates by insurers have caused many imaging centers to cut back services or close...and more women have mammograms annually instead of every two years.

Large Women and Mammograms

Matthew J. Reeves, PhD, State Chronic Disease Epidemiologist, Michigan Dept. of Community Health, Lansing, MI.

Getting an annual mammogram and breast exam from your doctor are particularly important for larger women.

A study of almost 3,000 women with breast cancer found that among women who detected their own cancer, the tumors were larger and more advanced among overweight women.

The findings suggest that larger women are less likely to find small lumps by self-examination techniques than smaller women, making it more important for them to get regular mammograms.

The best chance of detecting breast cancer at an early stage for women of all weights is to obtain regular mammograms along with regular exams by your doctor.

Antiperspirants and Mammograms

Daniel Kopans, MD, director, Breast Imaging Division, Massachusetts General Hospital, and professor of radiology, Harvard Medical School, both in Boston.

Antiperspirants can interfere with mammography. They contain aluminum and/or other metals that can be mistaken for suspicious calcium deposits. Deodorants don't interfere—because they contain no metal.

Other substances that interfere with mammography: Lotions, oils, powders and zinc oxide, often used by women with large breasts to treat chronic irritation.

Incontinence and Exercise Connection

Ingrid Nygaard, MD, professor of obstetrics and gynecology, University of Iowa, Iowa City. Her study of 18 women 33 to 73 years of age was published in *The Journal of Reproductive Medicine*, 8342 Olive Blvd., St. Louis 63132.

One in three women experience incontinence while working out.

Helpful: A tampon worn in the lower vagina—to support the urethra. Fifty-eight percent of women who tried this remedy reported no urine leakage during aerobic exercise. Wet the tampon to ease insertion—and to prevent vaginal dryness.

Urinary Incontinence Advance

Jane Miller, MD, associate professor of urology, University of Washington Medical Center, Seattle.

A disposable urethral insert significantly reduced incontinence in 98% of women who participated in a study. When inflated, the balloon-tipped device rests at the neck of the bladder, blocking the flow of urine. To urinate, the woman pulls the attached string to deflate the balloon, then removes the device. The insert must initially be fitted by a doctor.

Sold under the name *Reliance Urinary Control Insert Device*, the device is now available in most drugstores.

Osteoporosis Advance

Robert R. Recker, MD, professor of medicine and director, Osteoporosis Research Center, Creighton University School of Medicine, Omaha.

A prescription drug called *alendronate* (Fosamax) cut the incidence of vertebral fractures by nearly 50% among women with osteoporosis. During a three-year study, only 18% of women on alendronate suffered more than one fracture, compared with 68% of women given a placebo.

A Mile a Day...

Study of 238 postmenopausal women by Elizabeth Krall, USDA Agricultural Research Service, Washington, DC.

Walking as little as a mile a day can delay the development of osteoporosis for up to seven years.

Background: Most women lose 3% to 6% of their bone mass annually during the five years surrounding menopause.

A study found that following a walking regimen will delay osteoporosis significantly. Women who walked regularly took four to seven years longer to lose as much bone as women who did not walk at all.

Cancer and Chemotherapy

Bernard Fisher, MD, distinguished service professor of surgery, University of Pittsburgh.

All breast cancer patients can benefit from chemotherapy. For years, chemotherapy has been the standard treatment for all *node-positive* tumors and *node-negative* tumors that are *estrogen-receptor negative*.

But *node-negative, estrogen-receptor-positive* tumors traditionally have been treated with the drug *tamoxifen* (Nolvadex) alone.

Finding: After five years, 90% of patients with such tumors who underwent chemotherapy were cancer-free. Only 84% of the patients who were taking tamoxifen alone remained cancer-free after five years.

Weight Loss May Not Be Good for Some

Jean Langlois, ScD, senior epidemiologist at the National Institute on Aging, Bethesda, MD.

Women over age 50 who lose a lot of weight increase their risk of hip fractures. A study of women age 67 and older found that those who lost 10% or more of their weight after age 50 doubled their chances of breaking a hip.

Physicians suggest that overweight 50-year-old women should strive to reach an appropriate weight and then stay at that level, because heart disease, associated with being overweight, is more dangerous than hip fractures. But they should take calcium and vitamin D supplements to help strengthen bones and prevent osteoporosis.

Hot Summer Days And Premature Labor

Shoghag Lajinian, MD, assistant professor of obstetrics–gynecology, State University of New York Health Science Center, Brooklyn. Her analysis of New York City's heat index and admissions for preterm labor was presented at a meeting of the American College of Obstetricians and Gynecologists, 409 12th St. SW, Washington, DC 20090.

Hot summer days can trigger premature labor. Women were twice as likely to begin contractions on the hottest days of the year as on the coldest.

Theory: Heat and dehydration boost the body's production of the hormones *oxytocin* and *antidiuretic hormone*. These compounds play a role in inducing contractions.

Self-defense: Women at risk—those between 24 and 36 weeks of pregnancy—should stay out of the heat and drink plenty of liquids to prevent dehydration.

Depression–Osteoporosis Link

David Michelson, MD, medical officer, National Institute of Mental Health, Bethesda, MD. His study of bone density in 48 women, average age 41, was published in *The New England Journal of Medicine*, 10 Shattuck St., Boston 02115.

Depression raises a woman's risk of osteoporosis. Bone density in young women who had suffered depression was 6% to 14% lower than in women who had never been depressed.

Theory: Depression boosts synthesis of the stress hormone *cortisol*, which has been linked to bone loss.

Breast-Feeding Benefit

Burris Duncan, MD, professor emeritus of pediatrics, pediatrics department, University Medical Center–Arizona Health Sciences, Tucson. His study of 1,013 infants was published in *Pediatrics*, 141 Northwest Point Blvd., Elk Grove Village, IL 60007.

Breast-fed infants experience fewer ear infections than those who are bottle-fed. Infants who nurse exclusively during their first four months have half as many ear infections as bottle-fed babies…and 40% fewer infections than those who were breast-fed but had supplemental feedings prior to four months. At least some of the beneficial effects last a full year, even if breast-feeding is stopped.

Pregnancy and Smoking

Carolyn Drews-Botsch, PhD, associate professor of epidemiology, Emory University, Rolling School of Public Health, Atlanta. Her study of the mothers of 221 children with mental retardation and 400 other mothers in a control group was published in *Pediatrics,* 141 Northwest Point Blvd., Elk Grove Village, IL 60009.

Pregnant women who smoke as few as five cigarettes per week are 50% more likely to give birth to children with mental retardation. The more a woman smokes during pregnancy, the greater the likelihood that her child will have mental retardation. Smoking during pregnancy has been linked to low birth weight, higher infant mortality and lower intelligence in children. This is the first study to link smoking and mental retardation. If these numbers are accurate, mental retardation could have been prevented in one-third of the children whose mothers smoked during pregnancy.

Folic Acid's Role in Pregnancy

William F. Rayburn, MD, chief of maternal–fetal medicine and professor of obstetrics and gynecology, University of Oklahoma College of Medicine, Oklahoma City.

Folic acid supplements are worth considering for all women of reproductive age. This B vitamin helps prevent brain and spinal column defects in newborns. To prevent such defects, women should begin taking 400 micrograms a day at least one month prior to conception…and continue for at least three months afterward.

Problem: If women start taking folic acid supplements *after* learning they are pregnant, it may be too late for the nutrient's beneficial effects in preventing birth defects.

Morning Sickness Self-Defense

Miriam Erick, MS, RD, senior dietitian manager at Brigham & Women's Hospital, Boston, and author of *Take Two Crackers and Call Me in the Morning: A Real-Life Guide for Surviving Morning Sickness.* Grinnen-Barrett.

Avoid smells that commonly trigger nausea—coffee, perfume/cologne, rotting garbage, pet foods, hot foods, body odors.

• **Don't watch food commercials on TV.**

• **Be wary of public transportation and driving in stop-and-go traffic.** Jerky motion can add to nausea.

• **Avoid visual motion**—such as a fast-paced music video—which can increase nausea.

• **Drink at least 10 cups of water or liquids daily** or eat foods with high water content, since adequate hydration reduces nausea.

Pregnancy and Thinking

T. Murphy Goodwin, MD, professor of obstetrics and gynecology, University of Southern California Medical Center, Los Angeles.

Pregnancy dulls women's thinking. In a study, women scored as much as 20% lower on intelligence tests during their last month of pregnancy than they did after giving birth.

Weakest areas: Remembering new information and tracking more than one piece of information at a time.

The Truth About "Post-Baby Blues"

John Studd, MD, DSc, consultant gynecologist, Chelsea and Westminster Hospital, London. His study of 61 women with postpartum depression was published in *The Lancet*, 32 Jamestown Rd., London NW1 7BY.

Because of a drop in estrogen levels following childbirth, one in 10 new mothers experiences depression. Sadness can last for months, and severe cases can lead to suicide.

Good news: Estrogen skin patches eliminated depression within three months in 80% of new mothers. Most of those who wore *placebo* patches stayed depressed for at least four months.

Bladder Pain Relief

Vicki Ratner, MD, an orthopedic surgeon in private practice in San Jose, CA. An interstitial cystitis sufferer, she is cofounder of the Interstitial Cystitis Association, 110 North Washington St., Ste. 340, Rockville, MD 20850.

Bladder pain caused by the mysterious disorder *interstitial cystitis* (IC) can be controlled with an oral medication called *pentosan polysulfate* (Elmiron). Sufferers say the pain is like having broken glass inside the bladder. The only drug previously approved to treat IC, *dimethyl sulfoxide* (DMSO), had to be administered into the bladder via a catheter. It was inconvenient and unpleasant.

Study: Pentosan helped about 38% of sufferers who took it three times a day. Ninety percent of the 500,000 people who have IC are women.

How Reliable Are Pregnancy Ultrasound Exams?

Sheryl Burt Ruzek, PhD, MPH, professor of health education, Temple University, Philadelphia.

Although they can provide valuable information about a developing fetus, ultrasound scans are prone to misinterpretation. For example, doctors often identify anatomical defects where none actually exist...or fail to spot actual defects.

Anorexia and Older Women

Paul L. Hewitt, PhD, associate professor of psychology, University of British Columbia, Vancouver, Canada. His study of 10 million death records over a five-year period was presented at the International Congress of Psychology in Montreal.

Only 25% of those who die of this eating disorder fit the stereotype of the young, overachieving woman.

Reality: Four out of five of those who die of anorexia nervosa are 45 years of age or older.

Female Athletes and Knee Injuries

Laura Huston, MS, researcher, department of orthopedic surgery, University of Michigan, Ann Arbor, who led a study of 140 men and women of varying fitness levels.

Female athletes suffer eight times more knee injuries than male athletes.

Reason: In female athletes, the quadriceps (the muscles at the front of the thigh) are generally stronger than their hamstrings (the muscles at the back of the thigh). This imbalance stresses the knee, causing injury.

Simple self-defense: Strengthen hamstrings by jumping rope for a few minutes three times a week.

Bone Density Study

Ethel Siris, MD, professor of clinical medicine, College of Physicians and Surgeons, Columbia University, New York City.

Bone thinning is grossly undiagnosed in women over age 50. In a recent study of more than 200,000 seemingly healthy women age 50 or older, 40% were found to have low bone density. Seven percent suffered from full-fledged osteoporosis. In the following year, the women with low bone density suffered broken bones at twice the rate of those with normal bone density. Those with osteoporosis did so at four times the rate.

Women and Calcium

Ethel Siris, MD, professor of clinical medicine, College of Physicians and Surgeons, Columbia University, New York City.

Few women get enough calcium. The recommended intake is 1,000 mg for women 25 to 50 years of age and for women over 50 who take estrogen. For women 50 or older who are not taking estrogen and for all women over 65, 1,500 mg is recommended. Eight ounces of milk (or yogurt) contains about 300 mg of calcium.

Getting Enough Minerals

Barbara S. Levine, RD, PhD, director, Calcium Information Center, New York Hospital–Cornell Medical Center, New York City.

Women taking calcium to ward off osteoporosis should be sure to get enough magnesium, too. The body aims to keep the two minerals in balance. Without enough magnesium, calcium is simply excreted. .

Surprising: Up to 70% of women are magnesium-deficient.

Helpful: If you're already taking calcium supplements, ask your doctor about adding a magnesium supplement (200 mg a day)...or about eating more magnesium-rich foods like green, leafy vegetables, whole-grain breads, fortified cereals, soybeans, tofu, milk or yogurt.

Incontinence and Smoking

Richard C. Bump, MD, associate professor of obstetrics and gynecology, Duke University Medical Center, Durham, NC. His study of 606 women was published in the *American Journal of Obstetrics and Gynecology*, 11830 Westline Industrial Dr., St. Louis 63146.

Women smokers—even those who had kicked the habit—were two to three times more likely to suffer from incontinence than women who never smoked.

Theory: Harsh, persistent coughing permanently damages pelvic muscles that control urine flow. Animal studies have found that nicotine constricts the bladder, causing unintentional urine leakage.

How Women Can Outwit The Sneaky Malignancy That Killed Gilda Radner

M. Steven Piver, MD, director and founder of The Gilda Radner Familial Ovarian Cancer Registry at Roswell Park Cancer Institute, Elm and Carlton Streets, Buffalo, NY 14263. He and Gilda Radner's former husband, actor Gene Wilder, are the authors of *Gilda's Disease.* Broadway.

In the autumn of 1985, comedienne Gilda Radner began experiencing fatigue, abdominal cramps, intestinal gas and distension and shooting pains down her thighs.

Gilda consulted gynecologists, gastroenterologists, holistic doctors—even an acupuncturist. All of these experts reassured her that her symptoms were harmless.

The doctors were wrong. Gilda's symptoms got worse. Finally, on October 23, 1986, after extensive testing, she was diagnosed with ovarian cancer.

Over the next three years, Gilda underwent four operations, plus agonizing bouts of chemotherapy and radiation. Nothing worked. She died on May 20, 1989.

Gilda's story is tragic. Even more tragic is the fact that her case of missed and delayed diagnosis is typical of ovarian cancer.

Many of the 26,000 American women diagnosed with the disease each year go months or even years without a diagnosis. The longer it takes to get a correct diagnosis, the smaller the chance of survival.

RISK FACTORS

Ovarian cancer is a sneaky and often deadly disease—one doctors frequently fail to consider when rendering a diagnosis. It is easily confused with many other conditions, including uterine fibroids and colitis.

None of Gilda's doctors suspected ovarian cancer until it was too late, even though she had all the classic risk factors. *Gilda...*

●**Ate a high-fat diet.** Dietary fat has been implicated in many cancers, including cancer of the breast, ovaries and colon.

●**Was childless.** Some cases of ovarian cancer are associated with ovary damage caused by

137

years of repeated ovulation. The more times a woman ovulates, the greater her risk.

- **Used fertility-boosting drugs.**

- **Used personal hygiene products containing talcum powder.** Many soaps, deodorants, condoms and contraceptive diaphragms contain talc. Asbestos-like talc particles travel through the cervix and then line the uterus and fallopian tubes, slowly poisoning the ovaries.

- **Had several relatives with ovarian or breast cancer.** The gene for ovarian cancer can be inherited from the mother's or father's side.

THE FAMILY CONNECTION

Women can inherit a predisposition to ovarian cancer *even if none of their relatives had the disease.* That is, women with a family history of certain other types of cancer (breast, colon or prostate) are at increased risk for ovarian cancer.

GENETIC TESTING

It's now possible to be tested for BRCA1 and BRCA2, two of the genes that predispose women to breast and ovarian cancer. In most cases, however, testing is pointless unless you have at least two close relatives with ovarian cancer.

Even then, genetic testing is of limited value. Knowing that you're at increased risk for ovarian and breast cancer causes anxiety...and it doesn't really help you prevent either disease, unless you have your ovaries and breasts surgically removed.

TELLTALE SYMPTOMS

Ovarian cancer is often thought of as a disease that produces no symptoms until it's too far advanced to be cured. That's untrue—although the symptoms tend to be "nonspecific" and thus easy to misinterpret.

In addition to the abdominal and gastrointestinal symptoms Gilda experienced, she also experienced fever and back pain.

Any woman who experiences one or more of these symptoms for three or more weeks should consult her primary-care doctor or gynecologist. Do *not* wait for the doctor to think of ovarian cancer as a possible diagnosis. Ask to be checked for it right away.

In addition to a pelvic exam, this checkup should include...

- **Blood test for CA125.** This protein is elevated in about 50% of cases of early ovarian cancer and about 95% of cases of advanced ovarian cancer.

- **Vaginal ultrasound exam.** By placing the probe *inside* the vagina, rather than on the abdomen as is traditionally done, the doctor can obtain a better picture of the ovaries.

If the doctor uncovers anything suspicious, he/she should perform a transvaginal sonogram using color-flow Doppler technology (an advanced form of ultrasound).

He should also perform a CT scan of the abdomen and/or a laparoscopy. That's a surgical procedure in which the doctor inserts a viewing scope through a small incision in the abdomen.

GETTING EFFECTIVE TREATMENT

The key to surviving ovarian cancer is getting a prompt diagnosis...and aggressive treatment by a doctor specializing in the disease. For referral to a *gynecologic oncologist* in your area, contact the Gynecologic Cancer Foundation at 800-444-4441, *www.wcn.org/gcf.*

Most cases of ovarian cancer are treated via removal of the ovaries, plus chemotherapy.

Recently, it was found that women who take a combination of the drugs *paclitaxel* (Taxol) and *cisplatin* (Platinol) live almost three times longer (38 months) than women who undergo standard chemotherapy (25 months).

When the disease is diagnosed early, the five-year survival rate approaches 95%. When it is diagnosed in later stages, survival is reduced to 5% to 30%.

HOW TO PROTECT YOURSELF

In addition to eating a low-fat diet and avoiding talc, women should take these precautions...

- **Get regular checkups.** Women without a family history should have an annual pelvic exam, starting at age 18. Women with a family history of ovarian cancer should have a pelvic exam, CA125 test and a transvaginal ultrasound twice yearly, starting at age 25.

- **If you use birth control, consider taking the Pill.** Oral contraceptives prevent damage to the ovaries that occurs during the childbearing years.

Women who take the Pill for four years have a 40% reduction in their risk for ovarian cancer. Ten years of use cuts the risk by 80%—and the protection lasts for 15 years after you stop taking it.

In women with a strong family history of ovarian cancer, use of the Pill can reduce their risk to that of women who do not have a family history of the disease.

●**Get pregnant...and breast-feed your children.** Pregnancy and breast-feeding interrupt ovulation, cutting your risk by 40%.

●**Consider surgical sterilization.** Having your "tubes tied" stops ovulation, reducing risk by 71%.

●**If you have a strong family history of ovarian cancer,** consider having your ovaries removed. If you're over 40 and scheduled for a hysterectomy, it's prudent to have your ovaries removed along with your uterus—even if you don't have a family history of the disease.

Any woman with two or more close relatives who had ovarian or breast cancer should consider enrolling in The Gilda Radner Familial Ovarian Cancer Registry. Call 800-682-7426... or visit *www.ovariancancer.com.*

Weight-Loss Health Trap

Jean Langlois, ScD, epidemiologist, who published a study of more than 3,600 women, age 67 and older, National Institute on Aging, Bethesda, MD.

Women who become too thin can endanger their well-being.

Reason: Women who go to extremes to eliminate fat from their bodies often go too far. Researchers have found that in healthy women, body fat should be between 16% and 26% of total weight—with the ideal being about 20%.

Quick way to see if weight is in healthy range: Use the hip-to-waist ratio. Pass a tape measure around your body, and cross the navel. Jot down the result. Then pass the tape around your buttocks to measure your hips. Divide the waist measurement by the hip measurement. If the result is below 0.85, you are in

good shape. If it is higher than 1.0, you are heavy and need to lose weight.

Stretch Mark Help

Joshua L. Fox, MD, a dermatologic laser surgeon in Fresh Meadows, New York.

Ask a dermatologist or dermatologic laser surgeon about having stretch marks treated with a pulsed-dye laser. The marks won't disappear altogether, but they should become less noticeable. Several laser treatments may be required.

Risky Surgery

John M. Thorpe, Jr., MD, distinguished professor of obstetrics and gynecology, University of North Carolina at Chapel Hill School of Medicine.

Surgery to widen the vaginal opening during childbirth is rarely helpful. Called *episiotomy,* this common surgical procedure does not reduce the risk of vaginal or rectal tears. In fact, episiotomy increases the risk of tears. Yet episiotomies are still performed on the majority of first-time mothers in the United States. Many doctors who perform episiotomies routinely are unaware of the problems associated with the procedure. Episiotomy may be necessary in cases involving fetal distress or breech delivery.

Cervix-Sparing Hysterectomy

Ernst G. Bartsich, MD, associate professor, obstetrics and gynecology, New York Hospital–Cornell Medical Center, New York.

In an alternative to ordinary hysterectomy, only the top of the uterus is removed. *Supracervical* hysterectomy has been used to treat fibroid tumors, pelvic pain, persistent bleeding and endometriosis. It's less likely than ordinary hysterectomy to injure the bowel and/or bladder...or to cause vaginal prolapse (a shift in the position of the vagina), sexual dysfunction or the "sense of loss" that is common following ordinary hysterectomy.

Vaginal Douching Danger

Donna Day Baird, PhD, epidemiologist, National Institute of Environmental Health Sciences, Research Triangle Park, NC.

After 12 months of trying to conceive, about 90% of women who had never douched became pregnant—compared with only 73% of the women who douched more than once a week.

Also: Douching may increase risk of pelvic inflammatory disease and other infections by spreading germs to the upper reaches of the uterus and fallopian tubes.

Unfaithful Husbands and Cancer Link

Keerti V. Shah, MD, professor, Johns Hopkins School of Hygiene & Public Health, Baltimore.

Women with unfaithful husbands are more likely to contract cervical cancer. A study of more than 1,200 men and women found that women whose husbands have other sexual partners are five to 11 times as likely to develop cervical cancer as those whose husbands do not stray. Incidence was eight times greater for women whose husbands frequented prostitutes. Researchers theorize that the husbands contract the human papilloma virus (HPV) during their extramarital liaisons and bring it home to their wives. Genital HPV infections are known to cause cervical cancer.

Sex and Urinary Tract Infections

Thomas M. Hooton, MD, professor of medicine, University of Washington, Seattle. His six-month study of 796 women was published in *The New England Journal of Medicine*, 10 Shattuck St., Boston 02115.

Frequent sex raises a woman's risk for urinary tract infection (UTI)...as does using a diaphragm with spermicide.

Study: Women who had sexual intercourse three times a week were three times more likely to have a UTI than women who abstained from sex. *Theory:* Intercourse introduces vaginal bacteria into the bladder. Spermicide kills beneficial bacteria but leaves infection-causing ones unharmed.

UTI Warning

Amee Manges, MPH, epidemiology researcher specializing in UTIs, School of Public Health, University of California, Berkeley. Her study of 302 women with drug-resistant UTIs was published in *The New England Journal of Medicine*, 10 Shattuck St., Boston 02115.

About 18% of urinary tract infections (UTIs) are now resistant to the most commonly prescribed antibiotic, *trimethoprim sulfamethoxazole* (Bactrim)—up from about 10% five years ago. UTI symptoms include abnormally colored or bloody urine...frequent or painful urination... and pressure in the lower pelvis. If antibiotics do not clear up symptoms within two days, consult your physician about prescribing a different antibiotic. *To avoid UTIs:* Drink plenty of water... urinate frequently—and immediately after sexual intercourse...and practice good hygiene.

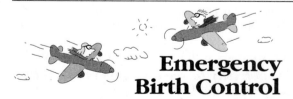

Emergency Birth Control

Roberto Rivera, MD, director, Family Health International, Box 13950, Research Triangle Park, NC 27709.

Taken shortly after "unprotected" sexual intercourse, oral contraceptives are a safe and reasonably effective way to prevent pregnancy. Emergency use of the Pill is roughly 75% effective at preventing pregnancy. Regular daily use of the Pill is 97% effective.

Caution: Emergency contraception should be initiated only under a doctor's supervision.

Safest Birth Control Pills

James McGregor, MD, professor of obstetrics and gynecology at University of Colorado Health Sciences Center, Denver.

Triphasic birth control pills are safest because they deliver *lower doses of estrogen* by weight to the body than earlier versions of the Pill. Pills that provide more than 35 micrograms of estrogen have been associated with increased probability of blood clots and stroke, particularly in older women.

Another benefit: The newer pills, which deliver varying hormone levels appropriate to the phases of the body's natural menstrual cycle, also cause less spotting in many women. Physicians prescribe an initial formulation that takes into account the patient's age and other factors—including susceptibility to acne. Physicians may vary the dosage after observing its side effects until the optimal formulation is determined.

Yeast Infection Relief

Study of 46 women with recurrent vaginosis by Eliezer Shalev, Central Emek Hospital, Afula, Israel, published in *Archives of Family Medicine,* Box 10946, Chicago 60610.

Yogurt relieves recurrent yeast infections. In a study, women who daily ate five ounces of yogurt containing live bacteria lactobacillus acidophilus had two-thirds fewer cases of recurrent vaginosis as before. This is the first study to demonstrate such positive effects from yogurt containing live cultures.

Theory: Bacteria present in the yogurt are believed to protect against infection either by maintaining an acidic environment in the vagina or by producing compounds such as hydrogen peroxide that kill harmful bacteria.

Ease Menstrual Cramps

Menstrual Cramps Self-Help Book by Susan M. Lark, MD, authority on women's health care in private practice in Los Altos, CA. Diane.

Avoid certain foods that can make menstrual cramping worse. Dairy products, fats, salt, alcohol, sugar and caffeine can all make cramping more severe.

Diaphragms and Cystitis Risk

Study of almost 800 sexually active women by researchers at University of Washington School of Medicine, Seattle, published in *The New England Journal of Medicine,* 10 Shattuck St., Boston 02115.

Women using diaphragms with spermicides for birth control change their bodies' internal environments in ways that allow the bacteria that cause cystitis to flourish. The more frequent the sex, the higher the risk.

If you have frequent bladder infections: Consider a different form of birth control.

More on Fertility Treatment

Zev Rosenwaks, MD, director, Center for Reproductive Medicine & Infertility, New York Hospital–Cornell Medical Center, New York.

The increasingly popular technique *intracytoplasmic sperm injection* (ICSI)—in which individual sperm are selected and injected directly into eggs—allows men with

141

low-quality sperm to become fathers. Fertility experts had worried that sperm selected by lab technicians might be more likely to carry genetic defects than sperm "chosen" by nature.

Finding: Only 2.6% of ICSI babies suffered birth defects. That rate is comparable to that for children conceived normally.

Treatment for Ovarian Cancer

David S. Alberts, MD, professor of medicine and pharmacology, University of Arizona, Tucson.

Doctors have begun administering the anti-cancer drug *cisplatin* via an abdominal catheter instead of via an arm vein.

Benefit: Women who use the abdominal route have a 24% lower death rate. They're also less likely to experience hearing loss, nerve damage and other side effects.

This approach should be considered for ovarian cancer patients who have a small amount of tumor remaining after initial surgery.

Powder Risk

Linda Cook, PhD, epidemiologist, Fred Hutchinson Cancer Research Center, Seattle, leader of a study of 313 women with ovarian cancer and 422 without it.

Women who use talcum powder in the vaginal area right after bathing increase their risk of ovarian cancer by 60%. Women using powder deodorant sprays have a 90% increased risk. *Reason:* Unknown.

Self-defense: Avoid these products.

Fertility Drugs and Ovarian Cancer

David L. Healy, MD, PhD, chairman, department of obstetrics and gynecology, Monash Medical Center, Melbourne, Australia. His nine-year study of 10,358 infertile women was published in *The Lancet*, 32 Jamestown Rd., London NW1 7BY.

Fertility drugs do not increase a woman's risk of ovarian cancer. Doctors have long thought that *clomiphene* (Clomid), *menotropins* (Pergonal) and other fertility drugs promote ovarian cancer. But a study found no evidence of increased risk. In fact, women who had taken fertility drugs had a slightly reduced cancer rate.

Theory: Infertile women pay more attention to their health. Thus, they're more likely to discover precancerous cysts earlier.

Ovary Removal Danger

Donna Kritz-Silverstein, PhD, associate adjunct professor of family and preventive medicine, University of California, San Diego. Her study of 1,150 women 50 to 89 years of age was published in *Circulation*, 560 Harrison Ave., Ste. 502, Boston 02118.

Women whose ovaries have been surgically removed face an increased risk of heart disease, although the risk may not become apparent for 20 years. In a study, total cholesterol levels of women who had undergone a hysterectomy involving removal of *both* ovaries (bilateral oophorectomy) were seven points higher than women whose ovaries were intact.

Self-defense: Before undergoing a hysterectomy, discuss with your doctor whether removing your ovaries is necessary.

7

The Healthy Family

What You Need to Know About Your Child's Health Care

Charles B. Inlander

Many parents will find themselves seeking answers to the same old questions about their children's health...

•How can I find a good doctor for my child? While a pediatrician is the most obvious choice, family practitioners often make equally good doctors for children.

Carefully interview different types of doctors, then pick one that meets your requirements...one with a pleasant, caring attitude...a willingness to talk directly with your child as well as with you...a clean, orderly office...and a good system for fielding after-hours phone calls. Make sure your child gets along with the

doctor and that the doctor accepts your health insurance plan.*

Caution: If the doctor belongs to a group practice, ask that you be allowed to make appointments specifically with him/her.

Ask if the doctor can provide you with educational materials regarding specific health issues. They're a big help when illness strikes —or during puberty.

•Does my child need an X-ray? In addition to being costly, X-rays, CT scans, magnetic resonance imaging and other diagnostic tests are typically frightening to children, risky and unnecessary.

They should be administered only if their findings will have a direct bearing on your

*To obtain a list of pediatricians in your community, send a self-addressed, stamped envelope to the American Academy of Pediatrics Pediatrician Referral, 141 Northwest Point Blvd., Elk Grove Village, IL 60007.

Charles B. Inlander, a consumer advocate and healthcare consultant based in Fogelsville, PA. He was founding president of the nonprofit People's Medical Society, a consumer health advocacy group in Allentown, PA. He is author of numerous books, including *Take This Book to the Hospital With You.* St. Martin's.

child's treatment. If your child has a cough, for example, a chest X-ray is generally unnecessary—unless the doctor has reason to suspect a serious lung ailment. Before agreeing to any test, question the doctor thoroughly to make sure it is necessary. *Key questions...*

- **What's the name of the test?**
- **Why is it necessary?**
- **What will it reveal that you don't already know?**
- **What will happen if the test is not performed?**
- **What are the possible side effects?**
- **Is a less-invasive test available?**
- **Will the test results change your method of treatment?**
- **Are childhood immunizations safe?** Most states require that all children be immunized against the following diseases—diphtheria, pertussis (whooping cough), tetanus, measles, mumps, rubella (German measles), poliomyelitis and Haemophilus influenza type B (bacterial meningitis). Experts are also now recommending varicella (chicken pox) and hepatitis B.

These vaccinations are typically administered between the ages of two months and 16 years. They are generally quite safe.

Exception: Pertussis. Half of all children who receive this five-dose vaccine develop fever, and, in rare cases, children have developed mental retardation or another permanent disability. However, because pertussis is such a serious disease, it is still prudent to have your child immunized.

To minimize risk: Insist that your child receive the *acellular* pertussis vaccine. It's less likely to cause dangerous reactions than the old vaccine, which remains in use.

The pertussis vaccine should never be given to any child who is over age six, who has a fever or has already had pertussis. Any child who experiences fever, shock, persistent crying, convulsions or neurological problems after the first pertussis shot should not receive any of the additional pertussis boosters.

- **My child has recurrent throat infections. Should his tonsils be removed?** Tonsillectomy is neither necessary nor particularly effective at curing recurrent ear or throat infections, even though doctors often urge surgery.

When it's appropriate: Only if the tonsils become so swollen that they interfere with the child's breathing, or if lab tests indicate the presence of abscesses behind the tonsils. In all other cases, it's best to treat such infections with antibiotics.

- **What about chronic ear infections?** Ear infections (otitis media) are common among children of smokers. If you smoke—stop. New mothers should avoid bottle-feeding their children. Research suggests that breast-feeding helps prevent earaches. Beyond this, there's no real consensus on treatment.

The American Academy of Pediatrics recommends use of oral antibiotics (usually amoxicillin), although some research casts doubt on their effectiveness. The surgical insertion of drainage tubes through the child's eardrums (tympanostomy) can cause serious complications, including severe infections and hearing loss.

Conservative approach—to discuss with your doctor: At the first sign of pain, give your child acetaminophen (Tylenol) or another non-aspirin painkiller. *Also helpful:* A heating pad held against the ear.

- **Do children's hospitals offer better pediatric care than general hospitals?** The standard of care in children's hospitals is no better than that in general hospitals with good pediatric sections. If your child requires inpatient surgery, pick a hospital that performs that surgery on a routine basis.

Are Your Immunizations Up-to-Date?

Timothy McCall, MD, an internist, medical editor of *Yoga Journal* and author of *Examining Your Doctor: A Patient's Guide to Avoiding Harmful Medical Care.* Carol. *www.drmccall.com.*

Most of us make sure our kids get immunized against infectious diseases like measles, mumps and polio. But we aren't so good at protecting ourselves. Each year, more than 60,000 adults in the US die of diseases that vaccines could have prevented. Compare that to fewer than 1,000 children a year.

About 20,000 adults die of influenza each year. Current guidelines call for everyone 65 or older to get a flu shot every fall, just before the influenza season starts. The guidelines also recommend flu shots for individuals with chronic diseases like heart or kidney disease, diabetes or HIV infection. Evidence suggests that flu shots may also benefit healthy individuals under age 65.

Flu shots don't always work in elderly or chronically ill people, whose immune systems tend to be weaker. If you have an elderly or chronically ill friend, coworker or family member, be sure to get vaccinated yourself. By doing so, you'll make sure they won't catch influenza from you.

One important vaccine that few people seem to know about is for the bacterium *pneumococcus*. Each year, 500,000 Americans get pneumococcal infections, primarily pneumonia. Forty thousand die from them.

I think everyone over 65 should get the pneumococcus vaccine. So should younger people with chronic heart or lung conditions, liver disease or diabetes—and people who have had their spleens removed.

People infected with the AIDS virus should get the pneumococcus vaccine as soon as they learn they're infected. As their immune system declines, the vaccine is less likely to be effective. Unlike the flu shot, the pneumonia vaccine usually needs to be given only once in a lifetime. Even so, only 14% of those at high risk have received it.

The other vaccine many adults overlook protects against two infections—tetanus and diphtheria. Current recommendations call for everyone to have a tetanus/diphtheria booster once every 10 years.

It used to be that people only got tetanus shots if they sustained a "dirty" cut and went to the emergency room. Recently, scientists discovered that many older people—some of whom haven't had a tetanus booster in decades—have lost protection against this potentially fatal disease.

Consequently, the recommendations have changed. Now all primary-care doctors should see to it that their patients are up-to-date with their tetanus shots, whether they cut themselves or not.

Some vaccines not recommended for the general public are appropriate for people at increased risk of particular infections. German measles (rubella) is of particular concern for women of childbearing age. It can cause severe birth defects.

Women who *might* become pregnant who have not had the rubella vaccine should have their blood tested for rubella antibodies. If no antibodies are present, they should have the vaccine right away—and avoid becoming pregnant for at least three months.

Hepatitis B causes fewer deaths than AIDS—around 5,000 a year in the US—but is almost 10 times easier to catch. Still, only about 10% of people at risk for hepatitis B have been vaccinated. IV drug users, sexually active gay men and anyone exposed to blood (health-care workers, dialysis patients, etc.) should get this safe and effective vaccine. The vaccine is also a good idea for sex partners of people with hepatitis B.

Vaccines are one of the great success stories of modern medicine.

Healthy Toll-Free Calls

Matthew Lesko, coauthor, *Free Stuff for Seniors.* Information USA.

Many groups provide free health information by phone…

● **Eldercare Locator** gives referrals for home-delivered meals, transportation, legal assistance, housing options, more. 800-677-1116.

● **Partnership for Prescription Assistance patient assistance programs**—find out if your income makes you eligible for free—or nearly free—prescription drugs from manufacturers. 800-762-4636.

● **Special services for veterans.** 800-827-1000.

● **Social Security questions**, duplicate cards, more. 800-772-1213.

● **Medicare information and problems.** 800-633-4227 (800-MEDICARE).

The Highest Life Expectancy

Study by Bruce Schobel, corporate vice president and actuary, New York Life Insurance Co., and Robert Myers, retired chief actuary, US Social Security Administration.

The world's highest life expectancy is in Japan. A Japanese boy born today can expect to live almost 76 years...a Japanese girl, almost 82 years. An American boy can expect to live 72 years...an American girl, 79 years. *Possible reasons:* Access to high-quality health care, low-fat diet, high standard of living.

Flu Self-Defense

The late Steven R. Mostow, MD, former chairman, department of medicine, Rose Medical Center, Denver.

Get a flu shot. It is 70% effective at stopping each year's bug.

●**See your doctor immediately if you feel yourself coming down with the flu.** He/she can prescribe *amantadine* (Symmetrel) or *rimantadine* (Flumadine), or the newer drugs *oseltamivir* (Tamiflu) or *zanamivir* (Relenza), medications that minimize discomfort and prevent complications such as bronchitis, ear infection or pneumonia.

●**Keep a positive attitude.** Negative emotions depress the immune system, making you more susceptible to illness.

Remedy for Low Back Pain

Louis Kuritzky, MD, assistant clinical professor of health and family medicine, University of Florida, Gainesville.

Most cases of low back pain are best treated with activity—walking, swimming, bicycling, etc.—*not* medication, rest or physical therapy. Nine out of 10 low back pain sufferers get better on their own, whether or not they receive treatment.

Preventing Back Injuries

University of California at Los Angeles study of 36,000 workers at The Home Depot in California from 1989–1994.

Back injuries can be prevented with the use of back-support belts (corsets). Despite earlier evidence to the contrary, the latest research concluded that use of the belts reduced low-back injuries by about a third. The biggest benefits were for men under age 25 and over age 35, and those doing material handling jobs.

Declaring War on Asthma

Richard N. Firshein, DO, assistant professor of family medicine at New York College of Osteopathic Medicine, and medical director of the Paul Sorvino Asthma Foundation, both in New York City. He is author of *Reversing Asthma: Reduce Your Medications with This Revolutionary New Program.* Grand Central Publishing.

The incidence of asthma has risen dramatically in recent years. In 1980, five million Americans were diagnosed with asthma. This year the number will be closer to 20 million—in part because of rising levels of ozone and other airborne pollutants.

What's the best way to prevent asthma? To treat it? For answers, we spoke with asthma specialist—and asthma patient—Dr. Richard N. Firshein.

CAUSES OF ASTHMA

Most doctors view asthma as simply a breathing problem caused by obstructed airways. To reduce this obstruction, doctors tend to rely on bronchodilators, adrenaline and other prescription drugs.

Trap: Drugs have severe side effects, including headache, nausea and rapid heartbeat... and they do *not* control the chronic inflammatory process that underlies asthma. Medication is one part of a comprehensive asthma program.

ASTHMA SELF-TEST

1. Are you breathing wrong? Proper breathing technique involves using the diaphragm to expand the belly. Asthmatics tend to breathe from the chest, lifting their shoulders as they inhale.

2. Do you need more than one breath to finish each sentence when speaking? Many asthmatics need to breathe in mid-sentence.

3. Do you have a rapid pulse? If so, you may be responding to a lack of oxygen or may have an underlying allergy.

4. Do you make a wheezing sound as you breathe? Wheezing is usually a sign of inflammation, narrowing of the airway or excess production of mucus.

5. Are you often anxious? Fear of suffocation gives many asthmatics chronic anxiety.

6. Are you in pain? Because they use the wrong muscles to breathe, asthmatics often have abdominal, back or chest pain...or tenderness in the ribs.

If you answered "yes" to three or more of these questions, see a doctor right away for a medical exam.

LIFESTYLE INVENTORY

As part of your medical exam, you and your doctor should review several key issues...

- **Allergies and intestinal complaints.**

- **Medication.** Discuss all prescription and over-the-counter drugs you take. Many drugs can exacerbate asthma, including hormones, antibiotics, antidepressants, antifungals, acid-blockers and antihypertensives.

- **Home environment.** Discuss where you notice symptoms most...how your home is heated and cooled...what sort of floor coverings you have...and what household cleaners you use.

- **Work environment.** Are you exposed to cigarette smoke, industrial chemicals, copier dust and other lung irritants? Is your office well-ventilated?

- **Dietary practices.** Deficiencies in magnesium, vitamins C and A and other antioxidant nutrients are contributing factors in many cases.

- **Immune status.** Do you suffer from frequent colds? Do you wake up tired after a full night's sleep? If so, your immune system may be compromised.

If this review finds a potential source of trouble, your doctor may want to test your blood or skin for allergies...evaluate nutrient levels in your body...test your immune response...and/or analyze your digestive tract.

Once the doctor understands the factors involved, he/she can help you plot a program to keep your symptoms in check.

ASTHMA-PROOFING YOUR HOME

Every asthmatic needs a "safe room"—someplace to go during an asthma attack. For most people, the best choice is the bedroom. *Here's how to prepare your safe room...*

- **Dust frequently** with a specially treated cloth that prevents dust from scattering.

- **Remove all carpeting.**

- **Encase your mattress, box spring and pillows in airtight vinyl covers.** This helps get rid of dust and dust mites, which can trigger an asthma attack.

- **Eliminate water leaks** and other sources of humidity.

- **Consider purchasing** a *high-efficiency particle-arresting* (HEPA) air filter. *Cost:* $150 and up.

- **Consider getting rid of houseplants.** While plants themselves are not a problem, plant soil often contains mold, which can trigger an asthma attack.

AVOIDING TRIGGER FOODS

People are often surprised to learn that what they eat affects their breathing. For some, asthma is caused by unsuspected allergies or sensitivities to "trigger" foods—eggs, shellfish, nuts, seeds, soy, etc. For others, the culprit is pesticide residues or food additives.

Since no two people are alike in this respect, your doctor may order skin tests to identify specific triggers.

ANTIOXIDANTS TO THE RESCUE

Asthma is sometimes a result of lung damage caused by *free radicals.* These renegade molecules are found in polluted air and are produced by the body during vigorous exercise.

By consuming more antioxidants—which neutralize free radicals—many asthmatics notice a swift reduction in symptoms.

Antioxidant foods: Broccoli, cauliflower, squash, carrots, garlic and onions.

Many asthmatics are helped by taking a daily capsule of fish oil or—if they're sensitive to fish—flaxseed oil. Oils found in fresh salmon, tuna and mackerel have an anti-inflammatory effect on the lungs.

Ask your doctor about taking grape seed extract...and a daily supplement containing magnesium (250 mg)...vitamin A (4,000 IU)...vitamin C (1,000 mg)...and vitamin E (400 IU).*

Magnesium reduces elevated levels of calcium, which can cause the breathing muscles to spasm.

Magnesium-rich foods: Tofu, spinach and beets.

For severe asthma, intravenous magnesium may be required.

THREE BREATHING STRATEGIES

●**Belly breathing.** Lie on your back on a mat, with knees bent and feet slightly apart. Place a hardcover book on your lower stomach, with the binding touching the bottom of your rib cage.

Breathe in through your nose. As you do, lift the book as high as possible using your stomach. Keep your chest relaxed and motionless.

As you exhale, use your abdominal muscles to squeeze every last bit of air from your lungs. Repeat slowly, taking about four breaths per minute.

●**Blowing out the candle.** Take a deep "belly" breath. Then exhale, pursing your lips firmly and blowing through them as forcefully as you can. Imagine that you're blowing out candles on a birthday cake.

●**"Breathing through."** If your breathing starts to accelerate because of emotional stress or an incipient asthma attack, shift over to belly breathing.

Notice any tension in your jaw, shoulders, chest or neck. Allow those body parts to relax.

Let your feelings "flow"—even if they're negative. Don't try to stop them with short, shallow breaths or clenched muscles.

*Due to the possible interactions between vitamin E and various drugs and supplements, as well as other safety considerations, consult your doctor before starting a vitamin E regimen.

Can't Stomach a Roller Coaster Ride?

Charles Kimmelman, MD, professor of otolaryngology, Manhattan Eye, Ear and Throat Hospital, New York, quoted in *Men's Health*, 33 E. Minor St., Emmaus, PA 18098.

Roller coasters are less fun as we age because the balance mechanism in the inner ear becomes less tolerant of excessive motion.

Solution: Take an over-the-counter motion-sickness medication before riding...eat a gram of powdered gingerroot—available at drugstores and natural-food shops...or wear a Sea Band, available at sporting-goods stores. This helps control nausea by stimulating an acupressure point on the inside of the wrist.

Easier Ways to Get Dressed

Richard B. Dewey, Jr., MD, assistant professor of neurology, University of Texas Southwestern Medical Center, Dallas.

Help for people with arthritis, Parkinson's disease or other disorders affecting coordination and flexibility...

●**Have a family member or tailor replace buttons and zippers** with Velcro fasteners wherever possible.

●**Have a shoemaker stick Velcro strips onto shoes** to make them easier to fasten.

●**Choose clothing that closes in front.**

●**Take off clothes from the more rigid side of the body first.**

●**If you must button clothes,** use a button hook.

●**Lower closet rods** to make clothes easier to reach.

GERD: A New Name For an Old Problem

Timothy McCall, MD, an internist, medical editor of *Yoga Journal* and author of *Examining Your Doctor: A Patient's Guide to Avoiding Harmful Medical Care.* Carol. *www.drmccall.com.*

In what may be a sign of the never-ending quest to give simple medical problems complex names, many doctors are now regularly diagnosing *gastroesophageal reflux disease* (GERD). In the old days, we called this ailment hiatal hernia or esophageal reflux—or simply heartburn.

Whatever the name, GERD is what happens when stomach contents leak upstream into the esophagus, the muscular tube linking the mouth to the stomach. Typical symptoms include a burning sensation in the lower chest and an acid taste in the mouth.

The condition can be disabling, and severe cases can even lead to esophageal cancer. Luckily, most cases can be controlled with lifestyle modifications, drugs and—in some extreme cases—surgery.

The first line of treatment for GERD is dietary modification. This involves avoiding foods known to trigger reflux. These include chocolate, coffee (including decaf), peppermints and other mints, citrus fruits and spicy or fatty foods. Drinking alcohol and smoking also promote reflux.

Certain medicines make GERD worse. These include the asthma drug *theophylline*, anti-inflammatory drugs like aspirin and ibuprofen, tricyclic antidepressants like *amitriptyline* (Elavil) and calcium channel blockers, which are used to treat heart disease and high blood pressure.

If you have GERD and are taking any of these drugs, ask your doctor about substituting another drug.

Anything that pushes on the belly encourages stomach acid to "backwash" into the esophagus. Tight clothing can do it. So can being overweight or even eating too much at a time.

When you're standing or sitting, gravity tends to keep stomach contents from moving upstream. For this reason, people prone to GERD should avoid lying down after eating, and should not eat or drink anything—even a glass of water—for a couple of hours before going to bed. Some people benefit by elevating the head of the mattress with a foam wedge or by placing the headboard on wooden blocks.

If lifestyle modification fails to bring relief, the first line of drug therapy for GERD is antacids. They bring quick relief by coating the esophagus and helping neutralize stomach acid. The next option is an over-the-counter (OTC) acid blocker, such as *Zantac 75* or *Pepcid AC*. If these drugs don't help, ask your doctor about prescription-strength versions. *Tagamet*, a similar drug, is no more effective than Zantac or Pepcid and is more likely to interact with other drugs.

Cisapride (Propulsid) and other prescription drugs that promote "motility" (movement of food through the gut) can also be helpful. These drugs can be used alone or in combination with other drugs. The prescription drug called *omeprazole* (Prilosec) also appears to be very effective against GERD.

The last resort for controlling GERD is usually surgery. In one procedure, called *fundoplication*, the surgeon wraps the upper portion of the stomach around the lower end of the esophagus. This operation can be very effective—although it isn't always and symptoms may recur years later.

If you go this route, be sure to ask your doctor about laparoscopic techniques. They require smaller incisions and afford faster recovery than conventional surgery. Check the surgeon's track record, too. Some have much better luck than others.

Test Your Knowledge About the Common Cold

William Schaffner, MD, chairman of the department of preventive medicine at Vanderbilt University School of Medicine, Nashville is a fellow of the Infectious Diseases Society of America, and a liaison member of the Advisory Committee on Immunization Practices of the Centers for Disease Control and Prevention.

The average American gets more than 100 colds in his/her lifetime, and scientists have amassed lots of information about the common cold. But misinformation still is widely circulated as fact. *Take the following quiz to see how much you really know about the common cold...*

•*True or False?* **Colds are mainly spread by coughs and sneezes.**

False: The viruses that cause colds usually are spread by hand-to-hand, hand-to-nose or hand-to-object contact. The *rhinovirus*, the most common cold virus, flourishes in mucous membranes. Someone infected with the virus rubs his nose or eyes, picking up the virus on his fingers. He then touches you or deposits the virus on another surface (doorknob, telephone, etc.). The virus can survive for 24 to 48 hours, so it can be readily picked up by the next person who comes along.

•*True or False?* **People with colds are highly contagious before they experience symptoms.**

True: You're most contagious in the 24 hours before symptoms start. You may feel healthy, but the virus is incubating—and spreading. Colds often are transmitted during this period because people who are infected aren't yet staying home—and other people aren't avoiding them the way they would someone who is coughing or sneezing.

•*True or False?* **Antimicrobial soap kills cold viruses.**

False: Antimicrobial soap kills bacteria, not the viruses that cause colds. The best protection against colds is to wash your hands often with warm, soapy water. It takes about a minute of washing to remove viruses from your hands.

Waterless alcohol-based hand sanitizers can be helpful when soap and water aren't available. Hand sanitizers such as Purell and Nexcare kill cold viruses, as do disposable alcohol towelettes.

•*True or False?* **Being cold increases the risk of getting a cold.**

False: Generations of moms have said, "Bundle up or you'll catch a cold"—but the best current evidence indicates that Mom was wrong.

In one well-regarded study, scientists divided volunteers into a "warm" group and a group that was damp and chilled. They exposed people in both groups to cold viruses. There was no difference in the incidence of subsequent colds between the two groups.

Opposing view: In a study recently reported in *Journal of Family Practice*, scientists did find an increase in colds in volunteers who soaked their feet in icy water for 20 minutes. This wasn't a controlled experiment, however. The scientists didn't know, for example, if the volunteers who got sick had more contact with people who already had colds than those who didn't get sick.

Cold weather brings an increase in colds, but being cold doesn't seem to be a factor.

•*True or False?* **Vitamin C has been proven to reduce the duration and/or severity of colds.**

False: Ever since the publication of Linus Pauling's book *Vitamin C and the Common Cold*, millions of Americans have attempted to prevent and/or treat colds by taking enormous amounts of vitamin C—as much as 1,000 milligrams (mg) every few hours. Since then, many studies have looked at the connection between colds and vitamin C. Most have been inconclusive—and many showed no benefit at all. In large doses, vitamin C inhibits the effects of *histamine*, a body chemical that causes sniffles and other cold symptoms. Yet there's no evidence that reducing histamine in this way has any effect on cold symptoms—and studies have not shown that it prevents colds.

Caution: Vitamin C is cleared through the kidneys. Taking large amounts can cause the vitamin to crystallize and result in kidney stones. Drink more water than usual if you decide to take extra vitamin C—and don't exceed 250 mg to 500 mg daily.

•*True or False?* **Yellow or green mucus indicates a serious infection.**

False: People who develop yellow or greenish mucus often rush to their doctors to ask for antibiotics because they believe that discolored mucus indicates a serious bacterial infection.

Colds can cause either clear, watery mucus or mucus that's thick and discolored. The coloration means that there's inflammation and more white blood cells. These immune cells are present in both viral and bacterial infections. Discolored mucus isn't a useful way to distinguish one from the other—and it doesn't mean that your cold is more serious or that it will last longer.

•*True or False?* **We get fewer colds as we get older.**

True: There are approximately 200 different viruses that cause colds. Each time your immune system is exposed to one of these viruses, it develops antibodies that make you immune to that particular strain. By the time you reach your 60s or 70s and have a lifetime of colds behind you, you have developed immunity to many—but not all—of the circulating cold viruses.

•*True or False?* **Stress increases the likelihood of getting a cold.**

False: There are theoretical reasons to think that emotional stress could increase the risk of getting a cold, but it has never been shown conclusively.

Studies have shown that chronic stress decreases the immune system's ability to suppress infections. But stress is ubiquitous —nearly everyone reports having stress in the days or weeks before a survey—so it's difficult to link it with illness.

•*True or False?* **Hot tea eases cold symptoms.**

True: Black and green tea both contain theophylline, a mild bronchodilator. Drinking tea when you have a cold may open the airways and make breathing easier. The heat and steam from the liquid also thin mucus and ease congestion.

Chicken soup also is a traditional remedy for colds—but don't expect too much. Though it provides extra fluids and the steam eases congestion, chicken soup cannot cure a cold, despite what many people think.

How to Avoid Irregularity

Adriane Fugh-Berman, MD, associate professor, complementary and alternative medicine, Georgetown University School of Medicine. She is author of *Alternative Medicine: What Works.* Lippincott, Williams & Wilkins.

How often should one have a bowel movement? In medical school, I was taught that "normal" people empty their bowels from several times a day to once a week.

I don't believe that anymore. Having a bowel movement more than once a day is okay. But having a bowel movement only once a week is definitely not normal—or healthful. Chronic constipation can lead to health problems.

First, chronic constipation promotes precancerous changes in colon cells. Presumably this is because these cells are exposed to bile acids and other toxins in intestinal waste for a longer-than-optimal period of time.

Constipation can also lead to hemorrhoids. People suffering from constipation often must strain to empty their bowels, and straining causes a buildup of pressure inside blood vessels lining the anal canal. Hemorrhoids are simply varicose veins in the anal canal.

What causes constipation? The most common causes are a lack of fiber in the diet… insufficient consumption of water…and a sedentary lifestyle.

Constipation is also a side effect of certain medications. These include codeine and other opiate painkillers…tricyclic antidepressants such as *amitriptyline* (Elavil)…*pseudoephedrine* (Sudafed) and other decongestants…and Maalox and other aluminum-based antacids.

Calcium can also be the constipation culprit. If you're taking calcium supplements, you should be taking magnesium supplements as well. Taken at about half the dosage of the calcium, magnesium helps counteract the constipating effect of the calcium.

Now for curing constipation. You've already heard that boosting your intake of dietary fiber can help make you regular. But I want to stress that you also need lots of water. In fact, eating more fiber without simultaneously increasing your intake of water can make constipation worse instead of better. I recommend drinking at least eight eight-ounce glasses of water each day.

Dietary fiber is found in fruits, vegetables and whole grains. If eating more high-fiber foods (and drinking more water) doesn't work for you, consider trying Metamucil or another over-the-counter psyllium seed product. Psyllium seed is a "bulking agent," and not a true (cathartic) laxative. Yet it's very effective against constipation.

Unlike laxatives, psyllium can safely be taken on a daily basis. Daily use of laxatives can lead to "lazy" bowels and to even worse constipation—not to mention dehydration and life-threatening imbalances in the body's sodium-potassium balance. Laxatives should be used only for occasional trouble.

One of the few laxatives recommended by conventional and alternative practitioners alike is tea made from the herb *senna*, which is available at health-food stores. Senna tea is quite effective, but I've found an even more potent remedy—*sennaed prunes*.

To make sennaed prunes, pour enough boiling water over a cup of prunes to cover them. Drop in a senna tea bag. Remove the tea bag after five to 20 minutes—the longer the bag stays in, the stronger the tea. Refrigerate the prune-senna mixture overnight before eating.

By the way, while caffeinated coffee has laxative properties, ordinary black tea contains *tannins*, compounds that cause constipation.

Mosquito Prevention

Bernice Lifton, a resident of Pasadena, CA, who has researched natural ways of eliminating pests. She is author of *Bug Busters*. Square One Publishers.

To mosquito-proof your property, eliminate any water-collecting places where they may breed.

Examples: Sagging gutters can accumulate water—so have them checked. Fix leaky outdoor faucets…put drainage by air conditioners so puddles do not gather underneath. Empty birdbaths every three days. If you put drinking water outside for pets, change it daily.

Also: Get rid of old tires and abandoned toys…and put away kids' wading pools that aren't being used.

Cuts and Scrapes

Alfred Lane, MD, professor of dermatology, Stanford University, Stanford, CA.

Many doctors advise patients to keep wounds dry to avoid infection. But in a study of premature babies, cuts treated with a petroleum-based ointment (*Aquaphor*) healed quicker and were less likely to become infected than those not treated. Researchers say the same treatment should also help adults' wounds.

No More Snoring

Gary Zammit, PhD, director of the Sleep Disorders Institute, New York.

Researchers believe snoring is caused by the vibration of soft tissues in response to turbulent air flow within the upper airway. Nasal strips, sold in drugstores, are narrow pieces of springy plastic encased in adhesive strips. When fastened to the outside of the nose so that the nostrils are opened up, the strip opens up the constricted passage, reducing the turbulence.

Caution: Their value for more serious disturbances, like sleep apnea, has not been demonstrated. If you suspect sleep apnea, seek expert evaluation. This condition can cause serious consequences.

Children and Sex

Jan Faull, child development and behavior specialist, Seattle, writing online in *Family Planet.*

Talking to children about sex should not be a one-time talk—and not strictly anatomical. The topic will come up as a child grows older. When a child asks a straightforward question, answer directly and honestly in an age-appropriate way, using the correct names for body parts. Then respond to any follow-up questions.

Bottom line: Be glad your children come to you with questions—otherwise, they will go elsewhere to learn about sex. If you do not answer perfectly the first time, you can always restate your answer later.

No More Mumbling

Ann Mitchell, licensed speech pathologist with the Rehabilitation Center, Falls Church, VA.

If you tend to mumble, take a deep breath and exhale slowly while counting out loud …continue counting at a steady rhythm, leaving about half a second between the numbers. Most adults can reach between 15 and 20 before they need to inhale. If you can't get past 10, you need to practice taking deeper, more controlled breaths as you speak.

Spring Allergies?

Peter B. Boggs, MD, an allergist in private practice in Shreveport, LA, and former president of the American College of Allergy, Asthma and Immunology, Arlington Heights, IL. He is author of *Sneezing Your Head Off? How to Live with Your Allergic Nose.* Patient Education Publishers.

If you suffer from seasonal allergies—as 22 million Americans do—both established and new treatments can relieve your allergy symptoms without putting you to sleep or forcing you to stay indoors.

HOW ALLERGIES START

Allergies occur when you inherit a genetic disposition to form allergic antibodies upon coming into contact with normally benign substances.

If one of your parents has an allergy, you have a 30% chance of being allergic, too. If both parents suffer from allergies, your risk jumps to 50% to 75%. If neither parent has allergies, your chance is only 13%.

You inherit and pass along only the propensity for allergies, not the specific allergies themselves.

Example: If your mother is allergic to cats, you may not develop the same allergy—but you may be allergic to pollen instead.

Still, having allergy-provoking genetic material isn't enough to prompt sniffling and sneezing. You must also be exposed to various allergens, such as dust mites…tree, grass or weed pollen …animals…mold…feathers…insect stings…and certain foods. The allergens are so widespread that they're really impossible to avoid.

Example: The most common causes of hay fever during early spring are tree pollens. Later in the spring, grass pollens are typically to blame. And in the fall, weed pollens spur many people to suffer allergic reactions.

HOW YOUR BODY FIGHTS BACK

After you come into contact with an allergen, your body regards it as a foreign object. When your body next detects this substance, your immune system launches an all-out attack to get rid of it. During this offensive, chemicals such as histamine, leukotrienes and prostaglandin D2 are released.

These chemicals—and the ensuing nasal inflammation—are responsible for the allergy symptoms of congestion…runny nose and eyes …sneezing…and itching in the nose, throat, eyes and ears.

TRADITIONAL TREATMENTS

•**Avoid allergy triggers.** This is the single most effective and inexpensive means at your disposal to ward off allergy symptoms. *Here's how to do it…*

•**Avoid outdoor activities between 5 a.m. and 10 a.m.** That's when pollen counts are highest.

•**Shower and change clothes when you come in** from working or playing outdoors. Pollen can cling to clothing and rub off on furniture.

•**Close windows and doors and run an air conditioner in the house and car** to filter pollen from the air you breathe. Avoid window and attic fans, which are notorious for drawing pollen into the house.

•**Antihistamines and decongestants** are the mainstays of seasonal allergy treatment. They're very effective for relieving symptoms quickly.

•**Antihistamines** don't prevent the allergic reaction, but they stop its symptoms, such as sneezing and watery eyes, by interfering with the action of histamine.

A slew of nonprescription and prescription antihistamines is available today. They are generally effective but may cause drowsiness or dizziness. *Caution...*

•**Don't take antihistamines at all** if you have glaucoma, a persistent cough or an enlarged prostate.

•**Decongestants**—available with and without a prescription—relieve nasal stuffiness by constricting blood vessels in the nose. They can cause dizziness or nervousness and can make it hard to sleep. *Cautions...*

•**Don't use decongestants** if you have heart or thyroid disease, high blood pressure, diabetes or an enlarged prostate, without discussing it with your physician.

•**Don't use over-the-counter (OTC) decongestant sprays** for longer than five days. They may actually cause increased stuffiness.

•**Steroid nasal sprays.** Prescription steroid nasal sprays—such as Beconase, Flonase, Nasacort, Rhinocort and Vancenase—reverse swelling in the nose and block the allergic reaction.

When you spray these steroid nasal sprays into your nose once or twice a day, they also stop the twitchiness that plagues allergy sufferers—and makes the nose more likely to react to allergens and irritants such as cigarette smoke and other pollutants.

These steroid sprays work well when combined with antihistamines and decongestants. However, if you can't tolerate those drugs, they can also be used alone.

Important: Start using a steroid nasal spray one or two weeks prior to the allergy season. This will help to prevent the inflammatory process before it begins. Many sufferers use nasal sprays daily for several months at a time. Steroid sprays cause few side effects if used at recommended doses.

•**Allergy shots.** If your allergy symptoms are severe...you have asthma...you get frequent ear infections...or you don't respond to oral or nasal allergy drugs—immunotherapy is another option.

Procedure: You'll be given a series of shots that contain progressively larger doses of allergen extracts.

You'll likely build up immunity to these allergens. You may, however, still need to take oral or nasal drugs to help control your allergic symptoms.

MEDICATIONS

•**Allegra** is a nonsedating prescription antihistamine.

•**Astelin** is a nasal antihistamine spray. It's available only by prescription. Astelin works within a few minutes after spraying, lasts 12 hours, doesn't cause drowsiness and has few side effects.

•**Claritin Reditabs** dissolve almost instantly when placed on the tongue. This means that they can be taken by children and adults who otherwise cannot take pills.

•**Nasalcrom** is a nonsteroidal nasal spray that has been used for years and is now available without a prescription.

Nasalcrom is extremely safe and effective at preventing the allergic reaction from taking place, reduces inflammation in the nose and doesn't cause drowsiness.

Most sufferers use it three to four times a day, starting a week or two before the allergy season begins.

•**Zyrtec** is another prescription antihistamine. It may cause some drowsiness—though not as much as OTC antihistamines—and is safe and effective.

Hepatitis B Vaccine And Preteens

Ann M. Arvin, MD, professor of pediatrics and microbiology/immunology and chief of the division of infectious diseases, Stanford University School of Medicine, Stanford, CA.

The hepatitis B virus (HBV), which can be transmitted sexually or via use of intravenous drugs, is 100 times more prevalent (and far more infectious) than the AIDS virus. All children 11 to 13 years of age should be vaccinated—whether or not their parents think they are sexually active or involved with drugs.

Kids Get Ulcers, Too

Mark A. Gilger, MD, associate professor of pediatrics and gastroenterology, Baylor College of Medicine, Houston.

Causes include infection with the bacterium *Helicobactor pylori*...reaction to certain drugs...stress caused by serious injury, infection or disease.

Symptoms parents should look for: Recurrent abdominal pain...awakening in the night with abdominal pain...recurrent vomiting ...vomiting blood. Most ulcers are treatable with antacids...and curable with antibiotics.

Young Children Don't Need Pillows

Jay Berkelhamer, MD, senior vice president, medical affairs, Children's Healthcare, Atlanta, and former president, American Academy of Pediatrics (AAP).

Kids up to age two or three seem to sleep better without them. And pillows and other soft bedding can be dangerous to very young children—they may contribute to the suffocation of as many as 1,800 infants each year.

Music and Babies

Jayne M. Standley, PhD, professor of music therapy, Florida State University, Tallahassee. Her study of 20 premature infants was published in *Pediatric Nursing*, E. Holly Ave., Box 56, Pitman, NJ 08071.

Music helps premature babies grow stronger. When lullabies were played in a hospital neonatal unit, preemies' blood-oxygen levels (a key measure of health) went up. When the music stopped, their blood-oxygen levels fell.

Your Baby's Diet

Study by researchers at the University of Illinois, Urbana-Champaign, IL.

When your baby refuses new foods, try again tomorrow.

Reason: It's natural for a baby to reject unfamiliar tastes. But most babies will eventually learn to like most foods. In a study, when babies were offered pureed peas or green beans for 10 consecutive days, they ate twice as much on the tenth day as they had on the first.

What Never to Feed Young Children

Martha V. White, MD, director of pediatric allergy and research, Institute for Asthma & Allergy, Wheaton, MD.

Peanuts are easily aspirated into the lungs ...and peanuts are one of the most common—and dangerous—foods to which one may develop an allergy.

Most at risk: Those from high-risk families —where both parents or one parent and a sibling are food-allergic. Even trace quantities can trigger an attack in peanut-allergic individuals.

Example: A boy began wheezing when a jar of peanut butter was merely opened nearby.

Helpful: Alert teachers and other caregivers to the food allergy...have the child wear a Medic-Alert bracelet (call 888-633-4298 for information)...older children should be taught to use spring-loaded syringes of epinephrine to ward off attacks after inadvertently ingesting a food to which they are allergic.

Exercise Benefits

James F. Clapp, MD, professor emeritus of reproductive biology, Case Western Reserve University, Cleveland, whose study of 65 newborn infants was published in the *American Journal of Obstetrics and Gynecology,* 11830 Westline Industrial Dr., St. Louis 63146.

Babies are more alert and less fussy if their mothers exercised regularly during pregnancy. *Note:* Always check with your doctor before starting any exercise program.

Prevent Infant Tooth Decay

Steven Grossman, DDS, co-chief of pediatric dentistry, Lenox Hill Hospital, New York.

Make sure your child's teeth are treated with fluoride...avoid sweet substances on pacifiers...use plain water in his/her bottle at bedtime...clean teeth and gums with a washcloth after feeding...brush his teeth once a day starting at age two or before...begin regular dental checkups as soon as the child's 20 baby teeth have erupted.

Lead and Obesity

Rokho Kim, MD, MPH, instructor of medicine, Harvard Medical School, Boston. His study of 79 young adults was published in *Environmental Health Perspectives,* 14600 Weston Pkwy., Ste. 100, Cary, NC 27513.

Exposure to lead during childhood can lead to obesity and shorter stature in adulthood. The greater the exposure between ages seven and 20, the greater the future weight gain.

SIDS Fact

E.A. Mitchell, MD, professor, department of pediatrics, University of Auckland, New Zealand, writing in *The Lancet,* 32 Jamestown Rd., London NW1 7BY.

Sleeping with an infant can put the baby at increased risk of Sudden Infant Death Syndrome (SIDS). The reason isn't known—but may be related to airway obstruction or rebreathing air that a parent has exhaled.

At greatest risk: Infants whose mothers smoke. A mother who smokes may safely breast-feed and comfort her child in bed but should not let the baby sleep with her.

Getting Kids to Eat Fruits and Vegetables

Tufts University Health & Nutrition Letter, 196 Boston Ave., Ste. 2100, Medford, MA 02155.

Kids eat more fruits and vegetables when healthful produce is part of meals instead of side dishes.

Helpful: Add pureed cooked vegetables to ground-meat dishes like meatloaf and hamburgers...substitute shredded carrots, zucchini or chopped spinach for some or all of the ground meat in lasagna or a casserole...add pureed or shredded vegetables and fruits to homemade muffins, cookies, cakes and quick breads...use pureed cooked apples or pears as a sauce for poultry, and whole pineapple chunks or rings to top baked or grilled chicken breast...mix unsweetened applesauce or fresh apples into hot cereal.

Kids and Sunglasses Safety

Stephen Miller, MD, director, clinical care center, American Optometric Association, St. Louis.

Children should wear sunglasses at the beach, pool or wherever sunlight will be reflected into their eyes.

Reason: A young child's eyes have less light-filtering pigment than an adult's eyes do, and are therefore especially vulnerable to cumulative eye damage from the sun's damaging UV rays.

Best: Lenses made of impact-resistant plastic or polycarbonate and that block 99% to 100% of both UVA and UVB rays.

The Value of Imaginary Friends

Jerome L. Singer, PhD, professor of psychology and child study, Yale University, New Haven, CT.

Imaginary playmates are the product of a child's needs and imagination. Two-thirds of preschoolers have them—and those who do tend to be more independent, cooperative with teachers and peers, happier and less aggressive than kids who do not have them. These playmates help children share ideas and feelings with adults that they might not otherwise feel comfortable expressing. Parents should accept imaginary companions—but not too enthusiastically. Kids need to feel that they retain complete control over imaginary friends.

Sleep and Behavior

Rafael Pelayo, MD, assistant professor, Sleep Disorders Clinic, Stanford University, Stanford, CA.

Too little sleep can lead to behavioral problems in children. Sleepy children tend to subconsciously look for things to stimulate them. This can lead to disruptive behavior.

Bottom line: A hyperactive child may actually be suffering from sleep deprivation.

Guidelines: Eight to 12 hours of sleep a day from toddlerhood through adulthood.

Helpful: To get children to adjust to an earlier bedtime, move bedtime back by 15 minutes each day.

Poison Alert

Mark Wortman, *Yale Children's Health Letter*, Yale University School of Medicine, New Haven, CT.

Top causes of poisoning in kids: Household cleaning products...analgesics such as aspirin, acetaminophen and ibuprofen...cosmetics and personal-care products...household plants that are toxic if ingested.

Important: If you suspect poisoning or exposure, call your pediatrician or state Poison Control Center immediately.

Kids and Caffeine

Study of 400 New York City preschoolers, reported in *Eating Well*, 823A Ferry Rd., Box 1010, Charlotte, VT 05445.

A study of 400 preschoolers found that 10% of them drink enough cola and iced tea every day to down an adult's caffeine equivalent of two cups of coffee.

Possible result: Jumpy and inattentive children.

Better: Drinks that are "caffeine-free."

Secondhand Smoke And Kids

Nancy J. Haley, MD, whose study was conducted while she was with the American Health Foundation, Valhalla, NY. Her study of more than 500 children, ages one to five, was published in *The New England Journal of Medicine*, 10 Shattuck St., Boston 02115.

Children who are exposed to tobacco smoke are three-and-a-half times more likely to develop respiratory illnesses—especially upper-respiratory problems—than ones who are not exposed. Children exposed to secondhand smoke have significant concentrations of a nicotine derivative in their urine. The more smokers in a child's home, the greater the concentration of nicotine by-products in the child's body and the greater the likelihood of respiratory problems.

Kids and Dehydration

Oded Bar-Or, MD, director, Children's Exercise and Nutrition Centre, McMaster University, Hamilton, Ontario.

Kids are more vulnerable to dehydration than adults. Youngsters don't sweat as much as adults, so they cannot cool their bodies as efficiently.

Problem: By the time a child feels thirsty, he/she is probably already at the beginning stages of dehydration.

Symptoms: Apathy…light-headedness…fatigue…nausea.

Helpful: To encourage kids to drink enough, offer them diluted fruit juice or sports drinks.

Avoid: Undiluted fruit juice and sweetened carbonated beverages, since their high sugar content can cause stomach cramps.

Skin Care for Kids in Puberty

Neal Schultz, MD, dermatologist in private practice in New York.

Eat plenty of fresh fruits and vegetables…drink lots of water…get regular exercise and fresh air…get plenty of sleep…keep skin clean by washing with gentle soap and water …use sunscreen to protect against the sun's harmful rays.

Don't Forget This Person

How Was Your Day, Baby? A Childcare Journal for Working Parents by Melanie Goldish, a working mother in Hoffman Estates, IL. Tracer Publishing.

Take your caregiver to the pediatrician, too, when your baby has an appointment. He/she will have observed your baby closely and may have important information to tell the doctor. It can also be useful for the caregiver to hear what the doctor has to say.

Balloon Danger

Frank Rimell, MD, a pediatric otolaryngologist at the department of pediatric otolaryngology, University of Minnesota, Minneapolis. His study of more than 600 children who died or underwent endoscopy for removal of objects that were choking them was published in the *Journal of the American Medical Association*, 515 N. State St., Chicago 60610.

Children under the age of three are the most likely to choke on common objects—but balloons can be dangerous to kids of all ages.

Other dangerous items: Hot dogs, nuts, seeds, vegetable and fruit pieces.

Troubling: Some children can choke on objects that pass federal small-parts hazard tests aimed at keeping dangerously small items out of young children's hands.

Self-defense: Watch children carefully. Only allow young kids to play with items that are significantly bigger than the minimum size allowed under US rules, which is about the diameter of a toilet paper roll. And look for child-safety warning labels on toy packages.

Children and Choking

David H. Darrow, MD, DDS, associate professor of otolaryngology and pediatrics, Eastern Virginia Medical School, Norfolk.

Most common objects that kill: Balloons and hot dogs.

Most common objects inhaled: Seeds… nuts, particularly peanuts.

Most common objects stuck in the throat: Coins. A child who inhales a foreign object into the bronchi and lungs will commonly have an episode of coughing, followed by wheezing. A child with an object stuck in his/her throat will complain of pain when swallowing and have severe vomiting. If you suspect your child has inhaled or swallowed an object, bring him to an emergency room for treatment.

How to Help Your Child Have a Great Time at Camp

Bruce Muchnick, EdD, a licensed psychologist in private practice, Glenside, PA. His work includes psychotherapy with children and adults, management consulting and a "subspecialty" in camp psychology. Dr. Muchnick advises camp owners, directors, camping professionals and parents throughout the year and works with camp staffs during the summer.

Summer camp is more than a country vacation for children. At camp, kids learn to appreciate the outdoors, develop companionship and pick up skills that enhance self-reliance, cooperation and interdependence. These skills will remain with them throughout childhood and into adulthood.

Camp also serves as a kind of refuge where children can unburden themselves of the pressures at home. Camp frees them, gets their creative juices flowing and renews their sense of being kids.

To help your child have a successful time at camp this summer…

●**Learning to let go** allows children to develop autonomy and a stronger sense of self. It also gives parents a chance to take care of themselves and get to know each other again. When children return, parents can feel refreshed and be available and accessible to them again.

●**Prepare for camp together.** Decisions about camp—like where to go and what to pack—should be a joint venture, keeping in mind your child's level of maturity. If your child feels part of the decision-making process, his/her chances of having a positive experience will improve.

●**Don't buy a whole new wardrobe.** Camp is more rugged than life at home. A child doesn't need new clothes…and having well-worn clothes and familiar possessions will help ease the transition. This is especially important for first-time campers.

●**Talk about concerns.** As the first day of camp approaches, some children experience uneasiness about going away. Children should be encouraged to talk about these feelings. Ask your child about his feelings rather than acting on what you think his feelings may be. Communicate confidence in his ability to handle being away from home and remind him about successes he has experienced in other situations.

●**Have realistic expectations.** Camp, like the rest of life, has high points and low ones. Not every moment will be filled with wonder and excitement. At times, your child will feel great while at other times he may feel unhappy or bored. And kids may not always get along well with each other.

Solution: Encourage your child to have a reasonable and realistic view of camp by discussing—in advance—both the ups and downs. Camp experiences will provide opportunities for problem solving, negotiating, increased self-awareness and greater sensitivity toward others. Don't send your child to camp feeling pressured to succeed. The main purposes of camp are to relax and have fun.

WHEN YOUR CHILD IS AT CAMP

●**Don't call within the first two weeks** if your child will be away at camp for the whole summer. It takes that long to adjust to being away…and a call from home may disrupt the process. It's hard to get an accurate sense of how a child is managing over the phone—this can be unsettling for you and your child, so it's best not to call at all.

●**Communicate in writing.** Summer camp offers kids and parents the chance to develop a rarely practiced skill—letter writing. Write as often as you want. Keep in mind that this is your child's connection to home and family.

Your letters should be upbeat. It's fine to write that you miss your child, but don't include things like *The house is so quiet without you.*

Better: Ask specific questions in your letters about your child's activities…bunk life…friends, etc. This will help him organize his letters home.

●**Packages are appreciated every now and then.** But don't send food—it's disruptive if some kids in the cabin receive food packages and others receive nothing. Receiving food packages may be contrary to camp policy. If your child asks you to sneak food packages, don't. Even if you think a rule is silly, breaking a camp rule might interfere with your child's sense of right and wrong.

Better: Send postcards, cartoons, newspaper and magazine articles, comics, game books, puzzles and other items that can be shared with friends.

Example: Tell your child...*I understand that you're hungry. That's why you have three great meals each day and snacks. I'll send you some comic books. Hope you enjoy them. Why don't you share them with your bunk?*

● **Don't make major changes at home.** This is not the time to redecorate his room or get rid of his pet snake. When kids return from camp, they like their rooms and their lives to be the same as when they left.

● **Help your child cope at camp.** Most kids need a few days to adjust to life at camp and being away from home. During this time, many experience homesickness. They miss familiar surroundings, parents, pets and friends.

Most kids cope with these concerns and—with the help of camp staff—build support systems. If your child's letters contain urgent pleas for you to bring him home, resist the temptation to rush to camp. Avoid making deals, such as *Give camp one more week. If you're still unhappy, we'll bring you home.*

Better: Support your child's efforts to work out problems with the help of the director and the camp's staff.

Communicate your love and confidence in your child's ability to work through problems. Remind him, if necessary, that he has made a commitment for the summer. Overcoming homesickness and upsets in the cabin and learning to care for oneself are important challenges faced at camp.

Important: If you sense legitimacy in your child's complaints, talk candidly with the camp director. Allow the director and staff an opportunity to apply their expertise in helping kids adapt to the routines of camp life. Follow up with another call a few days later. Most adjustment difficulties can be worked through.

● **Trust your instincts.** The occasional child who is truly not enjoying anything, having a

miserable time and not adjusting to camp life at all should be allowed to return home after a reasonable amount of time and effort.

Keep in mind that some kids feel guilty when an experience like camp does not work out for them. They may feel that they have let their parents down.

If your child leaves camp, let him know he has not failed and there will be other summers with other adventures.

WHEN YOUR CHILD COMES HOME

After a summer of fun, adventure and freedom, fitting back into the family and assuming responsibilities may be a challenge for some kids.

Strategy: Give him time and space for this reentry process. Support the positive changes you observe. Reintroduce "house rules" with patience and awareness that your child has done some maturing over the summer.

Safety Standards for Children's Camps

Reported in *Parents*, 375 Lexington Ave., New York 10017.

Is playground equipment well-maintained and age-appropriate? Are campers required to wear protective gear, such as helmets and pads, when playing sports? Are lifeguards certified by the YMCA or the Red Cross? Does the camp have a full-time health manager on-site who is certified in CPR and first aid and can administer medicines? Is there a nearby hospital for emergencies? Are camp vans and buses equipped with seat belts?

Warts and Children

Karl Beutner, MD, PhD, associate clinical professor of dermatology at the University of California at San Francisco.

About one in six school-age children will have warts at one time or another. While there are treatments, it isn't necessary to do anything. Often the warts will clear up by themselves. In children, 66% clear up in two years without treatment.

Treatments: Over-the-counter medications containing salicylic acid, which will get rid of warts within 12 weeks and is the least frightening treatment…or a dermatologist can freeze them with liquid nitrogen…lightly burn them with an electric probe…cut them off…or prescribe topical acids that are stronger than over-the-counter ones. The most effective treatment depends on the age of the patient, the number of warts and their locations.

Helping Your Kids Relax

Playwise: 365 Fun-Filled Activities for Building Character, Conscience and Emotional Intelligence in Children by Denise Chapman Weston, MSW, licensed play therapist, North Attleboro, MA. Penguin Group.

Teach kids to breathe deeply—important to developing the relaxation habit. When blowing bubbles, have your child take deep breaths, then breathe slowly into the wand. Or tape a four-inch strip of crepe paper to the bridge of child-sized sunglasses so it hangs in front of your child's nose—have him/her blow on it to see how long he can keep it off his face. Or have him pick a short song to sing or hum in a single breath. Or have him inhale and exhale into a harmonica—and see how long he can keep it going.

Anxiety Disorders In the Family

Vanessa E. Cobham, PhD, clinical psychologist, School of Psychology, University of Queensland, Brisbane, Australia.

More than 80% of anxious children have at least one parent who has a personal history of anxiety.

Good news: Cognitive-behavioral therapy is often helpful for such children—but only if the parent also undergoes therapy. For referral to a cognitive-behavioral therapist in your area, contact the American Psychological Association at 800-964-2000, *www.apa.org.*

How to Stop a Child's Bed-Wetting

Marla R. Ullom-Minnich, MD, a family physician in private practice in Moundridge, KS.

Reward the child for dry nights…have him change the sheets himself when he has an accident…have him practice holding his urine during the day for longer and longer periods of time.

Also helpful: A mattress pad that sounds an alarm when the child wets it. *Cost:* About $100.

Bed-Wetting Prevention Alert

Rudi A. Janknegt, MD, head, department of urology, University Hospital, Maastricht, The Netherlands. His 24-week study of 66 bed wetters was published in *The Journal of Urology,* 1000 Corporate Blvd., Linthicum, MD 21090.

Anti-bed-wetting nasal spray is often ineffective when the bed wetter has a cold or flu. Congestion keeps the medication, *desmopressin,* from being absorbed.

Good news: Desmopressin *pills* are 90% effective at stopping bed-wetting—even if the child or adult is congested.

ADHD Relief

Timothy Wilens, MD, associate professor of psychiatry, Harvard Medical School, Boston.

Attention deficit hyperactivity disorder (ADHD) can often be controlled with *desipramine* (Norpramin). In a study, 68% of adult ADHD sufferers treated with this antidepressant experienced significant reduction in 12 of 14 symptoms (including short attention span). None of the ADHD sufferers given a placebo showed improvement. Desipramine is the only nonstimulant drug shown in controlled trials to be effective against adult ADHD. Stimulants, including *methylphenidate* (Ritalin) and *dextroamphetamine* (Dexedrine), remain the "first-line" drugs for ADHD.

Ear Infections

Matti Uhari, MD, professor of pediatrics, University of Oulu, Oulu, Finland.

Childhood ear infections can be prevented with sugarless gum sweetened with *xylitol.*

Study: Only 12% of kids who chewed the gum five times a day came down with ear infections. This compares with 21% who chewed gum sweetened with ordinary sugar (sucrose).

Theory: Xylitol blocks growth of *Streptococcus pneumoniae*, a bacterium thought to cause 30% of ear infections.

Childhood Ear Infection?

Elizabeth Barnett, MD, assistant professor of pediatrics, Boston City Hospital. Her study of ear infections in 484 children three months to three years of age was published in *Pediatrics*, 141 Northwest Point Blvd., Elk Grove Village, IL 60007.

A single injection of the antibiotic *ceftriaxone* (Rocephin) works as well as 10 days of oral medication. Nearly two-thirds of all kids have at least one ear infection by their first birthday. Although oral antibiotics remain the first choice, an injection may be appropriate for children who are vomiting and can't keep medication down...children who refuse to take an oral medication...and children who are enrolled in a day care center that won't dispense medications. Parents should discuss with a pediatrician the best option for their child.

Restless Legs Syndrome... Almost Five Million Sufferers...How to Tell If You're One and What to Do About It

Arthur S. Walters, MD, clinical professor of neurology at the University of Medicine and Dentistry of New Jersey–Robert Wood Johnson Medical School in New Brunswick. An expert on sleep disorders, he is the editor of *Sleep Thief, Restless Legs Syndrome* by Virginia N. Wilson. Galaxy Books.

If you have trouble sleeping because of a burning, tingling or "creepy-crawly" sensation in your legs, you may be suffering from *restless legs syndrome* (RLS).

This neurological disorder affects 2% of the population—some so severely that they're unable to sit still long enough to travel in an automobile or airplane or see a movie.

RLS isn't dangerous, but it can seriously disrupt your sleep and your quality of life.

TELLTALE SYMPTOMS

RLS sufferers generally have more leg discomfort when sitting or lying down than when standing. The leg discomfort is especially bad at night, making it hard to fall asleep.

Some sufferers kick during sleep. All have an almost uncontrollable desire to move their legs around.

RLS can strike at any age, but most cases occur after age 40. It often gets worse over time. There is no known way to prevent RLS.

One-third to one-half of all cases of RLS seem to be inherited. RLS can also be caused by nerve damage in the legs—typically the result of diabetes, kidney disease or a pinched nerve in the back...a deficiency of iron...or, theoretically, a deficiency of the neurotransmitter *dopamine*.

CONTROLLING SYMPTOMS

Some RLS sufferers derive relief from iron supplements. The typical dosage is 300 mg three times a day—but check with your doctor first to make sure supplements are right for you.

Others swear by supplements of vitamins E and B-12 and folate. My most severely affected patients, however, generally do *not* benefit from vitamin supplements.

What about nondrug therapies? *Two seem to be particularly helpful...*

●**Revise your sleep schedule.** Try to sleep when your RLS symptoms are least pronounced. You may be able to work out a flextime arrangement with your employer to accommodate this schedule.

●**Avoid caffeine and alcohol.** They make RLS worse.

CONSULTING A DOCTOR

If symptoms persist, consult a doctor who has experience treating RLS patients. Unfortunately, RLS is often misdiagnosed as anxiety, stress, depression or garden-variety insomnia. Doctors often have a difficult time recognizing RLS, because patients seldom display the telltale leg symptoms in the doctor's office.

Once properly diagnosed, however—either by a primary-care doctor or a neurologist specializing in sleep or movement disorders—RLS can be effectively treated.

Well-controlled clinical trials indicate that 80% of RLS sufferers experience relief from long-term use of one or more of the following drugs...

●*L-dopa*, *pergolide* **(Permax) or *bromocriptine* (Parlodel).** These drugs boost dopamine levels. *Potential side effects:* Nausea, vomiting, light-headedness and fainting and "rebound" of symptoms into daylight hours.

●*Clonazepam* **(Klonopin) and other benzodiazepines.** *Potential side effects:* Drowsiness and mental dullness.

●**Acetaminophen with codeine, *oxycodone* (Percocet) and other opiates.** *Potential side effect:* Constipation.

Benzodiazepines and opiates can be addictive, but the risk is small if the drugs are used under close medical supervision.

FOR MORE INFORMATION

Check the Restless Legs Syndrome Foundation Web site for publications that can be downloaded or emailed to you for free. *www.rls.org.*

Puberty Fact

Marcia E. Herman-Giddens, DrPH, adjunct professor of public health, University of North Carolina, Chapel Hill.

American girls reach puberty as early as eight years of age. At age eight, nearly half of African-American girls and 15% of white girls are starting to develop breasts and/or pubic hair.

Theory: Puberty may be partially triggered by estrogen-like compounds now found in everything from pesticides to plastic wrap.

Drawstring Danger

Dorothy A. Drago, MPH, product safety consultant, Wakefield, MA. Her study of drawstring accidents was published in *Archives of Pediatrics & Adolescent Medicine*, Box 10946, Chicago 60610.

To reduce children's risk of accidental strangulation, remove all drawstrings from the necklines and hoods of their jackets and other outerwear...and cut waist and bottom drawstrings to three inches. Between 1985 and 1995, eight American children suffocated when their drawstrings snagged on playground slides or school bus handrails or doors.

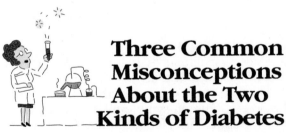

Three Common Misconceptions About the Two Kinds of Diabetes

David M. Nathan, MD, director of the Diabetes Center at Massachusetts General Hospital in Boston and author of *Beating Diabetes.* McGraw-Hill. He is chairman of the Diabetes Prevention Program (DPP), a study examining whether Type 2 diabetes can be prevented.

Diabetes is the most common chronic, serious ailment in the US. It's the leading cause of both blindness and kidney failure. It can cause nerve damage that requires amputations. And diabetes greatly raises the risk for heart disease and stroke.

Despite the wide swath diabetes cuts through our society, many people harbor misconceptions about the disease...

Misconception #1: Diabetes is a disease that *kids* get—and if you didn't get it then, you needn't worry about it now.

Misconception #2: Diabetes is an *old* person's disease—and middle-aged people needn't worry about it.

Misconception #3: When older people get diabetes, it's mild.

TWO TYPES OF TROUBLE

Both kinds of diabetes involve elevated blood sugar levels, along with abnormal metabolism of fat and protein.

Type 1 diabetes appears most often by young adulthood. But this type (once called *juvenile-onset* diabetes) accounts for only 5% to 10% of diabetic patients.

Type 2 diabetes strikes 8% to 10% of adults at some time in their lives. While Type 2 usually develops after age 45, half of all people with the disease develop it before age 60.

Background: Blood sugar is normally regulated by insulin, an enzyme synthesized by beta cells in the pancreas.

In Type 1 diabetes, an auto-immune reaction destroys the *beta cells*, leaving the body unable to make insulin. Without insulin injections, death may occur in a matter of days.

In Type 2 diabetes—which is often associated with obesity—the beta cells fail to make enough insulin. Because Type 2 diabetics may not need insulin shots, many people wrongly assume that the disease isn't serious.

The onset of Type 1 diabetes is usually obvious. Common symptoms include extreme thirst, frequent urination, blurred vision or unexplained weight loss.

With Type 2, glucose levels rise so slowly that these symptoms take longer to show up... or develop so gradually that they're noticed only after complications start to occur.

Half of the people suffering from Type 2 diabetes don't even know they have it. And—the longer diabetes goes untreated, the greater the risk of complications.

TESTING GUIDELINES

The current testing guidelines issued by the American Diabetes Association urges all Americans age 45 or older to be screened for diabetes at least once every three years.

The screening test recommended by the guidelines is simpler and less unpleasant than the old oral *glucose-tolerance* test. That test—given after an overnight fast—required the patient to drink a sweet syrup, followed by a blood test two hours later.

The *fasting plasma glucose* test also requires an overnight fast. But the patient doesn't have to drink the sweet liquid or wait two hours.

With the old guidelines, anyone whose fasting blood sugar level was 140 or higher—or whose sugar level two hours after the drink was 200 or higher—was said to have diabetes.

With the current guidelines, the cutoff is 126. Research shows that complications start to develop when blood sugar rises above that level.

GETTING THE BEST TREATMENT

From diet and exercise to new drugs, there are now several ways to control Type 2 diabetes and associated problems like high blood pressure, elevated triglycerides, low HDL (good) cholesterol, etc.

Caught early, Type 2 diabetes can often be controlled with diet and exercise alone.

Eighty percent of Type 2 diabetics are overweight. Once these patients lose weight—even as little as a few pounds—blood sugar level and metabolic state improve. So do blood pressure and cholesterol levels.

Unlike Type 1 diabetics—who must carefully monitor the balance of carbohydrates to other foods at every meal—Type 2 diabetics can mainly concentrate on cutting calories.

The best way to do this is to cut back on saturated fat...and to boost consumption of grains, fruits and vegetables.

What about eating less sugar? That's less important for Type 2 than Type 1 diabetics. However, since reducing sugar consumption can help keep blood sugar under control, it's worth doing.

Exercise reduces the body's insulin needs by boosting the cells' sensitivity to insulin. To get started, go for a 20-minute walk each evening

...or take the stairs instead of the elevator at work, while shopping, etc.

Caution: If you aren't used to physical activity, check with your doctor first.

When diet and exercise aren't enough to do the job, it's time for drug therapy. *There are now a variety of medications that can help control Type 2 diabetes...*

• **Sulfonylureas** (SFUs) stimulate the pancreas to make insulin. Side effects can include *hypoglycemia* (low blood sugar) and weight gain.

• **Biguanides,** including *metformin* (Glucophage), reduce the amount of sugar released by the liver. This lowers blood sugar to levels similar to those achieved with SFUs—but without the side effects of hypoglycemia or weight gain.

• **Alpha-glucosidase inhibitors,** including *acarbose* (Precose), slow digestion of carbohydrates and block their absorption.

Because their effect on blood sugar isn't as powerful as that of SFUs and biguanides, these medications are generally better suited for mild diabetes.

INSULIN INJECTIONS

When oral drug therapy fails to control diabetes fully, insulin injections can dramatically lower glucose levels.

Most patients who learn to give themselves insulin injections are surprised at how simple and painless the process is.

Type 2 diabetes rarely requires the frequent injections needed to control Type 1—once or twice a day is often enough.

Cold Sore Relief

Spotswood Spruance, MD, professor of medicine, University of Utah School of Medicine, Salt Lake City.

People with cold sores used to have to wait for them to clear up.

The prescription antiviral agent *penciclovir* (Denavir) speeds healing of cold sores.

Bonus: Penciclovir ointment reduces the span of time during which the virus that causes cold sores is contagious.

Kegel Exercises Beat Incontinence in Women

Consumer Reports on Health, 101 Truman Ave., Yonkers, NY 10703.

Kegel exercises strengthen the pelvic-floor muscles surrounding the openings of the urethra, vagina and anus.

What to do: Contract pelvic muscles for five seconds, relax for five seconds. Repeat 12 times—eight times a day.

To identify your pelvic muscles: Practice interrupting urine flow during urination.

How to Stop Recurring Hemorrhoids

Bruce Yaffe, MD, an internist and gastroenterologist in private practice, 121 E. 84 St., New York 10028.

Stay regular by consuming about 30 grams of dietary fiber and at least 48 ounces of water per day.

Also helpful: Take an over-the-counter stool softener like *Colace* or a bulking agent laxative such as *Metamucil*...don't strain or hold your breath while defecating...clean the rectum with moistened wipes instead of dry toilet paper...and soothe the area with zinc oxide paste, petroleum jelly, cold compresses or an over-the-counter ointment such as *Balneol.*

If hemorrhoids are inflamed: Try warm baths, and wear cotton underwear and loose, nonbinding clothing.

Keeping Wounds From Scarring

Alan Engler, MD, assistant clinical professor of plastic and reconstructive surgery, Albert Einstein College of Medicine, and a plastic surgeon in private practice, in New York City.

Don't wash the wound with hydrogen peroxide. Lubricate it with petroleum jelly or a topical ointment such as *bacitracin*.

● **Bandage the wound to minimize exposure to air.** Change the dressing once or twice daily.

● **Avoid exposure to sunlight.** It can cause skin to darken.

Pediatrician's Home Remedies

Norman Weinberger, MD, pediatrician in private practice in Norwalk, CT. He is a senior attending physician at Norwalk Hospital and on the faculty at Yale University School of Medicine. Dr. Weinberger is author of *You Just Don't Duct Tape a Baby: True Tales and Sensible Suggestions from a Veteran Pediatrician.* Grand Central.

Here are some of the problems my own adult kids ask me about their children—and what I suggest they do...

THE COMMON COLD

● **Make a cup of decaffeinated spice tea.** Add lemon and honey, and wait until it cools slightly. The tea is soothing and hot, which will combat stuffiness and open up the nasal passages. The honey in the tea can help soothe a sore throat as well. The lemon soothes and coats the throat with vitamin C.

● **Make old-fashioned chicken soup**—or use low-sodium canned soup. Not only will it make your child feel better, but making the soup keeps you too busy to worry.

● **Offer fun fluids.** The more fluids a sick child can drink, the better it is. The fluids help clean out the child's system.

Make colorful Jell-O water by doubling the amount of water in the Jell-O recipe...offer enticing flavored ices...or watered-down Gatorade.

FEVER

Fever is not usually as scary as most parents believe it to be. It is a sign that the body is fighting infection.

If you're concerned, take your child's temperature and make sure to tell the doctor how and when you obtained it.

If a high fever is not responding to acetaminophen (Tylenol), try a warm bath, which will dissipate body heat.

There is no reason for the water to be cold. Besides being unpleasant for the child, a cold bath can be dangerous. I have seen a really cold bath send a feverish child into shock. Alcohol rubs should also be avoided.

RASHES

Make sure you can tell your doctor...

● **When the rash began.**

● **Where on the body it began.**

● **How long it took to spread.**

● **Whether or not it itches.**

● **What color it is.**

● **Whether the bumps are flat,** raised or fluid-filled.

Do a little investigative work on your own, too. Did you just change laundry detergents? Often, it's a simple case of a reaction to a new food, lotion or sunscreen with PABA.

SUNBURN

For sunburn relief during winter vacations, try tea bags. Let the bags steep in boiled water for five minutes. Then, after they cool, remove from the water and apply the wet bags to the skin.

8

Reduce Stress, Lengthen Lives

You Can Make Stress Work for You

Kenneth Pelletier, MD, PhD
Stanford University School of Medicine

S tress is an unfortunate fact of life. But possessing a healthy sense of control—a confidence in your ability to influence the course and destiny of your life —can help you influence stress by shortening its duration or avoiding it altogether.

How to reduce the different types of stress in your life...

STRESS AT WORK

Career demands cause a specific type of stress called *job strain*. It occurs when a job makes high psychological demands but allows little or no control, autonomy or discretion over tasks.

Strategy: Be more proactive, and try to divide your workload into blocks of manageable time. Schedule difficult tasks during your best hours. Set aside an hour or two each morning, if possible, when you don't take phone calls. Use that time to conquer your paperwork.

Examples: If you're constantly racing to meet deadlines, place a colored dot on one of the numbers on the clock in your office. Whenever the clock shows that hour, take deep breaths—in order to let go of cumulative stress and clear your mind. If you work at a computer all day, give your eyes and mind a break by periodically looking into the corner of the room—or out the window.

STRESS AT HOME

The time you spend with your family is the time for self-healing. But all too often, family members find that despite their physical closeness, they feel alone or isolated because there isn't any *positive interaction*.

Strategy: Enhancing family bonds is the key to managing stress and a happier, healthier life. Reduce external distractions by turning off the TV or radio *at least* once a week, and using

Kenneth R. Pelletier, MD, PhD, clinical professor of medicine at the University of Arizona School of Medicine in Phoenix. He is author of *Sound Mind, Sound Body*. Fireside.

that time for conversation or for an activity the entire family can enjoy.

Examples: Take a walk…go to the park… visit the library. Schedule weekly family councils to discuss problems and concerns or to celebrate family members' achievements.

STRESS AND PERSONAL OBLIGATIONS

Stress at home is not always caused by family problems, and in fact is often due to an overload of bills, errands and household chores.

Strategy: Ask yourself, *Is it worth dying for?* Often, we assign trivial tasks (such as getting to the cleaners before closing time) too much importance. The key is to prioritize what needs doing and focus on getting it done, instead of focusing on what can wait (which leads to more stress).

You may also want to consolidate errands and do the most important ones together.

To reduce accumulating bills, try to identify what you absolutely *need*, not what you *want*, relative to your level of income and debt.

STRESS AND YOUR PARTNER

Relationships take time, commitment and energy. Such efforts and demands can be particularly stressful when other areas of your life make similar demands. However, we can turn shortcomings or insecurities into assets and strengthen our ability to reach optimal health by acknowledging them to our partners and to ourselves.

Strategy: Isolate blocks of time to discuss issues of concern to both you and your partner. Instead of assuming one party is "right" and the other "wrong," place yourself in the other person's shoes and rehearse his/her perspective.

Most arguments occur during transitional periods of the day—when we get home from work, for instance. So take time to allow tensions to dissipate by changing clothes, taking a shower or walking outside before confronting or devoting attention to each other.

RELAXATION SECRETS

Truly successful people are not overburdened by stress. This is largely due to the fact that they perceive stress as an opportunity for learning…believe that they have control over their lives and destinies…and invest in altruism,

recognizing the need to see beyond their personal needs and devote time to helping others.

Research has shown that *attitude* toward oneself and the world is the key to managing stress. So, enjoying what is happening "now" can enable you to stay in the moment and release your mind from built-up concerns and tensions.

While stress-management skills are only part of a total lifestyle program to stay healthy, they can also allow the body and mind to relax and let go of accumulated tension.

EXERCISES THAT HELP TO MANAGE STRESS

Exercise I: While seated in a balanced, comfortable position, tense and then relax each muscle group. Focusing on your left arm and hand, silently say to yourself, three times, *My left arm is heavy and warm.*

Repeat with your right arm, and then move your attention to your head and face, imagining a cool breeze.

End the exercise by raising hands to chest while slowly inhaling and stretching your legs as you exhale.

Exercise II: Visualize a place, preferably outdoors, where you feel safe and undistracted. Allow that place to become as real as possible by paying close attention to details, such as the time of day, the colors, smells and sounds.

Imagine that whatever it is you want to change appears before you, and then transform the image in a positive way. Gradually allow the image to disappear and return back to your safe place.

Stress Avoidance Secrets: Proven Strategies

Robert M. Sapolsky, PhD, professor of biological sciences and neuroscience at Stanford University, Stanford, CA. He is author of *Why Zebras Don't Get Ulcers: A Guide to Stress, Stress-Related Diseases and Coping.* Holt.

As the pace of American society continues to accelerate, the incidence of psychological stress keeps climbing. Stress is *not* just an annoyance. It has been linked to adult-onset diabetes, ulcerative colitis, atherosclerosis, high blood pressure and other serious ailments.

Yet we all know individuals who are *stress-resistant*—lucky folks who never seem "stressed out" despite the competing demands of career, family, etc.

To learn the secrets of stress resistance, we consulted Dr. Robert Sapolsky, a Stanford biologist and MacArthur "genius" grant recipient who has been studying stress for more than 15 years.

TWO SIDES OF STRESS

When confronted by a threat to its physical well-being, the body undergoes what is known as the *stress response*. It temporarily abandons its long-term "building projects"—growth, tissue repair, immune function, etc.

Instead, it floods the bloodstream with glucose, protein and fat from reserves in the liver and fat cells. Heart rate, blood pressure and breathing rate skyrocket. These physiological changes can save your life by giving you extra speed or strength…or a more focused mind.

Problem: The stress response occurs not only when we are confronted by *physical* danger, but also in situations that simply make us *feel* anxious—from getting stuck in traffic to having an argument with a spouse or coworker.

Research on both animals and humans suggests four effective strategies for limiting the toll taken by chronic stress…

A SENSE OF CONTROL

Having a sense of control over one's situation reduces the stress response. This has been shown in studies of humans exposed to a loud, intermittent noise.

Individuals who *believed* they could stop the noise by pressing a button felt less stress than subjects without this option—even though the sense of control was illusory.

But reducing stress is not as simple as saying, *Take as much control as possible.* In the case of an automobile accident, a diagnosis of a terminal disease or another uncontrollable event, suggesting that an individual can control the situation only adds feelings of guilt and inadequacy to stress.

In extreme situations it's usually better to *deny* personal responsibility for the problem—by identifying an *external* source of control.

Example: No one could have stopped the car in time.

Control is most helpful in coping with *moderate* stressors—traffic jams, supermarket lines, setbacks at work, etc.

If your boss gives you a tedious project, for example, look for areas in which you can exert control. Perhaps you could choose the members of your team, plot out a schedule for the project, etc.

PREDICTABILITY

Imagine asking your dentist, *How much longer will you have to drill?* It's much less stressful to hear, *Three minutes*, than it is to hear, *I don't know.*

Studies show that animals and humans given a warning signal before being subjected to a stressor experience less stress.

Caveat: This "early warning" must come far enough in advance to allow the subject to prepare…but not *too* far ahead.

With rats, flashing a warning light 10 seconds before the administration of an electrical shock reduces the stress response. A light that flashes one-half second before the shock has no effect.

When the light is flashed *five minutes* before the shock, rats experience more stress than if no light is flashed.

How can humans predict their stressors? By getting accurate, specific information.

Examples: Listening to the traffic report on the way to work…reading about treatment options for a serious illness…setting aside a specific time each day to speak with coworkers who otherwise might interrupt your workday.

HAVING AN OUTLET

A rat exposed to shock feels less stress if it's given an *outlet* for its nervous energy—the opportunity to run on an exercise wheel or gnaw on wood.

Humans benefit from outlets, too. Most people know what helps them relax—whether it's playing the clarinet, working out or practicing meditation. Each has been shown to lower blood pressure and adrenaline levels.

Most important: Create a change in tempo from the rest of the day. Pursuing your favorite activities three times a week has a greater effect on stress than saving all your outlets for the weekend.

CONTACT WITH OTHERS

As a threat to health and longevity, social isolation is second only to low socioeconomic status. Isolated people have a higher mortality rate than even smokers, obese people and hypertensives.

Implication: You can defuse stressful situations via physical contact with another person—holding hands, hugging, etc.

Exception: An Ohio State University study found that spouses in bad marriages had drastically suppressed immune systems.

People living alone needn't despair—health benefits can accrue from contact with a lover, close friends, fellow members of a church or synagogue, etc.

How to Turn Stress Into Strengths

Bruce Munro, PhD, director of behavioral medicine at the Institute of Stress Medicine–Jackson Hole, Box 279, Wilson, WY 83014. He is coauthor, with the late Dr. Robert Eliot, of *From Stress to Strength: How to Lighten Your Load and Save Your Life.* Bantam.

Feelings of stress are triggered by our natural survival mechanisms. Though few of us will encounter saber-toothed tigers in our daily routine, many of us are as stressed as our caveman ancestors when we're doing battle with the paper tigers of the modern workplace.

Much of our stress has to do with a mismatch between expectations and reality. As life's pressures mount and your burdens increase, the resulting pressures can have a catastrophic impact on your health. Cardiovascular damage is the most common result of stress—high blood pressure, heart attacks and strokes can be directly related to the amount of stress in your daily life.

Good news: There are steps you can take to diminish stress—even in the most difficult situations. How you react is your choice, far more than you realize.

Here are ways of identifying and controlling stress that can change your reaction pattern and lengthen your life…

HAVE A SOUL MATE

We know that up to age 70, marriage reduces the risk of premature death and disability by about 50%. We don't have studies about living together, but presumably it works the same way. Having a friend, lover or companion to share your life and your feelings is one of the most important health insurance policies you can have.

Also helpful: Owning a pet, which enables you to interact emotionally. Caring for your pet will also distract you and prevent stress from building up.

MAKE FRIENDS

Do you have someone—other than your mate—who is genuinely interested in you… who will empathize with you…and listen to you and your troubles anytime?

Such strong friendships are especially important for men—because men aren't naturally as good at making friends as women are. Early training to be competitive hampers their efforts at friendship.

Example: When a group of women have lunch together, they all usually share in the conversation. At a table of men, however, what you normally see is one man talking at the others—and every man in the audience is just waiting for his turn to seize the floor.

Real friends are made one at a time, usually through shared activity. If you're a man, you may have to make a special effort to cultivate friendships—but it's worth the time and energy.

If you have friends who enjoy you as you are and with whom you can act naturally, you have a second ring of protection. They add more time and enjoyment to the length of your life.

RELIGIOUS CONNECTION

People who have religious connections that are *fulfilling* also have a health advantage.

Note that I said fulfilling. It's how you feel about your religious connections that counts, not how anybody else feels about them. Even if you go to religious services because you think you should—or if you're doing it for the sake of appearances or for your kids—that counts.

If your spiritual beliefs are a source of support to you—if your participation in prayer or meditation or religious services is nourishing—then you've reduced your odds of dying before 70.

AVOID PERFECTIONISM

Most successful people think they have to do everything perfectly. Perfectionists are hard on themselves and are horrible to work for. Because nothing they do is good enough, they project their dissatisfaction and put the blame on you. Nothing you do will ever be good enough, either.

How do you tell whether you're a perfectionist? If you find yourself frequently saying, *I should…I must…I have to.*

Solution: Prioritize your perfectionism. Pick two or three things in your job or your life, and focus your perfectionism on them. Constantly remind yourself that it is fine to do other things in a less-than-perfect manner.

BE ASSERTIVE

A person who is unassertive is a people-pleaser—someone who doesn't like to say "no" for fear others won't like him/her. If you feel you have to say "yes" to too many things, you'll get overloaded.

Unassertive people are usually angry *inside.* When overloaded, they blow their tops. Others feel this anger and become uncomfortable …then they push the unassertive person away.

Be assertive to make your work life go well. If there are problems at work, decide what needs to be changed and how. Then talk to your boss. Tell him you need feedback to do your best work.

THE VALUE OF VALUES

My definition of values is knowing just what you want to guide your life. A person who has no values and who doesn't know where he's going or doesn't care what he's doing will never make any progress.

Hans Selye, the physician who created the field of stress study, once said that *no wind blows in favor of a ship without direction.*

Being aware of what guides you can have a profound impact on every aspect of your life. Benjamin Franklin was a loser in his 30s. He simply couldn't get his life together. Finally, he hit on the strategy of writing what he wanted out of life. He referred to his list frequently. By means of this process he was able to make great advances and increased his contributions to American life.

Helpful: Write down 30 or 40 things you want on 3" x 5" cards, one item to each card. Go over the list, and choose the six items that are most important to you. Carry those cards around with you during the day, and refer to them at least twice a day to see how much you've been able to accomplish on each task.

DIVERSIFY YOUR LIFE

It's important not to focus only on one or two areas of intent. All of us need a variety of diversions, so that if one interest area becomes stressful or goes sour, there will be others that are doing well and can take up the slack.

People who lead stressful lives narrow the focus of their lives to just one or two areas. But if one of those areas develops a problem, there's a danger that they won't have other interests to fall back on. If a person has a range of interests, the others can sustain him through whatever reorganization is done.

Examples: Volunteer work is particularly life-enhancing. Not only does it distract you from dwelling on your own anxiety, but it also enables you to channel your energy in a positive way. Aerobic exercise conditions our bodies and creates a sense of well-being. It releases natural chemicals (hormones) that create optimism and improve our resilience and our resistance to stress and illness.

HUMOR LENGTHENS YOUR LIFE

We have to be able to laugh at ourselves and at humorous situations. If you've lost this ability, you're in trouble.

Helpful: Try watching comedies on TV or going to see funny movies. Laughter is very powerful medicine. I prescribe a daily dose until you've regained your sense of enjoyment in life.

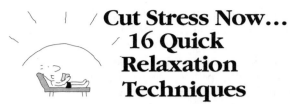

Cut Stress Now... 16 Quick Relaxation Techniques

Ed Boenisch, PhD, former adjutant general of the Wyoming National Guard. He is coauthor of The Stress Owner's Manual. Impact.

Practice the six-second release exercise. Anywhere, anytime you feel tense, inhale deeply for two seconds, then exhale for four seconds.

Say to yourself, "I'm relaxing." Let your shoulders and jaw drop. A wave of relaxation will flow downward.

●**Watch less TV.** Do not aimlessly channel surf. Do not watch violent or depressing shows.

Look through the television listings, and carefully select programs to watch. Emphasize uplifting, educational programs—those on the Discovery Channel and PBS, for example.

●**Don't take work home**...or take home to work. "Decompress" as you make the transition from one part of your life to another—so distress from one doesn't spill into the other.

Sing along with the radio...take a walk... nap...soak in a tub.

●**Look for humor in every situation.** Take yourself lightly and your work seriously. Read fun things—comics, cartoons, jokes— and share them with others.

●**Cultivate a "can-do" attitude.** As Norman Vincent Peale once said, "You are not what you think you are...but, what you think, you are."

●**Stop assuming the worst.** If someone cuts you off on the highway, don't automatically assume that the person is out to get you. Maybe he/she is rushing to the hospital to see a loved one who is desperately ill.

●**Take a 10-minute break.** At least once every hour, get up from your chair, stretch and move around. Doing so will help prevent stiffness and tension.

●**Listen to relaxing music.** Spend your day listening to instrumental classical or New Age music.

Good choices: George Winston, David Lanz, Enya, The Narada Collections.

●**"Box" your worries.** Categorize your worries into things you can/cannot control and things that are important/unimportant. If something is important and you can do something about it, take action. If it's unimportant and/or you can't do anything about it, let the worry go.

●**Take a one-minute vacation.** Pause to enjoy life's small, fleeting pleasures—the fragrance of a flower...the burbling of a brook... the tranquil beauty of freshly fallen snow...the cozy aroma of a wood fire. Notice and try to enjoy whatever is around you.

●**Practice "dot therapy."** Place adhesive dots wherever you need a cue to relax—on your car's rearview mirror...on your telephone handset...on your computer monitor.

Whenever you spy a dot, do the six-second release exercise.

●**Get an aromatic high.** Bring flowers to work. Spray perfume into the air. Light a scented candle. Floral fragrances reduce anxiety (even in the dentist's office)...cool, menthol-like scents boost energy...lavender is relaxing.

●**Boost your ego.** Carry a 3x5-inch card on which you've written all your good points. Whenever you start to feel overwhelmed, look at the card.

Ask those who care about you to contribute to your list.

●**Set realistic goals**—and envision yourself reaching them. If you're a salesperson, visualize yourself closing a deal with the client you're scheduled to see that day. You'll be less anxious when you go into the meeting.

●**Pet a dog or cat.** Doing so tends to lower heart rate and blood pressure—your own and those of the animal being petted.

●**Choose to be happy.** Abraham Lincoln once said, "Most folks are about as happy as they choose to be."

Each day, make a conscious effort to emphasize the positive and disregard the negative. Choose happiness day after day, and it soon becomes a habit.

Just Relax!

Janice Kiecolt-Glaser, PhD, professor of psychology at Ohio State University in Columbus, and a leading authority on mind–body medicine.

Dozens of studies have shown that emotional stress impairs the immune system. Relaxation reduces this stress, helping boost immunity. In one study, men and women who were taught relaxation techniques had a significant increase in the activity of natural killer-cells—a key marker in immune-system health.

Relaxation Can Control Seizures

Epilepsy: A New Approach by Adrienne Richard, an epileptic who uses mind–body techniques instead of anticonvulsants, and Joel Reiter, MD, neurologist, Santa Rosa, CA. Walker & Co.

An epileptic who practices deep diaphragmatic breathing daily in meditation may be able to stop a seizure from taking control.

Helpful: A partner can focus the epileptic on the relaxation techniques. If someone reminds him/her to relax and breathe deeply, the epileptic can switch into the relaxation technique and minimize the seizure's effects.

Quick Stress Buster

Jon Kabat-Zinn, PhD, founding director, Stress Reduction Clinic, University of Massachusetts Medical School, Worcester, MA.

A five minute session lowers blood pressure, reduces levels of stress hormones and boosts feelings of well-being.

What to do: Sit comfortably, straight and tall …become aware of your breathing…visualize a mountain scene, noticing all the details… imagine changes taking place, the sun arcing across the sky, violent storms whipping up… focus on the mountain's stillness and calm

throughout these events and carry this calm with you all day.

Sleep vs. Stress

Angela Clow, PhD, professor of psychophysiology, lecturer and coauthor of a study of 42 people at the University of Westminster, London.

Sleeping later reduces stress. In a study, people who woke up after 7:21 a.m. had lower blood levels of the stress hormone *cortisol* than those who woke up earlier. This was true even if they were woken suddenly at a later time…or went to bed later than usual. *Possible reason:* The body's natural "clock."

Cholesterol Levels Are Affected by Stress

Catherine M. Stoney, PhD, professor of psychology, Ohio State University, Columbus. Her studies of 127 airline pilots and 100 medical students were presented at the International Congress of Behavioral Medicine, Washington, DC.

In men, levels of LDL (bad) cholesterol rose 5% during periods of high stress. Women showed no stress-related rise in LDL. In another study, students who scored high on tests to measure conscientiousness had HDL (good) cholesterol levels about 4% higher than those who scored lower.

Good for Your Heart

James A. Blumenthal, PhD, professor of medical psychology at Duke University Medical School, Durham, NC.

Learning better responses to stress is good for your heart. This conclusion comes from experimental findings that people whose hearts are less able to pump blood in response to mental stress have three times more chance of a heart attack or heart surgery within five years than those whose hearts are better able to pump blood. Regular exercise and reacting to stress in a more relaxed way, perhaps by breathing deeply, are ways to head off the negative effects of stress.

Fight Stress Anytime, Anywhere

Alice Domar, PhD, assistant clinical professor of obstetrics and researcher, Deaconess Hospital and Harvard Medical School, Boston, and author of *Healing Mind, Healthy Women*. Delta.

If you practice simple breathing exercises, you can fight stress anytime, anywhere. *Reason:* When people are upset they tend to take quick, shallow breaths.

Much better: Deep abdominal breathing. Make a conscious effort to relax your muscles and take deep breaths. Practice this form of breathing regularly, several times a day. Switch to it whenever you feel stressed or tense. It relieves anxiety and makes it easier for you to cope with whatever problem is causing your tension.

Plants and Stress

Ashley Craig, PhD, professor of health sciences, University of Technology, Sydney, Australia.

Houseplants help reduce psychological stress. In a study, brain wave activity was measured as 31 volunteers stared for two minutes at a plant, an abstract sculpture or a white panel.

Result: Those who stared at the plant experienced a 20% increase in alpha waves. These electrical signals are a sign of relaxation. Those who looked at the sculpture had no change in alpha wave activity.

Presumably, their inability to "figure out" the sculpture prevented relaxation. People who looked at the white panel also experienced a rise in alpha waves—but the effect of looking at the plant was far more powerful.

Top Stress Reducer

Karen Allen, PhD, associate professor, department of physiology and biophysics, Boston University School of Medicine, and leader of a study of 480 people under stressful conditions.

The top stress reducers are dogs. People who were facing stressful situations had the lowest heart rates and blood pressure if they were with their dogs—even lower than those of people who were with their spouses.

Possible reason: Dogs are perceived as completely nonjudgmental.

Music and Stress

Cheryl Dileo-Maranto, PhD, professor of music therapy, Temple University, Philadelphia, and past president, World Federation of Music Therapy.

Music is a quick stress reliever. Listen to music for 10 to 20 minutes. *Helpful:* Sit in a comfortable chair, away from disturbances, with lights dimmed. Choose music you know well, instead of a new piece that might keep you alert...but avoid melodies that cause tension or remind you of anything unpleasant.

Instrumental music is preferable to songs with lyrics. *Reason:* The latter may distract you from relaxation and stimulate cognitive activity. If thoughts of the day's problems intrude, keep bringing your mind back to the music.

Writing Helps

Energy Secrets for Tired Mothers on the Run by B. Kaye Olson, nurse and stress consultant, Lansing, MI. HCI.

Write down your nagging worries...make two columns on a sheet of paper, one labeled "Worries I can do something about" and the other "Worries I can't do anything about." Accept problems you can't change... and find solutions for those you can control.

Wonderfully Simple Stress-Busters

Charles B. Inlander, a consumer advocate and health-care consultant based in Fogelsville, PA. He was founding president of the nonprofit People's Medical Society, a consumer health advocacy group in Allentown, PA. He is author of numerous books, including *Take This Book to the Hospital With You*. St. Martin's.

The toll that stress takes on our nation's health and finances is daunting. *Surveys by the National Institute of Mental Health and other groups reveal that…*

• **Stress contributes to fully half of all illnesses in the US.**

• **At least 70% of all visits to the doctor** are for stress-related or stress-induced illness.

That's the bad news. *The good news is that there are simple steps you can take to relieve and prevent stress…*

• **Laugh more.** Laughter is one of the healthiest antidotes to stress. When we laugh, blood flow to the brain is increased, endorphins (hormones that give a sense of well-being) are released and levels of stress hormones drop dramatically.

Research at Loma Linda University showed that watching filmed comedy shows lowered blood pressure and reduced the risk of other cardiovascular problems.

The late author Norman Cousins put this research into practice to fight a crippling and irreversible form of arthritis. He rented funny movies each day, and laughed as much as possible. *Result:* His disease went into remission and he outlived all medical expectations.

• **Be more sociable.** When we're under stress, our instincts tell us to withdraw from the action and isolate ourselves. Nothing could be worse, according to stress experts.

Reason: Isolation allows us to concentrate more on our own problems, and perpetuates negative thinking—intensifying stress, rather than resolving it.

Research shows a clear link between isolation and failure to cope adequately with stress, along with a heightened vulnerability to illness.

When you feel stressed, respond by calling friends, or being around young children—they have a way of making you forget your worries.

Doing volunteer work is also a good stress-buster. A 10-year University of Michigan study found that men who did not do volunteer work had twice the death rate of men who volunteered once a week.

• **Be more decisive.** Indecision prevents you from taking action—reducing your sense of being in control, and thus intensifying stress.

How to overcome indecisiveness: First, write down the problem—and a list of your options. Include the option of doing nothing. Next, try *lateral thinking*—in which you consider unusual alternatives and their pros and cons.

Helpful: Be ready to compromise. There's hardly any decision that can't be modified at a later point.

• **Learn to be more assertive.** Many people incorrectly associate assertiveness with hostility or aggression. But assertiveness simply means expressing your feelings, letting others know your beliefs and opinions…and acting on your own behalf.

Psychologist James Mills, PhD, author of *Coping with Stress* (Wiley), suggests these ways to become more assertive…

• **Speak up** when you feel it's warranted.

• **Initiate conversations** with others.

• **Concentrate on making your wishes and needs known to others.**

• **Make an effort to seek out and initiate friendships.**

• **Don't be afraid to disagree** with others.

• **Give out—and accept—compliments.**

• **Ask for information.**

• **Tell someone else about yourself.**

• **Break the stress–sleeplessness cycle.** On average, an adult needs between seven and eight hours of sleep a night. Lack of adequate sleep can make a person moody, angry and more vulnerable to illness and stress. *To beat sleeplessness…*

• **Develop a regular bedtime routine,** which will signal your mind that it's time to sleep.

• **Avoid alcohol, caffeine and tobacco—** all of which have negative effects on sleep.

• **Do something calming before going to bed.** And avoid doing things that may have an agitating effect. For example, don't watch a violent movie too soon before going to bed.

• **Don't use your bedroom for anything but sleeping and sex.**

• **Before retiring,** allot some extra time just to relax.

• **Give yourself pep talks.** If you're inclined to blame yourself for your problems, you may be guilty of negative self-talk, which causes stress.

Better: Talk positively to yourself. Tell yourself, "Good job" or "You handled that tough situation well." Practice in front of a mirror, if necessary. Eventually this positive talk will become an automatic response.

• **Reward yourself.** Rewards are a critical component of stress management. Those who reward themselves after completing a task by purposely engaging in something pleasurable, realize a boost in their immune systems that can last for several days.

Simple stress management technique: Schedule at least one pleasurable activity every day to reward yourself.

• **Write down pent-up emotions.** If you're under emotional stress, simply recording your feelings in a journal or diary can help relieve the problem—even when it involves marital or job difficulties.

This is especially true if you have trouble talking about worries or emotional issues, or if you have no readily available person to listen. The key may be the simple act of disclosure.

• **Slow down.** Try moving, talking and behaving in a more relaxed manner. You'll probably feel some of your stress start to ebb away. *Stephan Rechtschaffen, MD, cofounder and chairman of the Omega Institute for Holistic Studies, also offers these tips on slowing down...*

• **Drive 10 miles per hour slower** than you usually do.

• **Pause at the table before you start eating.** When you eat, chew your food more slowly than usual.

• **When you get home in your car,** wait five minutes or so in your driveway before going inside. Listen to the radio, or just relax and ease into the transition.

• **Take a shower when you get home from work.** It will help relax you, and also signals a change from your work environment.

• **Let the phone ring a few times before you answer it.** Racing across the room to grab the phone triggers more stress.

9

Hospital and Surgery Awareness

How to Have a Healthier, Happier Hospitalization

Theodore Tyberg, MD
Kenneth Rothaus, MD
New York Hospital–Weill Cornell Medical Center

How can you be sure of receiving the best possible care during a hospital stay? The first step is to become an informed patient. Being knowledgeable about your condition and treatment makes you more relaxed and confident—and therefore more likable.

Though it's not something they like to admit, doctors and nurses tend to provide better care to patients they like.

Of course, there's a fine line between being knowledgeable and being obnoxious. Try not to cross that line...but do not *let* yourself be ignored or mistreated.

Here are other strategies for ensuring you'll receive top-flight care...

BEFORE ADMISSION

● **Make sure hospitalization is necessary.** Schedule an appointment with your doctor to discuss your condition and the treatment options. Many procedures that once required hospitalization can now be done safely on an outpatient basis.

Examples: Hernia repair, cataract removal and breast biopsy.

● **Have your doctor explain the treatment you'll receive.** Find out how long the operation and recovery will take...and discuss scenarios that might unfold during your hospital stay.

A surgeon may decide *during* coronary angioplasty, for example, that you need bypass

---

Theodore Tyberg, MD, associate professor of medicine, and Kenneth Rothaus, MD, assistant professor of surgery, both at New York Hospital–Weill Cornell Medical Center. Dr. Tyberg and Dr. Rothaus are the authors of *Hospital Smarts: The Insider's Survival Guide to Your Hospital, Your Doctor, the Nursing Staff—and Your Bill!* Prentice Hall.

surgery. You and your surgeon should agree before you're wheeled into the operating room how the various scenarios are to be handled.

Do *not* expect your doctor to provide a detailed, step-by-step explanation of your treatment. If you'd like the details, ask him to steer you to relevant articles or books. The hospital's medical library may be open to patients.

●**Meet every doctor who will be involved in your care.** If you're scheduled for surgery, you'll want to meet the surgeon and the anesthesiologist. *Key questions to ask...*

●**Are you board-certified?**

●**How many cases like mine do you handle in a year?** If the number is 25 or fewer, ask your doctor why. Consider finding a new doctor or hospital.

●**Is this hospital appropriate for my condition?** For common medical problems and low-risk surgical procedures, a community hospital is fine. But teaching hospitals have more experience with serious conditions and complex, high-risk procedures.

Example: A woman was rushed to her community hospital emergency room with a severe headache...and was diagnosed with a brain aneurysm. The neurologist there had treated this life-threatening ailment only three times. After a couple of phone calls, the woman's husband had her transferred to a teaching hospital where 20 brain aneurysm repairs are done each year.

●**Learn hospital routines.** Call the hospital a week or so before your admission to inquire about admitting procedures, parking regulations, charges for telephones and televisions, etc.

Ask about the discharge routine. Will you be in a wheelchair? On crutches? Will you need an escort? Must you follow a special diet or other restrictions after you go home? Confirm details with your doctor.

●**Appoint a health-care advocate.** It's the job of this trusted friend or family member to speak on your behalf should you be unable to speak (during recovery from surgery, for example). Pick someone who is level-headed—*and assertive.*

To give your advocate more authority, sign a legally binding proxy. Obtain a proxy form from the hospital's patient services department—or from your lawyer.

If you have a living will, your advocate must make sure the doctor respects your wishes. Doctors tend to ignore living wills unless the patient advocate insists otherwise.

●**Pack wisely.** Take pertinent medical records, a list of allergies you have and a supply of the drugs you routinely take. Don't forget books and magazines and a list of telephone numbers of friends, family and doctors.

What about clothing? Bring slippers and a bathrobe. Pajamas aren't necessary—you'll receive a clean hospital gown at least daily. Leave jewelry and other valuables at home.

DURING YOUR STAY

●**Take an active interest in your care.** When unfamiliar people enter your room, ask who they are and what they're going to do. Consent to tests and procedures only *after* you've discussed them with your doctor.

Each time you see your doctor, ask what will happen next...and when to expect the next visit. Save questions about food, mail, etc., for a nurse or another nonphysician staff member.

●**Guard against mistakes involving drugs, food, etc.** Remind the staff of your condition and the treatment you expect. Have someone identify each drug before it's administered.

Examples: "Is this the blood thinner?" "Another IV bag! What's in that one?"

If your doctor tells you not to eat before surgery and housekeeping delivers a food tray, ask a nurse for an explanation.

A patient of ours who had surgery recently put a sticker on her leg that said, "Operate on this one." No one in the operating room thought this silly.

●**Insist that the staff wash their hands and don rubber gloves.** This is especially important if you have a fresh surgical incision. Don't be afraid to say, "I'd rather you wear gloves."

●**Don't suffer in silence.** Let the staff know about any discomfort—it might be symptomatic of a condition that needs attention.

Signs of a Good Hospital

John J. Connolly, EdD, former president, New York Medical College, Valhalla, and author of *How to Find the Best Doctors, Hospitals, HMOs for You and Your Family.* Castle Connolly.

● **Accreditation**—by the Joint Commission on Accreditation of Healthcare Organizations.

● **Board-certified doctors.** At least 70% of staff doctors should be board certified.

● **Salaried "chiefs."** The chief of each medical department (medicine, surgery, pediatrics, etc.) should be paid for extra time spent overseeing the department.

● **Registered nurses.** At least 60% of the nursing staff should be RNs.

● **Well-maintained facilities.** Unclean and/ or poorly maintained facilities may pose health and safety hazards.

● **Up-to-date equipment.** The best hospitals have the latest MRI machines, surgical lasers, mammography equipment, etc.

Hospital Rankings

Jesse Green, PhD, senior director, clinical evaluation and outcomes research, New York University Medical Center, New York City.

How reliable are the hospital rankings published each year by *U.S. News & World Report?*

Not very. The survey is based on three basic criteria—the hospital's human, physical and financial resources…the type of care it offers… and patient outcomes. But there are no objective data on these measurements.

Example: To rank hospitals by type of care, board-certified physicians are simply asked to name the top five hospitals in their various specialties. As you might expect, the doctors tend to pick hospitals they know.

Result: A small group of prominent hospitals—the "usual suspects"—get high scores.

Bottom line: Instead of revealing which hospitals are best, the survey reveals which hospitals are best regarded.

Shrewder Hospital Stays

An Insider's Guide to Understanding Your Hospital Bill by Nancy Collins, RN, and Jan Sedoris, RN, hospital bill auditors. Eggman Publishing.

Keep a detailed log of treatments, drugs, services and supplies so you can later compare it with your itemized bill to ensure you're not being overcharged. If you're unable to maintain the log, ask a friend or family member to do it. *Also:* The log lets the staff know that you intend to keep informed of your situation.

Common mistakes found on hospital bills: Same supplies billed by more than one department, unrequested personal supplies— such as toothpaste—and charges for services not rendered, such as hours of physical therapy.

How to Win the Hospital Game

Charles B. Inlander, a consumer advocate and health-care consultant based in Fogelsville, PA. He was founding president of the nonprofit People's Medical Society, a consumer health advocacy group in Allentown, PA. He is author of numerous books, including *Take This Book to the Hospital With You.* St. Martin's.

Except for elective surgery, we usually cannot control when hospitalization for an ailment or operation will be necessary. But if a hospital stay is necessary, there are steps you can take to minimize the risk of injury and infection—and maximize your comfort and care.

BEFORE YOU GO

● **Be sure you need the treatment.** All procedures—and hospital stays—involve risk. Get a second opinion from another specialist before having any procedure. If the second doctor disagrees with the first doctor, get a third…or fourth opinion.

Example: If your first doctor suggests a bypass, but two or three other cardiac specialists

179

feel your condition can be treated effectively with medication and diet, you would probably be wise to accept the recommendation of the majority.

- **Ask your surgeon how many such procedures he/she performs each year.** An adequate number depends on the procedure.

  Example: If you need a bypass, look for a surgeon who has done 100 bypass operations within the last year.

- **Ask the doctor what his surgical success rate is.** Ask him how that compares with national figures for the same procedure. And confirm this with the medical director of the hospital.

- **Make sure the hospital your doctor chooses is the best one for your condition.** Different types of hospitals do different types of procedures well.

  In general, local community hospitals are fine for uncomplicated procedures such as gallbladder removals, births, hysterectomies, etc.

  But for a more serious procedure—such as open-heart surgery or a transplant—you're better off at a hospital that is affiliated with a major university *and* that has top specialists with extensive experience in the type of medical care you require.

- **Have all your preoperative tests done as an outpatient prior to admission**—preferably several days in advance. You don't want to be admitted to the hospital only to discover that a blood test or an X-ray indicates your surgery should be postponed. This unnecessarily prolongs your hospital stay, which would also increase your costs.

- **Meet with your anesthesiologist or nurse-anesthetist *before* you are admitted.** Give him a list of all the prescription and over-the-counter drugs you are taking. Tell him about any medical conditions you may have.

IN THE HOSPITAL

- **Cut needless hospital costs by bringing everything you require**—including tissues, hand and body lotions, vitamins and medications for chronic conditions. Make sure these items do not appear on your bill.

  If possible, have a friend or relative visit you each day for companionship and to speak up for you if you are not able to. Studies show that patients who ask the most questions—or who have family members who ask questions—get better care and have better outcomes than those who don't.

- **Understand that you can say *no* to anything.** One of your most important rights as a patient is your right to refuse services and treatment you don't want or understand.

  Example: If you are getting a good night's rest without taking a sleeping pill, you can refuse the sedatives that are routinely administered to patients.

- **Question all tests.** Patients are sometimes given routine tests that are unnecessary, such as X-rays or blood tests—or tests that are meant for other patients.

  Key: Ask your doctor to tell you about every test in advance. If you were not advised of a test, ask the person who was sent to administer it whether your doctor ordered it…why the test is being done…and what the risks are.

- **Reduce your risk of medication mishaps.** Ask your doctor to show you the drugs he is prescribing for you while you're in the hospital. Note the shapes, colors and sizes.

  If a nurse tries to give you an unfamiliar pill or liquid, refuse to take it until your doctor has been contacted and has identified and approved the medication.

  Also ask your doctor what each pill is for and how often it should be administered. Keep a list so you don't forget.

- **Curb your risk of infection** by politely asking everyone who touches you—doctors, nurses, technicians—to wash their hands in the sink in your room. Unwashed hands are the leading cause of infections in hospitals, since doctors and nurses commonly move from room to room carrying germs.

  If you must receive fluids intravenously, ask that the IV bag be mixed by the pharmacy staff—not by a nurse or technician. IV bags that are opened by nurses or technicians have higher risks of being contaminated with microorganisms circulating in the hospital.

- **Insist that your bathroom be cleaned and disinfected daily,** especially if you share a room.

NEGOTIATE YOUR RIGHTS

- **Ask the staff to rearrange their schedules to fit your needs.** If your doctor wants blood taken every eight hours, ask the technicians to draw your blood at 11 p.m., when you are just going to sleep, and again at 7 a.m., when you wake up, rather than at 8 p.m. and 4 a.m.

If the housekeeping staff routinely cleans your room at 2 a.m.—this is not uncommon—ask that they come back between 7 a.m. and 9 p.m.

●**If you don't want to be disturbed by interns and medical students** marching into your room during their rounds, tell the nurse or a patient representative (a hospital employee who acts as an arbitrator between you and the hospital) to note your wishes on your chart.

●**If your medication does not sufficiently control discomfort,** ask a nurse to call your physician and get approval to increase your medication.

Also helpful: Ask about less expensive, alternative methods of pain control that may be available at the hospital, including acupuncture, relaxation techniques and biofeedback.

How to Survive a Hospital Stay

Charles B. Inlander, a consumer advocate and healthcare consultant based in Fogelsville, PA. He was founding president of the nonprofit People's Medical Society, a consumer health advocacy group in Allentown, PA. He is author of numerous books, including *Take This Book to the Hospital With You.* St. Martin's.

Some US hospitals are among the best in the world. Others are very, very good. But that doesn't mean that they are risk-free.

Better ways: You can greatly reduce the chance that something will go wrong in a hospital. To get special attention from doctors and nurses, take a few straightforward precautions and make use of inside information about the way hospitals operate. *Survival tactics...*

INFECTION SAFEGUARDS

Ten percent of hospital patients contract an infection after being admitted, adding $4,000 to $10,000 to a typical bill.

Examples: About 300,000 patients a year contract pneumonia in US hospitals. Other common hospital infections attack the urinary and respiratory systems. Staph infections are also a big problem.

Chief reason: Hospitals house a high percentage of infected people, many of whom have weakened immune systems. *Precautions:*

●**Make sure that all hospital staff members wash their hands before they touch you.** Don't be afraid to ask. It's your right.

●**Also ask personnel to put on a fresh pair of gloves** before touching you.

●**If you have a catheter, insist that hospital personnel monitor it at least three or four times a day.** A faulty catheter is an open door to infection.

THE TEAM APPROACH

Since you probably won't be at your most alert during a hospital stay, ask friends to help you monitor the treatment you receive.

Best: Ask three or more friends to stay with you in around-the-clock shifts.

Their very presence will help keep doctors and nurses on their toes, increasing chances that you'll receive above-average attention.

Myth: Guests are allowed to see you only during visiting hours.

Reality: Hospitals *hope* patients believe this, but visitors are *legally* allowed to see you at any time of day as long as they don't interfere with your treatment or that of any other patient in the room.

If your hospital stay is for more than a couple of days, consider making it more pleasant by decorating your room with some pictures from home or other familiar objects.

Leave valuables home. Many people have access to your room, so there's high risk of theft.

ATTENTION TO MEDICATION

With hundreds of patients receiving multiple medications each day, there's a great likelihood of a mistake in the type of medication you're given, in its dosage or in the frequency that it's administered.

The average error rate is 2% to 3%, meaning that in a 300-bed hospital there can be six medication errors an hour. *Precautions...*

●**Each time you receive medicine,** check to see if it's the same type you got on the last occasion. If it isn't, insist that hospital personnel check and double-check their instructions.

•**Similarly, ask staff members to justify any change** in the frequency of medication that you might notice.

•**Ask your doctor if the food you're served will have an adverse effect on your medication.** If it will, have him/her arrange for the appropriate diet.

REJECT THE UNKNOWN

If you don't understand a procedure or treatment, don't permit it until you *do*. Most hospitals will send in senior staff members to give you a proper explanation.

Myth: The release form you sign on entering a hospital means that you give up virtually all your rights.

Reality: You give up no rights whatsoever. You can accept or reject any type of treatment as well as any doctor who's assigned to you.

Exception: In life-or-death emergencies, hospitals are obligated to give you the appropriate treatment.

Above all, if you suspect that a doctor, nurse or other staff member is incompetent or negligent, call it to the attention of hospital authorities.

If hospital administrators don't correct the situation, ask for advice from an attorney who specializes in malpractice. If necessary, change doctors or even hospitals.

Many patients don't realize that they have the right to fire their doctor at any time and to leave the hospital whenever they wish.

SURGICAL SAFEGUARDS

If in the hospital for surgery…

•**Make sure that everyone involved in your surgery knows precisely what it's all about.** If you're having a cataract removed from your right eye, for instance, remind nurses, attendants, the anesthesiologist and the surgeon exactly which eye is to be operated on.

Some patients even use a marker to highlight the correct body part with an arrow or a circle. The measure might sound extreme, but it doesn't hurt to play it safe.

•**Choose a surgeon who frequently performs the operation.**

Rule of thumb: About 100 coronary by-passes a year and a higher frequency for more

common operations, such as appendectomies. This is no guarantee of getting a competent surgeon, but it's an easy way to weed out those who lack experience.

•**Meet with your anesthesiologist before the operation.** The meeting alone can help you get better treatment because it makes you stand out as a real person. You'll no longer be the "gall bladder in room 305" but a person whom the anesthesiologist knows by name.

At the meeting, ask the anesthesiologist how many times he has performed your type of procedure. If he is inexperienced, ask for another anesthesiologist. Also tell him about all your medical conditions, including allergies —they can have an effect on anesthesia.

PURSUING DISPUTES

Not every mistake in a hospital is reason for a lawsuit. But if the error causes serious damage and you suspect negligence or (in rare cases) intent, check with an attorney.

Retain a lawyer who does nothing but malpractice work. Ask for recommendations from your regular attorney, the local bar association or from the American Association for Justice (800-424-2725 or 202-965-3500, *www.atla.org*).

Reputable malpractice attorneys can assess your chances of a successful lawsuit.

What I Learned About Doctors And Hospitals On My Way to Recovery

Evan Handler, actor and writer in New York. He is author of *Time on Fire: My Comedy of Terrors*. Holt.

By the time I was 24 years old, I had already played leading roles in five Broadway productions and three major movies. Then in 1985, just as I was up for a part in a film with Dustin Hoffman and Warren Beatty, I was diagnosed with leukemia…and told that my chances for survival were slim.

For the next five years, I learned a great deal about hospitals and doctors. I was in and out of four hospitals, and I saw more than 100 doctors as I underwent repeated courses of chemotherapy and a bone-marrow transplant.

Now I am considered cured of the disease. I like to believe that part of the reason for my medical success was my intense curiosity and assertiveness during my treatment.

Here's what I learned about the medical system—and what anyone can do to ensure the best possible care for any serious illness…

●**Fight medical mediocrity and carelessness.** Someone dealing with a health crisis hopes to have a kindly doctor, like the ones shown on TV. But reality rarely lives up to that expectation.

Hospitals are large bureaucracies that are set up to care efficiently for many patients. Unfortunately, most are not designed to help individual patients flourish. The result is that any departure from conformity is often discouraged by administrators, doctors and staff—even when the standard procedure could *put your health at risk.*

Example: During my hospitalization, I had serious adverse reactions to several drugs routinely prescribed, including medications to combat the dangerous side effects of chemotherapy. So my doctors prescribed other drugs. Though this fact appeared on my bedside medical chart, *it was overlooked.* When nurses brought the standard medications to my room, I would have to remind them to check my chart—and request one of the alternative drugs that I could tolerate.

This meant delays while a doctor was summoned to write a new order…the pharmacy filled the prescription…and new tests were run. More than once, I was yelled at by nurses for the "trouble" I was causing—by insisting on medication that wouldn't make me sicker.

Don't be intimidated. It isn't easy to stand up for yourself when you're sick, vulnerable and dependent on others, so get support wherever you can.

When I was too weak to challenge the nurses' errors, my girlfriend did it for me. My refusal to conform may have made me unpopular—but it helped me survive.

●**If you have the time, it pays to shop for a doctor and a hospital.** My treatment began at one of the country's most renowned cancer centers. Yet I encountered conditions there that appalled me—ranging from a chronic shortage of bed linens to repeated examples of staff arrogance and insensitivity toward patients. There were even technicians who overlooked safe hygiene practices, such as properly sterilizing the catheters inserted into my body.

It doesn't have to be this way, as I realized only after visiting other, equally respected cancer centers. Many hospitals discourage comparison shopping—yet it's your right as a medical consumer to compare institutions and choose one you believe is right for you.

Self-defense: Get lists of medical centers and doctors from hotlines that specialize in your illness. Seek recommendations from everyone you know, especially people who work in the health care field. Call and visit medical centers. Interview doctors—dozens if necessary.

Consider not only the reputation of the person or facility, but the attitude with which you are treated as a potential patient. Are calls returned promptly? Are doctors and staff reluctant to answer questions…or are they generous with information?

Example: Be wary of any doctor or administrator who implies that, *Our facility is the only appropriate one for you. You would be foolish to accept any other. We are your only hope.*

Knowing what I now know, I would say to any doctor I was considering, *I want to work with someone who is willing to let me be a partner in the treatment. I don't want to be told what procedures may be "planned for" me. I want to know about the range of possible treatments, hear your recommendations and make my own decisions. I don't want interns and residents showing up every day to administer procedures and tests that I haven't been informed about.*

Look for the doctor who responds, *Of course —I wouldn't dream of anything else*—rather than the one who sputters…won't look you in the eye…or replies defensively, *Look, do you want to get well or not?*

●**Get the information you need about your illness and treatment.** The more you know about your condition and the treatment options, the easier it is to stand up for your rights.

While having faith in your doctor is important, you must always assume that there are other effective ways of dealing with your problem. You must be assertive.

Since accessibility to information about your illness is rare to nonexistent at most hospitals, it's up to you to do the research.

Strategy: Look for alternative treatments and medications by calling hotlines that specialize in your illness. Visit medical libraries and read journal articles yourself—or have a family member or friend do it for you. Do a search on the Web to see what you can find out. Call or visit a number of major medical centers known to treat your condition. You never know when you might discover information with which your doctor is not yet familiar.

There are also many medical professionals out there who would be willing to discuss options with you—even though they aren't personally treating you. Keep calling until you find them.

• **Choose your words carefully at hospitals.** Midway through my treatment at the hospital, I decided to "fire" the cancer specialist with whom I had been working—and request another doctor. I didn't feel he was treating me with the respect and consideration I needed or allowing me to adequately participate in decision making. I also found his brusque manner and pessimistic outlook to be frightening and depressing.

Many patients don't realize that they have the right to change doctors—even when they're already in the hospital. The usual procedure is to make an appointment for a consultation with another doctor and explain to the new doctor that you are considering changing physicians. Then continue this approach while interviewing doctors until you find one with whom you feel most comfortable.

Important: When making the request, avoid specific criticisms about your first doctor. Instead, stick to the message, *We have trouble communicating.* Otherwise, you run the risk of creating a "political" mess that could affect your care, since most doctors are highly collegial and easily offended in this situation.

• **Explore alternative treatments.** I wouldn't recommend that people force themselves to try methods with which they're uncomfortable. But I'm glad I explored a variety of nontraditional therapies, from visualization and meditation to hypnotherapy and psychic healing.

I entered into this investigation in a receptive frame of mind—coupled with a healthy dose of skepticism. I viewed these techniques as tools to maximize my potential to heal, not as rigid formulas that guaranteed certain results.

To the rescue: With the help of family and friends, I sought out stories of unexpected healings. I read news accounts and books about alternative therapies, talked to people who had successful recoveries, attended a week-long retreat on guided imagery and other ways of coping with illness. I even had friends of friends recommend psychic healers.

I'm still a skeptic about many of these alternative therapies, but I believe that stimulating my emotions helped me cope with stress, which in turn affected my vulnerability to illness…and my ability to heal.

Don't Let Them Throw You Out Of the Hospital

Timothy McCall, MD, an internist, medical editor of *Yoga Journal* and author of *Examining Your Doctor: A Patient's Guide to Avoiding Harmful Medical Care.* Carol. *www.drmccall.com.*

In an effort to boost their bottom lines, HMOs and other managed-care plans are dramatically reducing the lengths of their patients' hospital stays. To remain competitive, many traditional insurers are adopting similar tactics.

From bypass surgery to cancer chemotherapy, the length of hospital stays has shortened dramatically. For bypasses, stays of two weeks were common just a few years ago. Now it's down to four days. Women having hysterectomies get as few as two days in the hospital.

This isn't all bad. There's good scientific evidence that hospital stays were *too long* in the past. Under the old system, doctors and hospitals had a financial incentive to keep patients hospitalized as long as possible. Under the new world of managed care, doctors can be penalized—or even fired—if their patients stay longer than the HMO deems necessary.

Unfortunately, the logic used by HMOs seems to be, "If cutting a little was good, then cutting more is better." Despite having already made dramatic reductions, HMOs continue to trim hospital stays.

Take the case of childbirth—the leading cause of hospitalization. In 1970, women having normal deliveries stayed an average of four days. By 1992, it was two days. A few years later, however, some California plans were hustling mothers out of the hospital after only eight hours.

In response, laws were passed mandating that insurers pay for two-day stays for normal deliveries and four days for C-sections. Unfortunately, these laws don't help people who are hospitalized for other reasons.

How can you prevent your loved ones or yourself from being thrown out of the hospital too early? *Be assertive.* Keep in mind that in calculating when to send you home, managed-care plans rely on best-case scenarios. Be prepared to explain why your case may not fit that definition.

If your specified number of days is up but you don't feel well enough to go home, tell your doctor (or have a family member do so for you). Though they don't always tell their patients, doctors have the ability to challenge the discharge decisions of insurance companies and hospital "utilization reviewers." If necessary, make your case to the hospital ombudsman.

The major determinant of whether it's okay to go home early is your medical condition. Any fever should be resolved. You should be able to take food by mouth. You shouldn't be so confused or lightheaded that you risk falling when you walk to the bathroom. If you've had

surgery, you should be able to urinate on your own, and your pain must be controllable with oral medications.

The other important determinant is the situation at home. Is the environment conducive to healing? Will someone be there to take care of you? Will your insurer arrange for visiting nurses or other home care? Is there adequate backup if a problem arises? If these conditions aren't met, alert your doctor and insurance company.

Many people prefer to recover at home—if it's feasible. The surroundings are familiar, and there's more privacy. And given the risk of catching infections or developing other complications in the hospital, it makes sense to be discharged as soon as you can.

But the decision should be based on what makes sense *medically*—not on the HMO's bottom line. If you feel you're being taken advantage of, speak up. Tell whoever is trying to discharge you before you're ready that you'll hold them personally responsible if something goes wrong.

Cold Rooms and Heart Attacks

Steven Frank, MD, associate professor of anesthesiology, Johns Hopkins University School of Medicine, Baltimore.

Cold operating rooms can trigger heart attacks in surgical patients. Operating rooms are often kept cool for surgeons, whose scrubs can get hot.

Trap: The mix of anesthetic, low temperatures, cool intravenous (IV) fluids and an open incision can lower the patient's body temperature. In a study, patients given heated IV fluids and warmed with a forced-air heater suffered cardiac complications only 1% of the time. Patients who got the usual treatment suffered such complications 6% of the time.

Self-defense: Ask to be kept warm during surgery.

Common Hospital Billing Errors

John Connolly, EdD, former president, New York Medical College, Valhalla, and author of *How to Find the Best Doctors, Hospitals, HMOs for You and Your Family.* Castle Connolly Medical Ltd.

Up to 95% of hospital bills contain errors, and most of these errors favor the hospital. *Watch out for...*

•**Incorrect billing codes.** There are more than 7,000 five-digit codes for diagnostic tests, surgical procedures, etc. Don't trust the number. Look for the description of each procedure.

•**Duplicate billings.** These occur frequently with urine tests and other common tests.

•**Redundant or shoddy testing.** You should not pay for unclear X-rays, blood tests ruined because of inadequate samples or any test that has to be repeated because of a mistake by the hospital lab.

•**Unauthorized charges.** Hospitals sometimes charge your credit card without your approval. Always insist on advance approval. Don't pay for anything you didn't approve—even if you received the treatment.

•**Phantom charges.** Hospitals often charge for procedures that—while not performed in *your* case—are usually a routine part of patient care. Watch out for charges for tests that were ordered and then canceled.

•**Unrequested items.** Often, these carry confusing names so they'll slip by uncontested. A $15 "thermal therapy kit" may be a bag of ice cubes. A $5 "urinal" may be a plastic cup.

•**Unbundling.** Routine procedures are sometimes billed separately, and the sum of these parts is often greater than the whole.

•**Arithmetic errors.** They may be honest mistakes, but the hospital won't correct them unless you bring them to its attention. Don't pay the bill immediately upon your discharge from the hospital. Take it home and look it over carefully.

The Truth About Hospitals and Medication Mistakes

Charles B. Inlander, a consumer advocate and healthcare consultant based in Fogelsville, PA. He was founding president of the nonprofit People's Medical Society, a consumer health advocacy group in Allentown, PA. He is author of numerous books, including *Take This Book to the Hospital With You.* St. Martin's.

Medication mistakes can average 50 an hour in a medium-sized hospital.

Self-defense: Before taking medication at a hospital or having an IV started or changed, ask whether the doctor ordered it—and repeat your name to make sure that it is for you. If a loved one is unable to ask these questions—and friends or relatives aren't available 24 hours a day—pay for an attendant to do it. *Also:* If medication looks different or arrives at a different time, ask to see the doctor's order for the change.

Shorter Recovery Time

James A. Kulik, PhD, professor of psychology, University of California, San Diego. His study of 84 male bypass patients was published in the *Journal of Personality and Social Psychology*, 750 First St. NE, Washington, DC 20002.

Surgical patients go home faster when they're assigned to a semiprivate room.

Study: Bypass surgery patients were discharged an average of two days sooner when—before surgery—they shared a room with a postoperative bypass patient. This is compared with patients who had private rooms or who roomed with someone awaiting surgery.

Theory: Patients get better faster when they can talk with someone who has gone through the same experience.

Helpful: If you don't have a "post-op" roommate, seek out other patients in the hospital who have recently undergone the same surgical procedure.

Questions to Ask If Considering Heart Surgery

Julian Whitaker, MD, a trained surgeon who founded and runs the Whitaker Wellness Institute, which explores alternatives to surgery. Dr. Whitaker is author of *Is Heart Surgery Necessary? What Your Doctor Won't Tell You.* Regnery Publishing, Inc.

As far as I'm concerned, *90% of all heart surgery is unnecessary.* I recommend surgery to only 1% to 2% of patients with heart disease.

Opting for heart surgery isn't like taking vitamin C when you feel a cold coming on. You can't just "give it a try" and see what happens. You may sustain an enormous amount of unnecessary damage.

If heart surgery does not help you, it will harm you. Heart surgery hurts a lot, costs a lot and will weaken you for a long time.

Reality: Even necessary surgery can often be postponed while you try alternative therapies. The overwhelming majority of patients who are advised to undergo bypass surgery can afford to wait and are better off if they do.

Here are key questions that you should ask your doctor about heart surgery...and the answers I would give to my patients.

● **Why are you recommending surgery?** Any of the following situations is a good reason for bypass surgery...

● **Significant blockage in the left main coronary artery.** Since this artery is only one inch long, blockage can cut off the blood supply to the entire left side of the heart.

● **Significant blockage in three or more arteries,** *plus* decreased left ventricular function (how well the left ventricle of the heart is working), *plus* an ejection fraction (percentage of blood ejected from the heart with each heartbeat) of less than 50%.

● **Incapacitating chest pain** that won't respond to medication and that limits your activities.

There are few other justifications for bypass surgery.

● **What is my real statistical risk of death or other serious harm (including new arterial blockages) from the surgery itself? How does that risk compare with the risks of other therapies?** Heart surgery can kill you... whether you need the surgery or not. Ask your doctor to show you the results of the controlled trials in the US that are closest to your own situation.

In the two largest heart surgery studies to date, almost no group did better after surgery than groups treated in alternative ways. Furthermore, the death rate with nonsurgical techniques was lower.

● **What is the actual death rate?** The death rate for bypass surgery varies in the US from 0% to 52%, depending on the hospital. The national average is 3% to 5%. After age 65, there is a *one in three* chance of heart attack, coma, stroke, kidney failure...or death.

Even the common procedure of angioplasty—in which a catheter is inserted into an artery in the groin and "snaked" through blockages—has a 2% to 4% death rate and leads to emergency bypass surgery 5% of the time.

● **How long will the effects of my surgery last?** Heart surgery isn't always effective forever. Arteries treated with angioplasty reclose at a rate of 35% within six months. For about 70% of bypass patients, chest pain (angina) returns within five years.

● **Is there any way I can avoid surgery?** If your doctor flatly says *no,* beware. Alternative options are *always* worth at least a discussion.

Obtain a copy of a groundbreaking article by Thomas B. Graboys, MD, a cardiologist on the staff of Harvard Medical School (*Journal of the American Medical Association* 1987, 258: 1611–1614). Take Dr. Graboys's five-step checklist to your doctor to discuss whether you meet the criteria defined by this group of researchers, called the Lown Group (from the Lown Cardiovascular Center in Brookline, Massachusetts).

If all of the following apply to you, you probably *don't* need surgery...

● **Your left ventricle isn't impaired or damaged** and your ejection fraction is more than 50%.

●**Your angina may be caused by something that could be remedied without surgery.**

●**An extensive treadmill exercise stress test doesn't show exercise-induced arrhythmias.**

●**It is possible to institute a nonsurgical therapy program.**

●**Your left main coronary artery is not blocked by more than 70%.**

●**What steps can I take to reduce my need for heart surgery?** I call these measures the four pillars of therapy for reversing heart disease without surgery…

●**Diet.** Specialize in foods that are very low in fat. Fat should account for no more than 15% of your total daily calorie intake. This may be the most important step you can take. You'll lose weight, too, decreasing the stress on your heart.

●**Nutritional supplements.** Increase the amount of magnesium and potassium in your diet.

With your doctor's permission, take up to 1,000 milligrams of magnesium gluconate in pill form every day. Magnesium corrects heart irregularities, reduces cholesterol and helps control blood pressure. *Caution:* Dangerous for people with kidney failure.

Food sources of magnesium: Fresh fruits, deep green leafy vegetables, nuts, brown rice.

When potassium is depleted, the ratio of sodium to potassium rises—raising blood pressure. You can get enough potassium from foods. *Good sources:* Bananas, dried beans, lentils, oranges, tangerines.

●**Progressive exercise.** Exercise 20 minutes a day, three times a week. Little by little, increase the difficulty and the time spent. You'll lower your blood pressure, thin your blood and purge excess sodium by sweating. Ask your doctor to refer you to an exercise professional who can tailor a regimen to your situation.

●**Chelation therapy.** To reduce or eliminate angina pain, consider chelation therapy, which rids the body of harmful poisons. In each of 20 to 30 treatments—costing about $100 each—a synthetic protein called EDTA (ethylene diamine tetracidic acid) is administered intravenously. EDTA binds to the ions of toxic heavy metals and helps them dissolve in the blood.

Why this helps: Copper and iron are partially responsible for converting cholesterol into a damaging substance. Lead and mercury interfere with normal enzyme functions that help prevent plaque formation.

Many mainstream cardiologists disapprove of chelation therapy, an admittedly nontraditional technique. To explore the idea, contact the American College for Advancement in Medicine, 24411 Ridge Rte., Ste. 115, Laguna Hills, CA 92653. 949-309-3520, *www.acam.org.*

●**Maybe I'm one of the small percentage who really does need heart surgery. How can I tell?** People who really need surgery know they are very ill. They may have had a few heart attacks. Their symptoms may include severe chest pain that comes and goes, frequent shortness of breath, difficulty climbing stairs without resting, swollen feet and a host of other related warning signs.

●**I'd like a second opinion. Where can I get one?** *Always* get a second opinion about proposed surgery, whether your health insurance requires it or not.

Don't consult a surgeon who is your doctor's colleague. Surgeons who operate all day tend to think cutting is a good idea. Instead, ask the American College for Advancement in Medicine or another reputable alternative medical organization for the name of a physician in your area who practices preventive medicine with a specialty in cardiac disease.

How to Prepare for Outpatient Surgery

Charles B. Inlander, a consumer advocate and health-care consultant based in Fogelsville, PA. He was founding president of the nonprofit People's Medical Society, a consumer health advocacy group in Allentown, PA. He is author of numerous books, including *Take This Book to the Hospital With You.* St. Martin's.

The night before outpatient surgery, note any illness and report it to your doctor. He/she may want to postpone the procedure.

●**Do not eat or drink anything after midnight** unless your doctor approves.

●**Wear comfortable clothes** to the hospital.

●**Do not wear makeup,** which makes it harder for anesthetists to monitor changes in skin tone.

●**Bring any medications you use** so the anesthetist and the surgeon know exactly what you are taking.

●**Arrange for transportation after the surgery** and for help at home for as long as your doctor recommends it.

Secrets of Rapid Healing After Surgery

Mehmet C. Oz, MD, a heart surgeon and founder and executive director of the Complementary Care Center at Columbia–Presbyterian Medical Center, New York.

A top-flight surgeon may be the most important ingredient for successful surgery, but the surgeon's skill is just one of many factors that affect the speed and ease with which a patient recovers after an operation. *To speed healing…*

●**Approach surgery as if it were an athletic contest.** The surgeon is your teammate. Make sure he/she is a member of the American College of Surgeons (800-621-4111, *www. facs.org*). *Also, make sure that he answers "yes" to these questions…*

●**Do you encourage guest visits after surgery?**

●**Is it okay to wear headphones during surgery?**

●**Can my family bring in home-cooked meals?**

●**Would you mind if a massage therapist came in after the operation?**

●**Heed the surgeon's instructions about diet and medication.** Ask him about taking a daily vitamin supplement for seven to 14 days before an operation. This supplement should contain beta-carotene (up to 25,000 international units)…and vitamin C (2 to 3 grams [g]).

For heart patients, I also recommend 1 g a day of magnesium.

Caution: Stop taking vitamin E at least one week before surgery. It can cause the blood to thin.

●**Exercise regularly in the weeks prior to surgery.** I do *not* recommend vigorous exercise for someone about to undergo heart surgery. But gentle exercises like yoga or walking bring benefits without dangerously elevating the heart rate.

●**Lean on your loved ones.** Even before surgery, you may find it comforting to have family members present when treatment options are discussed.

Some family members prefer not to wait at the hospital during surgery. But they can find out ahead of time when you are expected to wake up—and plan to be there at that time.

●**Avoid hospital food, if possible.** When I'm ill, I don't want hospital food. I want my wife's cooking. Eating familiar food makes me feel better. When it's appropriate, I urge my patients to have some home-cooked meals brought in to the hospital.

Caution: Be sure home-cooked food does not violate any of your dietary restrictions.

●**Listen to tapes of soothing music during surgery.** Many surgical patients have at least some awareness even when under general anesthesia. The sound of surgical instruments at work or chitchat among the surgical team might be distressing—even though patients may not recall this distress afterward.

When I operate, I offer my patients tapes of soothing music to listen to through headphones …or let them bring in their own favorite music.

●**If you smoke, quit.** At the very least, stop smoking two weeks before surgery.

●**Practice stress management.** Several tried-and-true stress reducers can be adapted for use in the hospital…

●**Yoga.** Most patients can practice gentle yoga exercises within a few days after surgery. Yoga boosts strength and improves range of motion…and allows you to transcend your worries for a while.

●**Massage.** Some hospitals have massage therapists on staff. Others allow patients to make their own arrangements for in-room massage.

●**Hypnosis.** Self-hypnosis reduces not only presurgery anxiety but also postsurgical pain.

Ask your doctor or a hospital social worker to recommend a psychologist who is trained in hypnosis or other relaxation techniques.

Heart Surgery Recovery Fact

Thomas E. Oxman, MD, director of geriatric psychiatry, Dartmouth Medical School, Lebanon, NH.

Social support and religion help people survive heart surgery. Among people who had elective open-heart surgery, the risk of dying was four times greater for patients who did not participate in social groups, and three times greater for those without strong religious convictions. Patients with *neither* social support nor strong religious beliefs were 14 times more likely to die within six months of surgery as patients who had both.

Common Procedure May Be Unsafe

Alfred F. Connors, Jr., MD, chair, department of medicine, Metro Health Medical Center, Case Western Reserve University (CWRU), and professor of medicine, CWRU School of Medicine, Cleveland. His study of 5,700 critically ill patients was published in *The Journal of the American Medical Association*, 515 N. State St., Chicago 60610.

Called *pulmonary artery catheterization*, the procedure is used to diagnose and treat heart failure and other critical illnesses. It involves threading a catheter through a vein in the neck and into the heart.

Finding: Patients who underwent the procedure had a higher death rate and longer hospital stays than those who didn't receive it.

Self-defense: Before undergoing the procedure, patients should discuss its pros and cons with a doctor.

Shop Around First

Donald Palmisano, MD, JD, clinical professor of surgery and medical jurisprudence, Tulane University School of Medicine, New Orleans.

Shopping around for a hospital can result in better care and save you money on procedures that aren't covered or are only partially covered by insurance. Many doctors have admitting privileges at two or more hospitals. You can simply ask each hospital for a price estimate. If you are on a managed care plan and want to enter a hospital that is not in the plan, ask your doctor if he/she can help you negotiate for the hospital to accept whatever the managed care plan will pay. Because of increasing competition, some hospitals will agree.

Heel Surgery Danger

G. Andrew Murphy, MD, assistant professor, department of orthopedic surgery, University of Tennessee, Memphis.

Surgery for chronic heel pain can cause fallen arches and a feeling of weakness in the foot. Called *plantar fascia release*, the operation involves cutting a band of tissue at the bottom of the heel.

Better: A conservative approach involving painkillers, stretching and, if necessary, injections of cortisone. Surgery should be considered only if the pain persists for more than a year.

Transfusion Trap

Karen Shoos Lipton, JD, CEO, American Association of Blood Banks, 8101 Glenbrook Rd., Bethesda, MD 20814.

Patients who donate blood for their own use during surgery—a process called *autologous donation*—don't always get to use it.

Self-defense: Your doctor should notify the hospital's transfusion service upon your admission to the hospital. Just prior to transfusion, a recheck of the patient's blood type is necessary.

Anesthesia and Operations

Norig Ellison, MD, professor emeritus of anesthesia, University of Pennsylvania School of Medicine, Philadelphia.

Many operations can be done with local or regional anesthesia. These include cesarean section, knee repair, appendectomy, hysterectomy and many other procedures that used to require general anesthesia.

Benefit: Local or regional anesthesia—in which the patient remains awake—usually offers the best opportunity for a swift, uneventful recovery.

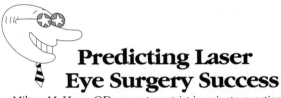

Predicting Laser Eye Surgery Success

Milton M. Hom, OD, an optometrist in private practice in Azusa, California.

Special contact lenses can help people who are considering vision-correcting laser eye surgery determine *in advance* whether the procedure will work for them. *Background:* Many ophthalmologists now use a 10-minute outpatient surgical procedure known as *laser in-situ keratomileusis* (LASIK) to correct aging-related vision trouble (presbyopia). Typically, LASIK is used to correct near vision in one eye, distance vision in the other. Some people can adapt to the resulting disparity between the eyes. Others can't. But by spending seven to 14 days wearing contacts that simulate the effects of LASIK, people can easily determine whether they would be able to adapt. The contacts can be fitted by an optometrist.

LASIK Surgery Warning

R. Doyle Stulting, MD, professor of ophthalmology at Emory University in Atlanta.

LASIK surgery to correct nearsightedness requires a highly experienced eye surgeon to minimize complications. LASIK corrects nearsightedness by using a laser beam to remove a thin layer of tissue from the cornea to flatten it. A study of 574 patients who had LASIK found that complications occurred about 5% of the time, and serious vision loss occurred in three cases. Complications were more frequent when the operation was performed by inexperienced surgeons.

Endoscopy...Is Your Doctor Competent?

Paul Jowell, MD, attending physician of gastroenterology, Duke University Medical Center, Durham, NC.

For years, gastroenterologists considered themselves competent at performing a given endoscopic procedure as long as they had performed it at least 50 times.

Now: Research suggests that adequate skill is achieved only when they've done the procedure at least 180 times.

Self-defense: If a doctor recommends endoscopy, ask about his/her experience level before agreeing to undergo the procedure.

To Reduce Blood Transfusion Risk

Neil Blumberg, MD, director, transfusion medicine, Strong Memorial Hospital, Rochester, New York.

Ask your surgeon if you're a candidate for *autologous donation* and/or *bloodless surgery*. Autologous donation involves donating your own blood for later use. That virtually eliminates your risk for blood-borne infection. Bloodless surgery involves the use of lasers and drugs to control bleeding during surgery. Since you lose less blood, you're less likely to need a transfusion.

All About the Latest Fat-Removal Technique

William P. Coleman III, MD, clinical professor of dermatology, Tulane University School of Medicine, New Orleans.

Ultrasound liposuction gets rid of even stubborn fat deposits—especially in the abdomen and in men's breasts. Like ordinary liposuction, the technique involves "vacuuming" fat out of the body using a long, thin tube (cannula) inserted through the skin. But ultrasound liposuction uses sound waves to *liquefy* fat cells before removal. *Cost:* $1,500 to $5,000—about the same as regular liposuction.

The Major Hospital Hazards and How to Avoid Them

Sheldon Blau, MD, clinical professor of medicine at the State University of New York at Stony Brook. He is coauthor of *How to Get Out of the Hospital Alive: A Guide to Patient Power.* Wiley.

Most people make an assumption when they check into a hospital. "I'm safe here," they think. "I can trust these people to take good care of me."

But mistakes do happen—sometimes with serious or even fatal consequences.

I've been a doctor for more than 35 years, but I didn't grasp just how dangerous hospitals can be until I was hospitalized for an angioplasty three years ago.

An artery ruptured during the procedure, and I had to have emergency open-heart surgery to repair it. Then I caught a nasty staph infection from an unsanitary catheter. To top it all off, I developed phlebitis in my arm from repeated needle sticks. The swelling took months to heal.

My experience was not unique. Something similar could happen to you. *But you can protect yourself if you know what to watch out for...*

•*Trap #1:* **Being mistaken for another patient.** This occurs more often than you might imagine. Once you get your room assignment, ask if another patient on the ward has a last name that's the same as or similar to your own. If so, ask to be moved to another ward. Such a request might raise a few eyebrows—but your life may be at stake.

As soon as you move into your room, post a sign with your name and room number directly over your bed. Ask a friend or family member to spend as much time with you as possible throughout your hospital stay—asking questions, insisting that you get proper care, etc.

Your "patient advocate" should make it clear that he/she expects to be consulted on all treatment decisions. During my hospital stay, my wife was at my side 24 hours a day. Her persistence saved my life.

If you're having surgery: It's not unheard of for surgeons to operate on the wrong side of the body, take out the wrong organ, etc. To avoid such errors, meet with your surgeon the night before surgery. Discuss the procedure in detail, including the exact body part being operated on.

For absolute safety: A few hours before surgery, use a felt-tip pen to write CUT HERE on the incision site.

•*Trap #2:* **Catching an infection.** One in five people catch some sort of infection while hospitalized. Each year, 80,000 patients die as a result of such *nosocomial* infections.

Biggest threats: Staph infections and pneumonia. Staph can be deadly, especially if you come down with one of the new antibiotic-resistant strains.

What underlies the high incidence of hospital infections in the US? Dirty hands and medical equipment are the usual culprits.

Only one out of four doctors consistently washes his/her hands between patients. An even smaller proportion wash their stethoscopes between patients. The American

Medical Association has issued a warning about "killer stethoscopes."

Self-defense: Wash your own hands frequently, and insist that all doctors and nurses wash their hands before touching you. Be polite, but don't worry about offending anyone.

Alert the staff immediately if your room seems dirty or if you run out of soap or paper towels.

Make sure that any equipment that comes into contact with your skin has been swabbed with alcohol (or covered with a fresh disposable plastic shield). This goes for stethoscopes, thermometers, otoscopes (used to check the ears), infusion pumps, hemodialysis equipment and urinary catheters.

Special danger: Intensive care units (ICUs). Because ICU beds are so close to one another, infection risk is far greater in an ICU than in a private or semiprivate room.

•*Trap #3:* Getting the wrong medication. A nurse might inadvertently give you the wrong drug…or give you the right medicine at the wrong dose, wrong time or through the wrong route.

Each year, tens of thousands of hospital patients die as a result of such medication errors.

Errors account for 40% of all adverse drug reactions in US hospitals, according to a Harvard study.

Self-defense: Learn the names, dosages and correct administration route of any drugs prescribed for you. Check this information with the nurse each time you're given a medication.

Learn the dosing schedule, too. Nurses sometimes fall behind schedule—and have to be reminded.

If you're given a pill or liquid (or intravenous fluid) that differs from what you've been getting, double-check with the nurse before taking it.

Alert the nurse *at once* if you experience any untoward reaction to a drug—pain or a burning sensation, shortness of breath, dizziness, confusion, tightness in your chest, numbness or itching. If you have any allergies, be sure they're listed on your medical chart.

Helpful resource: *The Johns Hopkins Handbook of Drugs* (Random House).

•*Trap #4:* Being robbed or assaulted. With all the hospital staffers, patients, family members, delivery people, etc., roaming the hospital, it's difficult for hospital security to keep track of everyone.

Especially dangerous: Emergency rooms (ERs). More than half of all hospital violence occurs in the ER. One in three ER patients is armed. One in four is on some kind of illicit drug.

If you're going to the ER, bring a companion. While there, don't talk to or stare at anyone who is tense, loud or belligerent. Quietly alert a security guard or desk attendant instead.

Hospital parking lots can be dangerous, too. If you feel nervous, ask a hospital security guard to escort you to and from your car.

If you're staying in a hospital room, inquire ahead of time about security arrangements. Before going to sleep, make sure that the bathroom light is on and that the nurse call button is within easy reach.

Safer Surgery

Karen Allen, PhD, associate professor, department of physiology and biophysics, Boston University School of Medicine, and leader of a study of 480 people under stressful conditions.

Operations go better when the patient is allowed to select the music played in the operating room. In a study, surgical patients who picked the playlist had lower heart rates and blood pressure than patients who were not allowed to pick the playlist.

Best Hernia Surgery Option

Robert Kozol, MD, chief of surgery, Veterans Administration Medical Center, Detroit. His two-year study of 62 hernia patients was published in *Archives of Surgery*, Box 10946, Chicago 60610.

Old-fashioned hernia surgery may be better than the new laparoscopic (keyhole) surgery.

Pros of keyhole surgery: It requires only a tiny incision…it causes less pain…it permits faster recovery…and the surgeon can fix a bilateral (double) hernia in a single procedure.

Cons of keyhole surgery: It requires general anesthesia, while open-incision surgery allows local anesthesia…it's harder to perform than open-incision surgery…and it's more expensive.

 # Coffee Drinker And Surgery Trap

Joseph Weber, MD, assistant professor of anesthesiology, Mayo Clinic, Scottsdale, AZ.

Coffee drinkers facing surgery can avoid postoperative headaches by having intravenous caffeine after surgery. Surgeons usually warn their patients to avoid coffee during the two hours prior to the operation. Consequently, these people are often experiencing caffeine-withdrawal headaches by the time they reach the recovery room.

Finding: Patients given intravenous caffeine after surgery had a lower risk for headache—10% versus 25% for those who didn't get caffeine.

Implication: Any coffee drinker scheduled for surgery should ask his/her doctor about postoperative intravenous caffeine.

Cataract Breakthrough

George Mintsioulis, MD, associate professor of ophthalmology, University of Ottawa Eye Institute, Ottawa, Canada.

A different type of cataract surgery makes for a faster recovery…reduces the risk of vision distortion…and improves eyesight right away instead of after the usual weeks to months.

Breakthrough: A *foldable* intraocular lens (IOL). Unlike conventional IOLs, which are made of a rigid plastic, the new lens can be slipped into place through an incision so small that no sutures are needed to close it. The patient generally does not even need an eye patch.

Information: Ask your ophthalmologist.

10

Health Secrets For Men

Hair Loss Prevention... Replacement...Regrowth

David Orentreich, MD
Mount Sinai School of Medicine

Men and women have battled hair loss for millennia. Ancient Egyptians tried slathering their bald spots with animal fat... while Julius Caesar wore his famous laurel wreath low to hide a receding hairline.

These measures may sound silly to us now. But the methods tried since then—from prescription lotions to spray-on fake hair—aren't much better at growing hair.

Is there any truly effective way to stop hair loss? *To find out, we spoke with hair specialist David Orentreich, MD...*

●**What causes hair loss?** By age 50, hair loss affects more than 50% of men and 25% of women. Most of them have what's known as *androgenic alopecia.*

In men, this hereditary condition (also known as male pattern baldness) causes hair to recede from the forehead back to the crown. In women, it causes the hair to thin all over the head.

At the root of the problem—literally—are the male hormones *testosterone* and *dihydrotestosterone.* Present in both men and women, these androgens cause hair growth to "switch off."

●**What about other causes?** The second leading cause of hair loss is *alopecia areata.* This poorly understood autoimmune disorder inflames hair follicles and causes bald patches on the scalp—and sometimes on other parts of the body as well.

Hair loss can also be caused by thyroid trouble, pregnancy and other medical conditions that upset the balance of hormones in the body.

Some cases of hair loss are caused by "cornrows" and other hairstyles that pull the hair too

David Orentreich, MD, clinical professor of dermatology at Mount Sinai School of Medicine and a dermatologist in private practice, both in New York City.

tight. Such hairstyles cut off blood flow to the follicles, causing the hairline to recede.

●**Don't certain medications cause hair loss?** Yes. Some diuretics, antidepressants and cancer chemotherapy agents can cause temporary hair loss.

Sometimes even discontinuing birth-control pills causes sudden shedding of hair.

●**What's the best way to treat hair loss?** That depends on what's causing your hair loss. Sometimes all it takes is changing a prescription or hairstyle...or getting treatment for an underlying medical condition.

If the culprit is alopecia areata, injections of the anti-inflammatory drug *cortisone* often help.

A dermatologist simply injects tiny amounts of cortisone in a grid pattern on the scalp. This blocks the immune reaction underlying the hair loss, allowing hair to regrow.

If you're afraid of shots, cortisone lotion—100 to 1,000 times more concentrated than what's sold over the counter—may work.

●**What about androgenic alopecia?** There is no cure for this form of baldness. Most of the time, however, aggressive treatment can keep the problem from getting worse.

I've learned that the hair loss drug *minoxidil* (Rogaine)—which boosts blood flow to the follicles—is not the miracle cure we had been hoping for.

Minoxidil lotion often works at first, but it soon loses its effectiveness. That's because poor blood flow to the follicles is only one piece of the puzzle.

The real problem is the presence of androgens. For that, you need an androgen-blocking drug. One such drug is *finasteride* (Propecia), a medication originally developed to treat prostate enlargement.

I've found that hair loss can often be stopped on a long-term basis by mixing minoxidil with finasteride and thyroid hormone or another drug that stimulates hair metabolism.

All the patient has to do is rub this three-drug "cocktail" into his/her scalp every day.

If a dermatologist has advised you to use minoxidil alone, ask about using it with these other drugs. Finasteride should not be used by men who are trying to father a child...or by women who are pregnant or trying to conceive.

●**What about growing new hair?** If hair loss is caught early enough, the three-drug cocktail may regrow enough hair that the problem is less noticeable.

This is especially true for women. Since their androgen levels are just 10% those of men, it's easier for finasteride to do its job.

When it comes to men who have been balding for more than 10 years or so, topical therapy is rarely enough. When my male patients tell me they want to regrow hair, I tell them that *oral* finasteride is their best bet.

Finasteride doesn't work in all cases, of course. When it does work, we still can't promise 100% regrowth. But since finasteride came on the market, I can do more for my patients now than ever before.

●**Are there any other options for regrowing hair?** You can always try hair transplants.

The basic hair-transplantation procedure was developed by my father, Norman Orentreich, MD, back in 1953. Although the surgery has been refined many times since then, the basic concept remains unchanged. We "harvest" healthy hairs from the back of the patient's head and transplant them to the bare areas up top or in front.

In the old days, the grafts were so large that they often left a sort of "clumpy" look. Now I use micro-grafts, which contain no more than two hairs each.

With micro-grafts, the appearance is so natural that after the transplant has grown in, the patient often can't tell exactly where it was. Several two- to four-hour procedures are required. *Cost:* $1,000 to $6,000 per procedure.

●**What about hair weaves?** A hair weave is really just a wig that's been sewn into your hair. Weaves often look good initially, but they are hard to maintain.

A transplant needs no special care. But a weave requires regular cleaning and tightening. That means frequent visits to the salon that installed the weave.

Make the Most of Less Hair

Anthony Palladino, barbershop owner, Beverly Hills, CA.

Have your barber help find a good style for you.

Surprising: If hair is cut shorter, it usually seems fuller. An all-around short cut makes hair look more evenly placed even if it is concentrated in the back and on the sides.

Other ideas: For a receding hairline, trim the forward part short while letting hair at your temples grow longer. For a bald spot, keep the back short and grow top-of-head hair long to cover the spot.

Domineering Men Die Sooner

Michael Babyak, PhD, researcher at Duke University Medical Center, Durham, NC, who conducted a study of 750 men over 22 years.

Men who exhibited such vocal characteristics as attempting to interrupt conversations and making quick responses were 60% more likely to die sooner than men who spoke quietly and were more laid back.

Theory: Socially dominating men need to be in control at all times. This increases levels of stress hormones in the blood, which can, over time, damage the heart and immune system.

Men and Their Metabolism

Susan Roberts, PhD, researcher at the Jean Mayer–USDA Human Nutrition Research Center on Aging at Tufts University, Boston.

As men age, their metabolism becomes less "flexible." A study comparing men in their 20s with those in their 60s and 70s found that when the men were fed an extra 1,000 calories a day, members of the younger group were able to naturally burn up some of the extra food, while the older group naturally burned up less and gained more weight. The research suggested that exercise may help older men burn off extra calories directly—and also indirectly—by improving the body's capability to speed up its metabolism.

Potbelly Risk

Eric B. Rimm, ScD, associate professor of nutrition and epidemiology, Harvard School of Public Health, Boston. His five-year study of 28,643 men 40 to 75 years of age was published in the *American Journal of Epidemiology*, 111 Market Pl., Ste. 840, Baltimore 21202.

Men with potbellies face a heightened risk of stroke.

Critical factor: The waist-to-hip ratio (WHR). In a study, men with the highest WHRs (above 0.98) suffered two to three times the number of strokes as men with the lowest WHRs (0.89). To calculate your WHR, divide your waist measurement by your hip measurement.

Almost All Men Can Become Fathers

Richard J. Sherins, MD, director, male infertility program, Genetic & IVF Institute, Fairfax, VA.

Men who have no viable sperm in their semen almost always have some unmoving sperm in their testicles. Those sperm can fertilize an egg if they are injected into it. This used to require expensive, painful surgery to obtain the sperm.

Now the sperm are aspirated through a thin needle in a procedure that is simple enough to be done in a doctor's office.

Infertility Factors

Emmett F. Branigan, MD, assistant professor of obstetrics and gynecology, University of Washington School of Medicine, Seattle. His one-year study of 95 couples with unexplained infertility was published in *The Journal of Reproductive Medicine*, 8342 Olive Blvd., St. Louis 63132.

Unexplained infertility is often the result of *leukocytospermia*, a condition in which the man's white blood cells adversely affect his sperm cells.

Good news: In a study, fertility rates increased *eightfold* when the man and the woman began taking the antibiotic *doxycycline*. Antibiotic therapy costs much less than in vitro fertilization, which costs approximately $12,000.

Infertility and Infections

Harry Fisch, MD, director of the Male Reproductive Center at Columbia–Presbyterian Medical Center, 944 Park Ave., New York 10028.

Many male infertility problems come from infections. Bacteria or infection-fighting white blood cells present in the reproductive tract can severely affect both the production and motility of sperm, causing fertility problems. Many of these infections can be simply and effectively treated with antibiotics.

Also: A low sperm count may be a temporary condition caused by a current illness…or it may be a long-term holdover from a sexually transmitted disease contracted years ago but never completely cured. Antibiotics may rapidly clear up this problem, too.

Tight Underwear and Male Infertility

Carolina H.J. Tiemessen, MD, fertility specialist, St. Elizabeth Hospital, Tilburg, The Netherlands. Her study of sperm quality in nine men was published in *The Lancet*, 32 Jamestown Rd., London NW1 7BY, England.

Tight underwear can contribute to male infertility. For six months, men wore "boxers" and loose-fitting pants and avoided hot baths, saunas and electric blankets. During another six-month period, the men wore briefs and did not avoid these sources of heat.

Result: The men had lower sperm counts and reduced sperm mobility during the "brief" period.

Theory: The tight fit raises the temperature in the scrotum, impairing sperm formation.

Premature Ejaculation Help

Janet Lever, PhD, professor of sociology, California State University, Los Angeles, and Pepper Schwartz, PhD, professor of sociology, University of Washington, Seattle.

Premature ejaculation is the most common male sexual problem. Most cases can be easily fixed through a start–stop technique in which a man becomes more aware of his own arousal pattern and learns to change his technique.

More information: Consult your internist or urologist.

Safer Alternative to Vasectomy Reversals

Harry Fisch, MD, director of the Male Reproductive Center at Columbia–Presbyterian Medical Center, 944 Park Ave., New York 10028.

Men who have had vasectomies but now want children no longer need to have the surgery for vasectomy reversal. Instead, a small amount of sperm-containing tissue can be removed using local anesthesia—a procedure that takes only about a minute in the doctor's office, compared with about three hours in the operating room for a vasectomy reversal. The sperm is then injected into the wife's eggs through in vitro fertilization. About 500,000 men a year have vasectomies, and 1% to 2% have them reversed—a percentage that is increasing.

Impotence Drug News

Harin Padma-Nathan, MD, professor of urology at the University of Southern California and director of the Male Clinic in Santa Monica.

The impotence drug *alprostadil* can now be administered effectively at home *without* injections. Formerly, the drug had to be injected, which was often a painful process.

Now, a slender plunger device gently inserts the medicine—in the form of a tiny pellet—into the urethra.

About two-thirds of men for whom the technique works in the physician's office can also use it successfully at home. The effect typically occurs within about five minutes and lasts about one hour.

Snoring and Impotence

Karl Doghramji, MD, director, Sleep Disorders Center, Thomas Jefferson University, Philadelphia. His study of 250 subjects was published in *Sleep Research,* Brain Information Service, UCLA School of Medicine, Room 43-367, Box 951746, Los Angeles 90095.

Chronic poor sleep caused by snoring may disturb blood flow to the penis. A study found that about half of all impotent men also suffered from sleep apnea. Whether or not snoring causes impotence is unclear. However, there seems to be a clear association.

Self-defense: Impotent men should be checked for snoring and sleep apnea syndrome. If both are present, treatments are available—usually at sleep disorders centers. For referral to a sleep disorders center near you, contact the American Academy of Sleep Medicine, One Westbrook Corporate Center, Suite 920, Westchester, IL 60154. 708-492-0930, *www.aasmnet.org.*

Curved Penis Help

Tom F. Lue, MD, professor of urology, University of California, San Francisco.

A curved penis can be fixed via surgery. The condition, called *Peyronie's disease*, occurs when erectile tissue on one side of the penis becomes scarred as a result of physical trauma—usually during intercourse—or a genetic disorder. In one procedure, erectile tissue on the opposite side is stitched together. The procedure, done under local anesthesia, takes about 30 minutes.

Strategies for Overcoming Impotence

Irwin Goldstein, MD, professor of urology at Boston University Medical Center. He is author of *The Potent Male.* Regenesis Cycle Publishing.

Impotence can be a tough problem—but *not* because effective treatment is unavailable. A host of treatments introduced in recent years mean that most men can get help for this ailment.

The problem is that impotence is such a source of shame that many of the 30 million American men suffering from it are unwilling to seek help.

To tell a doctor a secret that's never been shared with anyone—maybe not even his spouse—is too much for some men.

The only advice I have for any man too proud to seek help for impotence is this—*get over it.* After all, would you rather endure a few minutes of embarrassment in the doctor's office…or forgo sexual satisfaction for the rest of your life?

GETTING HELP

Your first step should be to find a urologist who specializes in the treatment of impotence.

University-affiliated specialists are more likely to be up-to-date on impotence treatments than those without such an affiliation.

Any man suffering from impotence should be accompanied to the initial appointment by his sex partner.

Doctors used to think that nine out of 10 cases of impotence stemmed from purely psychological factors.

Now it's clear that while performance anxiety and other psychological problems often play a role, the vast majority of cases have physiological causes.

Examples: Injured blood vessels in the groin...atherosclerosis of arteries in the penis.

For this reason, diagnosing impotence requires a physical exam by a doctor *and* a psychological evaluation.

If your doctor cannot refer you to a sex therapist, get a referral by sending a self-addressed, stamped, business-sized envelope to the American Association of Sexuality Educators, Counselors and Therapists, Box 1960, Ashland, VA 23005, or use the on-line locator at *www.aasect.org.*

A small percentage of men overcome impotence with the help of sex therapy...or following microvascular surgery to repair penile blood vessels damaged by groin injuries.

Treatments for Male Impotence

J. Francois Eid, MD, director, advanced urological care at NewYork-Presbyterian Hospital and in private practice, both in New York City.

Male impotence—or erectile dysfunction, as doctors prefer to call it—is one of the most common untreated medical disorders in the world.

In the US, as many as 20 million men may have problems getting or maintaining an erection.

The disorder's prevalence increases with age. Only 5% of 40-year-olds experience erectile dysfunction. The rate among 70-year-olds is somewhere between 15% and 30%.

Of the men affected, however, only one out of 20 seeks medical help. *That's unfortunate for two reasons...*

- **Consistent loss of erection is not normal at any age**—and can actually be a symptom of an illness.

- **With many effective treatments now available** and many more on the way, erectile dysfunction can almost always be treated successfully.

More than 80% of all dysfunction can be traced to a physical (organic) cause—usually an inability to keep blood trapped in the penis after it becomes erect.

A much smaller percentage of cases is psychological in origin. These patients tend to be younger and usually report no erection at all with a partner, though they may be able to become erect when they're alone—watching an erotic movie, for example. (When the dysfunction is physical, the patient will usually have at least a partial erection.)

TREATING ERECTILE DYSFUNCTION

While its incidence is highest among older men, difficulty maintaining an erection is not a normal part of aging. A healthy male with a willing partner can expect to have one or two usable erections a week well into his 80s.

An occasional loss of erection is nothing to worry about. But if it happens consistently, see a physician who's very experienced at treating erectile dysfunction—either an internist specializing in erectile dysfunction (i.e., it makes up at least half of his/her practice) or a urologist.

Main difference: Only a urologist can surgically implant a prosthesis.

WHAT TO EXPECT

The first thing the doctor should do is take a medical history, including all psychological and sexual aspects of the dysfunction.

He/she should also give you a full physical checkup to identify any underlying illness that might be present. Difficulty in getting or maintaining an erection is often a predictor of vascular problems elsewhere in the body, including heart disease. *Other factors that can affect your erection include...*

- **High cholesterol.**

- **Cigarette smoking** (which constricts the blood vessels leading to the penis).

• **Excessive alcohol intake.**

• **Diabetes** (as many as 60% of diabetic men may have erection problems at some point).

• **Certain prescription drugs,** particularly blood pressure and cardiovascular medications, and some tranquilizers and antidepressants.

• **Radiation therapy.**

• **Pelvic surgery.**

• **Stroke or neurological disease,** including Parkinson's, Alzheimer's and multiple sclerosis.

Addressing these underlying causes can often solve the problem. If the dysfunction is psychological, you'll probably be referred to a certified sex therapist. If the problem turns out to be a simple issue of communication with your partner, a therapist could help you resolve it relatively quickly.

When the dysfunction involves more deeply ingrained issues—for example, inhibition or performance anxiety related to upbringing, religion and social background—it tends to be more difficult and time consuming to treat.

IT'S ALL IN YOUR MUSCLES

Most chronic erection problems aren't in a man's head, however, but in his muscle cells. Ninety percent of physical dysfunction occurs because the penis loses flexibility and elasticity over time, until its ability to trap and store blood becomes impaired. No matter how much blood flows into the penis, it leaks back out.

This happens because the muscle cells in your penis become thinner with age, while their supporting network of collagen (connective tissue) is no longer renewed as quickly as when you were younger, and becomes less elastic. As a result, the muscles in your penis are unable to fully relax—which is necessary for them to keep blood trapped in the penis.

FIVE TREATMENTS

Five types of treatment are now used to combat erectile dysfunction. Your choice of therapy should come only after discussing each option in detail with your doctor, and with your wife or sexual partner.

For a good outcome, it's vital to treat erectile dysfunction as a couple's problem, and include your mate in all aspects of treatment. I believe a supportive partner is the most important factor in regaining a full, healthy sex life.

• **Oral medications.** *Sildenafil* (Viagra) was approved by the FDA in 1998 and represents a new milestone in the field of erectile dysfunction. Viagra works by increasing blood flow to the penis, as well as causing penile muscles to relax. It does not initiate an erection, but helps store penile flow in response to sexual stimulation by counteracting the chemical in the body that diminishes an erection.

The FDA has also approved *vardenafil* (Levitra) and *tadalafil* (Cialis), two other drugs to treat impotence.

In addition, two other oral medications are currently undergoing clinical trials—*apomorphine* and *Vasomax*—and will probably not be as effective as Viagra, Levitra or Cialis. *Yohimbine* (a vasodilator), another popular oral medication, is worthless, in my opinion.

The antidepressant drug *Trazodone,* taken one hour before sexual activity, has been found to prolong erections in men who are able to obtain, but not maintain, an erection during intercourse. Trazodone, however, is much less effective than Viagra or Levitra.

• **Topical cream.** *MUSE* (Medicated Urethral System for Erection), which contains a prostaglandin cream that's applied into the opening of the urethra just before intercourse, has also produced good results in clinical trials. This cream is a vasodilator, meaning that it causes blood vessels to widen—encouraging blood flow into the penis. However, patient response has been very disappointing. With the approval of Viagra, this method has become less popular.

• **Injection therapy.** Prior to FDA approval of Viagra, this was the newest form of treatment to emerge over the past 20 years, and is still the most effective treatment currently available. A drug is injected at the base of the penis 20 minutes before intercourse, using a very small needle. Like creams, the drug works by dilating the blood vessels. The result is usually a very natural, high-quality erection.

When it was first used in the 1980s, the injection of choice was a mixture of *papaverine* and *phentolamine*. The injections have some side effects, including scarring from repeated injections, and sometimes a painfully prolonged erection (solved by reducing the dosage).

Approved by the FDA in 1995, *prostaglandin E1* (Alprostadil), a substance that occurs naturally in penile tissue, is an injectable drug that can be self-administered at home. Tests show that scarring from prostaglandin E1 injections is minimal (occurring in only 1% of cases)—and the satisfaction rate is very high. This is currently the only FDA-approved method for penile injection.

Eight out of 10 men tested reported a usable erection and satisfactory intercourse. It also appears to work well for some cases of psychological dysfunction.

●**Vacuum device.** This is the least invasive method of all, involving no medication or surgery. A tube is placed over the end of the penis. The device creates a vacuum that encourages blood to flow in, creating an erection. A rubber ring is then snapped over the base of the penis.

While the success rate is very high with vacuum devices, only one-third of the men who buy them end up using them. *The complaints:* It's too cumbersome, while the erection that results can be a bit painful and is usually not quite as hard as normal.

●**Prosthetic device.** If injections, pills and creams don't do the job, you may want to think about having a prosthetic device implanted through a minor procedure in which a small opening in the skin is made between the testicles. This can be done using local anesthetic.

Currently the most popular device is an inflatable prosthesis, which includes a fluid reservoir and a small pump, which the patient activates to become erect. The prosthesis does not interfere with normal sensation or ejaculation. After implantation, the patient can't even feel it—or see it—and often his partner can't tell it's there. However, once the patient selects the prosthesis option, injection therapy or the vacuum device will no longer be appropriate. Fortunately, the prosthetic

device group of patients has an extremely high satisfaction rate.

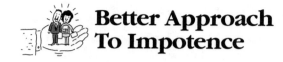

Better Approach To Impotence

J. Francois Eid, MD, director, advanced urological care at New York-Presbyterian Hospital, New York City.

A better approach to impotence is to treat the couple, not just the man. When partners are included in the process—from evaluation through treatment—the success rate increases dramatically over treating the man alone…no matter what treatment method is used.

Important: Solving the impotency problem does not miraculously solve any other problems in one's personal life. *Reality:* I see many couples who enjoy fabulous love lives even though the man is completely impotent… as well as many couples with awful personal lives for whom there is no impotence problem.

Impotence Predicts Heart Disease

Kenneth Goldberg, MD, director, Male Health Center, Lewisville, TX.

Twenty-five percent of men who see doctors for impotence caused by vascular problems have a heart attack or stroke within five years of the start of impotence. *Reason:* Sexual impotence is often caused by the same problems that cause heart trouble, including diabetes, smoking, high blood pressure and high cholesterol levels.

Hormones and Men's Health

Alvin C. Powers, MD, chief of endocrinology and diabetes at the Nashville Veterans Affairs Medical Center, and professor of medicine at Vanderbilt University Medical School, both in Nashville.

Four million American men suffer from low testosterone (*hypogonadism*), but only 200,000 receive treatment for the condition. Untreated, hypogonadism can cause impotence, depression, fatigue, excess body fat and osteoporosis. Many men fail to report these symptoms to their doctor.

Study: For six months, 227 men with low levels of testosterone were treated with the hormone. One group received it through a topical gel. The other used a patch, the most widely used form of supplemental testosterone.

Both groups had improvements in sexual desire and function as well as muscle strength. Bone loss slowed in both groups, too.

However, 66% of patch users reported skin irritation. Only 6% of gel users experienced such irritation.

The gel group also reported a greater increase in muscle mass and a decrease in body fat.

Implication: Testosterone gel is better tolerated and may be a more effective treatment than the patch.

Any man suffering from sexual dysfunction or depression should have his testosterone level measured. If the level is low, the doctor should consider prescribing testosterone.

FEWER PROSTATE SYMPTOMS

Many men over age 50 suffer from prostate enlargement. This noncancerous condition—*benign prostatic hyperplasia* (BPH)—causes frequent urination (particularly at night), often with decreased flow and dribbling.

Theory: Two contributing factors to BPH may be insufficient consumption of grains, beans and other isoflavone-containing foods… and excessive consumption of animal fat and protein.

Study: For three months, 29 men ages 50 to 75 took a daily supplement containing 40 milligrams (mg) of isoflavones (the amount in one cup of soy milk). The men experienced a 29% decrease in the frequency of nocturnal urination and a 10% increase in the rate of urinary flow.

More research is needed to compare this treatment with standard drug treatments and to determine its safety and effectiveness.

Saw Palmetto Benefits

Leonard S. Marks, MD, clinical professor of urology, University of California, Los Angeles, School of Medicine. His study of 44 men with benign prostatic hyperplasia was published in *The Journal of Urology*, 1000 Corporate Blvd., Linthicum, MD 21090.

The effectiveness of saw palmetto against urinary problems associated with an enlarged prostate has been proven in numerous studies in other countries. But in the first US study of its kind, saw palmetto was shown to shrink swollen prostate tissue, thereby relieving the frequent urge to urinate…difficulty urinating…and the inability to empty the bladder fully.

More good news: Saw palmetto had *no* effect on testosterone levels. That suggests that the use of this herb does not reduce sex drive. Diminished libido is a common side effect of certain drugs used to treat prostate enlargement.

Treatment for Prostate Problems

Muta M. Issa, MD, associate professor of urology, Emory University, Atlanta, and chief of urology, Veterans Affairs Medical Center, Atlanta.

Benign prostate hyperplasia (BPH) is a common, age-related condition in which the prostate swells, impeding the flow of urine through the urethra. A treatment called *transurethral needle ablation* (TUNA) involves heating the prostate with radio waves emitted by a needle-like antenna inserted within the gland. TUNA requires only local anesthesia, and is up to 70% less costly and just as effective as conventional surgery.

Recovery time: One day (compared to three to four days for conventional surgery).

For the Enlarged Prostate

John Kabalin, MD, assistant professor of urology, University of Nebraska College of Medicine, Scottsbluff. His study of laser prostatectomy in 227 men was presented at a meeting of the American Urological Association, 1120 N. Charles St., Baltimore 21201.

Men with enlarged prostates find it easier to urinate following laser surgery. *Laser prostatectomy* clears away unwanted tissue just as effectively as standard surgery, in which the surgeon uses a wire loop or scalpel to remove prostate tissue…yet it causes virtually no bleeding and requires less anesthesia. The laser "cooks" the part of the prostate that encircles the urethra. This tissue disintegrates and is passed in the urine.

Best Time For Prostate Test

William J. Catalona, MD, professor of urology, Feinberg School of Medicine and director of the Clinical Prostate Cancer Program at the Robert H. Lune Comprehensive Cancer Center, both at Northwestern University, Chicago.

A prostate-specific antigen (PSA) test is best performed at least 48 hours after having sex. Ejaculation can make a PSA reading jump. The test might then indicate possible prostate cancer. PSA readings return to normal 48 hours after ejaculation.

Prostate Test Schedule

H. Ballentine Carter, MD, associate professor of urology, Johns Hopkins University School of Medicine, Baltimore. His study was published in the *Journal of the American Medical Association*, 515 N. State St., Chicago 60610.

Men are typically advised to get their first annual *prostate-specific antigen* (PSA) test at age 50. But new evidence suggests that it's better to have the first test at age 40, followed by another at age 45 and then every other year starting at age 50. Experts believe this revised screening schedule should save lives by spotting tumors when they are still small and confined to the prostate gland, when treatment is most effective.

Best Treatments for Prostate Enlargement

Patrick C. Walsh, MD, distinguished service professor of urology at Johns Hopkins University School of Medicine, Baltimore. Dr. Walsh developed the nerve-sparing radical prostatectomy procedure for treating prostate cancer. He is coauthor of *The Prostate: A Guide for Men and the Women Who Love Them*. Grand Central.

Prostate cancer gets lots of media coverage—but prostate enlargement is far more prevalent.

Technically known as *benign prostatic hyperplasia* (BPH), the condition affects more than half of men over age 50…and 80% of men by age 80.

The prostate is a walnut-sized gland that surrounds the urethra at the base of the bladder. It produces one component of seminal fluid and helps propel the fluid through the urethra during orgasm.

For unknown reasons, the prostate often begins to enlarge around age 40.

The enlarged tissue presses against the urethra, often leading to urinary problems…

Mild symptoms: Difficulty in starting the flow of urine…a weak urine stream…stopping and starting during urination…and dribbling afterward.

Severe symptoms: An urgent need to urinate up to several times an hour…a constant feeling of fullness in the bladder…and frequent awakening at night to go to the bathroom.

DIAGNOSING BPH

Although BPH is unrelated to a man's risk of developing prostate cancer, it's prudent to see a urologist if you're experiencing any urinary difficulties.

Reason: BPH and prostate cancer produce similar symptoms. Also, untreated BPH can lead to urinary tract infection or even bladder or kidney damage.

After reviewing your symptoms and medical history, the urologist should take a urine sample to check for infection. Then he/she should perform a digital rectal exam to feel for prostate enlargement.

The doctor should also test your blood level of *prostate-specific antigen* (PSA). A high level suggests prostate cancer.*

For mild BPH, the doctor will probably recommend *watchful waiting.* That involves simply keeping an eye on your symptoms, with checkups at least once a year to make sure no complications have developed.

Caution: Antihistamines and decongestants can worsen your symptoms. If you have BPH, ask your doctor about avoiding these drugs.

PROSTATE MEDICATION

More aggressive treatment may be called for if your BPH is clearly getting worse…if the symptoms are causing moderate discomfort… or if you're having to restrict your life to deal with them (such as always having to be near a toilet). *Two classes of drugs are used to treat BPH…*

●**Alpha-blockers** such as *terazosin* (Hytrin) and *doxazosin* (Cardura). These drugs—also used to treat high blood pressure—relax the prostate muscle.

*The American Cancer Society recommends an annual PSA test for all men starting at age 50 (age 45 for African-American men and men with a father, brother or son diagnosed with prostate cancer younger than age 65). Caught early, prostate cancer may be curable via radiation and/or surgery.

●**5-alpha reductase inhibitors** such as *finasteride* (Proscar). It shrinks the prostate by blocking the prostate-stimulating effect of dihydrotestosterone.

In deciding which kind of drug is appropriate, it's important to understand that the prostate is made up of two types of tissue—*glandular tissue*, which enlarges, producing mechanical obstruction…and *smooth muscle tissue*, which squeezes the urethra shut.

Which drug is best for your BPH depends on which of the two kinds of tissue is the real culprit.

If your prostate is enlarged: Finasteride may help by shrinking it. It may need to be taken for six months to a year before symptoms begin to improve.

Side effects: Impotence occurs in fewer than 5% of men taking finasteride. Potency generally returns when medication is stopped.

If your prostate is of normal size: It doesn't help to shrink it. The treatment of choice is an alpha-blocker.

Side effects: Weakness, dizziness and drowsiness occur in up to 10% of men taking an alpha-blocker. To avoid these problems, ask your doctor about adjusting the dose and taking the drug at bedtime.

PROSTATE SURGERY

If drugs fail to bring relief, surgery can help. The "gold standard" for surgical treatment of BPH—the one considered most effective—is *transurethral resection of the prostate* (TURP).

In this procedure, the surgeon inserts a tiny lighted instrument called a *resectoscope* into the urethra. Excess tissue from the prostate's "inner ring" is chipped away bit by bit.

TURP is attractive to patients because it involves no incision…minimal postoperative pain…and a hospital stay of less than three days (followed by a week of rest at home).

If the prostate is of normal size, the surgical treatment of choice is *transurethral incision of the prostate* (TUIP).

As in TURP, a resectoscope is inserted through the urethra. But instead of chipping away tissue from the inner ring, the surgeon makes two tiny cuts in the muscular portion of the prostate. This relaxes its grip on the urethra.

Many men fear they'll become incontinent or impotent as a result of surgery. In fact, fewer than 4% of men who undergo TURP or TUIP experience such problems.

However, three out of four men who undergo TURP (and a slightly smaller proportion of those who undergo TUIP) experience retrograde ejaculation. In this condition, sperm liberated by orgasm go backward into the bladder instead of being ejected from the penis.

Retrograde ejaculation can render a man infertile. It is not dangerous, however, nor does it interfere with a man's enjoyment of sex.

MORE SURGICAL PROCEDURES

Two newer procedures destroy excess prostate tissue via heat administered via catheter…

• **Transurethral needle ablation** (TUNA) uses radio waves to produce heat.

• **Transurethral microwave thermal therapy** (TUMT) uses microwaves.

TUNA and TUMT have real advantages over TURP and TUIP. They can be done on an outpatient basis, for instance, and the risks of retrograde ejaculation, impotence and incontinence are smaller.

Prostate Cancer Drug

Glenn S. Gerber, MD, associate professor of surgery/urology, University of Chicago Pritzker School of Medicine.

The drug *mitoxantrone* (Novantrone) is highly effective at stopping pain caused by prostate cancer that has spread to the bones.

Study: Taken in combination with steroids, mitoxantrone significantly reduced pain in 38% of men with advanced cancer. This compared to 21% treated with steroids alone.

Also: The mitoxantrone group stayed pain-free for an average of eight months, compared to two months for the steroids-only group.

What's Better for Early-Stage Prostate Cancer— Radiation or Surgery?

Patrick Kupelian, MD, director of clinical research, MD Anderson Cancer Center, Orlando, FL.

Early-stage prostate cancer responds just as well to radiation as to surgery—even though doctors often consider surgery the treatment of choice. In a study, 75% of patients given radiation were cancer-free after five years. That's roughly equivalent to the 76% who were cancer-free after surgical removal of the prostate. In choosing between the two therapies, men should consider the side effects associated with each—rectal bleeding from radiation…and incontinence from surgery.

Special consideration: Because of the potential for heart trouble, older men may be unable to have surgery.

More Prostate News

Glenn S. Gerber, MD, associate professor of surgery/urology, University of Chicago Pritzker School of Medicine.

Surgery is extremely successful in treating early prostate cancer. A study of nearly 2,700 men between ages 48 and 79 with early prostate cancer who had their prostate glands removed surgically between 1970 and 1993 found that those with the least aggressive form of tumor had a 94% chance of surviving 10 years.

Those with *moderately aggressive* tumors had an 80% 10-year survival rate, while the comparable rate for men with the *most aggressive* tumors was 77%.

Researchers believe that in more recent years, the success rate has become even higher.

However, because surgery sometimes results in impotence and urinary incontinence, physicians sometimes suggest that elderly men with slow-growing cancer simply wait and see how the cancer develops before deciding to operate.

Testicular Cancer Self-Defense

Mark G. Seal, MD, assistant clinical professor of urology at the Medical College of Ohio, and a urologist in private practice, both in Toledo. He is author of *The Patient's Guide to Urology.* High Oaks.

Although it does not get much publicity, testicular cancer is the most common malignancy among men 15 to 45 years of age.

Doctors don't know how to prevent the disease. Fortunately, however, it's now easy to detect—and cure.

Thirty years ago, testicular cancer proved fatal for 90% of its victims. Today the *cure* rate is 90%—and that includes advanced cases.

To reduce the threat of testicular cancer, all men should examine their testicles on a monthly basis. Monthly self-exams should start at puberty and continue until age 50. Testicular cancer is rare among older men.

In addition, any man in this age group should make sure his doctor performs a testicular exam with each checkup.

Testicular cancer is especially common in men who have had an undescended testicle (whether or not it was surgically corrected)… and in men with a personal or family history of testicular cancer.

HOW TO PERFORM A SELF-EXAM

The best time to do a self-exam is while showering. Gently anchor your right testicle with your right hand, and run your left index finger over the testicle's front and side surfaces.

Next, use both hands to check the back of the testicle. Gently squeeze the soft tubular structure (epididymis) that runs up into your lower abdomen.

Repeat this process on the left testicle, using your left hand and right index finger. The self-exam should take only 15 to 30 seconds per side.

If you find a lump or an area of tenderness, tell your doctor right away.

Helpful: Before starting a program of monthly self-exams, have your doctor check out your technique. This will also give you a "baseline" against which you can compare future self-exams.

If you're shy about touching yourself—many men are—consider asking your wife or sex partner to examine you.

One in three cases of testicular cancer are discovered by the patient's partner.

Good news: Most scrotal lumps are benign. *Noncancerous causes of scrotal lumps include…*

• **Varicose veins of the scrotum** (varicocele). A varicocele feels a little like a bag of worms under the skin.

• **Sperm-filled cyst** (spermatocele). This consists of a pea-sized lump, clearly separate from the testicle.

• **Fluid buildup** in the scrotum (hydrocele).

• **Hernia.**

In examining a scrotal lump, your doctor will use his/her hands and check to see whether it can be "separated" from the testicle itself. If so, it's probably benign.

If the lump is intrinsic to the testicle, there's a good chance that it is cancerous. In such cases the doctor should perform blood tests to check for the presence of proteins associated with testicular cancer.

He/she may also do an ultrasound scan to see whether the lump is solid (possibly cancerous) or fluid-filled (probably benign).

TREATING TESTICULAR CANCER

Testicular cancer takes several forms. Treatment must be tailored to the particular form, although all cases necessitate surgical removal of the testicle, along with the attached structures (epididymis) and cord (blood vessels).

Chemotherapy and/or radiation therapy may also be appropriate, especially if the cancer has spread outside the testicle. One type of testicular tumor, called *seminoma*, is especially vulnerable to radiation.

Divorce and Men

The late David B. Larson, MD, MSPH, president, National Institute for Healthcare Research, Rockville, MD.

Divorce raises a man's risk of developing cancer.

Divorced men are 21 times more likely than married men to be admitted to a psychiatric hospital. Children of divorced parents are 30% more likely to die young than are kids whose parents stay married.

Breast Cancer Strikes Men, Too

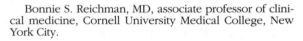

Bonnie S. Reichman, MD, associate professor of clinical medicine, Cornell University Medical College, New York City.

Each year 1,400 American men develop breast cancer.

At greatest risk: Men with a family history of breast cancer—male or female.

Warning signs: A typically painless breast mass on one side…a swollen, sore breast… puckered, scaly or irritated skin patches on the breast…a firm lump or thickness in the breast …a crusty or retracted nipple…discharge from the nipple.

Low-Fat Diets and Men

William J. Kraemer, PhD, professor of kinesiology, professor of physiology and neurobiology and professor of medicine, University of Connecticut, Farmington. His study of dietary and exercise routines of 12 men was published in the *Journal of Applied Physiology*, 9650 Rockville Pike, Bethesda, MD 20814.

Very low-fat diets can cause a drop in blood levels of testosterone, which is needed for muscle mass and strength.

At special risk: Wrestlers and other athletes who attempt to drastically reduce their fat intake.

Bottom line: The body needs a balance of nutrients—including fat.

11

Food and Nutrition Tips For a Healthier You

The New Superfoods

Joy Bauer, RD, CDN
Registered Dietitian and Certified Dietitian-Nutritionist

Some foods have received so much attention recently for their disease-fighting benefits that they have been dubbed "superfoods."

Wild salmon, for example, is rich in *omega-3 fatty acids,* which counter the inflammation associated with arthritis and help reduce levels of harmful blood fats (triglycerides) that can contribute to heart disease...and blueberries and blackberries contain antioxidants known as *anthocyanins* that help guard against memory loss.

But top nutritionists know there are lesser-known foods that are just as healthful as these popular superfoods. Adding these other foods to your diet not only gives you more variety in planning meals, but also broadens the range of nutrients you are consuming.

Common medical conditions and the best foods to relieve symptoms...

ARTHRITIS

Wild salmon's inflammation-fighting properties help guard against the pain associated with osteoarthritis and rheumatoid arthritis. *Other foods for arthritis...*

•**Pacific oysters** contain high levels of inflammation-fighting omega-3 fatty acids as well as the mineral *selenium,* which has antioxidant properties that may help prevent the cartilage damage that can lead to osteoarthritis. Other omega-3–rich foods include Atlantic mackerel (not king mackerel, which is too high in mercury) and sardines (fresh or canned). Wheat germ is another good source of selenium. Have one serving (three to four ounces) of oysters or other omega-3–rich fish three times per week. (Avoid raw oysters —they are often contaminated with harmful

Joy Bauer, RD, CDN, a registered dietitian and certified dietitian-nutritionist in private practice in New York City. Ms. Bauer is the nutrition expert for the *Today* show and nutritionist for the New York City Ballet.

bacteria.) Two tablespoons of wheat germ daily.

●**Pumpkin** is a rich source of *beta-carotene* and *beta-cryptoxanthin,* antioxidants that help reduce the risk for osteoarthritis and rheumatoid arthritis. Eat at least one-half cup daily of pumpkin (fresh or canned) or an orange-colored vegetable or fruit, such as carrots or oranges.

●**Onions** contain high levels of *quercetin,* an antioxidant that has powerful anti-inflammatory effects. Add onions to your meals every day, in whatever quantity you desire.

●**Fortified skim milk** has significant amounts of vitamin D. Vitamin D helps preserve cartilage and may reduce the risk of developing arthritis. Drink one to three cups daily.

EYE DISEASE

Spinach has achieved superfood status as a rich source of the antioxidant *lutein.* It helps fight cataracts (clouding of the lens that leads to progressive loss of vision) and macular degeneration (age-related damage to the central area of the retina) by protecting the eyes from the harmful effects of ultraviolet light. Although these conditions cannot be "cured," some foods can help slow their progression. *Foods for eye disease...*

●**Bell peppers** (any color) are rich in lutein as well as vitamin C, an antioxidant that may help reduce the risk for cataracts and macular degeneration by protecting cells from damage caused by free radicals (harmful molecules that can cause oxidative damage to the body's cells). Other good sources of lutein and vitamin C are summer squash, turnip and mustard greens, kale and brussels sprouts. Eat at least one-half cup most days of the week.

●**Sunflower seeds** are proven sources of the B vitamin *niacin.* This nutrient may help prevent cataracts by promoting blood vessel health, which improves circulation to the eyes. Sunflower seeds also contain the mineral *zinc,* which is critical for retina health. Add unsalted seeds to salads or eat as a snack every day—one serving is one-quarter cup in the shell (or one to two tablespoons shelled).

●**Asparagus** contains lutein as well as the antioxidant vitamin E, which protects against free radicals that can damage the eyes. Eat asparagus twice a week. One serving is about eight spears.

●**Sweet potatoes** are packed with beta-carotene, which may help reduce the risk for macular degeneration by curbing free radical damage. Other good sources are carrots, cantaloupe and apricots. Have at least one-half cup daily.

HEART DISEASE

Wild salmon decreases levels of harmful triglycerides and raises beneficial HDL cholesterol levels. *Other helpful foods...*

●**Rainbow trout** (wild or farmed) is rich in omega-3 fatty acids and can be substituted for wild salmon. Other good sources of omega-3s include anchovies, sardines, Atlantic mackerel, walnuts and flaxseed (ground). Have three to four ounces of fish three times per week... one-quarter cup of walnuts per day...or one to two tablespoons of ground flaxseed daily.

●**Wheat germ** contains cholesterol-lowering plant sterols, as well as magnesium (for healthy blood vessels) and vitamin E. Aim to have two tablespoons daily.

●**Psyllium seeds** (ground) provide the high levels of *soluble* (dissolves in liquid) *fiber* needed to reduce LDL "bad" cholesterol and lower blood pressure. Some whole-grain breakfast cereals are good sources of psyllium seeds. Eat three to seven half-cup servings weekly of cereal that contains psyllium seeds.

●**Garbanzo beans** are rich in soluble fiber as well as magnesium. Together, these nutrients can lower blood pressure and LDL cholesterol. Eat at least one-half cup per day.

●**Turnip and mustard greens** have high levels of the B vitamin *folic acid,* which reduces levels of homocysteine, an amino acid linked to heart disease. Other good sources of folic acid include beets and broccoli. Have at least one-half cup per day.

MEMORY LOSS

Blueberries and blackberries usually top the list of foods that help promote brain function. *Other memory-protecting foods...*

●**Apples (with skin)** are similar to blueberries and blackberries (fresh or unsweetened frozen)—they contain anthocyanins and quercetin, which are believed to slow the progression of age-related memory loss by promoting blood flow through vessels to the brain. Other good sources of anthocyanins and quercetin include red and black grapes, red cabbage and red onions. Have one-half cup three days per week.

•**Coffee** temporarily improves memory skills and reaction time, but only when it contains caffeine, which stimulates nerve cells in the brain's prefrontal cortex region. Drink two eight-ounce cups of caffeinated coffee daily.

•**Herring** and other omega-3–rich foods slow age-related memory decline because these fatty acids promote blood flow to the brain. Another good source of omega-3s is omega-3–fortified eggs. Have three to four ounces of herring or other omega-3–rich fish three times weekly…or two eggs three times a week.

•**Lentils** contain folic acid, which is believed to help memory by keeping blood vessels healthy and lowering homocysteine. Eat one-half cup (cooked) daily.

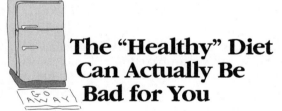

The "Healthy" Diet Can Actually Be Bad for You

Barry Sears, PhD, former staff scientist at the Massachusetts Institute of Technology, and president of Surfactant Technologies, a biotechnology firm in Marblehead, MA. He holds 12 patents for cancer treatments and dietary control of hormonal responses and is author of many books, including *The Zone*. HarperCollins.

Poor eating habits have led to an epidemic of obesity in the US. One in three adult Americans is now obese, as compared with one in four a little more than a decade ago.

Even people who follow the conventional wisdom for healthful eating—lots of carbohydrates, little fat and protein—often fail to lose weight. Why? Because, hormonally speaking, those guidelines are dead wrong.

When it comes to obesity, eating carbohydrates is a bigger problem than eating fat.

THE TROUBLE WITH CARBOHYDRATES

Modern humans are genetically identical to our Stone Age ancestors. Our digestive system, like theirs, evolved to handle a diet based on protein, fiber-rich vegetables and fruit.

Grains—the chief source of carbohydrates in modern diets—were unknown until the advent of agriculture, 10,000 years ago. That's only yesterday in evolutionary terms.

Problem: Carbohydrates cause a sharp rise in blood sugar levels. In response, the body makes more insulin, the hormone that lowers blood sugar levels and "tells" the body to store excess calories as *fat*.

Insulin also affects the body's synthesis of *eicosanoids*. These potent "superhormones" control virtually all physiological functions in the body—from the circulation of blood to digestion.

For optimum health, eicosanoids must be in balance. But high insulin levels cause the body to make more "bad" than "good" eicosanoids.

This can lead to platelet clumping, high blood pressure, reduced immunity and other potentially dangerous conditions.

A BETTER WAY TO EAT

Over the past 14 years, I have developed a simple yet precise eating plan that allows you to regulate levels of insulin and other hormones…and reach an ideal metabolic state.

Athletes call this state the "Zone," but in reality it is simply optimal control of hormonal function. You needn't be an athlete to realize the benefits. My program has been tested on heart patients, "ordinary" people and elite athletes, including professional football and basketball players.

All have reported greater mental focus and energy, better physical endurance, painless weight loss and improved cardiovascular function.

How do you reach the Zone? Treat food with the same respect you accord to prescription medications.

Specifically, you must regulate the *amount, proportion* and *rate of entry into the bloodstream* of all the nutrients you eat. And I mean *each time* you eat. Counting calories isn't necessary.

EATING IN THE ZONE

My eating plan has five major components…

●**Protein.** Besides serving as building blocks for every cell, dietary protein causes release of *glucagon*. This hormone works in opposition to insulin and works to maintain blood sugar levels.

To maintain proper glucagon levels, it's important to eat the right amount of protein.

Easy formula: At each meal, eat about as much protein as would fit in the palm of your hand. For most people, this translates into three to four ounces of low-fat protein.

Animal foods contain *arachidonic acid*, a fatty acid that the body uses to make "bad" eicosanoids. The fattier the meat, the higher the arachidonic acid content.

That's why it's best to stick to chicken, fish, wild game (or range-fed meats), tofu and other low-fat protein sources…and to avoid organ meats entirely.

●**Carbohydrates.** For optimal hormonal balance, each meal should contain the proper ratio of carbohydrate to protein—4 grams (g) of carbohydrate for every 3 g of protein.

Emphasize "favorable" carbohydrates like fiber-rich fruits, vegetables and legumes. Since these are absorbed into the bloodstream slowly, blood sugar rises slowly…and insulin production is moderate.

Avoid "unfavorable" carbohydrates, such as bread, rice, pasta, tropical fruits, dried fruits and fruit juices…and starchy or sweet vegetables, such as corn, potatoes, squash, carrots, peas and beets. These foods enter the bloodstream quickly, initiating a drastic insulin response.

If you do eat grains, concentrate on eating *whole* grains whenever possible. Their higher fiber content means slower absorption into the bloodstream.

What about dessert? An occasional treat is okay, as long as you balance your carbohydrate and fat intake by taking a "dose" of protein just beforehand—a few ounces of cottage cheese or sliced turkey, for instance.

●**Fat.** Though often treated as a dietary villain, fat in *moderate amounts* slows the rate of carbohydrate absorption, thus helping to moderate insulin response.

Fat also sends a satiety (satisfaction) signal to the brain, making you feel so full you'll *want* to stop eating.

Your ratio of grams of dietary fat to grams of dietary protein should be 1 to 3. Zone-favorable fats are largely monounsaturated—olive oil, canola oil, almonds, macadamia nuts, natural peanut butter and avocados.

Avoid butter, red meat and other sources of saturated fat.

●**Caloric restriction.** Have no more than 500 calories per meal. Too many calories from any source raises insulin levels.

●**Timing.** Except for the time you spend asleep, let no more than five hours pass between Zone-favorable meals or snacks.

This works out to three small meals and two snacks a day. If you eat breakfast at 7 a.m., have lunch no later than noon. If dinner isn't until 6:30 p.m., grab a mid-afternoon snack. Have a small snack at bedtime, too.

Vital: Snacks should respect the same 4 to 3 to 1 ratio of carbohydrate to protein to fat.

Examples: One ounce of hard cheese (or two ounces of cottage cheese) and half an apple… or one small muffin baked from a mix to which you added protein powder and substituted olive oil for butter.

Curative Curry?

Bandaru S. Reddy, PhD, chief, division of nutritional carcinogenesis, American Health Foundation, Valhalla, NY.

Rats exposed to a chemical that ordinarily causes colon cancer developed far fewer tumors when they were fed a diet high in *curcumin*. That's the ingredient that gives curry its bright orange color.

The tumors that did form in the curry-eating rats were less likely to grow and spread.

Grapefruit and Oranges Protect the Heart

Pamela Mink, PhD, MPH, senior managing scientist, Health Sciences, Exponent Inc., Washington, DC.

In a new study of nearly 35,000 women ages 55 to 69, researchers found that women who consumed the most *flavanones,* a flavonoid antioxidant found primarily in citrus fruits (such as grapefruit and oranges), had a 22% lower risk for death from heart disease than those who consumed the least.

Better than Butter

Alice Lichtenstein, DSc, professor of nutrition and director of the cardiovascular nutrition laboratory at the USDA Human Nutrition Research Center on Aging at Tufts University, Boston.

Although it's best to avoid butter entirely, a spread made of equal parts of butter and olive oil has about half the saturated fat of butter. It has lots of good-for-the-heart mono-unsaturated fats and few "bad" transaturated fats. Mix butter and oil in a food processor. Store in the refrigerator.

Eggs Can Be Part of A Healthful Diet

Barbara Retzlaff, MPH, RD, head dietitian, Northwest Lipid Research Clinic, University of Washington, Seattle.

Although they can be part of a healthful diet, eggs should be avoided by anyone with *combined hyperlipidemia* (elevated cholesterol and triglyceride levels). When patients with combined hyperlipidemia ate two eggs a day for three months, their total cholesterol levels climbed from 238 to 250...while LDL (bad) cholesterol levels rose from 149 to 162. In egg eaters who had elevated cholesterol alone, levels were unchanged. *Note:* Cholesterol below 200 is considered desirable.

A Most Expensive Hamburger

Neal D. Barnard, MD, president, Physicians Committee for Responsible Medicine, 5100 Wisconsin Ave. NW, Suite 404, Washington, DC 20016.

America's appetite for meat causes an additional $29 billion to $61 billion a year in health-care costs. Individuals who eat beef, pork, poultry or fish face increased risk for high blood pressure...heart disease...diabetes...gallbladder disease...obesity and osteoarthritis... food poisoning...and cancer of the colon, lungs, ovaries and prostate.

Protein and Kidney Disease

Ping H. Wang, MD, professor of medicine, University of California, Irvine.

Kidney patients have long been told to limit the amount of protein in their diet. An analysis of 10 studies involving 1,521 patients confirms that protein restriction does, in fact, significantly reduce risk of kidney failure or death in patients with nondiabetic kidney disease. It also slows progression of kidney disease in patients with insulin-dependent diabetes.

Two Are Better than One

Study of almost 6,000 adults, reported in *Tufts University Health & Nutrition Letter,* 196 Boston Ave., Ste. 2100, Medford, MA 02155.

People who live alone get fewer nutrients than those who live with others. People living alone are less likely to meet the recommended daily allowances of many nutrients.

But live-alones consume less fat, cholesterol and sodium—probably because people tend to eat less when they eat alone.

Foods Can Change Your Moods

Judith J. Wurtman, PhD, research scientist, department of brain and cognitive science, Massachusetts Institute of Technology, Cambridge. She is author of *Managing Your Mind & Mood Through Food* (Harper Perennial) and *The Serotonin Solution*, a weight-loss book for people who overeat because of stress (Ballantine).

Sweet and starchy carbohydrates boost the level of serotonin, a "stress-relief" chemical in your brain, making you feel relaxed and in emotional control. *Examples:* Bagel, pasta, baked potato.

Foods high in protein can help increase mental alertness when you are feeling tired. *Examples:* Fish, poultry and dairy products.

Food Danger Zones

Stephen P. Gullo, PhD, president, Institute for Health and Weight Sciences, New York, which offers one-on-one coaching to retrain eating habits.

Food trouble spots are places where you're most likely to overeat—or eat the wrong foods. Some people are tempted in movie theaters, others have trouble at the office.

Self-defense: Understand your weaknesses and guard against them. If you cruise the vending machines at work, break for a planned snack —eating healthful food like a banana.

Salt-Watchers

N. Nicole Spelhang, managing editor, *Mayo Clinic Health Letter*, 200 First St. SW, Rochester, MN 55905.

If you're trying to cut back on sodium in your diet, be aware of these salt facts: Sparkling bottled water has only 3 milligrams (mg) of sodium per 12 ounces, club soda has 75 mg… fresh turkey has less than 20 mg of sodium per ounce, but deli-variety turkey and ham each have more than 300 mg…even light soy sauce has more than 600 mg of sodium per tablespoon compared with 234 mg for a tablespoon of Worcestershire sauce.

 ## We Are What We Eat

Judith J. Wurtman, PhD, research scientist, department of brain and cognitive science, Massachusetts Institute of Technology, Cambridge. She is author of *Managing Your Mind & Mood Through Food* (Harper Perennial) and *The Serotonin Solution*, a weight-loss book for people who overeat because of stress (Ballantine).

Folk wisdom has long held that our moods are influenced by the food we eat. That belief is gaining support from scientific research.

Food-mood strategies can't cure clinical depression or other serious psychological disorders. Such problems call for professional help. But they can be used to boost alertness at work…increase your sense of relaxation at home…and make it easier for you to tolerate life's ups and downs.

Mood-altering foods aren't unusual or hard to find. You don't have to follow a long, complex regimen before seeing results. They are ordinary, everyday foods…and in some cases, their effects are felt within as little as 30 minutes.

HOW FOOD ACTS ON OUR MOODS

Research suggests that food affects mood by altering the brain's production of chemical messengers called *neurotransmitters…*

The neurotransmitters *dopamine* and *norepinephrine* have an energizing effect. When your brain is producing these chemicals, you're alert, highly motivated and have fast reaction times.

The main building block of these "alertness chemicals" is the amino acid *tyrosine*. Eating protein—which contains lots of tyrosine—raises tyrosine levels in the brain. This, in turn, boosts synthesis of dopamine and norepinephrine. *Result:* Greater mental energy.

The neurotransmitter *serotonin* has a calming effect. Its presence in the brain boosts concentration, relieves feelings of anxiety and—at night or if you're sleep-deprived—makes you feel drowsy.

To make serotonin, your brain needs a supply of the amino acid *tryptophan*. Like tyrosine, tryptophan is found in proteins. But eating more protein won't increase levels of tryptophan inside your brain. In fact, a high-protein diet *depletes* the brain's tryptophan supply.

Reason: Tryptophan must "compete" with tyrosine and other, more plentiful amino acids to enter the brain. It tends to be "crowded out" by them when you eat protein.

To increase the brain's supply of tryptophan, eat carbohydrates—*without protein*. Doing so triggers the release of insulin, which shunts some of the amino acids from the blood to other organs. Tryptophan, however, is left behind in the blood. With less competition from other amino acids, it can easily enter the brain.

BASIC FOOD-MOOD PRESCRIPTION

Because tyrosine and tryptophan can be dangerous when taken in pill form, it's best to use *food* to affect levels of these neurotransmitters.

Caution: The following principles are no substitute for eating a healthful, well-balanced diet. If you have diabetes, hypoglycemia or another diet-related condition, consult a doctor before changing your eating habits.

●**For greater alertness, motivation and mental energy...eat protein.** Just three to four ounces (less than half the size of a typical restaurant entrée) is enough to get tyrosine to the brain so it can be used to make dopamine and norepinephrine.

Best sources of protein: Fish, shellfish, skinless chicken, veal, lean beef and egg whites. Because these foods are essentially pure protein—with little or no fat or carbohydrates—they work especially quickly.

Other good sources: Low-fat dairy products, dried legumes, tofu and other soy products. These contain carbohydrates but are low in fat.

Avoid: Fatty foods, such as pork, lamb, fatty cuts of beef, most hard cheeses and other whole-milk products. High-fat foods divert blood from the brain to the digestive tract. They take a very long time to digest.

●**To relax and focus...eat carbohydrates.** As little as one to one-and-one-half ounces is all most people need. Overweight people and women during the two or three days just prior to menstruation may need up to two-and-one-half ounces.

Eating the carbohydrate without protein is crucial.

Reason: Protein will boost levels of amino acids that compete with tyrosine for entry to the brain. Instead of feeling calmer, you'll feel hyped-up. (If alertness is your goal, eating carbohydrates along with protein usually does not interfere with tyrosine's energizing effect.)

Best sources of carbohydrates: Gumdrops, licorice, marshmallows, jam and other sweets...grain-based foods such as bread, crackers, pasta, rice, popcorn and pretzels... and starchy vegetables such as potatoes.

Fruits and nonstarchy vegetables are not good materials for the brain's serotonin factory. A healthful diet includes plenty of both, but these are not the foods to eat when you need to feel calm or focused.

FOOD-MOOD STRATEGIES AND WEIGHT-LOSS DIET

Dieters often wonder whether these food-mood strategies lead to overeating—and to weight gain. *In fact, these strategies are more likely to promote healthful eating...*

Reason #1: Very small portions are needed to produce results.

Reason #2: The recommendations call for little or no fat. Not only is fat bad for you, but it also interferes with the food-mood effect.

MEALTIME POWER

For consistent results, use the food-mood principles to plan your meals and time your intake of proteins and carbohydrates...

● **Breakfast.** It should contain protein but little or no fat. *Options:* An orange, eight ounces of low-fat yogurt and a low-fat bran muffin…or cranberry juice and hot cereal with skim milk.

● **Morning snack.** A snack is OK for those who find it hard to eat even a light meal first thing in the morning…and those who eat breakfast so early that they feel hungry by mid-morning. It will keep these individuals from coming to lunch so hungry that they overeat and feel sluggish all afternoon. *Good choice:* A small can of grapefruit juice, two rice cakes and one slice of skim-milk mozzarella.

● **Lunch.** It should be high in protein to keep you alert…and low in fat and calories, so you won't have to expend your energy digesting a heavy meal.

Don't *begin* lunch with a carbohydrate. If you have a roll or pasta before the entrée arrives, for example, you'll be sending tryptophan to the brain. That will dull your mental edge. *Instead:* Start your meal with a salad, juice or consommé.

● **Afternoon snack.** Few people need a snack after an energy-boosting lunch—unless they're carbohydrate cravers. For reasons we don't understand, these people start to feel irritable and scattered at midday. A handful of crackers or jelly beans will help them feel calmer and more focused.

● **Dinner.** Make sure it's high in carbohydrates if you want to relax. If you need to keep your energy up for classes or volunteer work, your dinner should be high in protein.

● **Bedtime snack.** If you have trouble unwinding at bedtime, eat one-and-one-half ounces of carbohydrates 30 minutes before retiring. (That's the equivalent of five or six graham crackers.) Make sure the snack is low in fat and protein.

Warm milk at bedtime is a *bad* idea. *Reason:* Milk contains quite a bit of protein, which most people find energizing.

POWER EATING AT CONFERENCES

To avoid the exhaustion that plagues many conference-goers, bring your own light breakfast—or skip breakfast altogether. Avoid heavy coffee-shop meals. Easy choices include a mini-box of fruit juice plus eight ounces of yogurt, or a single-serving box of cereal with low-fat milk and a banana.

If a buffet breakfast is part of the program, skip the hot table, where the high-fat foods are clustered. Instead, stick with fruit, cereals and low-fat muffins. During the coffee break, have coffee or tea, but skip the pastries.

At lunch, don't touch your roll until after you've eaten the protein part of the meal. If the entrée is a large serving, eat only half.

Pack a carbohydrate snack (such as graham crackers or fat-free cookies) in case you need to revive yourself during mid-afternoon presentations.

At dinner, emphasize protein if you need to be "on," carbohydrates if you're ready to unwind—just as you would at home.

Better Pasta Buying

Maggie Riechers, editor, *Healthy Decisions*, Georgetown University Medical Center, 3800 Reservoir Rd., Washington, DC 20007.

Buy pasta packaged in boxes, not in cellophane, and store it in a cupboard—not in glass containers on the counter. *Reason:* Exposure to light quickly robs pasta of much of its riboflavin.

Added Fiber Helps

Bruce Yaffe, MD, an internist and gastroenterologist in private practice, 121 E. 84 St., New York 10028.

Fiber supplements are effective for people who don't get enough fiber in their diets. They improve regularity, as well as firm up the movements of those who suffer from loose stools. People who don't eat enough natural sources of fiber such as fruits and vegetables should consider taking a fiber supplement like Metamucil. Other sources of supplementary fiber are oat bran and Citrucel.

Important: Supplements like Metamucil need to be accompanied by lots of fluid.

Tomatoes and Prostate Cancer Link

Edward Giovannucci, MD, professor of medicine, department of nutrition, Harvard Medical School, Boston. The nine-year study of 47,000 men between the ages of 40 and 75 was published in *The Journal of the National Cancer Institute,* 8120 Woodmont Ave., Ste. 500, Bethesda, MD 20814.

Eating cooked tomatoes reduces the risk of prostate cancer by 50%.

A study of almost 50,000 men found that those who ate two or more servings of cooked tomato products a week had one-third less risk of developing prostate cancer than those who rarely ate cooked tomato products.

Fact: Approximately 10% of all men develop prostate cancer. Another study found that men who ate 10 or more servings of tomatoes each week benefited from the high content of *lycopene,* an antioxidant. Other antioxidants, such as beta-carotene and vitamin A, had no effect on the risk of prostate cancer. And cooked tomato products seemed to bring out more lycopene than raw ones.

While tomatoes are the best food source of lycopene, there is a variety of other cancer-fighting foods to include in your diet, such as broccoli, cabbage, soybeans and carrots.

Red Meat and Non-Hodgkin's Lymphoma

Brian C.H. Chiu, MS, department of preventive medicine, Feinberg School of Medicine, Northwestern University, Chicago.

Eating red meat increases the risk of developing non-Hodgkin's lymphoma. A study of more than 35,000 women showed that those who ate the most red meat were almost twice as likely as those who ate the least to develop this cancer. Women who ate the most animal fat also had one-and-a-half times the risk of developing the disease as those who ate the least.

Vegetarianism Can Mask Anorexia

David Herzog, MD, director, Harvard Eating Disorder Center, Massachusetts General Hospital, Boston.

People with eating disorders tend to spend a lot of time categorizing foods as "safe" and "unsafe." A vegetarian diet automatically rules out many unsafe foods—particularly the fatty, calorie-rich items.

Key question: Is your diet rigid and socially isolating? Most vegetarians can "get by" when eating in restaurants and at the homes of family and friends. However, eating disorder sufferers tend to withdraw from social situations in which food plays a central role.

Prevent Asthma, Cataracts, Gallstones and Heart Failure by Eating the Right Foods

Isadore Rosenfeld, MD, Rossi Distinguished Professor of Clinical Medicine at Weill Medical College of Cornell University, New York City. He is author of several books, including *Doctor What Should I Eat?* (Grand Central) and *Dr. Isadore Rosenfeld's 2005 Breakthrough Health* (Rodale).

Almost every major medical condition is either caused or affected by what you eat. Yet very few medical doctors are knowledgeable about nutrition. As a result, they rarely give nutritional advice—even when specific foods can help curb symptoms or correct underlying problems as well as or *better than* prescription medications.

Following are the best food treatments for four common diseases…

ASTHMA

This respiratory ailment affects up to 20 million Americans and is becoming increasingly common, presumably because of worsening air pollution.

Best foods: Chili peppers...fish...and coffee.

People who regularly consume hot sauces or chili peppers may have less frequent—and less severe—asthma attacks. *Capsaicin,* the chemical that makes peppers hot, may stimulate nerve endings to help keep airways open.

The fatty acids in cold-water fish, such as salmon, tuna and sardines, lower levels of *prostaglandins* and *leukotrienes,* chemicals that increase airway swelling.

Helpful: Three or more two- to three-ounce servings of fish each week can reduce the frequency of asthma attacks.

Doctors traditionally have advised people to drink one cup of strong coffee at the onset of asthma attacks if none of their usual medications are available. One of the active ingredients, *methylxanthine,* relaxes airway muscles.

Adult asthmatics who drink several cups of caffeinated coffee daily have 30% fewer asthma attacks than noncoffee drinkers. I recommend three to four cups a day, provided you don't have active ulcers or cardiac arrhythmias.

CATARACTS

A cataract is a clouding (opacity) of the lens of the eye, which results in impaired vision. Much of the damage is caused by free radicals, harmful oxygen molecules that are produced as a by-product of metabolism.

Best foods: Brightly colored fruits and vegetables—especially squash, spinach, broccoli, oranges, carrots and sweet potatoes. They're rich in vitamins C and A as well as beta-carotene, all of which reduce eye damage.

Helpful: Eat five or more servings daily.

CONGESTIVE HEART FAILURE

It occurs when an underlying condition—such as a viral infection, hypertension, a narrowed heart valve, etc.—inhibits the heart's ability to pump blood.

Best foods: Brown rice, spinach, oatmeal, legumes (such as beans and peas), potatoes and bananas. They're rich in magnesium and potassium, both of which improve cardiac function.

Warning: These minerals often are depleted by the use of diuretics—standard drugs for the treatment of heart failure.

Helpful: Eat two daily servings of magnesium- and potassium-rich foods.

Also: Eat four to six small daily meals instead of three big ones. Blood flow to the stomach following big meals increases energy demands on the heart.

Limit total daily sodium intake to less than 2,000 mg daily (a little less than one teaspoon). Excessive salt increases fluid retention and reduces the heart's pumping ability.

GALLSTONES

About half of the 20 million American adults who have gallstones don't have symptoms. In the remaining sufferers, these collections of solid crystals in the gallbladder or bile ducts may cause severe pain under the breastbone or in the upper right side of the abdomen, especially after meals.

The presence of such crystals can irritate the gallbladder and promote infection. Even a single, large stone developing in the gallbladder predisposes that organ to cancer.

Best foods: Fruits...legumes...and vegetables—anything that's low in fat. Fatty foods stimulate gallbladder contractions that can precipitate attacks.

Bonus: The fiber in plant-based foods interacts with bile in the gallbladder and reduces stone formation. A high-fiber diet may dissolve existing stones and also helps with weight loss.

Warning: People who are just 10% overweight are twice as likely to get gallstones as those who maintain a healthful weight.

Helpful: Get 35 g to 45 g of fiber daily. Eat at least five daily servings of fruits and vegetables, along with whole-grain pasta and breads, legumes and other high-fiber foods.

Good choices: One cup of baked beans (13 g of fiber)...one medium baked potato (4 g)...one large apple (5 g)...or one-half cup All-Bran (10 g).

Finish Your Cereal

Richard Wood, PhD, associate professor of nutrition, Tufts University Human Research Center, Boston.

Drink the leftover milk in your cereal bowl. *Reason:* Some of the vitamins and minerals in fortified cereals are dissolved into the milk while you eat.

Nonfat Pancake Recipe

Brand Name Fat-Fighter's Cookbook by Sandra Woodruff, RD, nutrition consultant, Tallahassee, FL. Avery Publishing Group.

Replace each tablespoon of oil in the batter with three-fourths as much nonfat buttermilk, nonfat yogurt, applesauce or mashed banana.

Example: If a recipe calls for two tablespoons of oil, use one-and-a-half tablespoons of your chosen fat substitute. *Also:* Replace each whole egg with three tablespoons of egg white or fat-free egg substitute.

Sparkling Waters May Be Sugary

Environmental Nutrition, Box 5656, Norwalk, CT 06856.

Some clear beverages are really sugary soft drinks—but are placed on supermarket shelves near plain bottled waters and fruit-flavored waters.

Self-defense: Read the label to see the calorie content. Water has no calories. Soft drinks can contain 50 or more calories per six- to eight-ounce serving.

Lactose Intolerance

Michael D. Levitt, MD, associate chief of staff for research, Veterans Affairs Medical Center, Minneapolis.

A study suggests that only a fraction of those who think they are lactose intolerant actually are. The others have simply been swayed by widespread publicity about the condition. In a study of 30 people who thought they suffered from lactose intolerance, all were able to consume up to eight ounces of milk daily with negligible problems.

Antioxidants And Fewer Health Problems

Maureen Callahan, MS, RD, of Clearwater, FL, who writes frequently about nutrition and health. She is co-author of *The Miracle Nutrient Cookbook: 100 Delicious Antioxidant-Enriched Recipes and Menu Suggestions for Optimum Health.* Fireside.

The foods we eat have a big impact on our health—both positively *and* negatively.

Study after study shows that antioxidants—disease-fighting chemicals that occur naturally in many foods—have certain properties that may boost the immune system. They also reduce the risk of health problems—particularly heart disease and cancer.

While the antioxidants beta-carotene, vitamin C and vitamin E are available in supplement form, researchers recommend we try to obtain them naturally through the foods we eat.

ANTIOXIDANT-RICH FOODS

It is most prudent to build a proper diet through a diverse combination of foods. There are several foods that contain all three antioxidants. *They include...*

● **Mangoes.** Mangoes contain 57 milligrams (mg) of vitamin C—almost the full Recommended Daily Allowance (RDA)—as well as ample amounts of vitamin E and beta-carotene. No other tropical fruit provides all three.

● **Sweet potatoes.** They are low in calories and loaded with beta-carotene and vitamins C and E. One to two sweet potatoes—with or without the skin—almost meets the RDA for all three nutrients.

OTHER GREAT SOURCES

● **Beta-carotene is commonly found in leafy green plants.** Most health organizations recommend eating at least five fruits or vegetables a day, which amounts to a diet containing 6 mg of beta-carotene.

Beta-carotene is "fat soluble"—meaning that you need to eat a small amount of fat with the beta-carotene in order to absorb it.

Scientists have not yet determined the exact amount of fat needed, but it is not a lot. This is one example of how fat in moderation is important to maintain good health.

•**Vitamin C.** The RDA for vitamin C is 60 mg. But researchers say that you need between 100 mg and 500 mg daily to fight off cataracts and other diseases such as cancer and heart disease. *Rich sources...*

•**One papaya** (188 mg).

•**Half a raw red, green or yellow pepper** (170 mg).

•**One cup of broccoli**—steamed or microwaved (98 mg).

•**10 to 12 strawberries** (85 mg).

•**8 ounces of orange juice** (124 mg).

Vitamin C is highly sensitive to heat and cooking. So when cooking vegetables, use a pressure steamer...or lightly steam or microwave.

•**Vitamin E** is one of the most potent antioxidants when it comes to preventing disease.

Studies show that the current RDA for vitamin E—30 international units (IU)—is probably too low to be able to offer much protection against disease. Some experts believe that anywhere between 100 and 400 IU of vitamin E daily might offer better protection.

Vitamin E is most commonly found in high-fat foods, such as vegetable oils (corn, soy and peanut) and nuts.

Other examples: Sunflower seeds... wheat germ...or peanut butter.

Vitamin E can also be found in some leafy vegetables—and in sweet potatoes.

Although some experts recommend complementing dietary "E" with supplements (contrary to advice regarding other antioxidants), be aware that the synthetic "E" in some supplements is not as effective as the form naturally occurring in foods.

A Good-for-You Frozen Treat

The Healthy Gourmet by Cherie Calbom, expert and speaker on diet and nutrition, Lake Ariel, PA. Three Rivers Press.

Freeze peeled bananas. Coat each in plain low-fat yogurt. Roll the coated bananas in chopped nuts and freeze again.

Control Your Cholesterol Without Drugs

Kenneth H. Cooper, MD, MPH, president and founder of the Cooper Aerobics Center, 12200 Preston Rd., Dallas 75230. He is author of numerous books on health and fitness, including *Controlling Cholesterol the Natural Way.* Bantam.

Cholesterol-lowering statin drugs are among the most widely prescribed drugs in the United States.

Although statins are safe for most people, they can cause diarrhea, muscle pain or liver damage in 2% to 10% of patients. These drugs also cost up to $1,800 for a year's supply and must be taken for life.

That's why I prescribe statins only when total cholesterol is about 240 mg/dL or higher...or when patients already have heart disease or a high risk of developing it due to smoking, high blood pressure or other coronary risk factors.

Drug companies don't advertise this, but many people can lower their cholesterol without taking medication.*

Best approach: Eat foods with anti-cholesterol properties. Along with basic lifestyle changes, the right diet can effectively lower cholesterol to safe levels.

Bonus: If you eventually need a statin to cut cholesterol levels even more, these foods will allow you to take the lowest possible dose.

THE DIET CURE

Even people with moderately elevated cholesterol (above 200) should be on a low-fat diet.

*Talk to your doctor about the best cholesterol-lowering regimen for you.

This means limiting total fat calories to 30% or less of your total fat intake. Saturated fats, found in butter, meats and baked goods, should account for no more than 10% of total calories.

However, low-fat diets are not the perfect solution. Even with such diets, cholesterol rarely drops more than 50 points, which is not enough for some people. Also, a low-fat diet reduces levels of beneficial high-density lipoprotein (HDL) cholesterol along with the harmful low-density lipoprotein (LDL).

To compensate, everyone with high cholesterol needs to eat "functional" foods daily. These are natural and laboratory-modified foods that inhibit cholesterol absorption or promote its excretion from the body. *I advise patients to eat both types of these foods to get the most cholesterol-lowering benefits…*

●**Traditional functional foods**. The soluble fiber in some grains, legumes and fruits dissolves and forms a gel in the intestine. This gel traps cholesterol molecules and prevents their absorption into the bloodstream. People who eat 7 grams (g) to 8 g of soluble fiber daily can lower total cholesterol 5% to 8%. *Best options…*

●Psyllium. It's an ancient Indian grain added to some breakfast cereals as well as commercial laxatives. In one study, as little as 3 g of psyllium daily lowered total cholesterol by 15% and LDL by 20%.

Many breakfast cereals, including Kellogg's All-Bran Bran Buds and multigrain cereals, contain psyllium. Or you can take three tablespoons of Metamucil daily, which is equivalent to about 10 g of soluble fiber.

●Oat and rice bran. New studies show that people who eat three ounces of oat bran daily can improve the ratio of "bad" LDL to "good" HDL cholesterol by 24%.

Rice bran lowers LDL almost as much as oat bran in those who eat approximately three ounces daily.

●Fish. Two to three fish meals weekly will lower LDL and triglycerides, fats that have also been linked to heart disease.

One study of 20,000 American doctors found that one meal of salmon, tuna or other omega-3-rich fish per week reduced the risk for fatal heart attack by 52%.

Fish-oil supplements are an option for people who don't eat fish, but they may not provide as many health benefits as fish. *Typical dose:* 1 g to 3 g daily.

●**Designed functional foods.** The trans-fats in traditional margarines raise cholesterol about as much as saturated fat does. Benecol, a cholesterol-lowering margarine, contains stanol esters, chemically modified plant extracts that lower cholesterol as effectively as some drugs.

Eating four tablespoons of Benecol (the equivalent of three pats) daily lowers LDL by up to 14%. Benecol is also available in gel tablets for people who want the convenience of supplements or don't eat margarine.

Helpful: A low-calorie version, Benecol Light, contains approximately 50% fewer calories. It can be spread on toast, bagels, etc., but it should not be used for cooking. You can cook with regular Benecol, however.

ADDITIONAL STRATEGIES

In addition to following a low-fat diet and eating functional foods, people with high cholesterol should consider…

●**Vitamins.** Certain antioxidant vitamins reduce heart attack risk by blocking chemical changes (oxidation) that cause LDL cholesterol to stick to arterial walls and promote atherosclerosis (fatty buildup in the arteries).

●Vitamin E. Take at least 200 international units (IU) of the natural form (d-alpha-tocopherol) daily, but consult your doctor first.

●Vitamin C. Like vitamin E, it inhibits oxidation of LDL molecules. People who get the most vitamin C in their diets or from supplements are less likely to die from cardiovascular disease than those who get smaller amounts. *Dosage:* 500 mg, twice daily, in supplement form.

●**Exercise.** We used to think that only vigorous workouts would elevate levels of beneficial HDL cholesterol.

New research: Walking or jogging at low to moderate intensity—for example, walking a mile in about 14 minutes—can raise HDL by as much as 9%.

I advise patients to walk briskly for 30 minutes at least three days a week, then after two weeks to add additional exercise, such as calisthenics and weight training.

Bonus: Combining a healthful diet with aerobic exercise can lower LDL by up to 20 points.

● **Weight loss.** It's not clear why, but many people who lose weight also reduce their LDL cholesterol levels. Total cholesterol typically drops by about 5% for every five to 10 pounds of weight loss.

● **Niacin.** High doses of this B vitamin (1.5 g to 3 g daily) can lower LDL by as much as 15% to 30% and raise HDL by 10% to 40%.

Niacin can be taken alone but is normally added if statins do not lower triglycerides or raise HDL sufficiently. But at high doses, niacin can cause side effects, such as flushing, liver problems and heart rhythm irregularities. Use it only under a doctor's supervision.

Better Breakfasts

Brand Name Fat-Fighter's Cookbook by Sandra Woodruff, RD, nutrition consultant, Tallahassee, FL. Avery Publishing Group.

The healthiest breakfast cereals have whole grain listed as the first—and therefore main —ingredient. *Reason:* Whole grains contain essential fatty acids, vitamin E and other important nutrients. Also check the nutrition label for sugar content. A prudent daily sugar limit is 50 grams (four grams equals one teaspoon). Look for low-fat cereals—not necessarily *no-fat* ones.

Creamy Dishes Without Cream

Brand Name Fat-Fighter's Cookbook by Sandra Woodruff, RD, nutrition consultant, Tallahassee, FL. Avery Publishing Group.

Replace the cream called for in the recipe with an equal amount of evaporated skim milk.

Alternative: Replace one cup of heavy cream with one cup of regular skim milk plus one-third cup of instant nonfat dry milk powder. These substitutions work in quiches, sauces, casseroles, custards, puddings and other traditionally high-fat dishes.

What You Should Know About Caffeine

Timothy McCall, MD, an internist, medical editor of *Yoga Journal* and author of *Examining Your Doctor: A Patient's Guide to Avoiding Harmful Medical Care.* Carol. *www.drmccall.com.*

Over the years, conflicting information has been written about the risks of caffeine. Studies have shown that drinking coffee has been tied to pancreatic cancer …high cholesterol…heart attacks…and birth defects.

Reality: The results of these studies have been called into question by health experts. That's because people who drink a lot of coffee tend to have other bad habits as well, such as smoking or not exercising—which may be the culprits.

CAFFEINE AND OSTEOPOROSIS

While caffeine in coffee, tea, cola, chocolate and some medications can cause jitteriness, trembling, irritability and insomnia, studies have not substantiated most of the claims about caffeine's negative *long-term effects*.

Exception: There appears to be a connection between consuming high levels of caffeine and osteoporosis—the thinning of bones that can lead to hip fractures, especially in older women. Risk factors for osteoporosis include being female, thin, white—particularly of Northern European ancestry—or Asian…not exercising…smoking…and having a family history of the disease.

Self-defense: If you are at high risk for developing osteoporosis, you should significantly reduce your caffeine intake and be sure to include enough calcium in your diet. In one study, women who drank at least one glass of milk per day were protected from the bone-thinning consequences of caffeine.

If you can't drink milk, take a calcium supplement. Calcium carbonate, sold in supermarkets, drugstores and health food stores, is an inexpensive and effective source.

Premenopausal women should take 1,200 mg/day...postmenopausal women, 1,500 mg/day. For best absorption, take no more than 500 mg at one time.

CAFFEINE WITHDRAWAL

People who are accustomed to drinking several cups of coffee a day may find that they develop headaches, difficulty concentrating, fatigue and depression if they eliminate caffeine from their diets.

If you decide you want to cut down on caffeine, it's best to do so slowly. Cut back by about 20% a week over a month—or more.

Slowly reducing the amount of caffeine in your system prevents withdrawal reactions. If headaches or other symptoms develop, increase your consumption slightly, then continue to slowly lower it over time.

Liquid Nutritional Supplements Are No Substitute for Real Food

Bonnie Liebman, MS, director of nutrition, Center for Science in the Public Interest, Washington, DC.

Liquid nutritional supplements, including brands such as Boost, Ensure, Resource and Sustacal, were originally created for the infirm and elderly. Today they're being promoted with slick commercials to active seniors as well as healthier, younger people who don't have the time to eat three square meals a day.

Reality: Most supplements contain a mixture of water, oil, sugar, soy, milk protein and added vitamins and minerals. *Better choices:* Fruits and vegetables, whole grain breads, yogurt. These old favorites also contain fiber as well as substances such as phytochemicals, which are believed to help prevent cancer and heart disease.

Distilled Water Is Safe to Drink

The late Richard P. Maas, PhD, associate professor of environmental studies, University of North Carolina, Asheville.

Distilled water provides an even higher degree of protection than other bottled waters for people with weakened immune systems who need to make extra efforts to avoid the *Cryptosporidium* parasite.

All About Food Allergies

Thomas Brunoski, MD, a physician in private practice in Westport, CT. Dr. Brunoski specializes in the treatment of medical problems with nutritional and allergy therapy rather than medication.

Every year, hundreds of people suffering from chronic health conditions—headaches, anxiety, asthma, heart disease, arthritis, mood swings and more—come to me for help.

One of the first questions I ask them is, *What do you eat?*

Reason: The most basic fact of our health is food, since every cell of our body comes from what we eat. Many people I see are making efforts to eat well, but their diets seem to betray them.

For many people, unsuspected allergies are present that can cause or aggravate a wide range of problems. If this seems likely, then I run a series of allergy tests to see what foods may be triggering their individual symptoms. Since it is almost impossible for a person to identify offending foods on his/her own, the findings are often surprising—not only to my patients but to me as well.

Once I discover which foods are making a patient sick—or worsening his condition—I'm able to prescribe a diet that can significantly improve that person's health.

The following are stories of just a few patients who have been helped by simply changing their diets.

ASTHMA AND ALLERGIES

A 30-year-old woman with a history of asthma told me her condition was getting worse, even though her doctor had prescribed four strong asthma medications. She had no energy, wheezed all the time and couldn't sleep because her coughing kept her awake. Her doctor told her that she might have to take oral steroid pills, which have unpleasant and harmful side effects.

Solution: First, I urged this woman to cut out all processed sugar. She could eat fruits since they contain fiber. Fiber binds sugar, releasing it over a longer period of time so that the body can digest it more slowly.

I explained that studies done in the 1930s at the Mayo Clinic suggested a link between sugar intake and asthma. These same studies found that a sugar-free diet helped control or even cure asthma in many children. (I also advised her to cut out caffeine, which seems to worsen asthma attacks.)

Because asthma is an allergic condition, I tested her for food allergies and found that she was sensitive to a variety of foods, including beef, milk, eggs, corn, tomatoes, wheat and peanuts.

Result: Within two weeks, the patient had stopped consuming sugar, caffeine and her specific "allergy foods," and she reported that she felt great. She had more energy…her sleeping had improved…and her husband was getting more sleep, too, since she wasn't waking him with her constant coughing.

During the past year, she has stopped using all asthma medications and hasn't had a single attack.

OSTEOARTHRITIS AND ALLERGIES

A middle-aged man came to me six years ago after being diagnosed with osteoarthritis. He suffered from pain in many joints and was taking over-the-counter and prescription pain medications, but his condition was worsening.

Solution: I advised him to cut out all junk food and start eating healthful meals, including salads. If there's such a thing as "miracle food," I'm convinced it is dark green salads—romaine, arugula and red leaf lettuce. These are loaded with vitamins, minerals and disease-fighting nutrients—flavonoids and retinoids.

I also tested him for food allergies and found he was strongly allergic to many things, including soybeans, oranges, potatoes, corn and onions. After following a diet devoid of these items for two months, the patient returned complaining that he felt better but still had pain.

I asked what he had been eating, and he replied, *Lots of chicken and broccoli.* So I did more tests and found that he was highly allergic to both of these foods. Broccoli was quite a surprise to me since I had never heard of anyone who was allergic to it.

Result: He stopped eating broccoli and chicken and started feeling better immediately. He also reported that he had little or no swelling in his joints. If he indulged his passion for these two foods, he felt achy the next day.

Eventually, I treated this man with oral immunotherapy (liquid allergy treatment that is administered under the tongue and that "desensitizes" people to particular foods or other allergens). Now he can eat both chicken and broccoli without trouble.

MIGRAINES AND ALLERGIES

A 27-year-old woman had migraine headaches once or twice a month. The symptoms were severe—extreme pain, nausea, vomiting and visual disturbances. She also felt fatigued much of the time. She mentioned that she had a childhood history of allergies, which is common in migraine patients. But she couldn't pinpoint any headache triggers—such as particular foods that might set off an attack.

Solution: Since sugar and caffeine are well-known migraine triggers, I advised that she eliminate them immediately. She also cut out processed foods since additives, including artificial dyes and preservatives—nitrites and sulfites—can cause a migraine attack. Testing revealed that my patient was allergic to a wide variety of foods. I suggested that she stop eating them as well.

Result: Within four weeks of starting her new diet, she hadn't experienced a single headache. One year later she remains headache-free. And with allergy desensitization, she is now eating the allergy-causing foods again—but no junk.

Spinach Pasta Contains Very Little Spinach

Reported in *University of California, Berkeley Wellness Letter*, Box 420148, Palm Coast, FL 32142.

One cup of cooked spinach pasta contains less than one tablespoon of spinach—which is just enough for color and a hint of flavor. The same is also true for other types of vegetable pastas.

Power Eating… Foods to Make You More Productive

Judith J. Wurtman, PhD, research scientist, department of brain and cognitive science, Massachusetts Institute of Technology, Cambridge. She is author of *Managing Your Mind & Mood Through Food* (Harper Perennial) and *The Serotonin Solution*, a weight-loss book for people who overeat because of stress (Ballantine).

Whether you're an early bird or a night owl, you can maintain a high level of energy all day by eating the right foods at the right times.

HOW POWER EATING WORKS

Protein foods, such as meats, fish, poultry, dairy products, beans and eggs, contain the amino acid *tyrosine*. This stimulates the brain to produce *norepinephrine* and *dopamine*, two alertness chemicals. When eaten alone or with carbohydrates, such as breads, cereal products, fruits and vegetables, protein foods boost mental alertness and energy.

Never *start* a meal with a carbohydrate if you plan to work after the meal, because it may trigger drowsiness.

Reason: Carbohydrates contain the amino acid *tryptophan*, which triggers production of *serotonin*, a calming chemical.

FOODS THAT ENERGIZE

All low-fat protein foods produce quick mood-modifying and energy-boosting results. *For most people, three to four ounces of the following work well…*

Low-fat, low-carbohydrate foods, such as shellfish, fish, chicken (without the skin), veal, extra-lean beef, beans and legumes. *Also good:* Low-fat cottage cheese, yogurt, milk or tofu.

WHAT TO EAT

The body's "biological clock" plays a big part in how food energizes us. This clock causes us to feel the most energetic and the least stressed during the first six hours after awakening.

From then on, our energy level slowly decreases until the end of the day—usually within one hour of normal bedtime—when we shut down mentally.

The key to maintaining high performance levels is to eat foods that are energizing when your biological rhythms are beginning to slow down. *Meal guidelines…*

●**Breakfast.** A nutritious breakfast or a snack before noon keeps you from overeating at lunchtime. For maximum results, eat within three hours of awakening.

Best: A breakfast rich in protein foods, high in vitamins and minerals and low in fat.

Example: One piece of fresh fruit sliced (or one-half to three-quarters cup of berries) mixed into eight ounces of plain yogurt…a bran muffin with one or two teaspoonfuls of jelly or diet margarine …one cup of coffee (black or with skim milk).

●**Lunch.** Your midday meal will either sustain your morning alertness or accelerate the drop in your energy level.

Best for you: A high-protein, low-fat, alcohol-free meal.

Examples: Three to five ounces of meat, poultry, seafood or fish…or eight ounces of low-fat yogurt or cottage cheese…or two ounces of low-fat cheese, such as mozzarella, ricotta or feta…or two eggs. *In addition:* One piece of sliced fruit (or one-half to three-quarters cup of berries) and two slices of whole-grain bread.

Myth: Pasta at lunch increases your mental and physical energy.

Reality: Most athletes load up on pasta before a prolonged endurance event because the body converts it to *glycogen*, which fuels the muscles…not the brain.

●**Dinner.** Your evening meal comes at a time when your biological rhythms are telling your body to shut down. To stay alert for evening projects, eat high-protein, low-carbohydrate foods.

Example: Four to five ounces of skinned, boneless, broiled chicken...one cup stir-fried mixed vegetables (broccoli, water chestnuts, onions, etc.) ...three-quarters cup of steamed rice and one fresh orange. Never begin with a carbohydrate—breads, crackers, deep-fried vegetables, etc.

Caffeine alert: Your brain cells are most sensitive to caffeine first thing in the morning. *Recommended:* Limit your daily intake to one or two cups of coffee or tea when you get up (the effects will last up to six hours) and another cup in the middle of the afternoon.

Important: Avoid caffeine after 4:30 pm if it keeps you awake at night. However, if you have to work late or are fighting jet lag, a cup of coffee with dinner may keep you going a little longer.

PREPERFORMANCE EATING

The foods you eat before giving a speech, presentation or other public performance can make or break it...

- **Never perform on an empty stomach.**
- **Eat sparingly**—if possible, two hours before your performance.
- **Choose low-calorie**, low-fat foods.
- **Drink enough coffee or tea** to maintain your body's usual level of caffeine during your performance. *Caution:* If you rarely drink coffee or tea, don't start now. It will only make you more nervous.
- **Drink little or no alcohol**...and do not drink any alcohol in the three hours before your presentation.

Cancer Self-Defense

Ronald W. Estabrook, PhD, O'Hara professor of biochemistry, University of Texas Southwestern Medical Center, Dallas, who led a study of more than 200 cancer-causing substances found in the diet.

The biggest cancer threats are eating too much fat...and too many calories...and drinking too much alcohol—far greater cancer threats than consuming "cancer-causing" foods.

Reason: Most carcinogens, whether natural or synthetic, are present at levels so low that they pose an insignificant cancer risk.

Self-defense: Eat a varied and balanced diet that includes plenty of fruits and vegetables. This type of diet is not only better for your body but also helps protect against natural carcinogens. And, of course, don't smoke.

Wasted Food Statistics

William Rathje, PhD, instructor and professor of anthropology and archeology, University of Arizona, and director of the Garbage Project, which studies landfills, quoted in *The ULS Report*, Box 130116, Ann Arbor, MI.

Households that buy the highest proportion of processed foods also waste the highest percentage of fresh foods...

- **Vegetables make up one-third** of all wasted food.
- **22% are baked goods** and 18% are fruits.

Little-Known Blood Clot Buster

John Folts, PhD, professor of medicine, University of Wisconsin Medical School, Madison. His study of 15 people was published in the *Journal of the American College of Cardiology*, 3655 Nobel Dr., Ste. 360, San Diego, 92112.

Purple grape juice prevents dangerous blood clots even more effectively than aspirin. *Flavonoids* in the juice reduce platelet "stickiness" by about 40%.

Researchers believe the same benefits can be derived from red wine and other kinds of grape juice—but not from grapes or "grape drink," which isn't 100% juice. The clot-fighting properties of grape juice are especially beneficial for certain heart patients.

Counting Calories

Soren Toubro, MD, associate professor of human nutrition, Royal Veterinary and Agricultural University, Copenhagen.

Counting calories is less effective at keeping weight off than eating a low-fat, high-carbohydrate diet.

Finding: Formerly overweight people who ate such a diet for one year regained less than one pound on average. Similar people who counted calories gained eight pounds. After two years, the calorie-counting group had regained 23 pounds each, those in the low-fat, high-carb group 11 pounds.

The Ultimate Summer Barbecue

Chris Schlesinger, head chef and co-owner of the East Coast Grill in Cambridge, MA. He is coauthor of *The Thrill of the Grill* and *License to Grill.* Morrow.

Come summer, everyone wants to cook out. But with steaks and burgers banned from many barbecues because of their high fat content, is there anything left that's really worth grilling?

Absolutely, says Chris Schlesinger, a Cambridge, Massachusetts-based chef who is noted for his grilling recipes. Poultry, seafood, vegetables and even fruit make great alternatives.

Here are Schlesinger's six rules for healthful grilling. Together, they make for a great cookout.

AVOID CHARCOAL BRIQUETTES

Briquettes contain petroleum-based compounds that can wind up in your food. Lump hardwood charcoal—sold in supermarkets and hardware stores—makes a better choice.

These irregular lumps of pure charcoal are easier to light than briquettes...and they're free of petroleum products.

Gas grills are easy to use, but food cooked over gas just doesn't taste as good as food cooked over hardwood charcoal.

BUILD A TWO-LEVEL FIRE

If you're not careful, grilled food can end up getting burned on the outside and still be raw on the inside. To avoid this, build a fire with a high-heat area for searing...and a low-heat area to continue cooking food through.

Build your fire on one side of the grill. Once the coals are red-hot, use tongs to move a *few* over to the other side. Let food get well-seared before moving it to the "cool" side.

USE A CHIMNEY STARTER

Lighter fluid certainly does the job, but a chimney starter costs less and is just as convenient.

Fill the base of the starter with crumpled newspaper, then place it on the grill's fire grate. That's the *lower* grate, not the one the food touches. Fill the top with charcoal and light the newspaper.

Once the coals are red-hot, spill them onto the fire grate. Use long, fireproof mitts when handling the starter. Reattach the grill (cooking surface). Wait until the coals are covered with gray ash before grilling. Chimney starters can be purchased at hardware stores.

AVOID OIL-BASED MARINADES

Easy-to-make spice "rubs" are tastier than traditional oil-based marinades, and they're fat-free.

All purpose barbecue rub: Mix one-third cup each of freshly cracked black pepper, kosher salt, lightly packed brown sugar, paprika and cumin. Add two tablespoons each of cayenne pepper, ground allspice and ground ginger. Using your hands, rub it onto poultry or seafood before grilling.

USE STEAK SPARINGLY

If you love steak but fear its high fat content, use it as an accompaniment rather than an entrée. For example, add small bits of steak to a salad. Throw in some grilled portobello mushrooms for a texture and flavor so meaty, even confirmed steak lovers find them satisfying.

TOP FOOD WITH SALSA

Salsas are just as tasty as traditional barbecue sauces—*and* much better for you. Try topping grilled chicken or swordfish with a mixture of chopped tomatoes, fresh cilantro and lime juice.

Dangerous Diets

Stephen P. Gullo, PhD, president, Institute for Health and Weight Sciences, New York City, and author of *Thin Tastes Better.* Dell.

Beware of diets that do one or more of the following...

●**Claim weight losses of more than one to two pounds per week.**

●**Promote *miracle* foods or supplements.**

●**Restrict or recommend large quantities of specific foods** to the detriment of a balanced diet.

●**Imply that you can lose weight—and keep it off—without making any lifestyle changes or exercising.**

●**Rely heavily on case histories, testimonials and anecdotes**—but offer no scientific research to back up those claims.

●**Typically promise a "money-back guarantee."**

Simple Dieting Trick

Charles R. Attwood, MD, a physician in private practice in Crowley, LA, and author of *Dr. Attwood's Low-Fat Prescription for Kids.* Viking.

Trim fat from your diet by remembering the simple acronym MEDICS.

●**M** is for meat...

●**E** is for eggs...and

●**D** is for dairy products.

Avoid or limit the first two and eat only non-fat versions of the third. *And minimize consumption of I, C and S...*

●**I** stands for *invisible fat* in nuts, soybeans, olives and vegetable oils.

●**C** is for condiments like ketchup, salad dressings, sauces and gravies.

●**S** is for cookies, candy, chips and other fatty snacks.

If You Need to Use Eggs...

Franca B. Alphin, MPH, RD, LDN, assistant clinical professor, dietitian and director of health promotion, Duke University Diet and Fitness Center, Durham, NC.

To cut cholesterol and fat in recipes calling for eggs, use two egg whites instead of one whole egg. That cuts out all the cholesterol and 5 grams of fat—yet the dish should taste basically the same. If the recipe calls for more than one egg, substitute two egg whites for the first egg and one egg white for each additional egg.

More About Flavonoids

Paul Knekt, PhD, head of laboratory, National Public Health Institute, Helsinki. His 26-year study of 2,748 men and 2,385 women 30 to 69 years of age was published in the *British Medical Journal*, BMA House, Tavistock Square, London WCIH 9JP.

Fruits, vegetables, red wine and tea are all good sources of these potent antioxidants. Recently, researchers suggested that flavonoid-rich diets cut the risk of heart disease.

Now: Flavonoid-rich diets appear to reduce the death rate from *all* causes. In a study, individuals who ate the most flavonoids had a 25% to 30% lower risk of premature death than those who ate the least.

Arthritic Knee?

Timothy E. McAlindon, MD, MPH, associate professor of medicine and chief of rheumatology, Tufts-New England Medical Center. His eight-year study of knee pain in 556 participants in the Framingham Study was published in *Annals of Internal Medicine,* 190 N. Independence Mall West, Philadelphia 19106.

In a study, people who consumed little vitamin D were three times more likely to have worsening of osteoarthritis of the knee than those who ingested high levels of vitamin D. The recommended daily allowance is 400 international units (IU). Dairy products, cod liver oil, salmon and sardines are good sources of vitamin D.

Cut Kidney Stone Recurrence

Robert A. Hiatt, MD, PhD, director, population sciences and deputy director, University of California, San Francisco, Comprehensive Cancer Center and professor of epidemiology and biostatistics at UCSF. His five-year study of 99 kidney stone patients was published in the *American Journal of Epidemiology,* 111 Market Pl., Ste. 840, Baltimore 21202.

Doctors have long urged kidney stone patients to adopt a low-protein, high-fiber, high-fluid diet. But a study suggests that the most important thing to do is to drink lots of water—six to 10 eight-ounce glasses a day.

Safer Meat Marinating

Reported in *University of California, Berkeley Wellness Letter,* Box 420148, Palm Coast, FL 32142.

Always marinate meat in the refrigerator rather than at room temperature.

Reason: Leaving the meat out allows bacteria to grow.

Do not put cooked meat back into an uncooked marinade or use it as a sauce unless you heat the marinade to a boil for at least one minute.

Reason: The used marinade could be contaminated by bacteria from the raw meat.

Cut the Fat

Cut the Fat! More than 500 Easy and Enjoyable Ways to Reduce Fat from Every Meal by the American Dietetic Association. Collins.

Put soups, broths, stews and baked beans in the refrigerator for 30 minutes before opening. Remove the lid, and skim off the solidified fat. This also works with *homemade* soups and stews—chill them and take out the fat that rises to the top.

Proven Diet for Arthritis Pain Relief

James Scala, PhD, a nutrition and health researcher for more than 30 years. Based in Lafayette, CA, he has taught nutrition at universities and medical schools in the US and abroad. He is author of several books, including *The New Arthritis Relief Diet.* Plume.

If you have arthritis and think drugs are your only hope, think again. When scrupulously followed, a surprisingly simple diet plan has reduced arthritis symptoms for people all over the world. At least 15 major clinical studies have shown that this dietary approach works effectively.

THROW AWAY YOUR NSAIDS

The study's subjects—most of whom had had arthritis for many years—reduced their use of nonsteroidal anti-inflammatory drugs (NSAIDs), common arthritis medications. That means many, if not most, could stop taking them completely...and all of the subjects could get along with less.

That's pretty spectacular because NSAIDs have potentially severe side effects that get more serious over time. For example, they raise blood pressure and increase the risk of ulcers by about 15%. With long-term use, they can cause harm.

If you go on this diet, your arthritis discomfort should begin to abate within a couple of weeks.

Important: It will be three months before the diet has its full impact.

REBALANCING YOUR BODY'S CHEMICALS

Your goal is to create a better balance between two *prostaglandins* (hormone-like substances that your body cells make) so that you favor the one that reduces inflammation instead of the one that increases it.

The best way to decrease the harmful prostaglandin is with *eicosapentaenoic acid* (EPA). EPA is an omega-3 fatty acid found almost exclusively in the oils of fish and sea animals. Fish is good for you. It provides the most protein for the least number of calories and possesses the most healthful form of fat.

Caution: Most fast-food and frozen cooked fish contain ingredients that counteract the healthful effect by burying it beneath unhealthful deep-fried breading.

In restaurants, order baked, poached or broiled fish. Lemon juice is a tasty butter substitute.

Consume all the omega-3 oils you can. In addition to their inflammation-reducing properties, they also inhibit the development of arterial plaque that leads to heart disease and stroke. *Good sources of omega-3 oils...*

●**Fish...**especially deep-sea cold-water fish. *Excellent:* Salmon, herring, mackerel. *Good:* Bluefish, smelt, tuna and whitefish. If fresh fish are unavailable, eat frozen, canned or farmed fish (catfish, farm-raised rainbow trout, perch, cod and pike).

●**Fish oil supplements...**sold in health food stores and drugstores.

●**Flaxseed oil...**sold at health food stores and grocery stores. This powerhouse oil, which your body converts to EPA, is tasteless, golden yellow and easily added to foods such as hot or cold cereal, salad dressing, tuna salad or juice. One tablespoon or three capsules of flaxseed oil is equivalent to a one-gram EPA capsule.

Goal: Get at least three grams of EPA every day (five is better) in protein-rich fish and in capsules as food supplements.

EATING STRATEGY

●**Eat like a vegetarian**—but without limiting the amount of fish.

●**Chicken (skin removed)** is acceptable in moderation.

●**Venison and rabbit** are OK, but avoid all other meat. If you must indulge—eat low-fat red meat no more than once a month.

●**Cut back on milk and eggs** except for skim milk and egg whites.

●**Seek low-fat protein** from vegetable products such as tofu.

A salmon a day: If you eat just one meal of salmon each day and no meat or animal products, you'll feel better.

Caution: The nightshade plants—tomatoes, potatoes, eggplant and red and green peppers—cause inflammation for many, but not all, people with arthritis. To find out whether nightshades affect you, note in a food diary whenever you eat one nightshade, then don't eat it for three or four days. If you get a reaction in your joints within eight hours, try the food again. Same result? Avoid that food indefinitely.

THE WEIGHT GAME

Losing weight isn't the whole antiarthritis pain story, but it's definitely an issue. Extra body weight makes arthritis worse...not only in weight-bearing body areas, like the hips and knees, but also in common sites like the hands. No one is sure why.

The same is true for inflammatory disease in general, including migraine headaches, Crohn's disease and multiple sclerosis.

VITAMINS, MINERALS, FIBER AND MORE

Take a multivitamin and up to 500 milligrams of vitamin C daily.

Every day, put color on your plate—in the form of red, orange and yellow vegetables.

Certain substances that occur in some foods or are produced by the body, are capable of stimulating an immune response against the membranes in the joints, exacerbating arthritis. To help your body excrete these substances, eat enough fiber to have a bowel movement every 24 to 36 hours.

Excellent sources of fiber: Whole grains, such as bran cereal and whole wheat bread... fruits and vegetables. In addition, it helps to take a powdered fiber supplement, usually made from psyllium seed husks. Be sure to drink a lot of water when taking fiber supplements.

Don't deep-fry...stir-fry instead. When you cook with oil, use olive oil or canola oil. Peanut and soybean oils are acceptable—but not as good. Avoid corn oil—it helps the body make the bad prostaglandin.

TRACKING EVERYTHING YOU EAT

Help your health care practitioner—someone with interest and expertise in nutrition—treat your arthritis with diet. Present the facts in a food diary. Record everything you eat and drink, the amount, the time and why you ate it (main meal, snacking, felt faint, social occasion).

Each morning and evening, describe how your arthritis feels.

Examples: Inflammation, pain, stiff hands, inability to open an applesauce jar.

At night, evaluate whether your diet was balanced that day…whether you ate enough of the right stuff, too little or too much.

Bottom line: We eat an enormous amount of food in our lifetime—one bite at a time. Make each bite work for you, not against you.

Fruit Juice Trap

Barbara A. Dennison, MD, associate professor of clinical pediatrics, College of Physicians and Surgeons, Columbia University, New York City. Her study of 116 two-year-olds and 107 five-year-olds was published in *Pediatrics*, 141 Northwest Point Blvd., Elk Grove Village, IL 60007.

Too much fruit juice can make kids fat. Children who drank more than 12 ounces of fruit juice a day were likely to be fatter and/or shorter than those who drank less.

Theory: Fruit juice is rich in calorie-dense simple sugars like fructose and glucose. Kids should consume no more than two six-ounce glasses of juice per day.

Eat Less Fat… Easy Ways

Men's Health, 33 E. Minor St., Emmaus, PA 18098.

Blot the grease on the top of pizza with a napkin. That will get rid of at least one teaspoon of fat.

●**Leave the last half-inch of take-out Chinese food in the container** so that you'll eat less sauce.

●**Make mashed potatoes with buttermilk—** or skim milk and butter-flavored seasoning—instead of using butter and whole milk.

●**Sauté meat and vegetables in fruit juice** or Worcestershire sauce instead of oil.

●**Do not drink alcohol on an empty stomach.** Alcohol increases food cravings and can trigger a high-calorie binge.

Other Calcium Sources

Barbara S. Levine, RD, PhD, director, Calcium Information Center, New York Hospital–Cornell Medical Center, New York City.

Broccoli, kale, bok choy and other leafy greens are calcium-rich…as are canned sardines and calcium-fortified orange juice, tofu and soy milk. If you worry about your calcium intake, ask your doctor about taking a daily calcium supplement.

Eat Healthier

Nikolaos Scarmeas, MD, is assistant professor of neurology, Columbia University Medical Center, New York City, and lead author of a study of 2,258 elderly patients.

The Mediterranean diet reduces Alzheimer's risk, we hear from Nikolaos Scarmeas, MD. Elderly patients who strictly followed the diet were 40% less likely to develop the disease than similar patients who did not.

Theory: The diet—which is high in monounsaturated fats (such as olive oil), produce, fish and legumes and low in meat and dairy—is associated with lower rates of cardiovascular disease and inflammation, both of which increase risk of Alzheimer's.

Ales, Beer and Alcohol

Nick Funnell, head brewer, Great American Restaurants, Centreville, VA.

Mild ales have less alcohol than normal beer, but more beer taste than nonalcoholic beers. Mild ales contain about 3% alcohol. Regular beer contains nearly 5%. Labels do not always point the way to less alcohol. Light beer is usually lower in calories but not much lower in alcohol content. Dark-colored beers may have stronger flavor than regular beers but not necessarily more alcohol.

Healthy Cheese Cooking

Skinny Italian Cooking by Ruth Glíck, recipe developer and member of the International Association of Cooking Professionals, Columbia, MD. Surrey Books.

For healthier cooking with cheese, substitute low-fat varieties—and cut back the amount used. Use shredded mozzarella instead of sliced—it goes further—or sprinkle cheese on top of a dish instead of mixing it in. *Fresh-grated* Parmesan has a distinctive taste, so a little goes a long way—one-quarter cup has only seven grams of fat.

Medication Trap

Jerry Avorn, MD, professor of medicine, Harvard Medical School, Boston. His study of 3,500 New Jersey Medicaid recipients was published in *The American Journal of Medicine*, 360 Park Ave. So., New York City, 10010.

Stiffness, tremors and other symptoms attributed to Parkinson's disease may actually be side effects of drugs used to treat dementia, psychiatric problems or gastrointestinal complaints.

Danger: Doctors who fail to recognize this may prescribe *additional* medication to control the symptoms. The new drug may exacerbate tremors—and produce hallucinations and/or psychosis.

Self-defense: Before a new drug is prescribed for anyone with Parkinson's-type symptoms, the doctor should take him/her off the initial drug to see if the symptoms subside.

More Fat-Free Food Traps

Martin Katahn, PhD, professor emeritus, Vanderbilt University, and Lee Fleshod, PhD, former director of Nutritional Services, Tennessee Department of Public Health.

Makers of fat-free foods often compensate for the lack of flavor by adding extra sugar—boosting total calories significantly.

The extra calories from sugar can both add to your weight and increase the level of triglycerides in your blood, which raise the risk of heart disease.

Also: Independent analyses of "fat-free" foods often find fat content far in excess of what can legally be labeled "fat free."

Treatments for Nail Fungus

Mary Ellen Brademas, MD, clinical assistant professor of dermatology, New York University Medical Center, New York City.

Infected fingernails and toenails can be cleared up faster and better with two types of oral medication. Much more effective than creams, these prescription drugs—*Lamisil* and *Sporanox*—are incorporated into the nail bed and kill the fungus as the nail grows out.

Reducing Heart Attack Risk

Martha L. Daviglus, MD, PhD, professor of preventive medicine at Northwestern University Medical School, Chicago. Her study was published in *The New England Journal of Medicine,* 10 Shattuck St., Boston 02115.

Eating just a small amount of fish may significantly reduce your chance of having a heart attack. A 30-year study of more than 1,800 men found that those who ate as little as seven ounces of fish a week had a 40% lower risk of fatal heart attack than those who ate no fish. Researchers believe that all kinds of fish are beneficial, including canned tuna and salmon. They advise people who wish to avoid heart disease to have at least two servings of fish a week in their diets.

Hidden Allergies... How to Identify The Causes

Janice M. Joneja, PhD, director of the allergy nutrition program at Vancouver Hospital and Health Sciences Centre in Vancouver, British Columbia. She is coauthor of *Understanding Allergy, Sensitivity and Immunity*. Rutgers.

Ever had a rash, stomach problem or respiratory ailment that defied diagnosis? You might have been suffering from a hidden food reaction.

Up to 1% of adults and 7% of children under age five have at least one food *allergy*—an abnormal immune system response triggered by exposure to "foreign" proteins.

Food allergies can produce severe symptoms. Severe cases can lead to anaphylactic shock.*

Leading causes of food allergy: Fish (including shellfish)...cow's milk...eggs...wheat (including bread and pasta)...peanuts...tomatoes...spinach...strawberries...raspberries...oranges...mangoes.

It's estimated that 5% to 50% of all adults suffer from a related problem called food *intolerance*. This adverse reaction does *not* involve the immune system—but it produces similar symptoms.

Many cases of food intolerance are caused by a lack of one or more digestive enzymes. This deficiency impairs the body's ability to break down certain proteins in food.

Leading causes of food intolerance: Lactose...sulfites...artificial colors...food additives like *monosodium glutamate...histamines* (compounds in fermented foods like cheese, sauerkraut, alcoholic beverages and vinegar)...*tyramine* (an amino acid in aged cheeses, yeast extract, wine, beer, raspberries and bananas)...and food preservatives like *benzoic acid* and *sodium benzoate.*

*A potentially deadly condition marked by a drop in blood pressure, anxiety, reddening and swelling of the face, sometimes hives, tightness in chest and throat, difficulty breathing. Anyone experiencing these symptoms needs immediate medical attention.

PINPOINTING FOOD REACTION

Food allergies and intolerances manifest themselves differently in different people. A food that might give one person a rash might give another stomach pain.

Predictably, doctors often have a hard time pinpointing the trouble. Misdiagnoses are very common.

If you suspect certain foods are making you ill, ask your doctor to refer you to a food-allergy specialist—someone experienced in the use of the "elimination and challenge diet."

This diet—the only surefire way to pinpoint food reactions—has two phases. During the four-week *elimination* phase, all suspect foods are off limits. Symptoms often begin to clear up during this phase.

During the ensuing *challenge* phase, lasting a few weeks to a few months, suspect foods are reintroduced one at a time. The patient watches carefully to see if symptoms return.

Here are four case histories illustrating the most common—and commonly overlooked—food allergies and intolerances...

CASE HISTORY #1

Jack, a 48-year-old salesman, had a long history of headaches, bloating, gas and abdominal pain. His symptoms usually began an hour or so after breakfast and lasted all day. He also complained of constant fatigue and was having difficulty concentrating.

Jack exhibited no signs of gastrointestinal disease and had regular bowel movements. He went on a diet that excluded wheat, rye, oats, barley, corn and milk products. (He took an 800-mg calcium supplement to make up for the lost calcium.) In addition, he ate no raw fruit or vegetables—only cooked or canned were permitted—and no whole nuts or seeds.

After four weeks, Jack was "challenged" with each of the above foods. It turned out he was allergic to wheat, raw fruits and vegetables and highly fermented foods (cheese, wines, beer).

Now that Jack avoids these foods, his symptoms have abated. His energy has increased threefold, he says.

CASE HISTORY #2

Mary, a 50-year-old nurse, was troubled by constipation, mood swings and leg cramps. She was also concerned about the poor condition of her nails and teeth.

She was taking a variety of medications—including herbal supplements and an antidepressant. Nothing seemed to help.

Mary's symptoms suggested an intolerance or allergy to several *different* foods. Indeed, an elimination diet revealed allergies to food additives, wheat and dairy products.

After giving up these foods for three months, her physical and emotional health improved. Within six months Mary was no longer constipated. She felt better than she had in 10 years.

CASE HISTORY #3

A 62-year-old telephone company employee named Virginia had a history of asthma and hay fever dating back to childhood. She was also bothered by stomach upset, flaky skin on her hands and feet...and a dangerously elevated cholesterol level.

Though she had been on a restricted diet, Virginia couldn't shake her symptoms. Then a series of elimination and challenge tests revealed sensitivity to certain nuts and seeds, wheat and and dairy products.

Within months of giving up these foods, Virginia's symptoms had disappeared, and her cholesterol level had fallen to normal.

CASE HISTORY #4

Rita, a 56-year-old computer worker, was plagued by diarrhea, gas and abdominal pain. She'd had these problems since childhood, but they had intensified over the past year.

When a thorough exam revealed no underlying illness, Rita was put on a diet that excluded grains, starches and sugar.

In the next four weeks, she reported only two episodes of diarrhea—and each occurred after she cheated on her diet. Subsequent challenges showed that she was affected adversely by foods containing refined sugar.

Having given up these foods permanently, Rita is now completely free of symptoms.

Diet and Alzheimer's Connection

William B. Grant, PhD, retired senior research scientist, NASA Langley Research Center, Hampton, VA, and director of the Sunlight, Nutrition and Health Research Center, *www.sunarc.org.*

High-fat diets may increase the risk of developing Alzheimer's disease. While this form of dementia has long been blamed on genetic factors, an analysis of dietary patterns around the world suggests that dietary fat may also play a role. *What the analysis found:* 5% of Americans over age 65 develop Alzheimer's. But Alzheimer's strikes only 1% of people over age 65 in China and Nigeria, where typical diets contain much less fat.

 # Social Drinking Facts

Jeff Cameron, MEd, an alcohol counselor with the early-intervention program DrinkWise, 157 Delhi St., Guelph, Ontario, Canada N1E 4J3.

Social drinkers average no more than 12 drinks a week...and no more than four drinks a day for men, three for women. Drinking more than that increases your risk of trouble. One drink equals one 12-ounce beer, five ounces of wine, 1½ ounces of spirits or three ounces of fortified wine.

To moderate your drinking: Abstain for at least two days each week. Doing so helps you think about your drinking and avoid habitual patterns. *Pace yourself.* Having more than one drink an hour raises your risk of becoming drunk. *Trace cause and effect.* What triggers your drinking? A visit from a friend? Watching sports? Plan strategies to drink less or not at all.

The Rest of the Story About Diet and Cancer...Fat vs. Fiber... And the Best Sources Of Cancer-Fighting Phytonutrients

Keith I. Block, MD, research assistant professor of medical dietetics and nutrition at the University of Illinois, and editor-in-chief, *Integrative Cancer Therapies.* Sage Publications.

Despite our nation's 30-year "war" on cancer, the US cancer rate keeps rising. Overall, the odds that you'll die of cancer are 6% *higher* today than they were in 1970, according to one estimate published in *The New England Journal of Medicine.*

Good news: Eating the right foods sharply lowers your cancer risk. That's true if you are cancer-free...or if you have had cancer and are trying to avoid a recurrence.

Consider people in China and other countries whose typical eating habits are healthier than ours. They have *far* less breast, ovarian, prostate and colon cancers.

DIETARY FAT AND CANCER

If you're like the average American, roughly 40% of your daily caloric intake is in the form of fat.

But your risk of developing cancer (or having a recurrence) climbs four- to eightfold for each additional 10 percentage points of calories that come from fat.

Example: If you eat a 30% fat diet, your cancer risk is up to eight times higher than if you were to consume a 20% fat diet.

To keep your cancer risk low, fat should account for no more than 15% of your calories. The fats you do consume should be monounsaturated or polyunsaturated. Good sources of such fats include salmon, cod, canola oil, olive oil and flaxseed oil.

Saturated fats—like those found in meats, whole milk products and palm kernel oils—should be avoided. Saturated fats weaken the immune system, letting tumors flourish.

THE IMPORTANCE OF FIBER

A diet high in fiber—the indigestible part of grains, fruits and vegetables—reduces your risk of developing cancer, especially colon cancer.

In Sweden, cancer rates are low despite the fact that most Swedes eat a high-fat diet. Researchers theorize that their consumption of rye bread, which is rich in fiber, protects them.

How much fiber should you eat? Twenty-five grams a day is good, but 40 grams is ideal. Be sure to eat both *insoluble* fiber (the kind in whole wheat products) as well as *soluble* fiber (like that found in oat bran).

To make sure that you get enough fiber, your daily diet should include...

● **Two to three cups of whole-grain foods** —breads, brown rice, oat products, high-fiber cereal, etc.

● **One-and-one-half cups of beans and other legumes.**

● **Four to five cups of fresh vegetables**, including leafy greens, cruciferous vegetables, root vegetables and fruits.

Avoid candy, cakes and other sweets that contain refined sugar. Refined sugar can suppress the immune system, leaving you vulnerable to cancer.

CANCER-FIGHTING FOODS

Virtually all forms of produce are good for you, but certain fruits, vegetables and grains have special cancer-prevention powers. They're rich in *phytonutrients*, compounds that have been shown to deactivate carcinogens and even shrink tumors.

Your diet should stress these phytonutrient-dense foods...

● **Cruciferous vegetables.** Broccoli, cauliflower, cabbage and brussels sprouts contain *indole-3 carbinol* and *sulforaphane*, compounds that regulate hormone levels in such a way as to lower the risk for breast cancer.

These compounds also help protect cellular DNA against attack by carcinogens, including those in tobacco smoke.

● **Citrus fruits.** Oranges, grapefruit, lemons and limes contain more than 50 different phytonutrients. These include *flavonoids*, which block carcinogens from getting inside cells.

•**Currants, blackberries, apples, grapes and plums.** These fruits contain *saponins* and *quercetin*. These flavonoids help neutralize carcinogens, inhibit tumor growth and protect cells against attack by *free radicals*—renegade molecules produced during normal metabolism that can turn cells malignant.

•**Yellow, red and dark-green vegetables.** They contain *carotenoids*, which protect cells against oxidation and break down cancer-causing chemicals.

Tomatoes are an especially rich source of phytonutrients, including *lycopene, glutamic acid* and *turmeric acid.* These compounds block the formation of cancer-causing *nitrosamines*, protecting against stomach cancer and prostate cancer.

•**Garlic, onions, leeks and shallots.** By increasing the activity of immune system cells called *natural-killer cells*, these foods help destroy tumor cells.

One-two punch: After carotenoid-rich vegetables break down carcinogens, garlic, onions, etc., flush them from the body.

•**Soy foods.** In addition to saponins, foods made from soybeans contain the isoflavone *genistein*, a phytochemical that tempers cells' response to cancer-promoting hormones.

Soy consumption has been linked to reduced rates of breast, colon and prostate cancer.

Substitute soy milk and soy cheese for dairy products. A fermented soy product called *tempeh* is high in protein and particularly rich in genistein. Its meaty texture makes it great for casseroles and vegetable stir-frys.

•**Mushrooms.** Shiitakes and reishis, popular in Chinese cooking, contain *beta-glucan* and other immunity-boosting phytochemicals.

•**Sea vegetables.** Dark-green seaweeds like *kombu* and *wakame* are chockablock with trace elements that keep the immune system strong. They also contain "chelating agents," which remove toxins from the body.

•**Green tea.** This traditional Japanese beverage inhibits formation of nitrosamines, prevents genetic mutations and blocks the creation of tumors.

•**Turmeric.** This spice, found in curries, contains a powerful antioxidant called *curcumin*. It has been linked to lower rates of colon cancer.

Best Low-Fat Nut

Leslie Bonci, MPH, RD, director of sports medicine nutrition, University of Pittsburgh Medical Center, PA.

Chestnuts have less fat than any other kind of nut. One ounce of dry-roasted chestnuts contains less than 1 gram (g) of total fat, less than 1 g of saturated fat and 70 calories (8% of which are from fat). An ounce of dry-roasted cashews—the second least-fatty nut—has 13 g of total fat, 3 g of saturated fat and 163 calories (72% of those from fat). *Other nuts, in order of increasing fat content:* Peanuts, almonds, pistachios, walnuts, pecans, hazelnuts (filberts), Brazil nuts and macadamias.

Your Diet and Your Immune System

Elinor Levy, PhD, associate professor of microbiology at Boston University School of Medicine. She is coauthor of *The 10 Best Tools to Boost Your Immune System.* Houghton Mifflin.

For you to stay healthy—and to recover quickly from illness—your immune system must be healthy, too.

What can you do to optimize immune function? Exercise and stress reduction help. But evidence suggests that the most important contributor to immune function is what you eat.

THE ANTIOXIDANT SHIELD

By now, you have probably heard about free radicals. These ubiquitous molecules cause cells to break down, speeding the aging process, promoting heart disease and cancer and weakening the immune system.

There's no way to avoid free radicals. They're produced within the body as a result of normal metabolic processes. *But certain antioxidant compounds destroy free radicals...*

●**Vitamin E.** This potent antioxidant forestalls the gradual decline in immune function brought on by aging. It boosts synthesis of antibodies and encourages reproduction of key infection-fighting cells called *lymphocytes.*

People who take vitamin E supplements mount a stronger immune reaction against invading viruses and bacteria. They also enjoy a reduced risk for cancer.

Good sources of vitamin E include whole grains, seeds and vegetable oils. Since it's impossible to get enough E for full protection against free radicals from dietary sources, I recommend a daily supplement containing 200 international units (IU) of vitamin E.

●**Carotenoids.** These antioxidants increase the numbers of lymphocytes and natural-killer cells. Supplements are available, but the best sources are fruits and vegetables—especially carrots, kale, tomatoes and cantaloupes.

●**Vitamin C.** It energizes the immune system to react more vigorously to cancer cells and microbes. Diets rich in vitamin C have been linked to reduced risk for breast, colorectal and prostate cancer.

The optimal intake of vitamin C is 200 milligrams (mg) a day. You can get more than enough through your diet. Good sources of vitamin C include citrus fruits, cantaloupes and green peppers.

Caution: Larger doses can cause stomach trouble, kidney stones and—in some people—problems with iron metabolism.

MINERALS

Minerals are needed for the synthesis of proteins, which are key components of all cells and enzymes in the body...

●**Zinc.** The most important mineral for immune function, zinc boosts the number of lymphocytes and helps natural-killer cells attack cancer cells.

The average person needs 15 mg of zinc a day. Higher dosages seem to impair immune function.

One serving of fortified cereal (check labels) provides all the zinc you need. Meats (especially cooked oysters) and whole grains are

also good sources. Zinc supplements generally are *not* necessary.

●**Iron.** An iron *deficiency* increases infection risk by weakening many different types of immune cells. Too *much* iron impairs immune function, too.

Women of childbearing age need 15 mg of iron a day. Men need 10 mg. Meats, beans and tofu are good sources.

Iron pills are a good idea *only* if a doctor has found you to be iron-deficient.

●**Selenium.** This mineral encourages growth of immune cells and stimulates production of antibodies.

Grains, nuts, seeds and fish are good sources of selenium. Because too much selenium can cause digestive and neurological problems, supplements generally are *not* a good idea.

LOW-FAT DIET

Excess dietary fat impairs your cells' ability to recognize viruses and bacteria, crippling your immune response. Even a diet that's *moderately* high in fat (41% of calories) *halves* the cancer-killing ability of immune cells.

Self-defense: Limit your intake of all fats to 25% of your total caloric intake. For most people, this means 44 grams (g) to 55 g of fat a day.

Avoid whole milk (8 g fat per eight ounces) ...margarine (11 g per tablespoon)...fatty meat (14 g in three ounces of lean ground beef)...and nuts (18 g per ounce of pecans).

IMMUNITY BOOSTERS

Research is beginning to confirm what traditional healers have long known—that certain foods and herbs boost immune function...

●**Shiitake mushrooms.** Studies in Japan show that these mushrooms boost immune function and inhibit viral multiplication. In Japan, a shiitake derivative called lentinan is used as a cancer-fighting drug.

Shiitakes are tasty in soups, stews and vegetable dishes. Eat two to six shiitakes a week.

●**Reishi mushrooms.** These Chinese mushrooms boost reproduction of lymphocytes and trigger production of chemical "messengers" that coordinate immune system activity. Eat two to four reishis per week.

●**Garlic.** Garlic is a good source of selenium and of certain compounds with anti-infection and anticancer properties.

Season food with garlic at least three times a week.

●**Echinacea.** This popular herb boosts the ability of immune cells to swallow up cells infected with viruses…and stimulates production of compounds that coordinate the immune system's response against yeast infections.

Echinacea extract should be taken for no more than three days in a row—when you have a cold or flu, or feel one coming on. The usual dose is 30 drops of echinacea tincture, twice a day.

Super Fat-Blocker

Arnold Fox, MD, an internist and cardiologist in private practice in Beverly Hills, CA. He is coauthor of *The Fat Blocker Diet: The Revolutionary Discovery that Lowers Cholesterol, Reduces Fat, and Controls Weight Naturally.* Macmillan.

In my 40 years of practicing medicine, I've seen every kind of diet aid you can imagine. But when it comes to producing lasting weight loss, I've never seen anything like *chitosan* (KITE-o-san).

This natural food supplement—made from the shells of lobsters—forms a gel in the stomach. This gel bonds with any fats that are present, forming fatty "clumps" that are indigestible. These clumps pass out of the body in the feces.

Animal studies have shown that chitosan taken before a meal blocks absorption of up to 50% of consumed fat.

One double-blind study in Italy found that people who ate a low-fat diet and used chitosan lost an average of 16 pounds…compared with seven pounds for those who followed a low-fat diet without chitosan.

I usually tell my overweight patients to set a target weight, then take 1,000 milligrams (mg) of chitosan 30 minutes before eating lunch and dinner. Once the goal is reached, they can stop taking the chitosan.

Taking chitosan does *not* give you permission to eat whatever you want. But it will give you an extra push in the right direction.

There's no evidence that chitosan causes any side effects—but consult your doctor before trying it just to be safe, especially if you're taking any other medications.

Caution: Avoid chitosan if you're allergic to shellfish, or are pregnant or breast-feeding. Don't take vitamins A, D or E within four hours of taking chitosan. If you do, the health benefits of these vitamins will be lost.

Chitosan pills are available at most drugstores.

Anticholesterol Supplement

James W. Anderson, MD, professor of medicine and clinical nutrition, University of Kentucky, Lexington. His study of cholesterol levels in 248 men and women was reported at a meeting of the American Academy of Family Physicians.

Anyone with elevated cholesterol levels should ask a doctor about taking Metamucil or another supplement containing the bulking agent *psyllium*. *Finding:* Total cholesterol levels of volunteers who added 5 grams (g) (one heaping teaspoon twice daily) of psyllium to their daily diets fell 4.7% after 24 to 26 weeks. LDL (bad) cholesterol levels fell 6.7%. *Bonus:* Psyllium fights constipation. *Caution:* Psyllium should not be considered a substitute for cholesterol-lowering medication.

Which Fruit Contains The Most Antioxidants?

Ronald L. Prior, PhD, scientific program officer, US Department of Agriculture, Arkansas Children's Nutrition Center, Little Rock.

Ounce for ounce, blueberries contain more of these disease-fighting compounds than any other fruit or vegetable.

Other rich sources of antioxidants: Concord grape juice, kale, strawberries and spinach.

12

Vitamins and Minerals Savvy

All You Ever Really Wanted to Know... Almost...About Vitamins and Minerals

Jeffrey Blumberg, PhD
Tufts University

Given the many conflicting vitamin studies, it's easy to see why so many people are confused about which supplements to take and, of course, which ones to avoid.

To clear up the confusion, we spoke with Dr. Jeffrey Blumberg of Tufts University...

●**Does beta-carotene prevent cancer...or cause it?** The body converts beta-carotene into vitamin A. But beta-carotene is also an antioxidant—which neutralizes "free radicals" in your blood. Left unchecked, these highly reactive compounds can damage tissues and cells and possibly lead to diseases such as cancer.

More than 200 studies suggest that beta-carotene does indeed play a role in *preventing cancer*. A Chinese study of 30,000 people showed a significant decrease in the incidence of cancer and mortality in those who took a combination of beta-carotene, vitamin E and selenium.

Conflict arose with the release of three major studies that contradicted established results...

●**Two widely reported studies** found that taking supplements of beta-carotene in the 30-to-50-milligram (mg) range may increase the risk of lung cancer. What wasn't mentioned in detail by the media was that those who developed cancer were heavy smokers, heavy drinkers and/or asbestos workers.

●**The other major trial** tracked 22,000 doctors and found that those taking 50 mg of

Jeffrey Blumberg, PhD, senior scientist and chief of the Antioxidants Research Laboratory at Tufts University, Boston. He is a leading vitamin supplement expert and has served on several national health advisory committees.

beta-carotene every other day for 12 years had no increased risk of cancer—but no decrease either.

However, this study tracked men in the highest socioeconomic group in the US—physicians who had full access to health care and were more likely than the average person to have healthy lifestyles. Evidence suggests a potentially modest effect of beta-carotene, which is unlikely to be readily found in a low-risk group.

Strategy: Because we are not certain whether large doses of beta-carotene increase the risk of lung cancer in smokers or heavy drinkers (those who have more than two drinks per day), people who smoke and/or drink heavily should avoid beta-carotene supplements. But nonsmokers who do not drink heavily can take between 10 mg and 20 mg of beta-carotene daily to reduce their risk of cancer.

● **Do iron supplements cause heart attacks?** One Finnish study showed a correlation between iron intake and increased risk of cardiovascular disease in older adults.

Reality: Several subsequent studies—most of which were conducted in the US—found absolutely no link between iron intake and heart disease.

Strategy: People age 50 or older who take a vitamin/mineral supplement containing the Recommended Daily Allowance (RDA) of iron—8 mg—need not worry that this minimal amount will trigger a heart attack.

Because people over age 50 do not need large amounts of iron anyway, it is best to steer clear of high-dose iron supplements—such as those containing more than 25 mg, which are wrongly promoted as "energizers" for the 50-plus crowd.

Women who are premenopausal should take 15 mg of iron per day...adult men should take 10 mg of iron per day.

● **Is folic acid only a must for pregnant women?** When taken during the weeks before conception and the first two months of pregnancy, folic acid helps prevent neural tube problems and other birth defects.

But folic acid is an important supplement for everyone. A major study suggested that folic acid might prevent more than 50,000 deaths from cardiovascular disease each year in adults.

Folic acid lowers blood levels of a toxic amino acid called *homocysteine*, which is produced in the normal course of cell metabolism. High levels of homocysteine significantly raise the risk of heart attack and stroke.

Folic acid may also protect against colon cancer.

Strategy: All adults need to consume 400 micrograms (mcg) of folic acid daily. Spinach and dark leafy lettuces, such as romaine, are good sources...but you would have to eat about two cups of spinach a day to get your 400 mcg.

Alternative: A multivitamin supplement containing 400 mcg of folic acid.

● **Does vitamin E prevent serious diseases?** Probably not at the current US RDA level—which is 30 international units (IU).

Numerous studies link considerably higher doses of vitamin E to a decreased risk of some forms of cancer and cataracts and macular degeneration.

A British study of 2,000 people who had suffered heart attacks found that those who took 400 IU or 800 IU of vitamin E daily for a two-year period had a 77% reduction in the incidence of a second attack.

Because it's almost impossible to get enough vitamin E from a low-fat diet (the richest sources are vegetable oils and nuts), supplements may be necessary.

● **Is it true that calcium is the most important dietary factor in preventing osteoporosis?** Almost every major health organization recommends that people get their RDAs of calcium. This mineral helps prevent osteoporosis and may reduce the risk of colon cancer and hypertension.

The problem is that calcium absorption depends on adequate levels of vitamin D in the body. The body manufactures vitamin D when it is exposed to sunlight. Vitamin D is also found in fortified milk and multivitamins.

As you age, your body becomes less able to manufacture vitamin D. About 80% of women over age 60—and almost as many older men—get less than two-thirds of the RDA of this nutrient.

Strategy: Make sure you get your daily dietary requirement of calcium—1,200 mg to 1,500 mg per day.

For those age 60 or older, a 400-IU vitamin D supplement daily is advisable.

•Does vitamin C prevent colds? While there is no sound evidence that vitamin C *prevents* colds, some studies show that daily 1,000-mg to 2,000-mg supplements can *lessen* the severity and duration of colds. That's because vitamin C has an antihistamine effect.

In addition, numerous studies link a lower daily intake of vitamin C to a decreased risk of some forms of cancer and heart and eye disease.

Strategy: A National Institutes of Health study suggests the current RDA of 60 mg of vitamin C is far too low—and that doses of 100 to 200 mg may be closer to our actual daily requirement for optimal health.

To lower your risk of serious diseases, consume between 250 mg and 1,000 mg daily in food or supplement form.

•Do chromium supplements aid in weight loss? Health food manufacturers claim that this trace mineral helps body-builders bulk up and the overweight shed pounds. The evidence for both claims, however, is weak.

Emerging research suggests that chromium may be an important player in the prevention of one of this nation's top killers—adult-onset or Type 2 diabetes—since chromium helps regulate glucose (sugar) levels.

Strategy: For people who are at risk for adult-onset diabetes because it runs in their families, studies suggest a 200-mcg chromium supplement daily. The average adult consumes only 25 mcg to 30 mcg a day, which may not be enough to ward off diabetes if you're at risk.

Important: Taking nutritional supplements can have health benefits, but too much of any nutrient can be dangerous to your health. Be sure not to exceed suggested dosages and to discuss any supplements with your doctor.

Which Mineral Supplements Should You Take?

Timothy McCall, MD, an internist, medical editor of *Yoga Journal* and author of *Examining Your Doctor: A Patient's Guide to Avoiding Harmful Medical Care.* Carol. www.drmccall.com.

Minerals—iron, calcium, chromium, zinc, etc.—are vital components of a healthful diet. But claims made about their health benefits extend far beyond the evidence. As with vitamins, it's important to remember the distinction between taking mineral supplements to prevent or treat dietary deficiencies and taking them in higher doses in an effort to improve health in other ways.

There's been a great deal of controversy over *chromium picolinate*. This dietary supplement has become very popular with body-builders and with people involved in weight-loss programs. But despite all the hoopla, there is little evidence that chromium picolinate is effective for these uses.

A study has raised questions about chromium picolinate's *safety*. When scientists exposed cells taken from the ovary of a hamster to high concentrations of chromium picolinate, they found that it caused severe chromosomal damage. This raised the possibility that the mineral supplement might be carcinogenic.

The industry that manufactures the supplement responded to this study within days, criticizing how the study was done and claiming that, when taken at the recommended dose, chromium supplements are completely safe. You have to wonder, though, if these critics might be more concerned with protecting their profit margins than your health.

There is less controversy about calcium, iron and zinc. Calcium supplements, especially when combined with vitamin D, exercise and/or hormone supplements, help prevent some of the normal bone loss that occurs as women enter menopause. It's even more important, however, to build strong bones in the first place by getting enough calcium when you're younger.

Adolescents and young adults—particularly women—should get 1,200 mg of calcium a day. Most get less than half of that amount. Elderly women should consume 1,500 mg a day. There is about 300 mg of calcium in a glass of milk or a cup of yogurt.

Those who don't get enough calcium in their diet should take a supplement. It's usually less expensive to buy a separate supplement like calcium carbonate than to try to get the full amount of calcium in a multivitamin.

Women of childbearing age, especially those who donate blood or have heavy periods, often need supplemental iron. Your doctor can give you a simple blood test that determines whether you are iron-deficient. It's best to have this test before you start taking iron. Too much iron in your system can pose a hazard to your health.

The average American gets only 80% of the recommended daily allowance of zinc, according to a study. If you suspect you're not getting enough zinc from your diet (good sources include shellfish, beef, beans and nuts), take a multivitamin that contains the recommended daily allowance.

Whenever you hear fantastic claims about the curative powers of mineral supplements, keep in mind that the multibillion dollar industry that manufactures them is behind a lot of the hype. As with vitamins, a balanced diet is the best way to ensure that you're getting the minerals you need. A simple multivitamin containing the *recommended daily allowances* of vitamins and minerals is safe, however, and provides insurance against dietary deficiencies.

Beware of higher doses. Until further studies sort out questions of effectiveness—and safety —their risks and benefits simply aren't known yet. In the meantime, it's your choice whether you want to be a guinea pig. Personally, though, I think I'll stay in the control group.

The Value of Herbal Ingredients

David Roll, PhD, professor emeritus of medicinal chemistry, University of Utah, College of Pharmacy, 201 Skaggs Hall, Salt Lake City 84112.

Don't pay extra for vitamin supplements with herbal ingredients. Herbal substances are of questionable value, and may interfere with vitamins in a manner that *blocks* your body from absorbing them. So you may wind up paying more for less.

Nutritional Supplements: What You Really Need For Optimal Health

Jeffrey Blumberg, PhD, senior scientist and chief of the Antioxidants Research Laboratory at Tufts University, Boston. He is a leading vitamin supplement expert and has served on several national health advisory committees.

Venture into any health-food store or pharmacy these days and you'll find yourself surrounded by nutritional supplements—from vitamins to bee pollen.

Is there any health benefit to taking supplements? Absolutely, says Tufts University nutritionist Dr. Jeffrey Blumberg.

Even if you aren't sick, says Blumberg, a few well-chosen supplements can make you much, much healthier…

Item #1: Few Americans get the Recommended Daily Allowance (RDA) for all nutrients. Only 9% adhere to the Agriculture Department's dietary guidelines.

Item #2: The RDA is based on the amount of each nutrient *needed* to prevent deficiency-related diseases—scurvy, beriberi, rickets, etc. Yet hundreds of studies confirm that risk of chronic diseases like cancer and heart disease can be minimized only by taking these nutrients at levels *in excess* of the RDA.

Item #3: It's virtually impossible to get sufficient quantities of some key nutrients from food alone—even with the most healthful diets.

KEY NUTRIENTS

•**Folic acid.** This B vitamin (also called folate) reduces blood levels of *homocysteine*. Research has linked high levels of this amino acid (a by-product of cell metabolism) to both heart attack and stroke.

Folic acid also guards against colon cancer and birth defects.

Since these defects occur in the first two months of pregnancy, any woman who even *thinks* she might become pregnant should take a daily supplement containing 400 micrograms (mcg) of folate.

Sources: Green leafy vegetables, whole-wheat bread, nuts, peas and beans. *RDA:* 400 mcg.

•**Vitamin B-6.** This vitamin works with folic acid to break down homocysteine. If all Americans upped their daily intake of folic acid and B-6, 50,000 fewer people would die annually of heart attack and stroke.

Sources: Meat, poultry, fish, liver, whole-grain products, most fruits and vegetables. *RDA:* 2 milligrams (mg).

•**Vitamin D.** This vitamin facilitates the body's absorption of dietary calcium. It's essential for healthy bones.

Sources: Fortified dairy products, fortified cereals and breads, liver, eggs and cod liver oil. Also synthesized in the skin during exposure to sunlight. *RDA:* 400 international units (IU).

•**Vitamin E.** Along with vitamin C and beta-carotene, vitamin E is a potent antioxidant. It neutralizes "free radicals," cell-damaging molecular fragments that circulate through the body.

Daily doses of vitamin E may reduce the risk of cancer of the esophagus, stomach and lung …and cataracts and other eye diseases.

Unfortunately, it's hard to get sufficient vitamin E from a healthful low-fat diet—so supplements are necessary.

Sources: Vegetable oil, wheat germ and nuts. *RDA:* 30 international units (IU).

•**Beta-carotene.** More than 200 studies have shown that this antioxidant plays a key role in preventing cancer.

Sources: Broccoli, cantaloupe, carrots. *RDA:* There is no RDA for beta-carotene.

•**Selenium** is another cancer-fighting antioxidant. A study in China involving 30,000 people found a dramatically reduced risk of cancer among individuals who took supplemental vitamin E, beta-carotene and selenium.

Sources: Fish, shellfish, meat, whole-grain cereals, dairy products. *RDA:* There is no RDA for selenium.

•**Vitamin C.** Studies have linked this antioxidant to reduced risk of lung, colon and gastrointestinal cancers. It may also help prevent heart and eye disease.

The typical American diet provides 120 mg a day of vitamin C. That's twice the RDA, but a National Institutes of Health study suggested that the RDA is *too low*. A daily intake of 250 mg is better.

Sources: Citrus fruits, green peppers, broccoli, cabbage, cauliflower, potatoes, tomatoes. *RDA:* 60 mg.

•**Calcium.** This mineral is crucial for preventing osteoporosis—and it's *not* just for older women. A high calcium intake—along with sufficient vitamin D—is important for all ages, to build bone tissue and retain it.

Adults need 1,200 to 1,500 mg of calcium a day. To get this much from food, you'd need to drink about five glasses of milk…or eat several servings of yogurt, cheese or broccoli. For most people, it's easier to take a daily supplement.

Sources: Dairy products, leafy green vegetables and beans. *RDA:* 800 mg.

THE THREE-PILL STRATEGY

All adults should take daily nutritional supplements with breakfast. This simple three-pill-a-day regimen provides high levels of the most critical nutrients—with minimal hassle.

Pill #1: **Multivitamin/multimineral.** It should contain 100% to 200% of the RDA for all vitamins mentioned above.

Check the expiration date on the bottle—pills lose potency as they age.

Pill #2: **Vitamin E.** Take a pill that contains 100 to 400 IU.* Or if you prefer, you can take a combination pill containing vitamins E and C, beta-carotene and selenium.

*Due to the possible interactions between vitamin E and various drugs and supplements, as well as other safety considerations, consult your doctor before starting a vitamin E regimen.

***Pill #3:* Calcium.** The average person gets only about 750 mg a day in calcium from food sources. Since this is about half the amount you need for healthy bones, take one 600- to 700-mg calcium pill each day.

Which Vitamins? Which Minerals? Here's What I Do

Timothy McCall, MD, an internist, medical editor of *Yoga Journal* and author of *Examining Your Doctor: A Patient's Guide to Avoiding Harmful Medical Care.* Carol. *www.drmccall.com.*

When speaking with patients, I try to base my recommendations on the scientific data. There aren't any definitive studies about the benefits of vitamin supplements yet, but I'm going to tell you what I do based upon the evidence there is.

Each month, dozens of reports come out on the subject of vitamins and minerals. Despite all the information, many gaps in our knowledge remain. We know, for example, that people who eat diets high in certain nutrients like beta-carotene and vitamin C have lower rates of some cancers. Does that mean that taking a dietary supplement containing these vitamins will reduce your risk for cancer? No one really can say for sure.

Many medical experts say it's wrong for doctors to recommend something to their patients before there's scientific proof of its effectiveness. The problem is, people can't wait. In the "real world," we often have to make choices based on incomplete information. Even if the hard science isn't in yet, people want to know what makes the most sense now.

Many experts fail to recognize that there can be serious consequences to *withholding* recommendations until the proof is in. *Consider this:* As a first-year med student in 1979, I asked a professor who had just given us a lecture on heart disease whether he would recommend a

low-fat diet to people at risk for heart attack. No, he replied, there wasn't enough evidence yet.

I thought to myself that maybe there wasn't enough evidence for him, but there was for me. By that point I'd already been eating a low-fat diet for a couple of years. I had been doing so based on the theory that dietary fat contributes to the buildup of cholesterol in coronary arteries—a theory that seemed to have been confirmed by several preliminary studies.

Think of all the heart patients who might have benefited if doctors back then had been willing to recommend a low-fat diet. After all, the risk of cutting down on fat is pretty small.

The situation is similar with vitamin supplements today. There are theoretical reasons to take antioxidants (including vitamins C and E and the mineral selenium). They gobble up free radicals, ubiquitous molecules that are thought to contribute to the development of both cancer and heart disease. And the evidence is that the risk of taking moderate doses of these vitamins is pretty small.

In that spirit, here are my educated guesses. Every morning, in addition to a multivitamin with minerals, I take 250 milligrams (mg) of vitamin C, 400 international units of natural vitamin E and 200 micrograms of selenium. Whenever possible, I buy inexpensive store brands.

Even though I take these supplements, I firmly believe that a healthful diet is more important. If you eat poorly, I doubt you can undo all the damage by popping a few vitamins. Accordingly, I've been a not-too-strict vegetarian for years, consuming mostly whole grains, fruits, legumes, vegetables, a little fish and some low-fat dairy products like yogurt. To me, the vitamins are like a little added insurance.

My educated guesses could turn out to be wrong, so by all means stay tuned. New evidence might suggest the benefits of some vitamins not previously understood—while discrediting others.

Like me, plenty of doctors take dietary supplements, even if they don't recommend them to their patients. In this case, you may want to do what we do—and not what we say.

Timed-Release Vitamin Alert

The Vitamin Revolution in Health Care by Michael Janson, MD, American College for Advancement in Medicine. Arcadia Press.

Avoid "timed-release" vitamin and mineral supplements.

Reason: They cost more but may actually be less effective than the plain variety. Many vitamins, such as vitamin C, work best when they're present in the blood in high levels. This can be difficult to achieve with timed-release pills because they dissolve too slowly. *Also:* Some vitamins may not dissolve in time or in the right place to be well absorbed by the intestinal tract.

Exceptions: Both vitamin B3, or niacin, which can cause a temporary flushing of the skin, and iron, which can cause constipation and indigestion, should be taken as timed-release versions.

Where Never To Store Your Vitamins

Michael Janson, MD, American College for Advancement in Medicine, and author of *The Vitamin Revolution in Health Care.* Arcadia Press.

Never store vitamins in the refrigerator. Each time you open the bottle, warm air from the outside will mix with the cold vitamins, causing condensation. Over time the pills will become sticky and may actually begin to dissolve. *Also:* Don't store them in the bathroom, where heat and humidity can shorten their shelf life.

Better: Store vitamins in a pantry or on the kitchen counter where they'll stay dry and at room temperature.

Exceptions: Supplements of intestinal flora, such as *lactobacilli* or *bifidobacteria.* These should be kept in the refrigerator.

Depression and Vitamin B Connection

Maurizio Fava, MD, professor of psychiatry, Harvard Medical School, and vice chair, department of psychiatry, Massachusetts General Hospital, both in Boston.

Depression that fails to respond to antidepressants may indicate a deficiency of the B vitamin *folic acid* (folate). In a study of 213 depressed people, the antidepressant *fluoxetine* (Prozac) was less effective in those with low folate than in those with normal folate.

Self-defense: If you don't respond to an antidepressant, ask your doctor to check your folate level.

Calcium Is Inexpensive

Timothy McCall, MD, an internist, medical editor of *Yoga Journal* and author of *Examining Your Doctor: A Patient's Guide to Avoiding Harmful Medical Care.* Carol. *www.drmccall.com.*

You can get the medically recommended dosages of calcium, multivitamins and vitamins C and E for as little as 12 to 21 cents a day.

Key: Buy store brands, which are often made by the very same companies that manufacture the more expensive, best-selling supplement brands.

Vitamin B-12 Alert

The late Victor Herbert, MD, JD, professor of medicine, Mount Sinai–New York University Health Systems and Bronx VA Medical Center, and editor of *Total Nutrition: The Only Guide You'll Ever Need.* St. Martin's Griffin.

Individuals over 50 years of age need to supplement their diets with at least 25 micrograms a day of vitamin B-12.

Take vitamin B-12 in tablets by itself—or combined with folic acid.

Don't take it in tablets that include other vitamins or minerals. *Reason:* When the pills dissolve in your stomach, the vitamin B-12 is destroyed.

Important: Do not take other vitamins prescribed for you by a health professional within one hour of taking vitamin B-12.

Vitamin C to the Rescue

Scott T. Weiss, MD, professor of medicine at Harvard Medical School, Boston.

Vitamin C may help prevent asthma, bronchitis and other lung problems. When researchers studied the diets and lung functions of over 2,500 people, they found that the people who consumed the most vitamin C had the best-functioning lungs. The difference in lung function between those whose daily diet contained an amount of vitamin C equivalent to that contained in 10 ounces of orange juice (99 milligrams) and those who had almost none was as great as that between nonsmokers and people who smoked a pack of cigarettes every day for five years.

Vitamin C and Arthritis

Tim McAlindon, MD, an associate professor of medicine at Boston University School of Medicine.

The progression of arthritis of the knee can be significantly slowed by vitamin C. An eight-year study of 640 people found that knee osteoarthritis progressed three times more slowly in those who consumed the most vitamin C than in those who ate the least.

Scientists offer two possible theories to explain this effect. One is that vitamin C's antioxidant properties mop up harmful free radicals that are released by the inflamed knee joint. The second theory is that vitamin C helps the body synthesize proteins that repair the arthritis caused damage. But either way—you win.

Possible Ulcer Protection

Joel A. Simon, MD, MPH, associate professor of medicine, general internal medicine, Medical Service, San Francisco Veterans Affairs Medical Center.

Vitamin C may be an effective way to prevent ulcers. People with high blood levels of ascorbic acid—the chemical name for vitamin C—were less likely to show signs of infection from *Helicobacter pylori,* a common cause of ulcers. Try to get 250 to 500 milligrams of vitamin C daily from foods and supplements.

Good food sources: Oranges, red bell peppers, strawberries.

Relief from Colds

Michael L. Macknin, MD, chairman, department of general pediatrics, The Cleveland Clinic Foundation.

Relieve symptoms and reduce the duration of colds by sucking zinc lozenges. They are available over-the-counter in drugstores.

Study: Cold sufferers were divided into two groups, one of which received zinc lozenges. This group reported that colds lasted an average of 4.4 days, compared with 7.6 days for the group receiving placebo lozenges. The group receiving zinc lozenges also reported suffering milder symptoms.

Dosage: The group took an average of five 13.3 mg zinc lozenges, totaling about 65 mg of zinc daily. The lozenges studied were zinc gluconate glycine (*Brand name:* Cold-eeze).

Vitamin C Danger

Sheldon Nadler, DMD, a dentist in private practice in New York City.

Chewable forms of vitamin C (ascorbic acid) may be bad for your teeth. Breath mints, chewing gum, etc., fortified with C are now being sold as easy ways to get your daily dose of this key nutrient.

Danger: Repeated exposure to any acid—including ascorbic acid—can corrode your tooth enamel. *Most damaging:* Habitual use of products containing more than 500 milligrams (mg) of vitamin C per piece.

Cold-Weather Wellness

John H. Weisburger, PhD, senior scientist at the American Health Foundation, Valhalla, NY.

To get the vitamin C you need for winter, keep up your fruit and vegetable consumption—preferably at the same high level you would over the summer months. Vitamin C, along with other vitamins, is necessary for optimal health…and studies show that it lowers the risk of heart disease and some types of cancer.

Best: A minimum of five servings—fresh or canned—per day.

Alternative: Two 250-milligram tablets of vitamin C every day—one with a high-fiber breakfast and one at dinner. But these dietary supplements don't give you the extra nutrients or fiber that fruits and vegetables do.

Bladder Cancer and Vitamin C

Barbara Bruemmer, PhD, nutrition analyst, division of clinical research, Fred Hutchinson Cancer Research Center, Seattle. Her study of 667 men and women ages 45 to 55 was published in the *American Journal of Epidemiology*, 111 Market Pl., Ste. 840, Baltimore 21202.

Bladder cancer risk can be cut by up to one-third by consuming lots of vitamin C, fruit and a daily multivitamin supplement.

What raises risk: Eating fried foods and smoking.

Vitamin C and Artery Link

Haruo Tomoda, MD, clinical professor of cardiology, Tokai University Hospital, Kanagawa, Japan. His study of restenosis in 101 angioplasty patients was published in the *Journal of the American College of Cardiology*, 3655 Nobel Dr., Ste. 360, San Diego 92112.

Vitamin C helps keep coronary arteries from clogging. Only 25% of angioplasty patients who took 500 mg of vitamin C a day suffered reclogging (a process called *restenosis*). But restenosis affected 43% of angioplasty patients who didn't take vitamin C. *Theory:* Vitamin C blocks restenosis by keeping oxidation of LDL (bad) cholesterol low. LDL cholesterol must be oxidized before it can attach to artery walls. Anyone who undergoes angioplasty should ask his/her doctor about vitamin C.

Vitamin D and Diabetes

Stanley Mirsky, MD, associate clinical professor at Mount Sinai School of Medicine, New York City.

Vitamin D may play a part in preventing diabetes. A Swedish study found that men with lower levels of vitamin D had higher blood pressure, higher triglyceride fat levels and higher insulin resistance, all factors associated with Type 2 or adult onset diabetes. Four eight-ounce glasses of milk have enough vitamin D to provide the RDA of 400 international units.

Adults and Vitamin D

Study of 250 women in their 50s and 60s by Bess Dawson-Hughes, MD, chief, calcium and bone metabolism lab, Human Nutrition Research Center, Tufts University, Boston.

Adults need more than the recommended allowance of vitamin D. In a two-year study, women who received the Recommended Daily Allowance (RDA) of vitamin D—from both diet and supplements—lost twice as much bone from their hips as did women who received 800 international units (IU) per day. Consider taking vitamin D supplements if you don't think you're getting enough of the nutrient from your diet, or if you don't get enough exposure to the sun, which allows the body to manufacture vitamin D on its own.

Vitamin E Protects the Lungs

Lindsey Dow, MD, consultant senior lecturer in care of the elderly, University of Bristol, England. Her study of 178 people 70 years of age or older was published in the *American Journal of Respiratory and Critical Care Medicine*, 61 Broadway, New York 10006.

Does vitamin E protect the lungs? In a study, the more of this antioxidant vitamin elderly people consumed, the better their lung function.

Caution: Researchers don't yet know exactly how much vitamin E is needed to improve lung function or if it is more beneficial when consumed in supplement form or in foods. Good sources include nuts, fresh vegetables and vegetable oil.

Vitamins vs. Birth Defects

Quanhe Yang, PhD, division of birth defects and developmental disabilities, National Center for Environmental Study, Centers for Disease Control and Prevention, Atlanta. His study of mothers of 117 babies was published in *Epidemiology*, 351 W. Camden St., Baltimore 21201.

Doctors have long urged pregnant women to take a daily multivitamin—to prevent limb deformities in their unborn children. *Study:* Taking vitamins during the month before conception cut the risk of such defects by even more. *Self-defense:* Any woman who *might* become pregnant should take a daily multivitamin containing folic acid.

Vitamin E, Aspirin and Stroke Connection

Manfred Steiner, MD, PhD, a professor of medicine at East Carolina University School of Medicine, Greenville, NC.

Aspirin's proven antistroke power is multiplied when it is taken with vitamin E. A study of 100 people who had suffered *mini*-strokes, often a precursor of *major* strokes, found that taking vitamin E daily together with aspirin produced a reduction of up to 80%, compared with aspirin alone, in the number of anchor strands that enable dangerous clots to form in blood vessels.

Vitamin E and Cuts

James M. Spencer, MD, director, dermatologic surgery, Mount Sinai School of Medicine, New York City. His three-month study was presented at a meeting of the American Society for Dermatologic Surgery.

Vitamin E *doesn't* help cuts and bruises heal faster—despite the common belief that it does.

Study: Fifteen volunteers applied vitamin E ointment to one-half of a wound twice daily. After three months, there was no difference in the rate of healing between the treated and untreated halves. And six of the volunteers dropped out, complaining of redness, swelling and skin irritation on the vitamin E side.

Vitamin E And Exercise

Kenneth H. Cooper, MD, MPH, president and founder of the Cooper Aerobics Center, 12200 Preston Rd., Dallas 75230. He is author of numerous books on health and fitness, including *Dr. Kenneth H. Cooper's Antioxidant Revolution*. Bookman.

Vitamin E can reduce muscle soreness and damage from vigorous exercise. Studies found the benefit when people took large doses of vitamin E during the 24 hours before—*and* after—they engaged in vigorous exercise.

Recommended dosage: 400 international units (IU)* daily for adults. Physicians believe this effect comes from the ability of vitamin E to combat DNA-damaging free radicals released by exercise. Other researchers are studying the relationship between exercise and other vitamins, including riboflavin (vitamin B2) and vitamin C.

Beta-Carotene Update

Bruce Yaffe, MD, an internist and gastroenterologist in private practice, 121 E. 84 St., New York 10028.

Don't discount beta-carotene—despite recent reports that have called into question its purported health benefits.

Reason: Two of the three studies reported were flawed.

Problem: They used only high-risk people …and the higher death rate in those who took beta-carotene was not statistically significant. In nonsmokers and nondrinkers, other studies have shown beta-carotene helps prevent stroke and heart disease.

Best: Get 15 milligrams (mg) of beta-carotene daily from vegetables and fruits—particularly sweet potatoes, carrots, spinach, cantaloupe and mangoes.

Folic Acid Danger

Mark Dykewicz, MD, professor of internal medicine, St. Louis University Health Sciences Center.

Synthetic forms of this vitamin can cause hives, breathing problems, cramps and itching.

Problem: The FDA is urging food producers to fortify bread, flour and pasta with folic acid…and many vitamin supplements now contain folic acid.

*Consult your doctor for the dosage that is appropriate for you.

Self-defense: Consult a doctor if you develop these symptoms after a meal—or while taking vitamins containing folic acid. (Stop taking the vitamins.)

Good news: You can get plenty of natural folic acid by eating dark green leafy vegetables, liver, nuts and wheat germ.

Folic Acid Benefits

Meir J. Stampfer, MD, professor of nutrition and epidemiology, Harvard School of Public Health, Boston, and the leader of one of the studies.

Folic acid may offer significant protection against heart attack and stroke. An inadequate intake of folic acid is associated with high blood levels of homocysteine, an amino acid which more than 20 studies have found increases the risk of stroke and heart disease.

Folic acid, a B vitamin, is found in dried beans, enriched whole-grain cereals, green leafy vegetables, peanuts, liver and orange juice. Researchers say that people eating five daily servings of fruits and vegetables receive enough folic acid (400 micrograms) to keep their homocysteine level down.

Magnesium Fights Migraines

Andreas Peikert, MD, neurologist, Munich–Harlaching Clinic, Munich, Germany. His 16-week study of 81 migraine patients was published in *Cephalalgia*, Henry Ford Hospital, 2799 W. Grand Blvd., Detroit 48202.

In a study, one group of migraine sufferers was given magnesium supplements, while a second group got placebos.

Result: 56% of the magnesium group reported fewer migraines, compared with 31% of the placebo group.

Caution: Magnesium supplements should not be taken by anyone who has kidney trouble.

Selenium vs. Cancer Facts

The late Larry C. Clark, MPH, PhD, associate professor of epidemiology, Arizona Cancer Center, Tucson. His eight-year study of 1,312 skin cancer patients 18 to 80 years of age was published in the *Journal of the American Medical Association*, 515 N. State St., Chicago 60610.

Selenium may help prevent cancer. An eight-year study of more than 1,300 people found that those who took 200 micrograms (mcg) of selenium supplements daily reduced their rates of colorectal, prostate and lung cancer by about half, compared with those who did not take the supplement.

Selenium is found in chicken, meat, seafood, grains, egg yolks, mushrooms, onions and garlic.

The average intake for US adults is only 108 mcg, so the supplement brings the total to approximately 350 mcg a day—considered a safe maximum. Don't overdo it, however—a daily intake of 1,000 mcg can cause side effects including hair loss and fragile nails.

Researchers conducted a study to determine whether selenium supplements prevent skin cancer.

What they found: Selenium did *not* affect skin cancer risk, but it *did* reduce deaths from cancers of the lung, colon, rectum and prostate. Skin cancer patients who took selenium developed 63% fewer prostate cancers, 58% fewer colorectal cancers and 46% fewer lung cancers. Ask your doctor about taking selenium supplements.

More Good Things About Selenium

Li Li, MD, PhD, assistant professor, division of cancer prevention and control, National Cancer Institute, Bethesda, MD.

Selenium may help protect the body against heart disease and cancer.

A study of 2,600 people in Finland found that the rates of both those diseases dropped by 60% as blood selenium levels rose from 60 to 103 micrograms per liter. The best sources of the mineral are seafoods, grains, muscle meats and Brazil nuts.

However, *don't* use selenium supplements without consulting your doctor first—it's easy to take too much, which is dangerous.

Chromium Picolinate Danger

Walter G. Wasser, MD, chief, division of nephrology, North General Hospital, New York City.

This popular weight-loss aid can cause kidney failure. *Case:* A 49-year-old nurse developed kidney failure after taking three times the recommended level of chromium picolinate for six weeks. *Bottom line:* Since the risk of chromium deficiency is small and the ideal dose is uncertain, there's no reason to take chromium supplements.

13

For a Healthy Sex Life

The Healing Power of Good Sex

Paul Pearsall, PhD
Henry Ford Community College

Sex involves more than procreation—or recreation. As countless studies have shown, an intimate, sexually satisfying relationship reduces the risk of heart disease...depression...migraine...premenstrual syndrome...and arthritis. It also boosts the immune system.

But sex is genuinely healing *only* if it transcends the mechanical, self-pleasure variety promoted by sex experts.

Indeed, the central goal of sexual healing should not be orgasm—but *connection with your partner.*

PHYSIOLOGY OF HEALING SEX

Healing sex brings a marked decline in bloodstream levels of *adrenaline* and *cortisol.*

These stress hormones provoke anxiety and reduce immune function.

In a study, women who were happily married had higher levels of natural killer cells and helper T cells than those in unhappy unions.

Healing sex is also a potent antidote for social isolation, which has been linked to serious illness and premature death.

A Yale study of 194 heart patients found that those without a spouse at home were twice as likely to die prematurely as those with a spouse.

HEALING SEX IS RARE

Most couples never experience sexual healing—because they're too quick to give up on their relationship. It takes at least *four years* to achieve the intimacy needed for sexual healing. Most couples split after only three years. Why do so many couples split? Because of lack

Paul Pearsall, PhD, professor of psychology at the University of Hawaii and member of the heart transplant study team at the University of Arizona School of Medicine. He is author of *A Healing Intimacy* (Three Rivers Press) and *The Pleasure Prescription* (Hunter House).

of intimacy. Intimacy doesn't just happen. You *make* it happen by treating your partner with care and genuine affection…and by taking the time to really connect, both in casual conversation and via sex.

Three factors are central to a sexually healing relationship…

●**Commitment.** Affairs and on-again-off-again sexual relationships are *not* healing because the two people never form a meaningful bond.

●**Consideration.** The bond between a couple must extend beyond the bedroom. Each partner must continually express tenderness and caring toward the other—by smiling… touching…being polite…giving compliments …and showing respect.

●**Honesty.** There must be no secrets within the relationship—only total connection and total confidence.

HOW TO FORGE A SEXUALLY HEALING RELATIONSHIP

●**Spend time together.** For at least five minutes a day, sit or lie together—just the two of you. Cuddle. Talk. Let your bodies synchronize.

●**Listen more, talk less.** Ironically, good relationships involve little talk. Partners communicate via their own private language— subtle body movements, gestures, expressions and a sense of connection that arises only between lovers who grow ever closer as a result of sharing crises.

●**Do something special for your partner.** If you spend your days apart, call periodically during the day and say something like, "Honey, I've been thinking about you. I can't wait to see you."

If necessary, set an alarm clock to go off periodically to remind you to place the call.

You come to feel love by behaving lovingly, so even the simplest acts of connection can translate to intense sexual feelings.

●**Have sex only when it feels "right."** Trust your senses. If you rely on your "sex sense" for a month, you'll soon see that when you do have sex, it is more fulfilling and sensual.

●**Seduce your partner.** Instead of dressing up in a sexy costume—as sex therapists often recommend—use "brain power."

Send your partner mental "messages" all day long. At night, lie still in bed and send him/her more "sex waves." You'll be surprised at how seductive your own brain can be.

●**Fantasize about your partner.** Put on some sensual music and lie in bed with your eyes closed. Use your brain—not a vibrator or your hand—and envision yourself making love to your partner.

You may become aroused—even experience orgasm—but mental sex can be surprisingly fulfilling even if you don't.

50-MINUTE SEXUAL FITNESS PLAN

My sexual fitness plan—which you can add to your weekly exercise regimen—contains three components…

1. Shared laughter. Twenty seconds of laughter produces the same cardiovascular benefits as three minutes of aerobic exercise, studies indicate.

Studies also indicate that a good laugh strengthens the immune system by lowering cortisol levels and raising endorphin levels. And—couples who laugh together become closer and more in tune with one another.

2. Shared crying. Watching a good tear-jerker enhances intimacy—and sometimes leads to sexual arousal. Tears, which contain stress hormones and other chemicals, may be nature's way of washing toxins out of the body.

3. Couple "erotorobics." The following suggested sexual exercises may seem strange, but they increase your ability to respond to intimate physical contact…

●**Simulated sex.** Go through the motions of intercourse—with your clothes on.

●**Genital massage.** This stimulates blood flow in that area.

●**Dancing to erotic music.** Use the muscles you would if you were having intercourse.

●**Flirting.** Arch your back, sway your hips and stick out your chest. And practice sexual gazing and sexual smiling. Both can make you feel more sensuous.

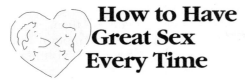

How to Have Great Sex Every Time

Edward W. Eichel, MA, a psychotherapist in private practice in New York City and the originator of the coital alignment technique. CAT is described in greater detail—and, yes, illustrated—in his book, *The Perfect Fit*. Signet. For more information on a CAT self-help videotape, call 212-989-1826.

Of all the concerns voiced by women undergoing sex therapy, none is more common—or emotionally distressing—than an inability to achieve orgasm during intercourse.

Only about 30% of women achieve orgasm regularly during intercourse (coitus).

Some women endure years of sex without a single coital orgasm. Typically, a woman relies upon a partner who "jumps through hoops" to bring her there, but never achieves the ideal.

Result: Sexuality, robbed of its playfulness and spontaneity, becomes more a chore than a pleasure.

TO THE RESCUE

A variant of the standard missionary position—known as the coital alignment technique (CAT)—not only helps the woman have an orgasm during coitus, but also boosts the odds that she and her partner will climax simultaneously.

Men who have long considered themselves sexually inadequate, as well as women who have worried they were frigid, can begin to experience sex with all its physical pleasure and emotional intimacy.

Bonus: Because good sex is usually synonymous with good communication, this improvement in a couple's sex life often carries over into other aspects of their relationship, bringing new levels of intimacy, contentment, and—important in this age of AIDS—commitment.

Unlike some other alternative lovemaking techniques, CAT is relatively straightforward. Couples have differed in the time necessary to master the technique, but with persistence, most have succeeded. Once mastered, it is remarkably effective—and quite reliable.

Study: Sexual response was measured in couples involved in committed relationships—before and after receiving CAT training. Prior to learning CAT, only 23% of the women reported achieving orgasm during intercourse on a regular basis. After CAT, that figure jumped to 77%. Before CAT, no women reported having regular simultaneous orgasms with their partners. Afterward, one-third of the women reported doing so.

Almost all participants reported at least some improvement in their sex lives following CAT training. In fact, the only participants who failed to benefit were those whose relationships were already jeopardized by nonsexual factors.

CAT BASICS

CAT encompasses five distinct elements, each designed to maximize contact between the penis and the clitoris, thus maximizing sexual response in both partners...

1. Positioning. The woman lies on her back. The man lies atop her, facing her much as in the conventional missionary position, but with his pelvis overriding hers in a "riding high" orientation.

His penis should be inserted into her vagina, with its shaft pressed firmly against her mons veneris—the soft fleshy mound covering the pubic bone above the vagina. She wraps her legs around his thighs, with her legs bent at an angle not exceeding 45 degrees and her ankles resting on his calves.

Important: He must let his full weight fall on her and must avoid using his hands or elbows to support his weight. While she may find this weight uncomfortable initially, it is essential to keep his pelvis from sliding back down off of hers.

2. Limited movement. Conventional intercourse involves a great deal of pushing, pulling and bracing of the arms and legs. CAT coitus focuses narrowly on the couple's pelvic movement. In fact, little additional movement is possible during CAT, given the partners' positioning. If additional movement is possible, the positioning is faulty.

3. Pressure-counterpressure. During ordinary intercourse, the man sets the rhythm while the woman moves little, if at all. In contrast, CAT calls for a rhythmic movement that is virtually identical for both partners.

Procedure: She performs an upward stroke, forcing his pelvis backward. He allows his pelvis to move, yet maintains a continuous counter-pressure against her pelvis (and her clitoris).

In the downward movement, the pattern of movement is reversed, with the man pushing downward and the woman maintaining the counterpressure against his penis. As her pelvis moves backward and downward, the penis shaft rocks forward against her mons veneris, sliding to a shallow position in the vagina.

Note: Although the force of pressure and counterpressure is quite intense during CAT, the partners' actual movement is surprisingly slight.

4. Full genital contact. Repeated thrusting of the penis into and out of the vaginal "barrel," typical of conventional missionary intercourse, affords little direct stimulation of either the clitoris or the penis.

Typical result: His orgasm, even if perceived as pleasurable, is far less powerful than it might be...and she, having gotten little if any clitoral stimulation, fails to climax at all. In CAT, the penis and clitoris are held tightly together by pressure and counterpressure...and the penile-clitoral "connection" is rocked up and down in an evenly paced, lever-like fashion. This vibratory motion all but guarantees orgasms for both partners.

Bonus: Orgasms produced by CAT differ significantly from those produced by conventional in-and-out sex. Whereas a conventional orgasm is limited to a pulsating sensation, a CAT orgasm combines this with a "melting" sensation.

Among participants of the study, 90% of all subjects said that CAT intensified their orgasms ...and 60% said that it increased their desire for more frequent sex.

5. "Passive" orgasm. In ordinary coitus, the man thrusts faster and more deeply as he becomes increasingly aroused, while the woman typically slows down or even stops moving altogether. At the moment of climax, the partners' movements often become disconnected and may fall completely out of sync.

Result: The orgasm is incomplete, almost "spoiled."

Better: CAT prescribes complete coordination of movement by the partners, up to and beyond the moment of climax. In other words, both partners make no effort to "grab" for orgasm, instead letting it "overtake" them.

The transition from voluntary motion preceding orgasm to the reflexive, involuntary movements typical of orgasm itself is thus fully coordinated. The possibility of incomplete orgasm is drastically limited.

Crucial: A conscious effort by both partners not to hold their breath or suppress natural sounds. Breathing freely and giving full rein to grunts, moans, spoken words and other vocalizations greatly facilitate orgasm—for the noise-maker and the listener alike.

Some couples report that the "reversed" CAT is an effective variation of CAT—if the man is much heavier than his partner.

Herpes Update

Anna Wald, MD, MPH, associate professor of medicine, University of Washington, Seattle.

Genital herpes can be spread even without the presence of genital sores. In a study of 110 women with genital herpes, 65% of women "shed" virus particles at some point, both with and without accompanying lesions.

To reduce risk: Use condoms unless you're sure your partner is uninfected. *Also:* Viral shedding can be reduced by taking the prescription drug *acyclovir* (Zovirax), *valacyclovir* (Valtrex) and *famciclovir* (Famir).

How to Perk Up Your Sex Life

Judith Seifer, PhD, RN, director of behavioral medicine at the West Virginia School of Osteopathic Medicine in Lewisburg. She is the host and co-creator of the *Better Sex Video Series.*

Remember the days when you had sex every other day—or even *daily?* Most couples make love less frequently as their relationships progress.

But your sex life needn't be dull—no matter how old you are or how long your relationship has lasted.

Here are the common problems that rob sex of its joy and satisfaction—and how to make things right...

LOSS OF DESIRE

Periods of low desire are usually linked to use of antidepressants or tranquilizers...depression...fatigue...or to disappointment, anger and other negative emotions that affect all relationships from time to time.

How can you boost your libido? First, make sure your partner doesn't think the problem lies with him. Admit that you have lost *your* desire.

If it's your partner whose sex drive has ebbed, gently encourage him/her to talk about it.

Good news: Talking about the problem usually leads to its resolution. If not, ask your doctor to rule out physical causes, such as the loss of estrogen during and after menopause.

Many menopausal women find their desire returns if they go on hormone-replacement therapy (HRT)...and researchers are evaluating testosterone-replacement therapy for men *and* women suffering from low libido.

IMBALANCE IN DESIRE

The old clichés are true. Women view intimacy in terms of acceptance, support and affection, whereas men think in terms of sexual intercourse. Many couples spend years struggling with this imbalance.

Mistake: Trying to get your partner to think the way you think.

Instead, look for ways to satisfy both the masculine need for intercourse *and* the feminine need to cuddle and talk. Embrace variety in your intimate encounters. Sometimes go for a quickie, sometimes go for a long, leisurely session. At other times, limit your touching to mutual massage.

IMPOTENCE*

Men who have persistent erection troubles —and their partners—come to view sex with anxiety and overwhelming seriousness. That makes good sex almost impossible.

*Impotence is defined as a "consistent inability to obtain or maintain an erection of sufficient rigidity to achieve satisfactory sexual intercourse." If a couple enjoys sex despite the man's inability to achieve an erection—that's not impotence.

Any man who is impotent in more than half of his sexual encounters should have a complete medical workup. He may have diabetes or heart disease.

Other common causes: Exhaustion, overeating, drinking, smoking, having high blood pressure and taking certain medications—such as antidepressants, antihypertensives and antianxiety agents.

Happily, most erectile problems are curable —thanks in part to an oral drug called *sildenafil* (Viagra)...the injectable drugs *papaverine* (Regitine) and *alprostadil* (Caverject)...and penile implants.

In many cases, a woman can give her partner an erection simply by performing oral sex ...or by gently pressing the fatty pad of her thumb on his perineum. That's the firm area beneath the scrotum. These techniques stimulate the prostate gland, which is intimately linked to sexual function.

Most important: Take sex less seriously. Over a lifetime, you'll probably be able to count earth-moving sexual encounters on one hand. Even the most passionate couples wind up having mediocre sex about 20% of the time.

VAGINAL DRYNESS

Women of all ages can experience inadequate vaginal lubrication. This problem can lead to pain during intercourse and—eventually—the desire to avoid sex altogether.

Usual causes: Hormonal imbalances brought on by pregnancy, breast-feeding, menopause or infrequent sex.

To boost lubrication, couples should devote more time to foreplay...and use a lubricated condom or a water-soluble vaginal lubricant like Erogel or Slip.

Any menopausal woman who is experiencing vaginal dryness should ask her doctor about HRT. Estrogen usually restores vaginal moisture. For women who do not want to go on HRT, topical preparations are available.

SEXUAL BOREDOM

If you've been having sex on the same day, at the same time, in the same room, in the same position for years, the real question is, "How could you not be bored?"

Don't blame your partner for your boredom. Find ways to put the zest back into your sexual encounters. *What to do...*

●**Have sex in an unusual place**—your car, another room in the house, the shower, etc.

●**Schedule sex for a different time of day.** If you ordinarily have sex at night, try getting romantic in the morning. Or—make a date for an afternoon tryst at a local hotel.

●**Look for ways to expand your sexual repertoire.** If you don't practice oral sex already, you might want to give it a try.

Couples over age 55 are 50% less likely to engage in oral sex than younger couples. That's too bad. *Fellatio* and *cunnilingus* can increase intimacy and enjoyment for *both* partners.

Fellatio can help a man to have an erection. And most women find that stimulation of the clitoris—with the tongue, fingers or a vibrator—is the most reliable way to reach orgasm.

Cunnilingus can prime older women for intercourse by helping them to lubricate. It can even be a sexually satisfying substitute for intercourse if impotence or another problem renders that impossible.

Other ways to expand your sexual repertoire...

●**Fantasy.** Sexual fantasies spice up your sex life by giving you—and your partner, if you feel comfortable sharing them—new ideas. If you fantasize about being tied up and tickled with a feather, tell your partner. It just might lead to a sensual, exciting experience for both of you.

It's okay to imagine you're having sex with someone else while you're making love with your partner. That's normal and healthy.

●**Aphrodisiacs.** The best aphrodisiac around today is *green oat straw*. Taken daily, this oral homeopathic remedy boosts desire by increasing levels of circulating testosterone in both men and women. It's available at health-food stores.

Oysters, ginseng, chocolate and alcohol and other recreational drugs do *not* boost sex drive.

●**Erotic videos.** Men aren't alone in their enjoyment of watching others have sex. According to the Video Retailer's Association, 40% of adult videos are rented by women.

A woman who is turned off by hard-core porn may want to explore soft-core porn, women's erotica or instructional sex tapes.

●**Sex toys.** Vibrators, dildos, massage oils, etc., can dramatically enhance your sexual pleasure. *Important:* To keep the man from feeling "replaced" by a vibrator, couples should use it to stimulate both partners.

Discreet sources for sex toys: Eve's Garden, *www.evesgarden.com,* 800-848-3837 or Good Vibrations, *www.goodvibes.com,* 800-289-8423. Request their mail-order catalogs or order online.

●**Masturbation.** Both men and women often find it highly pleasurable to touch themselves during sex with a partner—or to watch their partners touch themselves.

Masturbation is also a powerful tool for teaching yourself to achieve orgasm—so you can better guide your partner.

RENEWING YOUR COMMITMENT

For the next week or month, treat your partner in a romantic way—just like you would like to be treated.

Example: Call your partner at the office just to say, *I love you.* Leave love notes in his briefcase, or her lingerie drawer. Bring home flowers. Start touching one another often in an affectionate way.

For nine out of 10 couples, these simple gestures make a dramatic difference in psychological and sexual satisfaction.

Love and Sex After 60

Robert N. Butler, MD, president and CEO of the International Longevity Center in New York City. Dr. Butler is a former head of the National Institute on Aging. He is co-author of *The New Love and Sex After 60*. Random House.

While the myth persists that the joys of sex are just a memory for folks in their 60s, 70s and beyond, the truth is far different. As long as you and your partner are healthy and willing, *there's no age limit to sexual fulfillment.* We've seen 90-year-olds who lead active, satisfying sex lives.

Too many older people, however, are deprived of this vital pleasure by correctable physical problems, poor lifestyle and self-defeating attitudes.

Sidestep these obstacles and you're likely to find that sex is as good as—or better than—ever.

HOW SEX IS DIFFERENT

At age 75, you're not the man or woman you were at age 25—not physically, emotionally... or sexually.

For men, in particular, the sexual difference is largely a matter of *time*. It takes longer to become aroused...longer to reach a climax...and the refractory phase (time interval between arousals) is longer.

But the good news is that your lifetime of experience—and maturity—will enrich the quality of your sexual encounters. Where sex in young adulthood is athletic, even explosive, it's often self-centered.

Couples who have weathered the storms of life (or those who fall in love in their later years) have often become more sensitive to each other's needs. Sex becomes a matter of mutual giving and sharing.

Important: Don't judge yourself by a youthful standard. Appreciate what you have today—it's different, but not inferior to yesterday.

CLEAR AWAY OBSTACLES

If your sex life isn't satisfactory, illness, not age, may be responsible. Diabetes, depression or an underactive thyroid can rob you of sexual desire.

Inflammation of the prostate may make sex uncomfortable. These conditions are treatable.

Heart disease can have an *indirect* impact on sex. People who suffer from angina (chest pain) or have had heart attacks are often anxious about sex, or avoid it altogether. But the risk of harm is actually very low...less than 0.3% of heart attack deaths occur during sex. Check with your doctor.

After menopause, vaginal tissues grow thinner and natural secretions dry up. This makes sex painful for some older women. Estrogen replacement can correct the problem, but recent studies have called into question the safety of the long-term use of estrogen.

If you'd rather forgo hormones, an over-the-counter vaginal lubricant like Replens will also help restore the pleasure of sex.

Some medications may reduce sexual drive and impair performance (especially for men). Blood pressure drugs, antidepressants, tranquilizers and diuretics (water pills) are the most common culprits.

Almost always, your doctor will be able to prescribe an alternative medication that will work just as effectively and spare your sex life.

IMPROVE YOUR LIFESTYLE

●**Exercise.** If your stamina is limited, you can't bring much vigor to sex—yet another good reason to exercise regularly. Try to exercise for at least 20 to 30 minutes, three to five times a week.

Brisk walking is the best exercise for most older people. Start by walking rapidly until tired, then rest and return at a leisurely pace to the starting point. Gradually increase the distance and pace. *Good goal:* Two to three miles in 45 minutes.

If you've been inactive for years, or have heart disease, consult your doctor before starting any exercise program.

●**Get enough rest.** A well-rested body is more eager and able to perform sexually. Try for seven or more hours of sleep a day. Take naps or rest breaks in the afternoon if you need them. Get medical help for persistent sleeping problems.

●**Avoid alcohol.** Several drinks may relax you and put you in the mood for sex, but can diminish your ability to perform. Even small amounts of alcohol affect you more than when you were younger.

Better: Avoid alcohol altogether, or limit yourself to a single drink for several hours before having sex.

●**Don't smoke.** The sexual organs—both male and female—fill with blood when arousal occurs, and nicotine interferes with this process by constricting vital blood vessels. Men who smoke may also have lower levels of testosterone.

●**Stay sexually active.** If you don't have sex regularly, desire and ability will dwindle. Stay in shape without a partner by masturbating.

257

If it has been years since you've been sexually active, pay special attention to lifestyle factors, be patient (and ask the same of your partner)…and expect that it may take several months to get back in practice.

SET THE SCENE

You're never too old for a richer, more romantic, more exciting sex life. Habit tends to make sex dull and routine. *The antidote:* Flexibility, creativity and caring.

●**Create a romantic setting.** One couple has "dates" at home—they dress nicely, have a candlelit dinner and then retire to the bedroom, which they've made inviting with fresh flowers and soft lights.

A vacation to a new, exciting place is also a great way to recharge your sexual batteries.

●**Be willing to change and explore.** Try new positions and techniques. If you've never read about sexuality, this is a good time to start.

●**Be stimulating and stimulated.** As most men grow older, they need direct physical stimulation of the penis to attain an erection. For women, leisurely, loving foreplay, which includes stimulation of the clitoris, increases pleasure and promotes orgasm.

Watching erotic videos and sharing your fantasies can make sex more exciting for both of you.

Important: Communicate. Tell your partner what feels good—and what doesn't feel so good.

●**Timing is key.** Sex doesn't have to be just a bedtime activity—particularly if you're retired and have more time.

Feel free to have sex when you're both energetic and in the mood. Many people are most rested and relaxed in the morning (and men are generally most potent then). Or unplug the phone, lower the shades and treat yourselves to a matinee.

WORK ON YOUR RELATIONSHIP

Sex is just part of a mature relationship. Tender, generous feelings increase the pleasure, while anger and resentment get in the way.

Desire and sexual performance are especially sensitive to the emotional climate.

Strive to be responsive to each other's feelings and needs—and not just in bed. Bring resentments and disappointments into the open, and do your best to resolve them.

Don't take each other for granted, but make a sustained effort to be interesting and interested. If boredom has crept into your relationship, look within for the deeper feelings you have for one another…and express those feelings sexually.

Exercises May Relieve Impotence

E. Douglas Whitehead, MD, urologist and founding director, Association for Male Sexual Dysfunction, 24 E. 12 St., New York 10003.

Simple pelvic-muscle exercises called Kegel exercises—long known to control urinary incontinence in men and women—may also relieve impotence in some men. The most common cause of impotence is impaired circulation, which leads to inability to retain sufficient blood within the penis. Researchers say Kegel exercises may work as well as surgery.

Prescription Drugs That Affect Sex

Deborah Carson, PharmD, associate professor of pharmacy practice, Medical University of South Carolina, Charleston.

Many people don't realize that medication can affect their sex lives. *Some common drugs and their side effects…*

●**Antidepressants.** Tricyclics like Elavil and serotonin reuptake inhibitors like Prozac and Zoloft can dampen sexual desire and interfere with orgasm and/or ejaculation.

●**Ulcer drugs.** Tagamet and Zantac in large doses can cause impotence, loss of libido and breast pain or enlargement.

●**Diuretics.** Thiazides like Anhydron and Lasix can interfere with ejaculation…dampen sexual desire…and cause impotence.

●**Anti-anxiety drugs.** Tranquilizers like Valium and Xanax can cause impotence and reduced libido and can interfere with orgasm and/or ejaculation.

●**Beta-blockers.** Inderal and Tenormin can cause impotence and decreased sexual desire.

Caution: It can be hard to distinguish a drug's side effects from the underlying medical condition. Never stop taking a drug without first consulting your physician.

Medicines affect different people in different ways. Often a different medicine for the same condition will be less likely to inhibit desire.

Better Sex, Better Sleep

The Doctor's Guide for Sleep Without Pills by Peter Tanzer, MD, in private practice, Pittsburgh. Tresco Publishers.

Improved sexual relations bring relaxation and reduced stress—two keys to better sleep. For many people, regular nighttime sexual relations seem to create a sense of satisfaction, calm and well-being, reduce anxiety and depression and let the participants sleep better.

Warning: Some people find that sex causes insomnia instead of relieving it…and they should avoid sex near bedtime.

Women Are Just as Likely as Men to Initiate Sexual Contact

Monica Moore, PhD, professor, department of behavioral and social sciences, Webster University, St. Louis.

According to cultural myths, it is the male who is the sexual aggressor in male–female relationships. But because a woman's ways of flirting—like standing close to her target or using seductive glances—are more subtle, it is the man who is seen as initiating contact…even in situations when he is simply responding to an invitation.

Saying No to Sex

Shirley Zussman, EdD, sex therapist, New York, and former coeditor of the newsletter *Sex Over Forty.*

To say *no* to sex gently, start by telling your partner why you are not in the mood. Assure him/her you find him desirable and he is not the reason for your lack of desire. Consider nonsexual intimacy instead—snuggling, doing some activity together—so you can still be close without being sexual…and set a date to make love in the near future.

Example: On the weekend, if you are too tired during the week.

If your lack of desire is caused by a relationship problem, say so and try to work it out. Talk at a neutral time and place—not in bed.

Sex and Heart Attacks

James E. Muller, MD, former professor of medicine, Harvard Medical School, Boston. His study of 858 men and women who survived heart attacks was published in the *Journal of the American Medical Association*, 515 N. State St., Chicago 60610.

A study found that the risk of heart attack from sexual activity is only about two in one million. This compares with one in one million if the person did not engage in sexual activity during the prior hour. Heart patients who exercise regularly—meaning they simply walked briskly up a slight hill for 30 minutes a day—had no increased risk from sexual activity.

Sex Can Relieve Arthritis Pain

Warren Katz, MD, chief, division of rheumatology, Presbyterian Medical Center, Philadelphia.

Seventy percent of people in one study said their arthritis pain was relieved for up to six hours after intercourse.

Possible explanation: Sex triggers the release of natural cortisone and betaendorphins —two chemicals that relieve pain naturally.

Helpful: A warm bath or shower before sexual activity to relieve any initial stiffness.

Premature Ejaculation Drug

Stanley E. Althof, PhD, professor of psychology, Case Western Reserve University School of Medicine, Cleveland. His two-month study of premature ejaculation in 15 couples was published in the *Journal of Clinical Psychiatry*, 111 River Rd., Hoboken, NJ 07030.

Delay premature ejaculation with the prescription drug *clomipramine* (Anafranil). Taken six hours before sex, clomipramine delayed ejaculation from an average of only 81 seconds after vaginal penetration to as long as 419 seconds. Couples reported greater sexual satisfaction while the man was on the drug.

Lovemaking Is More than Sex

Real Moments for Lovers by Barbara DeAngelis, PhD, a specialist in human relations and personal growth, Los Angeles. Dell.

Limiting lovemaking to sexual times puts tremendous pressure on sex lives and misidentifies the type of connection that true lovers want. The physical connection of sex is only a part of true lovers' intimacy. *Better:* Try to seek real moments of love with your partner —moments to feel your love fully and rejoice in your relationship. Really making love means stirring up the feelings that constantly flow between you.

Drug for Genital Herpes

Bruce Yaffe, MD, internist and gastroenterologist in private practice, 121 E. 84 St., New York 10028.

Patients who have recurring episodes of these painful sores will get relief within six hours from *famciclovir* (Famvir)—a medicine that needs to be taken only twice a day when symptoms develop. Another drug—*acyclovir* —will also stop outbreaks, but must be used five times a day—and doesn't relieve the pain.

Dr. Ruth's Secrets of Great Sex

Sex therapist Ruth Westheimer, PhD, interviewed in *Investor's Business Daily*, 12655 Beatrice St., Los Angeles 90066.

Genuinely liking your partner…communicating well…being able to ask for what you want.

Sex Isn't Only for The Healthy

Robert N. Butler, MD, president and CEO of the International Longevity Center in New York City. Dr. Butler is a former head of the National Institute on Aging. He is co-author of *The New Love and Sex After 60*. Random House.

Generally, there is no medical reason why someone who is ill should abstain from sexual contact.

Example: Heart attack patients, after an initial recovery period, can usually safely have intercourse, and most actually benefit from it.

Helpful: Take preventive measures before making love, such as finding a comfortable position for both partners and taking nitroglycerin. Check with your doctor about appropriate precautions for your condition.

Better Communication

Sexual Healing: How Good Loving Is Good for You—and Your Relationship by Barbara Keesling, PhD, sex therapist, Los Angeles. Hunter House.

For greater intimacy, set aside a particular time for you and your spouse to practice asking *explicitly* what each other wants. Half the time, you do the asking...the other half, your spouse.

Benefit: No more second-guessing about what you or your partner wants.

Sex and Headaches

Fred G. Freitag, DO, associate director, Diamond Headache Clinic, Chicago.

Headaches associated with sex afflict about 3% of women occasionally.

Usual cause: Muscle strain of the neck and shoulders or rapid blood pressure increases from hormonal surges.

Self-defense: Stay in shape—sex requires stamina...take your time—extending foreplay lets hormone levels and heart rate rise gradually, not surge...change positions—certain positions cause more muscle strain and exertion than others.

Hysterectomies and Sex

Kristen H. Kjerulff, PhD, associate professor, Health Evaluation Sciences, Penn State College of Medicine, Hershey, PA, and leader of a two-year study of 1,100 women, published in the *Journal of the American Medical Association*, 515 N. State St., Chicago 60610.

Hysterectomies don't diminish women's sexuality. Most women who have hysterectomies report more sexual activity and greater pleasure after the operation than before it.

Probable reason: The symptoms that usually lead to hysterectomies—including pain and heavy bleeding—keep women from enjoying sex fully *before* the operation.

Sexual Frequency

Domeena Renshaw, MD, founder/director, Loyola University sexual dysfunction clinic, Maywood, IL.

Married couples today have sex less frequently than couples 60 years ago. Then, married men and women in their 30s had sex about three times a week. Now the average is about twice a week.

Possible reasons: Dual-career marriages and other elements of a high-pressure modern lifestyle.

Home HIV Test Kits

Frederick M. Hecht, MD, associate professor of medicine at the AIDS Program, University of California at San Francisco.

Home HIV test kits give results virtually as accurate as blood tests done at doctors' offices. After purchasing the kit, the buyer pricks his/her finger to take a blood sample and sends it to the company's lab. A code is given so that only the person with the code can obtain the results—which are available by phone within about a week. If the result is positive, the call is automatically directed to a company-provided counselor. *Cost of kit and lab work:* About $50.

Sensual Massage Made Easy

A Lover's Guide to Massage by coauthor Victoria Day, massage therapist and registered midwife, Bristol, England. Ward Lock, distributed by Sterling Publishing Co.

Start a sensual massage by putting oil on your hands and applying it to your partner with broad, easy strokes. Be very gentle at first, then feel through your fingers where to press harder. Keep your fingers relaxed. Use your whole palm and fingers for the massage. Keep strokes reliable and rhythmic, so the massage feels like a continuous sequence even though you move from one body part to another.

How to Find the Best Egg or Sperm Donor

Jonathan Scher, MD, obstetrician and gynecologist in private practice in New York, and coauthor of *Preventing Miscarriage: The Good News.* Collins.

Infertile couples seeking an egg or sperm donor should first contact an in vitro fertilization program or support group. These programs explain exactly how to proceed and what you need to find out about the donor. Trying to locate a donor by advertising is risky because of the unknown genetic background of the respondents. It may also cause future legal problems. The programs screen donors so you can specify factors such as preferred age, ethnic background and education. *Cost per attempt:* For sperm, about $200...for donated eggs, $1,000 to $3,000. Additional costs range from $6,000 to $10,000.

Questions that Keep Love Alive

Instant Insight: 200 Ways to Create the Life You Really Want by Jonathan Robinson, psychotherapist and seminar leader, Santa Barbara, CA. Health Communications.

Ask your partner: What helps you feel most loved by me?...Do you know what you do that makes me feel most loved?

Ask yourself: What act of love or kindness can I do for my partner this week?...What problems are we having that we are not talking about?...How can we talk about them?

Helpful: Plan to spend quality time together at least twice a week. Think about what you really love about your partner...and what fun things you can do together. Then work together to plan them.

Eminent Sex Therapist Reveals Her Secret Weapon Against Sexual Problems

Barbara Bartlik, MD, psychiatrist and medical sex therapist with the human sexuality program at New York Hospital–Cornell Medical Center in New York City. She studied with the late Dr. Helen Singer Kaplan, the renowned sex therapist, and was an associate in Dr. Kaplan's practice.

For most of us, erotica has long been taboo—an embarrassing vice. But as leading sex therapists have found, a new generation of "tasteful" videos and literature can be a powerful ally for couples struggling with sexual problems...or seeking to enrich their sexual relationship.

Even couples who find ordinary "porn" offensive often find that they enjoy—and benefit from—the new, sensitive erotica.

These materials—featuring interesting plots and caring, realistic relationships—are designed to excite *and* educate. *They have proven helpful in resolving several common sexual problems...*

SEXUAL ENNUI

The most obvious use of erotica is to spice up sex for couples who have fallen into a rut.

The late pioneering sex therapist Helen Singer Kaplan, MD, coined the term "hot monogamy" to describe couples who seek sexual adventure *within* marriage. This is done by using erotic toys, sexy lingerie, play-acting, reading and viewing erotica together.

PERFORMANCE ANXIETY

Old-style porn focuses exclusively on the sex act, emphasizing sexual prowess and anatomies of improbable proportions. That can exacerbate feelings of inadequacy in men (and women), contributing to impotence and performance anxiety.

Several more recent videos depict ordinary-looking people enjoying sex in the context of their broader lives. This gives viewers a more realistic standard against which to compare themselves, helping them overcome fears of inadequacy.

Some erotica depicts couples expressing passion *without* progressing to intercourse. Learning about noncoital ways to satisfy each other can remove pressure, rebuild confidence and curb anxiety—lessening performance concerns.

POOR COMMUNICATION

Many individuals find it hard to ask for what they want in bed—oral sex, anal stimulation, etc. They're simply unassertive...or they fear their partner will feel put down.

Erotica provides ways around this problem. One partner can say to the other, "Let's try what they did" or "I'd love it if we could do that."

In some videos, such as those in the *Femme* series (described on the next page), partners are shown giving each other suggestions and feedback in a sensitive, lighthearted way. Watching these "role models" can make talking about sex more comfortable.

SEXUAL INHIBITION

Even in our sexually liberated age, many adults come from restrictive upbringings that taught them sex is dirty and good people don't enjoy it. Many of these people never learned effective ways to give and receive sexual pleasure.

Erotica demonstrates a variety of ways to enhance foreplay and intercourse. And newer, plot-oriented tapes show people of all ages and from many walks of life enjoying sex. This can help viewers feel more comfortable with their own sexuality.

RELATIONSHIP CONFLICT

Pent-up anger or other conflicts with a partner can lead to loss of desire. This initiates a downward spiral in the relationship, since unsatisfying sex can lead to even more frustration.

To halt this spiral, couples must confront these conflicts directly—via honest conversation and perhaps counseling.

While couples are working out their difficulties, erotica can help reignite sexual interest, strengthening the bond between them.

LACK OF FOCUS

Some individuals have trouble focusing on their partners and find that they are unable to reach orgasm.

Typically, they're distracted by work pressures, concerns about body image or privacy, etc.

Erotica compensates for these distractions by "turning up the volume" of sexual excitement.

PROBLEMS THAT DON'T RESPOND TO EROTICA

Erotica is not helpful for...

- **Premature ejaculation.** Men with this problem need to focus on their own physical sensations, not images of others.

- **Sexual aversion.** For this problem, in which sex is extremely anxiety-provoking or distasteful, the partner or partners need to be exposed gradually to sexual activity.

- **Some individuals with a history of sexual abuse.**

Even minor problems sometimes require professional sex therapy. If the problem does not get better, seek professional guidance.

Helpful resource: American Association of Sexuality Educators, Counselors and Therapists, 804-752-0026, *www.aasect.org*.

WHERE TO GET EROTICA

Rent erotic videos at a neighborhood video store...or watch cable television.

Or browse through the classics of erotic literature in a bookstore's "sexuality" section. I recommend Anaïs Nin's *A Spy in the House of*

Love...Henry Miller's *Tropic of Cancer*...and D.H. Lawrence's *Lady Chatterley's Lover.*

If privacy is essential, consider using one of the following mail-order companies...

•**Critic's Choice Video & DVD**, 800-993-6357, *www.ccvideo.com.* Carries a selection of erotic videos, including the Playboy series.

•**Sinclair Institute,** 800-456-5683, *www. bettersex.com.* This video production company, started by former adult film star Candida Royale, features "female-friendly" erotic videos. It also carries the Better Sex Video series, featuring realistic couples in tasteful settings.

  # Get in Sync

Al Cooper, PhD, clinical director, San Jose Marital and Sexuality Centre, San Jose, CA, writing online in *Selfhelp Magazine, www.selfhelpmagazine.com.*

Synchronize your sexual desire with your partner's by finding out what is knocking you out of sync—an overcrowded schedule, pent-up resentments, concerns about your attractiveness or your partner's—or anything else. Make decisions that will allow you to plan when to get together.

Examples: Go to bed earlier or later...or take turns setting up lovemaking sessions, so each of you gets a chance to do it your way.

Sleep Positions and Relationships

David Fogel, MD, medical director, Human Sexuality Institute, Washington, DC.

The way partners sleep may provide a window into the state of their relationship. Changes in a couple's sleep position may signal anger, vulnerability, longing, forgiveness, worry or other feelings.

Caution: Not all sleep-position changes are meaningful. Some may simply be a result of a change in the room's temperature.

14

Growing Older— Healthier

The Key to Successful Aging

Joseph A. James, MD
Beth Israel Medical Center

The best news about staying in good physical health as you age is not the breakthroughs in medical technology, but in the way good doctors now treat their older patients.

Changed goals: For years, patients would go to a doctor to get treated for a specific problem. But if you visit an experienced physician today, he/she is much more likely to check on a full range of physical and mental functions, with the idea of preventing disease or illness from taking hold by nipping any health problem in the bud as soon as it's spotted.

SUCCESSFUL AGING STRATEGY

• **It's now recommended** that doctors see their older patients (generally 59 years old... and above) at least *three times a year*—and once a year make a full assessment of the patient's physical and mental status.

• **This assessment employs a multidisciplinary approach**—the doctor quickly refers the patient to an appropriate specialist if any preliminary test suggests a problem.

• **Preventive medicine is stressed,** including vaccinations and diagnostic tests.

• **The doctor is an active adviser on diet and exercise.**

• **If any medical problem *does* occur**— even a seemingly minor one—doctors will now treat it much more aggressively than in the past, when older patients were "expected" to become ill.

FINDING A GOOD DOCTOR

Many primary care physicians now have the equipment to make a full assessment right in their offices.

If you're looking for a doctor, seek out someone who treats a large number of older

Joseph A. James, MD, head of the Yarmon Division of Geriatric Medicine at Beth Israel Medical Center in New York City.

265

patients. For those who are age 70 or older and have several ongoing medical problems, I recommend seeing a geriatrician (a primary care doctor who specializes in age-related health issues).

FULL ANNUAL ASSESSMENT

Studies have shown that older people are significantly healthier from year to year if they have annual comprehensive assessments. This can be done by a doctor or a geriatric nurse practitioner. *The health assessment should include...*

• **An evaluation of your daily living activities.** How easy is it for you to dress, cook and shop for yourself? Are there any mobility or balance problems that need to be addressed?

• **Cognitive and psychological exam** that checks for any hint of early dementia, alcoholism (which may affect as many as one out of three people age 75 and older), side effects of medication or infection (both of which can cause delirium) and signs of depression, a common—and often undiagnosed—problem among seniors, and one that can be treated very effectively.

• **Nutritional risk evaluation.** This is very important. Many seniors don't eat the way they should, for a variety of reasons. Money can be an issue, or good shopping facilities might not be easily accessible. A physical disability such as arthritis could also make the act of cooking difficult.

The same is true of depression, or some other underlying medical problem. If there is a nutritional deficiency, nutritional supplements and more careful menu planning can help correct the problem.

• **Vision evaluation.** If a problem is diagnosed, the doctor should refer you to an ophthalmologist.

• **Hearing test**, using an audiometer. If any deficiency is spotted, you should be referred to an audiologist.

• **Urinary and bowel continence evaluation.** If there's even a slight problem, it's good to know about it. There are many things that can be done, either by your doctor or a urologist, to treat incontinence.

• **Basic dental evaluation.**

• **Full social evaluation**—including a look at how your support system of family and friends is holding up, what your general financial situation is, as well as key life decisions you'll be making—such as drafting a living will.

AGGRESSIVE SCREENING AND PREVENTIVE CARE

"Prevent it...or catch it early" is now the motto of doctors who cater to older patients. Your doctor should be making sure you are up to date on all important diagnostic tests and vaccinations, including...

• **Pneumovax vaccine.** Pneumonia can be fatal in older people, particularly those who live in cities. This vaccine is good protection against pneumoccocal pneumonia.

• **Tetanus vaccine.** This should be renewed every 10 years—something many adults forget.

• **A regular tuberculosis test.**

• **Annual mammogram,** to test for signs of breast cancer in women.

• **Annual prostate-specific antigen (PSA) blood test** to check for the signs of prostate cancer in men.

• **Flexible sigmoidoscopy.** This procedure checks for polyps in the colon, and should be done every three years.

• **Annual pelvic exam,** to check for signs of cervical or ovarian cancer in women.

• **Test for thyroid function.**

• **Annual evaluation of cholesterol** and triglyceride levels in the bloodstream.

• **Vitamin B-12 and folate evaluation**—for deficiencies that can lead to a decline in mental functioning.

• **Influenza vaccine shot** every autumn. This is important for all adults. Studies show that the flu vaccine curbs serious illness in all adult age groups.

AGGRESSIVE TREATMENT

While the tests listed above may seem expensive in the short term, they actually cost much, much less than the price of treating a serious illness further down the line.

This is why more and more HMOs and insurance companies are beginning to embrace the "whole-person" preventive philosophy—it saves them money.

Another part of this approach is to treat any illness, even a minor one, in an aggressive fashion.

Chronic problems like high blood pressure, diabetes, osteoporosis or mobility problems now get close attention from informed doctors. A wider range of treatments is now being used as well, including physical therapy and exercise and nutrition programs.

In the same way, swift aggressive treatment is now the rule for acute problems like respiratory infections or muscle or bone ailments. The view is that anything that takes away from your overall ability to live your daily life is a threat.

Finally, if you have any questionable health test results, expect your doctor to refer you to a specialist immediately. The older we get, the more important it is to get a qualified specialist's opinion—quickly.

Alzheimer's Self-Defense

Peter V. Rabins, MD, MPH, professor of psychiatry at Johns Hopkins University School of Medicine, Baltimore. He is coauthor of *The 36-Hour Day,* a guide for Alzheimer's caregivers. Johns Hopkins University Press. Contact the Alzheimer's Association (800-272-3900, *www.alz.org*) for more information.

Alzheimer's disease—the most common cause of progressive deterioration of mental function—now afflicts four million Americans.

For the latest on this devastating illness, we interviewed Dr. Peter V. Rabins, a leader in the field...

•**What causes Alzheimer's?** There are several theories. *Two of the most widely circulated ones, however, have been largely debunked...*

•**Aluminum.** Though high levels of aluminum are often found in the brains of Alzheimer's patients, there is no evidence that this metal causes the disease. It is safe to use aluminum pans and to drink from aluminum cans.

•**Zinc.** As with aluminum, there is insufficient evidence to indicate that an excess of dietary zinc causes Alzheimer's. But one study did find a link between zinc and the clumping of proteins in the brain, a condition associated with Alzheimer's.

In light of this study, I think it's prudent to stick to federal guidelines for daily zinc consumption—15 milligrams (mg) for men and 12 mg for women.

•**If aluminum and zinc aren't the problem, what is?** Heredity may be to blame. Researchers have identified several different genes for Alzheimer's, including three that cause the form that strikes before age 65.

Researchers have also found a gene that produces a protein called APOE4. A study published in *The Lancet* suggests that if you inherit a copy of this gene from one parent, you have a 35% chance of developing Alzheimer's by age 90.

•**Is heredity the sole cause of Alzheimer's?** No. *Studies suggest that some cases of Alzheimer's are associated with...*

•**Head trauma.** A history of head injury doubles the chance that you'll get Alzheimer's. Thus it's vitally important to use seat belts, purchase a car with airbags and wear a helmet when riding a motorcycle (or—better—avoid motorcycles entirely). It's also a good idea to avoid boxing and other sports that can lead to head trauma.

•**Head circumference.** Researchers found that people who get Alzheimer's tend to have smaller heads than those who don't. If this provocative finding is confirmed, doctors may someday be able to assess a patient's risk by measuring his/her head circumference and other risk factors.

•**Education.** Alzheimer's patients tend to have less formal education than those without the disease. Formal education may delay the onset of the disease by four to five years.

•**How is Alzheimer's diagnosed?** No single test can diagnose Alzheimer's with absolute certainty. Doctors make a probable diagnosis on the basis of physical, psychological and neurological exams.

First, we perform lab tests to rule out other possible causes of dementia. The list of dementia-causing ailments includes stroke, thyroid disease, liver and kidney disease, vitamin deficiency, depression and long-term use of tranquilizers, antiulcer agents, antihypertensives and heart medications.

If you must take one or more of these drugs, make sure your doctor has prescribed the lowest effective dose.

Next, we observe the patient for signs that the dementia is progressing slowly. Rapidly progressing dementia usually suggests a problem other than Alzheimer's.

Finally, we look for memory loss plus impairment in one or more areas of mental functioning, such as language, visual perception and the performance of everyday tasks. Alzheimer's involves a *combination* of deficits.

●**How can I assess my risk of developing Alzheimer's?** *Two experimental tests that have been in the news recently are the...*

●**Eyedrop test.** The patient's eyes are dilated with eyedrops. In individuals with Alzheimer's (or a predisposition to Alzheimer's), the drops cause the pupils to dilate significantly wider than in people who face little risk of the disease.

Problem: Not everyone with Alzheimer's has dilated pupils after getting the drops...and many people without Alzheimer's do.

●**APOE4 test.** Using this blood test, doctors can determine if you have inherited one or more copies of the Alzheimer's gene.

I'm not recommending this test for my patients—even those with symptoms or a family history of Alzheimer's.

All it can tell you is that if you inherit two copies of the gene, you're 2.5 times more likely to get Alzheimer's than someone who has not inherited this gene.

The real question, of course, is why anyone would *want* to know his risk of Alzheimer's—since there remains no effective means of preventing the disease.

●**What can I do to lower my risk?** Alzheimer's risk appears to be lower among people who take aspirin, ibuprofen or another nonsteroidal anti-inflammatory drug on a regular basis.

●**I read that mental activity helps prevent Alzheimer's. Is that true?** We don't know that for sure, but I encourage my friends, family and patients to stay mentally—and physically—active, just in case.

Reading, doing crossword puzzles or engaging in other mentally demanding activities stimulates your brain cells. This may enhance connections between the cells, slowing the rate of age-associated memory loss.

●**What about "smart foods" and "smart drugs"?** Some people have started taking so-called *cognition-enhancers*—drugs and nutrients such as deprenyl, DHEA, ginkgo biloba and acetyl-l-carnitine. Unfortunately, there is no substantial evidence that these agents prevent Alzheimer's.

●**Is Alzheimer's ever reversible?** Despite media reports of miraculous cures, there hasn't been a single documented case in which someone with Alzheimer's got better.

Of course, patients *mis*diagnosed as having Alzheimer's disease can experience a restoration of memory when the underlying cause—typically depression or another medical disorder or drug effect—has been controlled.

On Healthy Aging

Peg Krach, PhD, retired associate professor of nursing, Purdue University School of Nursing, West Lafayette, IN.

People who remain healthy past age 85 share several attributes. They remain socially active ...they are able to adapt to change and rebound from bad situations...they rely less on medication than their less-healthy peers...they view themselves positively, both physically and mentally...and they have frequent contact with friends and family.

Also: They accept age-related ailments gracefully and with few complaints.

Latest Findings on How to Live Longer

Michael F. Roizen, MD, dean of the School of Medicine at State University of New York Upstate Medical University, Syracuse. Dr. Roizen has published more than 150 peer-reviewed scientific papers and 100 textbook chapters. He is author of *RealAge* (Thorsons) and *The RealAge Makeover* (Collins).

Everyone knows that exercise and a well-balanced diet can slow the effects of aging—but that's only part of the story.

The "RealAge" concept is a scientific way of calculating a number that reflects your *overall* state of health rather than your calendar age.

Example: A 50-year-old could have the arteries and immune system of a typical 75-year-old. Or an 80-year-old who properly cares for his/her health could have the body of a typical 65-year-old.

What's new: Our scientific team has examined more than 33,000 medical studies to determine how lifestyle choices affect aging. *Here are the latest findings…*

USE NINE-INCH PLATES

RealAge reduction: 3.1 years.*

How it helps: The French, despite their traditional, high-fat diet, get heart disease much less often than Americans. Researchers previously attributed this exclusively to their high red wine consumption.

New finding: Food portion sizes in France are about half the size of those in America. Only 6% of adults in France are obese, compared with 18% in the US. How do the French do it? They use nine-inch plates rather than the 11- or 13-inch plates typical in the US.

My advice: Besides using a nine-inch plate, leave space between the different foods…eat slowly…and stop eating as soon as you feel full.

EAT FIBER EARLY IN THE DAY

RealAge reduction: 0.6 years.

How it helps: Plant foods are good for you, in part, because of their high fiber content. People who get 25 grams (g) of fiber daily have a RealAge that's up to three years younger than those who get the national average of 12 g daily.

*All RealAge reductions are based on a 55-year-old. If you are younger or older, reductions may be slightly more or less, respectively.

New finding: Eating fiber *early* in the day is particularly helpful because it prevents spikes in blood sugar (glucose) that can damage arteries and increase the risk for fatty buildup and heart disease.

My advice: Eat fiber at breakfast to slow the rate at which the stomach empties. It increases satiety, so you're less likely to snack and get excessive calories later in the day.

EAT FLAVONOID-RICH FOODS

RealAge reduction: 3.2 years.

How it helps: Flavonoids are plant chemicals that inhibit the effects of free radicals—molecules in the body that damage cells in the arteries, brain and immune system.

New finding: People who drink large amounts of green tea, which is rich in flavonoids, have lower rates of breast and prostate cancer. Other studies have linked green tea to reduced risk for heart disease.

My advice: Get 31 mg of flavonoids daily.

Best food sources: Green tea (8 mg per cup)…broccoli and strawberries (4.2 mg each per cup).

COMBINE VITAMINS C AND E

RealAge reduction: Up to 1 year.

How it helps: Vitamins C and E are antioxidants that prevent cell damage from free radicals…reduce cancer risk…and maintain the elasticity of arteries. Taken alone, however, each has very limited benefit in prolonging life.

New finding: Vitamins C and E are much more powerful when taken in combination. That's because each vitamin protects different parts of cells—vitamin C protects the watery parts and vitamin E the fatty parts.

My advice: Take 400 mg of vitamin C three times daily and 400 international units (IU) of vitamin E daily.

LAUGH MORE

RealAge reduction: 1.7 to 8 years.

How it helps: Laughing reduces stress—and people who are calmer have lower levels of heart disease and more robust immune systems, which can lower cancer risks. To calculate your RealAge, go to *www.realage.com*.

Mistakes Doctors Make When Treating Older Patients

Robert Butler, MD, professor of geriatrics and director of the International Longevity Center at Mount Sinai School of Medicine, New York City. He is the former director of the National Institute on Aging. In 1976, Dr. Butler won a Pulitzer Prize for his book *Why Survive? Being Old in America.* Johns Hopkins University Press.

The older you are, the more likely you are to have health problems that require first-rate medical care. As many seniors have learned, however, it can be hard to find a doctor suited to care for *their* special needs.

How can older people be sure to get good medical care? We put that question to Dr. Robert Butler, a well-known crusader for elder rights. *He explained how important it is to watch out for the common mistakes doctors make when treating elderly patients...*

Mistake: **Failing to appreciate the physical changes that come with age.** Most doctors now practicing know little about the aging body and its ills.

When we launched the geriatrics program at Mount Sinai in 1982, it was the nation's first.

A disease that causes one set of symptoms in a young person may manifest itself quite differently in an older person. Not all doctors realize that. And an unwary doctor can easily miss the diagnosis.

Example I: If a 30-year-old man suffers a heart attack, he is likely to experience severe chest pain. But chest pain is present in less than 20% of older heart attack victims. Instead, older victims may simply seem weak or confused.

Example II: An older person suffering from an overactive thyroid may exhibit apathy instead of hyperactivity, the classic symptom.

Mistake: **Urging older people to "take it easy."** This is awful advice. Even if you've been disabled by a stroke or another medical problem, leading an active lifestyle helps keep you healthy and happy.

Researchers at Tufts University have shown that even people in their 80s and 90s can develop big, powerful muscles with a program of weight lifting. Such a program can literally put a bedridden patient back on his/her feet.

Mistake: **Being too quick to blame health problems on old age.** Doctors often assume that health problems are inevitable in the elderly, exhibiting a defeatist "What can you expect at your age?" attitude.

They order fewer diagnostic tests and generally treat disease less aggressively in old people than in young people.

Example: An elderly woman seems confused and disoriented. *Assuming* that she has Alzheimer's disease, her doctor neglects to order tests that might show the real culprit to be an easily correctable drug reaction.

Mistake: **Not giving the patient enough time.** A good physician will take the time to ask about your work status and lifestyle as well as your medical problems...and, in general, make you *feel* taken care of.

At each office visit, the doctor should ask about the symptoms you have reported in the past. He should also review your response to medications...and ask about new problems.

If you have a *hearing problem*, don't be afraid to ask your doctor to speak up.

Your first visit to a new doctor should be devoted to taking a thorough medical history, and conducting a physical exam and lab tests. This can take more than an hour.

Once this comprehensive exam is completed, you won't need another exam for a year—unless there's a health crisis.

Mistake: **Failing to advocate preventive measures.** Some doctors seem to think, "Why bother trying to lower an elderly patient's cholesterol level. He's just going to decline anyway."

In fact, we now know that heart patients of *any* age can benefit from a program of dietary modification, lifestyle change and—if necessary—drugs or surgery.

Mistake: **Giving inappropriate prescriptions.** Doctors are too quick to order tranquilizers and antidepressants for their older patients, thinking—incorrectly—that psychotherapy is of no use. And they often fail to realize that older bodies respond differently to drugs.

Example I: It can take an elderly person twice as long to "clear" *diazepam* (Valium) from his body as a young person. A dose appropriate for a young person could make an older person drowsy.

Example II: Older people often must take several different drugs at the same time. If the doctor fails to consider all the drugs, dangerous interactions could result.

If you're not sure your doctor knows all the drugs *you're* taking, put all your medications (including nonprescription drugs) in a paper bag and bring them to your next office visit.

Treatments for Parkinson's Disease

Abraham N. Lieberman, MD, chief of movement disorders at Barrow Neurological Institute in Phoenix, and clinical director, National Parkinson Foundation, 1501 NW Ninth Ave., Miami 33136. He is coauthor of *Parkinson's Disease: The Complete Guide for Patients and Caregivers.* Fireside.

More than one million Americans have been diagnosed with Parkinson's disease—the progressive, degenerative brain disorder. An equal number are thought to have the condition—but don't know it.

One percent of people over 60 have Parkinson's, as do 2% of those over 70. But the condition can strike at any age.

There's no cure for Parkinson's. Drugs remain the mainstay of treatment, although surgery has become an option.

THE SYMPTOMS

Most people are first alerted to the possibility that they have Parkinson's by friends or family members who notice…

- **Tremor.** It's most apparent when the hand or foot is relaxed. Most Parkinson's-related tremors are more pronounced on one side of the body.
- **Slow movement** (*bradykinesia*). People with Parkinson's swing their arms less when walking and take longer to wash dishes, take out the garbage, etc.
- **Rigidity.** Muscles become stiff and resistant to movement.
- **Poor balance.** Because they have trouble telling when they're standing straight, people with Parkinson's are likely to fall.

WHAT CAUSES PARKINSON'S

Parkinson's disease stems from damage to the *substantia nigra*. This region of the brain produces the neurotransmitter *dopamine*, which is vital to the function of a second brain area called the *striatum*—which controls movement.

Just what destroys the substantia nigra is unclear. Heredity is apparently a factor. Recent studies suggest that pesticides may play a role as well.

The existence of clusters of Parkinson's disease—as on the island of Guam—suggests that environmental factors may also be involved. But which agents might be involved is unknown.

Bottom line: There is no known way to prevent the disease.

THE FASTEST TREATMENT

The principal treatment is with a drug called *levodopa* (Sinemet).

L-dopa is quite effective at controlling symptoms of Parkinson's. But there is a problem—fluctuating levels of the drug within the brain. When levels are low, Parkinson's symptoms return. High levels can cause tics, spasms and other side effects.

To maintain the right level, many Parkinson's patients take time-release L-dopa.

The drug *selegiline* (Eldepryl) helps maintain proper dopamine levels by blocking the action of an enzyme that ordinarily breaks dopamine down.

With or without selegiline, L-dopa works well for just so long. After five to 10 years, most patients have increased side effects and poorer response.

Doctors now have another drug in their anti-Parkinson's arsenal—*tolcapone* (Tasmar), though its usefulness may be limited by liver toxicity.

If you or someone you know is interested in participating in a clinical trial of Parkinson's therapies, contact the National Parkinson Foundation (800-327-4545, *www.parkinson.org*).

SURGERY

Surgery has been used to treat Parkinson's since the 1930s. But techniques have vastly improved since then.

The most common form of surgery is *pallidotomy*. In this procedure, the surgeon inserts a tiny probe through the skull, then applies electrical current to destroy a region of the brain called the *globus pallidum*.

Pallidotomy does not cure Parkinson's disease. But properly performed, the surgery dramatically reduces tremor and improves the ability to move. It can be extremely helpful for patients who respond poorly to medication.

Because the globus pallidum lies deep within the brain, pallidotomy is risky. Even with a good surgeon, there is a 1% to 2% chance of hemorrhagic stroke.

The procedure can also cause temporary or even permanent confusion and disorientation.

If you are thinking about pallidotomy, ask your neurologist for a referral to an expert neurosurgeon.

FETAL TRANSPLANT

Some surgeons have begun taking tissue from the brains of 9- to 12-week-old aborted fetuses and implanting it into the brains of Parkinson's patients.

This transplanted tissue starts producing its own dopamine, making up for the lack of dopamine in the patients' brains.

As with pallidotomy, fetal transplantation carries a small but significant risk of stroke. But fetal transplants are often extremely effective—especially in people under 60. (The older you are, the less likely the transplants will take hold and flourish.) Following surgery, some patients find that they no longer need medication.

Problem: Because fetal transplantation is considered experimental, the cost of the procedure—about $50,000—isn't covered by most health insurance.

And because of political objections to the use of fetal tissue, the operation is available only in certain states.

Good Samaritan Hospital in Los Angeles and the University of Colorado Health Sciences Center in Denver have the most experience with fetal transplants.

Vitamin Deficiency And Memory

Robert M. Russell, MD, associate director, Jean Mayer US Department of Agriculture Human Nutrition Research Center on Aging at Tufts University, Boston.

Memory loss in elderly people is sometimes caused by a vitamin B-12 deficiency.

Self-defense: If you're over age 60, have your B-12 level checked by a doctor. If it falls below 300, taking a B-12 supplement should fix the problem. Some people need an injectable form of the vitamin. Check with your doctor.

Vitamins Do Help

Study by National Research Foundations and Memorial University of Newfoundland reported in *Money,* 1271 Avenue of the Americas, New York 10020.

People over age 65 who take multivitamins daily were found to be sick with infection-related illnesses only *half* as often as people who did not take vitamins.

Colon Cancer Detection

Marion Nadel, PhD, an epidemiologist in the Division of Cancer Prevention and Control, the Centers for Disease Control and Prevention, Atlanta.

Everyone 50 and older should be screened for colorectal cancer. According to the advisory panel to the US Public Health Service, effective methods include fecal-occult blood testing and sigmoidoscopy (or both).

Stronger Seniors

Study of nursing home residents, ages 72 to 98—more than 80% of whom required a cane, walker or wheelchair—led by Maria Fiatarone Singh, MD, chief, nutrition and exercise physiology laboratory, the Jean Mayer US Department of Agriculture Human Nutrition Research Center on Aging at Tufts University, Boston.

Strength training for seniors improves mobility and counteracts muscle weakness and frailty—at any age. A study of 100 nursing-home residents, average age 87, found muscle strength more than doubled after 10 weeks of a progressive resistance training program for hip and knee muscles. Exercise had substantial benefits even for people using canes, walkers or wheelchairs.

Bottom line: Exercise helps people of any age become stronger and more mobile.

Owning a Dog Can Extend Your Life

Erika Friedmann, PhD, professor, University of Maryland School of Nursing, Baltimore.

A study of 369 heart attack sufferers found that those who owned dogs were far less likely to die within the first year than those who did not own dogs. Dogs make their owners feel wanted and needed. Dog owners also have to walk their pets regularly, and so are forced to get exercise, too.

Safer Lifting Now

Elizabeth Myers, PhD, assistant professor, Department of Orthopedic Surgery, Beth Israel Hospital, Boston.

People with brittle bones should be very careful about lifting.

Everyday activities like picking up grandchildren or lifting groceries out of the car can lead to painful compression fractures of the spine.

Researchers advise women with osteoporosis or others with fragile bones never to lift with outstretched arms or to bend from the waist while lifting.

Best way to lift: Keep arms as close as possible to the body and try not to bend at the waist.

How to Maintain Peak Mental Ability As You Get Older

Richard M. Restak, MD, clinical professor of neurology at George Washington University School of Medicine and Health Sciences in Washington, DC. He is author of *Older & Wiser* (Berkley) and *The New Brain* (Rodale).

Almost everyone experiences some decline in memory and reaction time after age 40. But a rich network of *neural connections*—links between brain cells that allow them to communicate—can help compensate for these losses.

A rich neural network may even help keep people from being incapacitated by Alzheimer's disease.

Extensive neural connections seem to act as a kind of *cognitive reserve*—allowing a person to function longer with the disease than someone whose mental resources were less extensive.

Good news: Brain cells can form new connections at *any* age. I'm 55 years old, and I've decided to take steps *now* to preserve mental function *later*.

DEVELOP A CONSUMING PASSION

When your brain is involved in a wide range of activities, more neural circuits are created and maintained.

Helpful: Cultivating an interest in something totally different from your customary pursuits. A lawyer might take up bridge...or an accountant might learn to play the clarinet.

It's also a good idea to take classes in unfamiliar subjects. Studies have shown that higher education early in life helps ensure proper brain functioning in old age. It seems likely that intellectual activity *later* in life builds cognitive reserves as well.

GET REGULAR EXERCISE

Every day, I walk a few miles at a moderate pace. In addition to keeping the heart and lungs healthy, exercise boosts blood flow to the brain, fueling it with oxygen and glucose.

Another excellent form of exercise is the gentle Chinese martial art *tai chi.*

TAKE SUPPLEMENTS—SENSIBLY

Cellular damage caused by *free radicals*—renegade molecules formed in the body as a by-product of normal metabolism—is thought to be a major cause of age-related mental decline.

To neutralize free radicals, I make sure to get enough of the antioxidant vitamins A, C and E.

I eat lots of fruits and vegetables...and take a supplement containing 10,000 international units (IU) of beta-carotene (the precursor of vitamin A)...1,000 milligrams (mg) of vitamin C...and 400 IU of vitamin E (in the form *d-alpha tocopherol,* which has the highest "biopotency").*

Since we tend to become deficient in zinc as we age, I also take a pill containing about 20 mg of this mineral every day. Zinc plays a key role in preserving the sense of smell.

•**Anti-inflammatory drugs.** The Baltimore Longitudinal Study also found preliminary evidence that taking nonsteroidal anti-inflammatory drugs (NSAIDs) such as *ibuprofen* might be protective against Alzheimer's.

Caution: Since NSAIDs can cause stomach trouble, they should be taken under a doctor's supervision.

•**DHEA.** Studies suggest that this hormone improves memory. But it increases men's risk for prostate cancer. We don't know if it poses any danger to women. More research is needed.

PREVENT STROKES

A stroke occurs when a blood clot or ruptured artery cuts off blood flow to the brain.

*Consult your doctor for the amount that is appropriate for you.

New research links stroke-induced brain damage with Alzheimer's.

To minimize your risk: Exercise regularly, eat a healthful diet, avoid smoking and keep your blood pressure under control.

If a stroke does occur, new drugs can help arrest the damage. They must be administered *within hours,* however, so seek medical attention *immediately* at the first sign of stroke.

The signs of stroke include numbness on one side of the body...difficulty speaking or understanding speech...sudden headache...dizziness or loss of balance...and blurred or decreased vision.

CONTROL STRESS

Chronic psychological stress causes the body to make excess *cortisol.* Over time, high levels of this adrenal hormone can cause deterioration of the *hippocampus,* a part of the brain that plays a critical role in memory.

We can't always control events, but we *can* control our response to these events. One strategy I use is to reframe *frustrations* as *challenges.* I ask myself, "What's the best course of action to follow at this time?" I also use words that have a calming rather than tension-producing effect—for example, *concern* rather than *worry.*

MAINTAIN FINGER DEXTERITY

French researchers found recently that older women who knit retain normal mental function longer than their nonknitting counterparts.

I don't knit, but I always carry a crossword dice game with me. Whenever I have a few minutes to spare, I play it.

MAKE PRACTICAL ADAPTATIONS

Memory aids—from making lists to carrying a palmtop computer—are great for helping offset age-related memory loss. But do *not* become so dependent on these helpers that you allow your own natural abilities to atrophy.

Example: If I'm carrying a list of things to do, I'll check it only *after* I've called up as many items as I can from my own memory.

Estrogen and Dementia

Sally A. Shumaker, PhD, associate dean for research, department of public health sciences, Wake Forest University School of Medicine, Winston-Salem, NC, and leader of a study of almost 3,000 women ages 65 to 79, published in *Journal of the American Medical Association*, 515 N. State St., Chicago 60610.

Estrogen-only hormone-replacement therapy (HRT) increases dementia risk in women over age 65. Earlier research showed that HRT combining estrogen and progestin increases dementia risk. The increased risk for estrogen-only therapy is small but measurable—estrogen could cause 12 additional women out of 10,000 to develop dementia.

Vitamin E and Aging

Marguerite M.B. Kay, MD, former Regents Professor of Microbiology and Immunology and Medicine at the University of Arizona, Tucson.

Vitamin E may help slow the effects of aging on the brain and immune system.

A study on mice found that when middle-aged and old mice were fed diets supplemented with vitamin E, normal age-related damage to vital proteins in their brain and immune system cells was delayed or prevented. Researchers believe that vitamin E, taken at the onset of middle age, will also slow damage due to aging in human brains and immune systems. The equivalent human dosage of vitamin E that was found effective in mice is about 400 international units (IU) a day.

Caution: Due to the possible interactions between vitamin E and various drugs and supplements, as well as other safety considerations, consult your doctor before starting a vitamin E regimen.

Consider Nursing Home Transfer Policies

Joseph Matthews, author of *Beat the Nursing Home Trap.* Nolo.com.

On occasion, nursing homes try to send residents to hospitals or other nursing facilities to deal with temporary medical problems that can be handled at the nursing home itself.

Note: Transfers to other facilities for medical reasons cannot legally be made without the consent of the patient or legal proxy. The consent of the patient's attending physician should also be obtained.

Fever Danger

Catherine Marco, MD, clinical professor, Medical College of Ohio, Toledo. Her study of 470 patients was published in *Annals of Emergency Medicine*, 360 Park Ave. S., New York City 10010.

Fever in an older person signals the need for hospitalization. In a study of patients 65 or older who went to the emergency room with a fever of 100 degrees or more, 76% were found to be seriously ill. Almost half showed no other outward sign of illness.

Blood Pressure Pill Benefit

Michael Murray, PharmD, senior scientist, Regenstrief Institute, Inc., Indiana University School of Medicine, Indianapolis, and leader of a study of 1,900 patients age 65 and older, presented at the 17th International Conference on Pharmacoepidemiology.

Blood pressure pills reduce risk of mental decline in older patients. People over age 65 who took blood-pressure–lowering medicine, such as diuretics and calcium channel blockers, for at least five years were 38% less likely to develop impaired thinking or dementia than those not taking the pills.

Exercise Improves Hearing

Helaine M. Alessio, PhD, professor of physical education, Miami University, Oxford, OH.

Research indicates that persons who are not physically fit improve their hearing when they begin regular aerobic exercise—and that persons who are fit are less susceptible to suffer a hearing loss as a result of exposure to loud noise.

Exercise vs. Alzheimer's

Robert Friedland, MD, professor of neurology, laboratory of neurogeriatrics, department of neurology, Case Western Reserve University, University Hospitals of Cleveland.

The risk of Alzheimer's is sharply reduced by exercise—both physical and mental. A seven-year study of 2,000 people over age 65 found that those who engaged in high levels of reading, physical exercise or just talking with friends reduced their risk of Alzheimer's by 38%.

Why: Physical and mental activities increase blood flow to the brain, which strengthens its resistance to disease and increases connections among nerve cells. The brain is like any other organ in the body—it ages better, with better function, when it is used.

The Mind/Body Approach to Arthritis

Margaret A. Caudill-Slosberg, MD, PhD, instructor of medicine, Dartmouth Medical School, Hanover, NH. She is author of *Managing Pain Before It Manages You.* Guilford Press.

If you suffer from arthritis, you probably already know that medication provides only partial relief.

Fortunately, arthritis—as well as headaches, back pain and most other forms of chronic pain

—can be managed via a set of mind/body techniques. These techniques cost nothing and can be self-administered. They are effective whether your pain is caused by a clearly identifiable disease or is of mysterious origin.

ACUTE VS. CHRONIC PAIN

Acute pain is the body's way of warning us that something is wrong. When we get this "warning signal," we take immediate action to protect ourselves.

Example: We drop a plate that's too hot to hold. Doing so helps us avoid additional injury and gives the injury time to heal.

With *chronic* pain, there is no hot plate to drop. With no obvious way to protect ourselves, we respond emotionally. We slip into depression…become unable to work…experience trouble with our relationships, etc.

The key to coping with chronic pain is to live well *despite* the pain.

KEEP A PAIN DIARY

Keeping a pain diary will help you look at your pain objectively.

What to do: Three times a day, rate the intensity of your pain, from zero (no pain) to 10 (the worst pain ever). Also—describe the sensation. Is it an ache? Burning sensation? Tightness?

Note what you are doing when pain strikes. Rate your distress—the frustration, anger, anxiety or sadness you feel in response to the pain.

Record what you did to alleviate the pain—took an aspirin, went for a walk, applied heat or cold, etc.

Your diary will help you pinpoint things that ease or exacerbate your pain…and clearly show the difference between the pain itself and your emotional response to it.

USE THE RELAXATION RESPONSE

In many cases, the psychological stress caused by pain is worse than the pain itself.

Stress causes muscular tension that can lead to new ills—headache or upset stomach, for instance. Stress also aggravates the fatigue that often comes with chronic pain.

By eliciting your natural "Relaxation Response," you can alleviate this emotional stress.

Technique: Pick a time when your pain is relatively mild, and find a peaceful place where you won't be disturbed. Sit comfortably or lie down. Use a heating pad, ice pack or pillows to make yourself comfortable, if necessary.

Focus on your breathing. With each exhalation, silently repeat a word or phrase of your own choosing. This can be something neutral, like "one"...or something uplifting, such as "God."

Or, count each inhalation and exhalation, starting over when you reach 10. When your mind wanders, gently bring it back to your focus word or phrase. Elicit the Relaxation Response for at least 20 minutes a day.

If you like, elicit the Relaxation Response while exercising. Just make sure your breathing and thoughts are synchronized with your movements.

PERFORM SELF-HYPNOSIS

Once you have mastered the Relaxation Response, add self-hypnosis. While deeply relaxed, close your eyes and imagine that your right hand is becoming pleasantly warm and heavy. Each time you exhale, imagine the pleasant sensation intensifying.

Now imagine a pleasant numbness that begins in your thumb, then moves to each finger with each exhalation. Feel it spread to your palm and the back of your hand, stopping at the wrist.

Place that numb hand on the painful area of your body, or imagine the numbness moving to that spot. When all the numbness has been "absorbed" by the painful area, return to your focus word.

End each session by returning the numbness to your right hand. Feel the normal sensations return to that hand, breath by breath.

PACE YOURSELF

Some chronic pain sufferers try to ignore their bodies—pushing on until the pain becomes unbearable. Others simply shut down, withdrawing from social and/or professional activities.

Better: Pace yourself. Learn to complete your daily activities and live as normally as possible.

To do this, you must...

•**Tune in to your body.** Use your pain diary and the Relaxation Response to become aware of subtle sensations that signal a flare-up.

•**Switch to a less demanding activity** when you feel pain building. If you're washing dishes when your pain worsens, sit down and use the time to pay bills. Go back to the dishes later.

CHANGE YOUR SELF-TALK

The meaning you ascribe to your pain makes an enormous difference in its effect on your life and your mood.

What does your pain mean to you? To find out, listen to your *self-talk*. That's the voice in your head that continually comments on and interprets your pain.

In individuals with chronic pain, self-talk is quite distorted. They tend to *catastrophize*—making a bad situation worse by engaging in exaggerated self-talk.

Example I: Instead of telling yourself you can bear a flare-up, you think, "This pain is unbearable."

Example II: Instead of acknowledging the many things you can still do despite your pain, you say, "My whole life is ruined."

Don't give in to such negative self-talk. Make a conscious choice to change it. Say your pain is too severe to keep a lunch date. You think, "My whole day is ruined."

Substitute a realistic interpretation. "This is unfortunate, but I can make other arrangements. I'll invite my friend to come here, and we'll send out for pizza."

PLAN FOR FLARE-UPS

No matter how well you manage your pain, there will be times when it becomes intense. To be ready for these episodes, keep a written list of strategies that make you feel better—things you can do to reduce the pain and ease your emotional distress.

Examples: Lying down...applying heat or ice...performing self-hypnosis...calling a friend ...or distracting yourself with a funny video.

HIGH-TECH HELP

Though medication can't stop chronic pain entirely, it can make your self-help program more effective. *Three drugs are especially effective...*

•**Gabapentin (Neurontin).** It seems effective for nerve pain caused by diabetes and post-herpetic neuropathy.

●**Fentanyl (Duragesic).** A new skin patch system delivers this potent painkiller continuously for three days.

●**Morphine (Duramorph).** The intrathecal pump constantly delivers morphine to the area around the spinal cord.

Risk Reducers

JoAnn E. Manson, MD, codirector of women's health at Brigham and Women's Hospital, Harvard Medical School, Boston.

The older a woman is at menopause, the less likely she is to die from heart disease —the leading cause of death in women. Studies show that the risk declines by about 2% for every year that menopause is delayed.

Other risk reducers: Cutting out cigarettes —smokers go through menopause earlier…regular exercise…maintaining a healthy weight…a low-fat diet.

Fainting Danger

J. King White, MD, cardiologist in private practice in Lake Charles, LA.

A fainting spell could signal a serious medical problem. One in five people faints at least once in his/her life.

Usual causes: Emotional stress, anxiety, the sight of blood, etc. But the older a person is, the greater the odds that a serious ailment is to blame—such as a heart disorder or a drug reaction.

To be safe: If you faint, see a doctor.

Best Shoes for Senior Citizens…

Steven Robbins, MD, associate professor of geriatric medicine, Center for Studies in Aging, McGill University, Montreal.

Those with hard, thin soles. Compared with going barefoot or wearing soft-soled tennis or running shoes, hard-soled shoes provide better "foot-position awareness," a sense that improves posture and helps maintain balance.

How to Guard Against Macular Degeneration

Neil M. Bressler, MD, professor of ophthalmology at the Wilmer Ophthalmological Institute of Johns Hopkins University School of Medicine in Baltimore.

Most people already know that diabetes and glaucoma can cause blindness. But one of the leading causes of vision loss is a breakdown of cells in the retina known as *age-related macular degeneration* (AMD).

This condition, which can be detected via a simple eye exam, causes four times more blindness in older adults than glaucoma or diabetes. One-quarter of people over age 65— and one-third of those over age 80—have early signs of the disease.

Scariest of all, AMD can rapidly progress from a minor vision problem to near total loss of "central" vision.

There's no way to restore vision loss caused by macular degeneration. But prompt treatment can often stop the disease in its tracks.

RETINAL BREAKDOWN

Macular degeneration gets its name from the *macula*. That's the exquisitely sensitive central region of the retina, the light-sensitive membrane at the back of the eye. The macula is what we rely upon for reading, driving, recognizing faces and other tasks that demand sharp vision.

Macular degeneration occurs when yellowish patches of material produced in the back of the eye called *drusen* begin to form behind a layer of cells in the macula.

In some cases, drusen cause no symptoms for 10 or even 20 years. But in some unfortunate individuals, drusen quickly give way to an abnormal proliferation of blood vessels and scar tissue within the macula itself.

WAVY LINES

It's at this point that symptoms often start to appear. Straight lines look wavy...or tiny blank spots appear in the center of your field of vision.

The course of the disease can vary. Some people with AMD lose the ability to read or drive within one year of the onset of symptoms. Others suffer comparatively minor vision loss—even after five or 10 years.

PREVENTION

Doctors have not yet found any way to eliminate the risk of developing AMD. *Preliminary research suggests, however, that the following two strategies may offer at least some degree of protection...*

● **Don't smoke.** Smokers seem to be more likely to develop the abnormal proliferation of blood vessels and scar tissue than nonsmokers. If you haven't yet kicked the habit, here's one more reason to do so.

● **Avoid heart disease risk factors.** The same factors that heighten the risk of cardiovascular disease—especially high blood pressure—seem to heighten the risk of losing vision from macular degeneration.

Let this reinforce your determination to cut your intake of saturated fat...control your blood pressure...get regular exercise...and avoid obesity.

EARLY DETECTION

Until doctors know more about prevention, the best way to protect your eyesight from AMD is via annual eye exams. The more conscientious you are about getting exams, the more likely you will be to catch AMD early—while it's still treatable.

Using a device called an ophthalmoscope, an ophthalmologist can easily see drusen and other retinal abnormalities that are the hallmarks of early macular degeneration.

There's no treatment for early AMD. But if the signs are there, it's vitally important to stay alert for the subtle changes in vision that suggest the disease is worsening.

Helpful: Check the vision of each eye separately every day. Some ophthalmologists suggest using an Amsler grid. Ask your eye doctor for one.

LASER SURGERY

Laser surgery is the only procedure proven to halt the progression of AMD.

This 15-minute outpatient procedure should help confine the troublesome blood vessels and scar tissue, thereby decreasing the risk of additional visual loss and protecting your remaining vision.

Laser surgery cannot restore the macula to its original state. Even if the operation goes well, odds are you'll find it impossible to read without low-vision aids that provide increased light and magnification.

After surgery, you'll need checkups—at one and three months later, and then every three or four months—for at least one year and possibly two. In about half of all cases, surgery must be repeated to take care of new areas of damage.

Important: Laser surgery is beneficial only when macular damage is limited to a tiny area—1.5 to 3 millimeters in diameter. That's why it's so crucial to see the eye doctor as soon as you notice symptoms. If you wait even a few weeks, it may be too late for effective treatment.

There's no good way to stabilize vision affected by larger areas of abnormal blood vessels and scar tissue. *But two ongoing clinical trials may change that...*

● **Study #1.** Doctors are evaluating the use of nonlaser surgical techniques to remove the damaged area and thus limit vision loss.

● **Study #2.** Doctors are trying to limit damage using *photodynamic therapy.* Dye injected into a vein in the patient's arm finds its way to the eye, where it concentrates in the abnormal blood vessels and scar tissue. Shining a harmless light into the eye causes a chemical change in the dye, rendering it toxic to only the diseased part of the retina.

For results of the study of photodynamic therapy with Visudyne, contact Novartis Ophthalmics at *www.visudyne.com*.

LOW-VISION AIDS

From high-power reading glasses and closed-circuit video systems to illuminated magnifying glasses, there are numerous visual aids to help you make the most of what vision you have remaining. These aids can make the difference in whether or not you can read or get around outdoors.

If your ophthalmologist isn't familiar with these devices, ask him/her to refer you to a low-vision specialist.

For more information on macular degeneration, send a self-addressed, stamped, business-sized envelope to the American Academy of Ophthalmology, Box 7424, San Francisco 94120.

Congestive Heart Failure And Blood Pressure Link

Daniel Levy, MD, director, Framingham Heart Study, Framingham, MA.

Controlling blood pressure is the best way to avoid congestive heart failure (CHF).

Trap: Doctors often overlook *isolated systolic high blood pressure*, the type most likely to cause CHF. In this form of high blood pressure, the first (systolic) number is 140 or higher... while the second (diastolic) number is below 90.

Implication: Patients with such blood pressure need close surveillance and may require treatment.

Alzheimer's Relief

Rachelle Doody, MD, PhD, associate professor of neurology, and Effie Marie chair in Alzheimer's Disease Research Center, Baylor College of Medicine, Houston.

While not a cure, *donepezil* (Aricept) may benefit up to 80% of Alzheimer's patients. The drug is able to slow the breakdown of the brain chemical *acetylcholine*, which is vital for transmission of nerve signals. Donepezil is the second Alzheimer's drug to receive FDA approval. Unlike the first, *tacrine* (Cognex), it cannot harm the liver. And it must be taken only once a day. Tacrine is usually taken four times daily.

PSA Testing: More Harm than Good?

Timothy McCall, MD, an internist, medical editor of *Yoga Journal* and author of *Examining Your Doctor: A Patient's Guide to Avoiding Harmful Medical Care*. Carol. *www.drmccall.com*.

One of the most common questions I get from my male patients is whether they should have the *prostate specific antigen* (PSA) test. This simple blood test, I tell them, can detect prostate cancer at an early stage. What isn't known is whether getting a PSA test will benefit *you*.

The American Cancer Society estimates there were about 218,900 new cases of prostate cancer in the US in 2007, and about 27,050 deaths. It's become the number two cause of cancer death in men. Lung cancer remains number one.

Prostate cancer is very common. It has been estimated that 40% of all men over age 50 have it. But only about 8% of men ever get symptoms, and only 3% die of the disease. In other words, four out of five men with prostate cancer never get symptoms and nine out of 10 will die of something else. In the past, most of these men never found out they had cancer.

The PSA test changed all that. Before the test went into widespread use—beginning in the mid-1980s—there were only about one-third as many cases diagnosed per year. Even so, the number of prostate cancer deaths was about the same as it is today.

This points out one of the biggest problems with PSA testing. We now have the ability to detect cancer not just in those destined to die of the disease but also in the majority who will never get symptoms. Unfortunately, it's impossible to differentiate between the two groups —at least so far.

The second big problem with PSA testing is that it's not clear that the standard treatments for prostate cancer—radical prostate surgery and X-ray therapy—save lives. Many doctors and patients assume that they do. But it's still unclear how effective these are, and no studies have compared one treatment to the other. Even so, the number of men undergoing prostate surgery has skyrocketed.

The side effects of radical prostate surgery, such as impotence and incontinence, are significant. Though surgeons in top prostate cancer centers report better results, a survey of men two to four years after the operation found that only 11% had had an erection sufficient for intercourse in the prior month. Almost a third wore adult diapers or clamps on their penises to control their urine. Radiation therapy also has significant side effects.

There are major disagreements among medical authorities about PSA testing. The American Cancer Society says men should have one every year starting at age 50 (earlier if they're African-American or have a family history of prostate cancer). The US Preventive Services Task Force does not recommend routine screening.

For my male patients over age 70 and for those whose life expectancy (due to other illnesses) is less than 10 years, I advise against PSA tests. The side effects of treatment simply outweigh the benefits. I tell younger men that a PSA test could save their lives—or it could cause them a lot of needless grief. Right now no one can tell you which.

I encourage my patients to learn as much as possible about prostate cancer. You might visit your local library. Remember, anything more than a couple of years old is outdated. If you (or the library) have access to the Internet, OncoLink (*http://oncolink.upenn.edu*) is a great place to start.

Given the uncertainties, whether to have the PSA test is a highly personal decision—one each man must make in consultation with his doctor. As with any medical decision that hinges mostly on value judgments, however, it should be your values—not your doctor's—that dictate what you do.

Avoiding Disabling Falls

Steven L. Wolf, PhD, professor and director of research, department of rehabilitation medicine, Emory University School of Medicine, Atlanta. For a good introduction to tai chi, order the videotape *Tai Chi: A Gift for Balance*, Dr. Tingsen Xu, Box 98426, Atlanta 30359.

Elderly people may be less likely to suffer disabling falls if they take up *tai chi*, the ancient martial art that blends meditation with slow, rhythmic movements. Tai chi improves balance by teaching better control of the body.

Caution: Elderly people should begin tai chi training only after a doctor has ruled out neurological problems.

Free Eldercare

Free eldercare services hotline can refer you to any of more than 4,000 local agencies that may help meet your needs. Help is available for problems involving medical care, taxes, the law, investments, housing, transportation and much more. The Eldercare Locator Service (*www.eldercare.gov*) is funded by the US Administration on Aging. Call 800-677-1116.

Dentist May Hold Key to Stroke Risk

Laurie Carter, DDS, PhD, director, oral and maxillofacial radiology, Virginia Commonwealth University School of Dentistry, Richmond.

Dental X-rays may identify people at high risk for heart attack and stroke. Hardening of the carotid arteries, which lead to the brain, can often be seen in a panoramic dental X-ray. This hardening of the carotids doubles risk of death from heart attack or stroke. *When X-rays are taken:* Ask your dentist to look for calcifications in the carotid arteries.

Stroke Sufferer Fact

David J. Ballard, MD, PhD, senior vice president and chief quality officer, Baylor Health and Hospital System, Dallas. While professor of medicine at Emory University in Atlanta, his study of 38,612 patients age 65 or older was published in *Stroke*, American Heart Association, 7272 Greenville Ave., Dallas 75231.

Stroke victims live longer when they're cared for by a neurologist. Ninety days after suffering a stroke, patients who had been treated by a neurologist had a 36% higher survival rate than those under the care of a family physician.

Alcohol and Disease... Stroke...Diabetes... And Cancer

Eric B. Rimm, ScD, a noted alcohol researcher and assistant professor of epidemiology and nutrition at Harvard School of Public Health in Boston.

The heavy toll of excessive drinking is all too obvious—from car accidents to liver disease, immune system problems and depression.

But the upside of alcohol is just as real. Drinking in moderation reduces the risk of developing serious illness.

Key: Knowing the level of drinking that is right for you.

HEART DISEASE AND STROKE

The evidence that moderate alcohol consumption cuts heart disease risk is very strong. More than 35 studies have shown that people who have one to two drinks a day are 25% to 40% less likely than nondrinkers to have a heart attack.

Moderate drinking seems to protect the heart by boosting blood levels of HDL (good) cholesterol...and by reducing concentrations of *fibrinogen*. That's a natural compound involved in blood clotting.

Alcohol's effect on the risk of stroke is more complex. *Ischemic* strokes (the most common kind) are caused by blood clots in the brain. One to two drinks a day protect against ischemic stroke the same way that they protect against heart attack.

Unfortunately, alcohol's anticlotting action may raise the risk for *hemorrhagic* stroke. This kind of stroke is caused by bleeding in the brain. Research has shown that people who consume three or more drinks a day are more likely than nondrinkers to suffer a hemorrhagic stroke.

Alcohol can raise or lower blood pressure, depending on how *much* you drink. If you're taking medication for high blood pressure, ask your doctor whether you should drink—and, if so, how much.

IS RED WINE SPECIAL?

You may have heard that red wine has special heart-protective powers. Red wine *does* contain antioxidants and other beneficial compounds not found in other alcoholic beverages. But an analysis of data from alcohol research around the world found that *all* forms of alcohol are equally effective at lowering the risk of heart disease.

To your heart, a drink is a drink. One drink equals four to six ounces of wine...12 ounces of beer...or 1.5 ounces of whiskey, gin or another "hard" liquor.

DIABETES

Moderate drinkers are 30% to 40% less likely than nondrinkers to develop adult-onset (Type 2) diabetes. This common condition is associated with blindness, kidney failure and heart disease.

Researchers don't yet have an explanation for this antidiabetes effect. One theory is that drinking with meals slows food absorption, which keeps insulin levels steady. Another is that alcohol makes cells throughout the body more sensitive to insulin.

CANCER—A DIFFERENT STORY

There's simply no question about it—drinking *raises* the risk for cancer.

Malignancies of the mouth and throat are especially common among drinkers. But these cancers are rare, and the increase in risk is negligible if you have fewer than four drinks a day.

There is evidence that as little as two drinks per day raise the risk for colon cancer. That's a *very* common malignancy.

Good news: A common B-vitamin called folic acid, or folate, can neutralize this extra danger.

For people who consume at least the recommended daily allowance (RDA) of folate, moderate drinking does *not* appear to raise colon cancer risk. The RDA for folate is 400 micrograms (mcg) per day.

Folate sources: Fresh vegetables, cereals, orange juice, vitamin supplements.

The link between alcohol and breast cancer is stark. Studies consistently show that two to three drinks a day increase a woman's risk for breast cancer by 30% to 40%. Whether lighter drinking has any effect is unclear.

Epidemiologists advise women to have no more than one drink a day. At this level, the benefits to the heart outweigh the increased cancer risk.

Exception: If you are at high risk for breast cancer (your mother or sister developed the disease, for example), it's probably prudent to limit your alcohol consumption to two drinks per week.

The media has reported research showing that red wine reduces the risk for cancer.

Lab studies did show that *resveratrol*, an antioxidant found in red wine, blocks DNA damage that leads to cancer, detoxifies carcinogens and prevents tumors from progressing. But there's no evidence that resveratrol has any effect on humans. Not one population study has linked red wine consumption to reduced cancer rates.

Implication: Taking grape extract, eating grapes or drinking grape juice for resveratrol is unlikely to cause you any harm. But there's no evidence it will help you.

THE BOTTOM LINE

There's compelling evidence that moderate drinking—up to two drinks a day for men, one a day for women—is better for health than abstaining. This level of drinking reduces deaths from all causes by 15%—in men and women alike.

If you already drink moderately, feel reassured.

If you're currently a nondrinker, should you start drinking? Not necessarily. You may be among the minority who cannot keep their drinking at a beneficial level. Once you exceed three drinks a day, your risk of disease and death becomes higher—not lower.

Concentrated bouts of drinking are a bad idea, too. Having all of your weekly quota of drinks on the weekend won't help your cholesterol…and it might raise your risk of suffering a stroke or a lethal heart rhythm disturbance.

And a healthy heart won't help you much if you wrap your car around a telephone pole.

How Effective Is Colon Cancer Drug?

Leonard Saltz, MD, assistant attending physician, division of gastrointestinal oncology, Memorial Sloan-Kettering Cancer Center, New York City.

Patients with advanced colorectal cancer may benefit from *irinotecan* (Camptosar). In a study, this injectable drug shrank tumor size by 50% or more in 23% of cancer patients who had failed to respond to other drugs. In patients with no prior chemotherapy, the response rate was 32%.

Smoking Kills 400,000 Americans Each Year… Here's How Not to Be One of Them

Harlan M. Krumholz, MD, professor of cardiology at Yale University School of Medicine in New Haven, CT. He is coauthor of *No Ifs, Ands or Butts*. Diane.

If you're trying to quit smoking—or know someone who is—here are eight strategies that will maximize your odds of success…

1. Forget about switching to "light" cigarettes. Some smokers switch to low-tar, low-nicotine brands, thinking that doing so will cut the levels of these toxins in their bodies. Or they switch to a light brand as a prelude to quitting altogether.

Switching does *not* help. Studies show that people who switch unwittingly compensate by inhaling smoke more deeply or frequently. Tar and nicotine consumption remain at the same levels as before.

2. Develop a concrete plan. Only about 2% of smokers who try to stop are successful on any given try. Most people fail several times before succeeding.

You must approach smoking cessation as you'd approach running a marathon or tackling any other major project.

Set a firm date for quitting. Plan what you will do *every day* when the inevitable cravings hit. If you backslide, try again.

3. Try nicotine-replacement therapy. Nicotine patches (Habitrol, Nicoderm, etc.) and nicotine gum (Nicorette) can double your odds of quitting successfully.

Both patches and gum are effective. Some people enjoy the oral sensation of chewing gum. Others find chewing a chore, and prefer to use the patch. It administers nicotine continuously throughout the day.

Do *not* smoke while wearing a patch or chewing nicotine gum.

Pregnant women should probably not use the patch or gum, though continued smoking is likely to be more harmful than nicotine-replacement therapy.

Some people find that the patch irritates their skin. If you're among them, alert your doctor.

4. Enlist friends and family. Many smokers try to stop in secret—because they want to avoid embarrassment if they fail. That's the opposite of what should be done.

Tell friends and family—even your doctor—exactly what you intend to do. Ask them to check up on you periodically to see how you're doing. Apologize in advance for how irritable you'll be as you go through nicotine withdrawal.

5. Join a support group. Meeting with fellow quitters for as little as 20 minutes a week can improve your chances of success.

To locate a support group in your area, contact your local hospital, the American Cancer Society (800-227-2345, *www.cancer.org*) or the American Lung Association (800-586-4872, *www.lungusa.org*).

6. Find ways to motivate yourself. Think how much healthier you'll be after quitting… how you'll live longer…or how much money you'll save. Over a 10-year period, a two-pack-a-day habit costs roughly $51,000.

7. Consider alternative techniques. There's scant scientific evidence that acupuncture, acupressure, hypnosis and other alternative therapies help people stop smoking. Yet many former smokers swear by them. If you do decide to give an alternative therapy a try, be sure to find a practitioner with legitimate training.

8. Ask your doctor about antidepressant therapy. There's some evidence that *fluoxetine* (Prozac) and other antidepressants make it easier to quit for certain patients. Yet doctors are often reluctant to prescribe these drugs for smoking cessation. They fear that smokers will shake their addiction to tobacco only to become dependent on the antidepressants.

If you've tried quitting several times without success, however, the risk of becoming dependent on an antidepressant may be outweighed by the dangers posed by continuing to smoke.

Another potentially useful medication is *bupropion* (Zyban). It's been used to treat depression for several years under the name Wellbutrin. Exactly how it works isn't known, but the drug is thought to affect the neurotransmitter *dopamine* that may play a role in nicotine addiction. Studies have found that the combination of nicotine replacement and Zyban is more likely to result in smoking cessation than either drug alone. Side effects include dry mouth and insomnia. People who have epilepsy shouldn't use Zyban as it can cause seizures.

Getting the Right Treatment

Stephen B. Soumerai, ScD, associate professor of ambulatory care and prevention, Harvard Medical School, Boston.

Elderly heart attack patients rarely get the right treatment. Heart attack survivors who receive beta-blockers are 43% less likely to die and 22% less likely to be readmitted to the hospital than similar patients who receive other treatments. Yet in a study of 5,332 elderly heart attack patients, only 21% of those who *should* have been prescribed beta-blockers actually got them.

Problem: Many doctors have exaggerated concerns about the side effects of beta-blockers, including depression, loss of libido and fatigue. These concerns are based on old studies that have since been refuted.

Rural Living and Longevity Link

Mark D. Hayward, PhD, director, Population Research Center and professor of sociology, University of Texas, Austin. His study, based on the National Longitudinal Study of Older Men, from 1966 to 1990, was presented at a meeting of the Population Association of America.

Men living in rural areas outlive their urban and suburban peers.

Theory: The rural way of life fosters tight relationships with family members, friends and neighbors. These social networks provide men with emotional support and assistance. There are no data on rural women.

Medical Care Self-Defense

Timothy McCall, MD, an internist, medical editor of *Yoga Journal* and author of *Examining Your Doctor: A Patient's Guide to Avoiding Harmful Medical Care.* Carol. *www.drmccall.com.*

To get the best medical care, you need to be informed and assertive. As a doctor, I'm in the unique position of hearing about and seeing the errors other doctors make most often during exams.

Here are some of the big mistakes doctors make and what you can do to prevent them…

Mistake: Prescribing drugs but not adequately explaining how to take them. If medicine isn't taken properly, it may not work —or it may have unexpected effects.

Helpful: After your doctor writes out a prescription, ask how much of the drug to take …how often…if you should take it on an empty stomach…what to do if you miss a dose…and what to do if you develop side effects. Then have the doctor write out a schedule for the drug so you'll know exactly when to take it each day and for how long.

Mistake: Recommending treatment without involving you in the thinking process or diagnosis. Urge your doctor to speak openly about what he/she thinks about your condition and the pros and cons of each treatment available. Be sure to take notes.

Important: When your condition requires elective surgery—or can lead to more serious complications—insist that you want time to think about the recommended treatment. This will give you time to research your ailment, seek a second or third opinion and consider alternatives.

Mistake: Coming to conclusions without considering the psychological factors in your life. The mind can have a profound effect on your immune system, yet many doctors overlook its impact.

Helpful: If there are important changes going on in your life that your doctor should know about, such as marital problems or job issues, be sure to mention them—even if your doctor forgets to ask.

Mistake: Prescribing the "latest" drug. Drug companies spend millions to influence the prescribing habits of doctors. Typically they try to get doctors to recommend brand-new drugs with high price tags and profit margins. What you want, however, is the best drug for your condition.

Helpful: Ask your doctor if there are any drugs that have been on the market longer than the one he is prescribing—and ask whether it would be acceptable to take those drugs instead. In general, older drugs have longer track records of safety and are usually cheaper.

Mistake: Giving you free samples of drugs that he normally would not prescribe. Most patients love getting free samples. But drug companies give most of these samples for the newer drugs that they're trying to promote. These are often drugs with which doctors aren't too familiar yet.

Helpful: Before accepting a sample, ask your doctor how good the new drug is and whether there is another drug that is established —or cheaper—in prescription form.

Antiaging Supplements: Dr. Ken Cooper Explains What Works... And What Doesn't

Kenneth H. Cooper, MD, MPH, chairman and CEO of the Cooper Aerobics Center, 12200 Preston Rd., Dallas 75230. He is author of numerous books on health and fitness, including *Dr. Kenneth H. Cooper's Antioxidant Revolution*. Bookman.

From DHEA (dehydroepiandrosterone) to melatonin, the market is now glutted with supplements purported to have antiaging properties. Do these pills do what their proponents say they do? Are they safe?

For answers, we went to Dr. Kenneth Cooper, the renowned exercise researcher and an early proponent of antioxidant supplements...

•**Of all the antiaging supplements, melatonin gets the most hype. Is it effective?** For occasional use to treat jet lag or insomnia, melatonin does seem to be safe and effective.

Melatonin has also shown promise against multiple sclerosis and certain forms of cancer, although research in these areas is in preliminary stages.

However, I am *against* the use of melatonin as an antiaging supplement. Most of the studies suggesting that it has antiaging effects have been done on animals. We just don't know if melatonin has the same effects on humans.

The safety of melatonin has never been fully established. Already there have been reports of troublesome side effects, including hangover and memory loss.

Since melatonin is a hormone, its long-term use might cause cancer—just as the long-term use of estrogen can raise women's risk for breast cancer. It's too early to know whether melatonin raises the risk for cancer. In the meantime, I'm not recommending it to my patients.

•**What about DHEA?** Short-term studies suggest that DHEA boosts the immune system, as its proponents claim.

But since DHEA stimulates the synthesis of sex hormones (testosterone in men and estrogen in women), it's only logical to think that it might also be promoting prostate and/or breast cancer.

Folks who take DHEA today might be inadvertently creating a time bomb with a 20-year fuse.

•**Is that also true for other hormones, like human growth hormone (HGH)?** Yes. A normal, healthy man who takes HGH and/or testosterone for their supposed antiaging properties may be upping his risk for prostate or testicular cancer and heart disease.

In my opinion, anyone who takes HGH or testosterone is playing with dynamite.

•**What about pycnogenol, the pine bark derivative?** There's no doubt that this mixture of bioflavonoids has promise.

Some studies show that its antioxidant properties are 60 times stronger than those of vitamin E. But until we know for sure that it's safe, I don't recommend pycnogenol supplements to my patients.

•**Are there any antiaging supplements worth taking?** I'm a firm believer in supplements containing vitamins C and E and beta-carotene.

Although these antioxidants are not usually thought of as antiaging supplements, they do slow the aging process by helping to prevent the diseases associated with aging.

These three antioxidants work by neutralizing *free radicals,* renegade molecules that cause the cellular damage that underlies aging.

Vitamin E is especially beneficial. It blocks oxidation of LDL (bad) cholesterol, thereby preventing formation of the arterial deposits that underlie heart attack. Vitamin E also prevents DNA damage, which is thought to be the first step in the development of cancer.

Since it's almost impossible to get sufficient levels of vitamin E from food sources, I tell my patients to take a daily supplement containing 400 international units (IU) of *natural* vitamin E (*d-alpha tocopherol*). Natural vitamin E is absorbed more efficiently than synthetic vitamin E.

However, due to the possible interactions between vitamin E and various drugs and supplements, as well as other safety considerations, consult your doctor before starting a vitamin E regimen.

•**What do vitamin C and beta-carotene do?** In addition to fighting free radicals, vitamin C now appears to be an effective remedy for mild arthritis pain. It's hard to get enough vitamin C from food, so I tell my patients to take a 500-milligram (mg) supplement twice daily.

Beta-carotene helps protect against heart disease, cataracts and certain cancers, including skin cancer.

I urge all nonsmokers to consume 25,000 IU of beta-carotene each day. You can get this amount in the form of a supplement...or from eating one and one-half average-sized carrots.

•**Anything else?** The mineral selenium seems to fight free radicals and help prevent cancer of the lung, colon, prostate and rectum. I would add 200 micrograms (mcg) a day of selenium to your vitamin/mineral "cocktail."

Finally, folic acid is now known to be critical for good health. It lowers bloodstream levels of *homocysteine,* a breakdown product of *methionine.* That's an amino acid that we get mostly from eating red meat and milk products.

Studies show a clear link between homocysteine levels and heart attack risk—even when cholesterol levels are low.

I tell my patients to take 400 mcg of folic acid a day in supplement form (800 to 1,000 mcg if heart disease is present).*

People over age 50 should take 50 mg of vitamin B-6 and 500 mcg of B-12 daily along with folic acid. Otherwise, vitamin B-12 deficiency can be masked.

Osteoporosis Risk Indicator

Michael Holick, MD, PhD, chief of endocrinology, Boston University School of Medicine, 609 Albany St., Boston 02118.

Prematurely gray hair is a risk factor for osteoporosis—loss of bone mass—in one's latter years.

Persons who have hair that went more than half gray by age 40 have been found to be

*High homocysteine levels are also thought to cause neural tube birth defects. That's why obstetricians recommend folic acid supplements for pregnant women—even women who *might* become pregnant.

four times as likely to develop osteoporosis as other persons without prematurely gray hair. The reason for this is not known.

Safety: If your hair went gray early in life, consult with your physician and consider increasing your calcium intake.

To Minimize Osteoporosis Risk

Barbara S. Levine, RD, PhD, director, Calcium Information Center, New York Hospital–Cornell Medical Center, New York City.

Most women *and* men need to boost their calcium intake. New federal guidelines call for adults over age 50 to get 1,200 milligrams (mg) of the mineral per day. That's the equivalent of four daily servings of low-fat milk, yogurt, fortified orange juice or other calcium-rich food. Adults under age 50 should get 1,000 mg per day...adolescents, 1,300 mg. Old guidelines recommended 800 mg a day for most adults. *Danger:* The average adult consumes only 500 mg to 700 mg a day.

How to Stay Safe in This Crazy, Crazy World

Louis R. Mizell, Jr., an expert on criminal tactics. He is author of *Street Sense for Seniors.* Berkley.

More than 4,000 Americans 55 years of age and older become crime victims in their homes every day.

Criminals target older people, expecting them to be less able to protect themselves and more likely to be poor witnesses.

Eighty percent of these crimes could be prevented if seniors learned more about criminal tactics and took a few simple steps to improve security. *Here are the facts about some of the most prevalent crimes and how to avoid them...*

HOME SECURITY

The idea that criminals will not enter an occupied house is a dangerous myth. Using force or trickery, crooks enter the homes of more than 500,000 people each year with at least one family member inside. *Most of these crimes would not occur if people took the following precautions...*

● **Don't open the door** unless you know who is on the other side. Every year, 15,000 seniors are victimized by the "push in" tactic when the criminal forces his/her way in. If you do not know the person, use a peephole and talk through the closed door.

Be aware that a determined criminal can push hard enough on a partially opened door to rip off most door chains that have not been professionally installed.

● **Don't trust people** just because they look respectable.

Example: In Miami, three little girls (one 10-year-old and two 14-year-olds) knocked at the doors of older people and melted their hearts with bright eyes and sweet smiles. After they were let in, one would slip into the bedroom and take cash and jewelry, while the other two distracted the victim. Before they were arrested, they had robbed 26 senior citizens.

● **Be wary of impostors.** More than 230,000 crimes per year are committed by criminals impersonating plumbers, gas and water inspectors, police officers, etc. Check the credentials of everyone who comes to your door *before* you open it. If you feel suspicious, call the organization he claims sent him.

● **Lock your door** whenever you leave your home, even if it's just to take out the garbage ...bring in the groceries...get the mail. Of the 3.2 million home invasions, 800,000 were the result of an unlocked door or window.

● **Keep your keys secure.** Someone who has your door keys has 24-hour access to your home, your family, your property and, of course, you.

● **Do not give your keys to anyone...** workers...home-care attendants...real estate agents...unless you know you can trust them and all their relatives and friends who may also gain access to your keys. Three hundred thousand crimes are committed by criminals who surreptitiously obtain our keys.

● **Don't keep your car ignition key** on the same key ring with your house keys.

● **Don't leave your garage-door opener in your unlocked car.**

CAR-JACKING AND DRIVEWAY CRIMES

In today's mobile world, criminals have learned a variety of ways to exploit vulnerable people in and out of their cars. Driveway crime is rampant.

Example: A top Exxon executive was kidnapped from his 200-foot-long driveway on his estate in northern New Jersey.

Do not drop your guard when you get to your driveway. Check the rearview mirror as you approach your home and as you drive onto your driveway. If someone is following, keep your doors locked and circle the block. If they are still behind, drive to the closest police station.

If you see anyone suspicious by your house, keep your doors locked and blow the horn. If an unfamiliar vehicle is in your driveway, get a description, take down the license plate number and call the local police department from a neighbor's house or from a cell phone. Keep your car doors locked and your engine running until you are certain there are no suspicious characters around.

Be aware of common ruses used by criminals to get you out of your car. *Two of the most common include...*

● **Bump and rob.** The criminal crashes into the victim's rear bumper...and robs her (victims are usually older women) when she gets out to inspect the damage.

● **Good Samaritan.** The criminal approaches his victim and points out that she has a flat tire (for which the crook is responsible). He then offers the victim a ride, and either robs or assaults her.

ATMs AND PAY TELEPHONES

Automatic Teller Machines (ATMs) and pay telephones provide *many* opportunities for criminals. At least 27,000 crimes, including kidnapping, murder, rape, car theft and robbery occur at pay phones each year. *To maximize security...*

- **Use machines and telephones that are in public view and well lit.**

- **Take along a companion** who can watch you from inside your locked car. If you do not have a car, have him stand 10 or 15 feet away to deter criminals.

- **Do not leave your car unlocked** or the keys in the ignition if you must go alone.

- **Face the street** when using the telephone.

- **Do your business quickly.**

- **Do not make withdrawals or deposits at the same place** or time every day.

- **Keep your PIN confidential.**

- **Be aware of your surroundings** and watch to see if you are being followed.

WISDOM

However safe you try to make your home, it will never be as secure as a bank. Do not keep large amounts of cash in your house. Word gets around.

Every year, thousands of seniors are the victims of robberies, losing hundreds of thousands of dollars.

Harry Lorayne's Cures For Absentmindedness

Harry Lorayne can memorize every person's name in a room of 500 people and recite from memory random pages of the latest issue of *Time* magazine. He is author of several books on memory, including the *Memory Power* package (book, audio and video cassettes).

It is no longer necessary to accept loss of memory or a poor memory as an inevitable part of growing older. Absentmindedness is caused by a lessening of interest in humdrum activities like making and keeping appointments, performing daily rituals and keeping track of affairs and possessions. It can happen to anybody, at any age.

The good news is that there are simple techniques you can use to sharpen your memory and remember where you put things, people's names...even errands you have to run.

WHERE DID I PUT THAT...

You'll never misplace anything again if you clearly focus on the *present* for the moment it takes to set something down or put it away.

Do this by creating a picture in your mind that connects the object to its new home in a silly or absurd way. It's the outlandishness of what you imagine that makes it interesting to your mind, which in turn makes you *aware*.

Example: On your way to mail a letter before the post office closes, you mindlessly toss your reading glasses on top of the TV. When you get back home, you can't remember where you put your glasses.

Better way: At the moment you put your glasses down on the TV, form a cockeyed mental picture. For instance, imagine the TV antenna poking through the lens of the glasses and into your eye. When you need your glasses, you'll automatically recall the unusual image, shudder and quickly retrieve them.

Why it works: This mind-jogging system, and others like it, cures absentmindedness and forgetfulness by grabbing the mind by the "scruff of its neck"—forcing it to pay attention for a split second.

The reminder principle: Such memory games exercise your mind the way walking exercises your body. You become more creative and imaginative while simultaneously improving your memory. Some other mind-jogging techniques...

DID I TURN OFF THE...

Last week, as you headed down the sidewalk, you couldn't remember if you'd turned off the stove.

The week before, it was the iron.

Tonight, you're lying in bed wondering if you remembered to set the alarm.

Memory joggers: To be sure later that you've actually done these things, visualize a silly picture in your mind as you do them.

Example: As you unplug the iron, imagine that you're pulling your iron-shaped head out of the electrical socket. As you set the alarm in the evening, imagine that the button is piercing your finger or that you're using the clock radio to sleep on instead of a pillow.

Later, when you begin to wonder if you've remembered to do these ordinary, mundane tasks, the extraordinary images that come to mind will assure you that they have been taken care of.

And don't worry—your mind won't incorrectly "remember" that you've done these things, even if you use the same silly image each day. "True memory" will ensure that you remember the truth about what you have and haven't done.

WHAT'S HIS NAME...

An easy way to remember names is to think of familiar words that sound like the name you're trying to remember. You have probably heard about all this before. But—it really works. *Try it...*

When you're introduced to a person, really *listen* to his/her name.

If you don't hear it the first time, ask to have it repeated. That will not only help you remember the name, it will also make the person feel good and let them know that you care about meeting him/her.

To remember a person's name, use your imagination.

What does the name sound like? What does it remind you of?

It's best to come up with your own words or mental picture, since your originally created image is more likely to remind you of the person's name than would an image or word suggested by someone else.

Example: The name "Dr. Carruthers" sounds like "car udders." One way to remember this person's name, then, would be to imagine a car with udders.

HIS FACE IS FAMILIAR, BUT...

Now take your mental picture to the next step. Look again at Dr. Carruthers's face. Which of his features jumps out at you? Does he have a high forehead? An unruly mop of hair? Crooked or capped teeth?

Whatever feature seems most prominent to you today is likely to stand out for you in the future. Once you've identified Dr. Carruthers's

dominant feature, connect it to your substitute words—in this case, "car udders," and your mental picture of a car being milked.

Example: You might picture Dr. Carruthers's long white sideburns being cars (or having cars driving out of them)—and picture the udders on the car. To remember Carruthers is a doctor, picture stethoscopes attached to those udders. Now you've connected Dr. Carruthers's name to his face in a way you're not likely to forget! You've forced yourself to listen to the name...and really look at the face—and one will remind you of the other.

FIRST THE DENTIST, THEN...

Let's say you have a bunch of errands to run. Instead of writing them down and bypassing your memory altogether (and possibly forgetting the list), link them to each other in this silly way...

Example: You have to see the dentist, mail a letter, pick up a gallon of milk and stop to get new tires for your car. One possible way to link these errands together would be to imagine the dentist pulling stamped envelopes out of your mouth. You're pouring millions of stamped envelopes out of a milk carton instead of milk...a car is drinking milk out of a gigantic milk carton—or a gigantic milk carton is driving a car.

Replay these silly pictures in your mind. Then, as you leave the dentist's office, replay them again. Almost without effort, you'll remember each and every one of your errands—because one must remind you of the other.

Pessimism Can Kill

Susan Everson, PhD, MPH, associate research scientist, Human Population Laboratory, Berkeley, CA, who led a 10-year study of 2,428 men ages 42 to 60.

Feelings of hopelessness can make you ill. A study reported extreme pessimism is more hazardous to your health than depression. Men who reported moderate-to-high levels of hopelessness died at rates two to three times higher than those who were not so pessimistic. They also suffered cancer and heart attacks more frequently.

Curing Aggression

Helen H. Kyomen, MD, assistant attending psychiatrist, geriatric psychiatry program, McLean Hospital, Belmont, MA.

Estrogen therapy helps curb aggression in women *and men* suffering from severe dementia.

Background: Because they tend to take drugs for other medical problems, many dementia patients cannot tolerate the drugs ordinarily used to calm physical and sexual aggression. But in a four-week study, all patients given estrogen pills were less disruptive. Estrogen has some risks—some men may develop enlarged breasts (*gynecomastia*). Consult your doctor before beginning this therapy.

Hip Fracture Reduction

Dennis Black, PhD, professor of epidemiology and biostatistics at the University of California, San Francisco.

Alendronate, an osteoporosis drug, cuts the risk of hip fracture by half. The drug is sold under the brand name Fosamax. A three-year study of 2,027 osteoporosis patients who took the drug daily found that it reduced their chance of a hip fracture by 51% compared with those who took placebos. Fosamax is an alternative to estrogen, which is thought to also be effective in reducing fracture risk.

How to Boost a Flagging Memory

Adriane Fugh-Berman, MD, associate professor in complementary and alternative medicine, Georgetown University School of Medicine, Washington, DC. She is author of *Alternative Medicine: What Works.* Lippincott, Williams & Wilkins.

Do you—or does someone you love—keep losing keys, forgetting names or having other memory lapses? If so, you may be worried that the culprit is Alzheimer's disease or another incurable form of dementia. While it's a good idea to consult a doctor, the odds are that it is simple forgetfulness—which can be treated.

In some cases, memory problems—especially those associated with aging—stem simply from a lack of mental activity. If your job isn't particularly stimulating—or if you're retired—you might consider keeping a journal, joining a book discussion group, playing chess or Scrabble, doing crossword puzzles, etc.

Physical exercise is also a memory-enhancer. Aerobic exercise boosts circulation throughout the body—and that includes the brain. Increased blood flow to the brain has been shown to increase mental function.

Another way to ensure adequate blood flow to the brain is to eat a low-fat diet. The arteries that feed the brain are tiny to begin with, and any narrowing that occurs as a result of eating a fatty or cholesterol-rich diet drastically reduces oxygen flow. Blood flow problems can lead to tiny strokes, which are now believed to be the cause of much age-related memory loss.

These strokes—which generally produce no obvious symptoms—are typically caused by chronic high blood pressure and/or high cholesterol. So be sure your blood pressure and cholesterol are under control.

While there's no magic memory pill, the following supplements are safe...and beneficial for many people. They can be taken individually or in combination. For absolute safety, use them under a doctor's supervision.

● **Antioxidants.** Vitamins C and E and the mineral selenium all may help prevent memory loss. I usually tell my patients to take 400 international units (IU) of vitamin E a day,* along with 1,000 milligrams (mg) of vitamin C and 100 micrograms (mcg) of selenium. It's also a good idea to eat lots of fruits and vegetables. They contain lots of other antioxidants.

● **Phosphatidylserine.** This fatty substance was found to be helpful in preventing further deterioration in people with memory problems. In some cases, memory *improved* after several months of phosphatidylserine therapy.

*Consult your doctor for the amount that is appropriate for you.

I usually recommend 200 to 300 mg per day. Be patient—it may take three months before you notice any improvement.

Some alternative practitioners recommend a related substance called *choline* (or *lecithin*, which contains 10% to 20% choline). Neither choline nor lecithin looks anywhere near as good as phosphatidylserine, and they can cause unpleasant side effects.

●**L-acetyl carnitine.** This form of the amino acid carnitine plays a key role in energy production in the body. It seems to help both Alzheimer's patients and those with mild mental deterioration. The usual dose is 500 mg to 1,000 mg three times a day.

●**Ginkgo biloba.** Like vitamin E, ginkgo helps thin the blood, boosting circulation inside even the tiniest capillaries—including those that feed the brain. Ginkgo also acts as an antioxidant, protecting the brain against attack by free radicals.

Ginkgo has been found to be effective in slowing the progression of Alzheimer's disease.

15

Taking Care of the Outer You—Your Skin

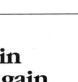

Make Your Skin Look Young Again Without Surgery

Joseph P. Bark, MD

It used to be that a face-lift was the only way to deal with skin that was wrinkled, sun-damaged, sagging or scarred. However, this is no longer true.

Today, while surgery is still required for serious problems, there are numerous safe, inexpensive *nonsurgical* techniques for rejuvenating your skin. *Here's a look at your options…*

ALPHA HYDROXY ACIDS

Glycolic, lactic, citric and other *alpha hydroxy acids* (AHAs) are found in a growing number of cosmetics. Excellent moisturizers, they also seem to minimize wrinkling, sun damage and acne—if used on a daily basis.

More effective: *Prescription* AHA products, which contain higher concentrations of the acid. These products are available from your dermatologist.

SUNSCREENS AND MOISTURIZERS

Sunscreens don't just prevent skin damage. They also help fade *existing* fine wrinkles.

Moisturizers keep skin soft and supple and *temporarily* improve its appearance. But they neither prevent nor reverse wrinkles. In fact, wearing moisturizer without sunscreen can raise your skin's vulnerability to sun damage.

VITAMIN A DERIVATIVE

Tretinoin (Retin-A) is a potent drug originally developed as a treatment for acne. Doctors may prescribe this vitamin A derivative to fade fine lines around the eyes…and to get rid of stretch marks and liver spots.

It's surprisingly effective when used on a regular basis, although it can take a year or more for the effects to become apparent.

Joseph P. Bark, MD, a dermatologist in private practice and a staff physician at St. Joseph Hospital in Lexington, KY. He is author of Your Skin: An Owner's Guide. Prentice Hall.

Tretinoin makes the skin appear smoother by thickening its outermost layer and "compacting" the layer of dead skin cells.

Caution: Tretinoin can cause redness and dryness…and can raise your susceptibility to sunburn. Because of the possible risk of birth defects, it's inappropriate for pregnant women.

Another formulation of tretinoin, Renova, is the first drug developed specifically for wrinkle removal. It reduces fine facial lines, brown spots and surface roughness just as effectively as ordinary tretinoin—and it's less likely to irritate the skin.

CHEMICAL PEELS

Chemical peels involve the application of concentrated AHAs (40% to 70% acid vs. 0.5% to 10% acid for over-the-counter AHA products). Peels are administered in a doctor's office.

A series of light *glycolic acid* peels helps remove damaged skin and improves the appearance of crow's feet and minor acne scars. The peel may cause stinging, as well as slight pinkness for a day.

Deeper peels, using *trichloracetic acid* (TCA) or *phenol*, are needed to obliterate wrinkles around the mouth, eyes and forehead, to correct irregular pigmentation and to eliminate liver spots.

The effects of a peel last for several years. However, peels may cause considerable pain, as well as persistent redness, skin tightness and scarring. Phenol peels are inappropriate for people with heart or kidney disease…or with dark skin.

Warning: Recovery from a TCA or phenol peel isn't pretty. Crust-like scabs that appear immediately after the peel can take up to two weeks to heal. During this period, it's essential to avoid the sun.

DERMABRASION

This procedure involves use of a rotating wire brush to "sand" off the upper two layers of skin, smoothing its appearance. Results last for several years.

Dermabrasion is good for removing acne scars, pockmarks and small wrinkles around the lips. For severe blemishes, two procedures, six to 12 months apart, may be necessary.

Caution: Dermabrasion can cause infection, scarring, variations in skin tone and extreme sun sensitivity. As with peels, the skin crusts over. And be advised that full recovery can take up to several months.

Also as with peels, dermabrasion works best for people with light complexions.

LASER PEEL

In this procedure—a new alternative to dermabrasion and chemical peels—the doctor uses a laser to "shear off" the epidermis. Laser peels are less likely than chemical peels to cause scarring and overlightening. They are also more precise.

Although crusting and redness still occur with a laser peel, recovery is usually faster. Laser peels are particularly effective against wrinkles around the eyes, age spots, scars and facial discoloration.

COLLAGEN INJECTIONS

Doctors can inject you with a natural protein called *collagen* to plump up facial skin and help fill in severe (cystic) acne scars and deep wrinkles.

Effects are immediate and will last for four to eight months, until the collagen is resorbed. Then a new round of injections need to be administered.

Infection and sun sensitivity at the injection site can occur following the injections. And allergies to collagen can cause excessive firmness and purple discoloration. This can last up to six weeks.

To make sure you're not allergic: Have two collagen allergy tests prior to receiving the injections. Do *not* have the injections if you have rheumatoid arthritis, Graves' disease, lupus or another autoimmune disorder.

Instead of collagen, some doctors have begun injecting fat "harvested" from elsewhere in the body (buttocks, back, etc.). Because the injected material is part of the body, there's no danger of allergic reaction. Unfortunately, it's not clear just how long fat injections last.

Low-Fat Diets May Reduce Skin Cancer Risk

Homer S. Black, PhD, professor of dermatology, Baylor College of Medicine, Houston. His two-year study of 76 patients was published in *The New England Journal of Medicine*, 10 Shattuck St., Boston 02115.

Skin cancer patients who were put on a diet that derived no more than 20% of calories from fat developed 70% fewer precancerous skin lesions (actinic keratoses) than similar patients whose diet remained above 36% fat. *Implication:* If you've had one skin cancer, adopting a low-fat diet can help you prevent a recurrence.

Help for Unsightly Scars

Tina S. Alster, MD, clinical professor of dermatology and pediatrics, Georgetown University Medical Center, Washington, DC. Her study of laser therapy on 16 heart surgery patients was published in *The Lancet*, 32 Jamestown Rd., London NW7 1BY, England.

Red, raised scars (*keloids*) left on the chest following heart surgery can be made less visible—and less itchy—when treated with light from a pulsed-dye laser. The results from laser treatment appear to be long lasting, with no scar recurrence within the first year following treatment.

Does Your Hair Protect You from the Sun?

Zoe Diana Draelos, MD, clinical associate professor of dermatology, Wake Forest University School of Medicine, Winston-Salem, NC.

A full head of hair does *not* offer full protection against skin cancer of the scalp. Scalp skin is just as vulnerable to sun damage as skin elsewhere on the body. When cancer does occur on the scalp, it's often very aggressive.

Self-defense: If you are bald or have thinning hair, rub SPF-15 sunscreen on your scalp… and wear a hat with a four-inch brim that goes all around the head. Even if you have a full head of hair, it's best to use conditioner or hair spray that contains a sunscreen.

Vitamin C vs. Wrinkles

Sheldon R. Pinnell, MD, professor emeritus of dermatology, Duke University Medical Center, Durham, NC.

A prescription skin cream containing 10% vitamin C significantly reduced wrinkling and age spots in patients who used it for eight months. The vitamin "instructs" skin cells to produce new collagen, plumping the skin slightly. Called *Cellex*, the cream delivers 20 to 40 times the amount of the vitamin than can be absorbed from pills.

Skin Cancer— How to Protect Yourself

Perry Robins, MD, chief, Mohs micrographic surgery, New York University Medical Center, and founding president of The Skin Cancer Foundation, 149 Madison Ave., Ste. 901, New York 10016. He is author of *Sun Sense*, which can be ordered through this foundation, 800-SKIN-490, *www.skincancer.org*.

The US is facing a growing epidemic of malignant melanoma, the deadliest form of skin cancer.

In the past 20 years, there has been a dramatic increase in the number of new cases reported.

Why the increase? We don't know exactly to what degree sunscreen really protects us, and not enough people are using it.

These are the most common questions I'm asked about skin protection and skin cancer…

●**Do you continue to recommend that people wear sunscreen?** Absolutely. Over the past 20 years, countless studies have shown sunscreen to be effective at preventing both sunburn *and* skin cancer.

Of course, sunscreen is *not* 100% effective. And wearing it does not give you complete freedom to bask in the sun all day.

● **What type of sunscreen is best?** Look for a sunscreen that offers protection against *both* forms of ultraviolet light—UVA and UVB.

UVB rays pose a greater threat of sunburn and skin cancer than UVA rays do. However, UVA rays can still be harmful if you are in the sun for prolonged periods of time.

Your sunscreen should have a sun protection factor (SPF) of at least 15…and if you plan to go swimming, it should also be water-resistant. With an SPF-15 sunscreen, you can remain burn-free for 15 times longer than you would with unprotected skin.

In regions where the sun's rays are particularly strong—such as in the South—use *sunblock* in addition to sunscreen.

Problem: Sunblock, which uses zinc oxide, talc or another opaque material to create a physical barrier to keep out rays, is messy and unattractive. Consequently, it is not appropriate for covering large areas of skin. I recommend using it only on two high-risk spots—the nose and the rims of the ears.

Avoid lotions containing mineral oil, cooking oil or cocoa butter. These products merely lubricate the skin. They do not block out harmful rays.

● **How should I apply a sunscreen?** Apply it liberally to all areas of skin that will be exposed to the sun. Do so at least 15 minutes before heading outdoors, so that it has a chance to be absorbed.

Pay special attention to easily overlooked areas—feet, earlobes, a bald spot, the backs of your hands, the tops of your ears, the nape of your neck and the tip of your nose.

Reapply at least once every three hours for as long as you're in the sun. Even with water-resistant sunscreen, it's prudent to reapply after going into the water or perspiring heavily.

● **I stopped sunbathing years ago. Do I still need sunscreen?** Yes. Your skin is at risk anytime you venture into sunlight—whether on the beach, in your backyard or on a brief walk. Sunscreens are *not* just for the beach!

In spring, fall and summer, applying sunscreen should become part of your daily routine. Rub it on just after your morning shower.

For office workers, a single morning application will suffice. If you work outdoors, reapply sunscreen frequently during the day. Even in winter, it's a good idea to wear sunscreen if you plan on being outdoors for more than a few minutes.

● **What else can I do to protect myself?** First of all, don't get too much sun too soon. On your first day in the sun, limit your exposure to just a few minutes. On each successive day, increase the length of exposure by a few minutes. If repeated exposure to the sun is inevitable, your goal should be to tan gradually rather than burn. A tan offers some protection by absorbing UV rays. *Other helpful strategies…*

● **Wear UV-blocking sunglasses.** Look for lenses that block at least 95% of UVB rays, 60% of UVA and 92% of visible light. Check the manufacturer's label…or look for the words "Z-80-3 Standard." A good pair of sunglasses will help protect your eyes from sunlight-induced cataracts.

● **Avoid sun exposure between the hours of 10 a.m. and 3 p.m.** The sun's rays are strongest during this period.

● **Always wear a wide-brimmed hat.** It should provide shade for your ears, forehead and neck.

● **At the beach, use an umbrella.**

● **What if I burn easily?** People who are fair-haired, light-skinned and blue- or green-eyed are *twice* as likely to develop skin cancer as dark-haired, dark-skinned, brown-eyed people are.

And—people who have a family history of skin cancer are at increased risk.

There are no special rules for these people to follow, except to be *extra* diligent in protecting their skin. For fair-skinned people, wearing a hat and using sunscreen every day are not just good ideas—they are absolutely *essential.*

● **What if I develop skin cancer?** Malignant melanoma is generally curable—if caught in its early stages, when it's very shallow. The deeper a melanoma gets, the more lethal.

To improve your chances of spotting a skin cancer in its earliest stages, give yourself a *total-body skin exam* at least once every three months. Look for any new growth or change in your skin. *Start today.*

•How do I perform this examination? You will need a hand mirror, a full-length mirror and a blow-dryer.

Begin with your head and neck, where 80% of all skin cancers occur. Examine your face, nose, lips and mouth, and your ears—especially the rims and lobes.

Use a blow-dryer to part your hair section by section. Standing with your back to the full-length mirror, use the hand mirror to examine the back of your scalp and neck. It may be better to ask a friend or family member for help.

Then continue downward, examining your back, hands, fingers, buttocks, genitals, thighs, ankles—right down to your toes.

The exam should take no more than 10 minutes.

Consult a dermatologist right away if you notice…

•A skin growth that increases in size and/or appears pearly, translucent, tan, brown, black or multicolored.

•A mole, birthmark or beauty mark that changes color, grows in size or thickness, changes in texture or becomes irregular in outline.

•A spot or growth that itches, hurts, crusts, scabs over, erodes or bleeds.

•An open sore or wound that persists for more than four weeks—or which heals and then reopens.

A Day Without Sunshine?

Wilma Bergfeld, MD, director of clinical research in dermatology, Cleveland Clinic Foundation, Cleveland.

Total sun avoidance is not healthful for you. The human body needs some sun exposure to synthesize vitamin D—merely five to 10 minutes a day is enough. And only a little skin need be exposed—even just a toe is enough.

Sunscreens Are Effective For Three Years After Purchase

Barbara A. Gilchrest, MD, professor and chair of the department of dermatology, Boston University School of Medicine, 609 Albany St., Boston 02118.

After that, some chemists say they may still be effective for another year—but there is no way for you to safely test them.

Self-defense: Discard unused sunscreen after three years. *Important:* Discard sunscreen immediately if it appears runny or starts to smell strange. This can happen if it's left in a hot car for too long.

Our Skin Would Change Very Little Over Time

Joseph P. Bark, MD, a dermatologist in private practice and a staff physician at St. Joseph Hospital in Lexington, KY. He is author of *Your Skin: An Owner's Guide.* Prentice Hall.

The most exposed areas of the body—particularly the face, scalp and arms—are the most likely to develop spots, dryness, wrinkles and skin cancer.

THE BEST GENERAL PROTECTION

•Use sunscreen. It's cheap and available without a prescription. If men used sunscreen instead of aftershave, they'd prevent many skin problems. Use a sun protection factor (SPF) of 30 or 50 (preferably 50) whenever you go out in the sun.

•Don't smoke. Smoking yellows the skin, dries it out and greatly increases wrinkling, especially around the mouth.

DRY, ITCHY SKIN

Complaints of dry skin are extremely common after age 50—for good reasons...

●**Less oil.** Some oil glands in the skin stop producing the oil needed for lubrication.

●**Winter itch.** In low-humidity areas such as the desert Southwest, and during the winter months elsewhere, water evaporates from the skin very quickly.

●**Overwashing.** We are a nation of clean freaks. We routinely wash away the oil layer that normally acts like plastic wrap, sealing in moisture. *Better:* Bathe every other day and don't scrub too hard. *Recommendations...*

●**Bathe, don't shower.** A shower equals an infinite number of rinsings. Sloshing around in the tub removes less oil.

●**Don't use bath oil.** Most goes down the drain. The residue will make the tub slippery, encouraging a fall. Instead, step out onto an absorbent mat and apply moisturizer while your skin is still wet, sealing in water. Pat dry.

Good moisturizers: Domol, Lubriderm, Hermal, Moisturel, mineral oil and the cheapest of all—Crisco solid. Crisco is great for itching, too. Rub it on gently with your fingertips.

●**Use tepid water.** Just as hot water flushes grease from dirty dishes, it flushes protective oils from your skin.

●**Choose a mild soap.** A major cause of dry skin is the daily use of harsh soap. *Good mild soaps:* Basis...Lowila...unscented Dove.

HARMLESS SPOTS

●**Liver spots.** The only connection between the liver and flat, dark brown "liver spots" (usually on the backs of the hands) is their color—although the liver was once wrongly considered their cause. "Age spots" is a more accurate term. I prefer to call them "birthday presents." These brown flat spots (called *lentigines*—the singular is *lentigo*) don't darken in the sun, as freckles do.

If you don't like the way your age spots or lentigines look, a dermatologist can freeze them individually with a quick spray of liquid nitrogen (it stings briefly) and they peel off over a week or two.

●**Seborrheic keratoses.** These look like drops of tannish to deep brown candle wax with superficial cracks ("splits"). They're hereditary, genetically timed to appear in later life. Seborrheic keratoses, which are extremely common, start small but can quadruple in size. *Prime sites:* The chest, back and temples.

If you have seborrheic keratoses that are flaky, itchy or unsightly, don't scratch or cut them off. A dermatologist can freeze them with liquid nitrogen. The crust that forms will fall off in two to three weeks.

WRINKLES

Wrinkles are harmless but can be reduced if they bother you. Sleep creases run vertically from scalp to chin and become more prominent on the sleeping side. To minimize sleep creases, vary your sleeping position. *Other ways to de-wrinkle...*

●**Retin-A** (tretinoin). This superb prescription cream is a good bet for keeping your skin fine and smooth as you age. *Caution:* Retin-A makes the skin much more sensitive to sunlight. Use sunscreen.

Caution: Many drugs besides Retin-A—most commonly the diuretics (water pills) taken for high blood pressure, heart problems and swollen legs—cause skin rashes or increase the burning effects of the sun. Results may be immediate or delayed for months—or years. If your skin gets red, a drug you're taking might be the culprit.

●**Collagen treatments.** Leather from cattle is chemically processed, broken into its component parts until it forms a thick gel and is then injected into the skin. The injections act like bricks that reassemble a "wall" under the skin to replace the collagen lost with age, especially in postmenopausal women.

Typical site: The upper lip. Lacking the support of a fat layer, the mouth folds in on itself.

The collagen treatment: Your dermatologist first tests a patch of skin on one arm. Thirty days later he tests near your hairline...to test for an allergic reaction. If no redness or itching results in two weeks, you'll have one collagen treatment (or possibly two, a few weeks apart). Benefits last for six to eight months. *Cost:* Several hundred dollars.

Mad cow disease isn't an issue with collagen, which is made from select herds.

●**Laser treatments.** These one-time treatments, done in the doctor's office, are especially effective for wrinkles above the lip and crinkly lines around the eyes. Treatment involves an extremely well-controlled quick burnoff of the outer layer of skin (epidermis) in a precisely defined area. The skin contracts and looks smoother.

What to expect: Some pain...weeks of healing...months of redness. Be aware that in some cases there may be permanent loss of skin color in the treated area, which will be more obvious the darker your natural skin color. The lighter your skin, the more pleasing the results. *Cost:* About $3,500 to $6,500.

BEWARE OF SUN SPOTS

For many types of skin cancer, having one spot or lesion increases the risk of recurrence. If you have ever had skin cancer, report faithfully to your dermatologist for follow-up visits.

"Sun spots," or actinic keratoses, are scaly red spots on exposed areas of the skin. They're generally harmless—but if left alone, up to 20% eventually turn into squamous cell skin cancers. Although this typically takes three to 10 or even 20 years, the potential for a malignancy makes it crucial to have them removed promptly.

Most common sites: The nose...face... tops of the ears...backs of the hands and arms.

How to tell if you have one: Close your eyes and run your fingers gently over your face. If you feel a scaly bump under the skin but can't see it, have it checked out. Actinic keratoses don't become visible for a while. They usually start out smaller than a pencil eraser (less than six millimeters in diameter) and get wider and more elevated over time, evolving to a button-like texture with a hard (indurated) base.

MELANOMA

This sometimes lethal form of skin cancer is dangerous at any age, but becomes increasingly likely over time, since its presence is closely related to accumulated exposure to the sun. Melanomas are flat to bumpy in texture, usually without cracks on the surface, and brown to black in color.

Bottom line: Any unrecognizable bump on your face—especially if it has any pigmentation at all—should be checked out by a dermatologist. If a biopsy reveals that it's a melanoma, or the doctor can definitely identify it as such, it must be removed immediately.

Melanoma Watch

Marianne Berwick, PhD, head of the Epidemiology and Cancer Prevention Program and chief, division of epidemiology, University of New Mexico, Albuquerque.

Inspecting your skin thoroughly can significantly reduce your risk from melanoma. A study of 1,200 people found that those who closely examined the skin over their entire bodies had a 63% lower rate of dying from melanoma. Dermatologists use the *ABCD* rule to identify suspicious moles and freckles— asymmetric shape, irregular borders, unusual color, diameter bigger than a pencil eraser's.

Sunlight Is Not the Only Threat to Skin

Pearon G. Lang, Jr., MD, professor of dermatology, Medical University of South Carolina, Charleston.

Skin cancer has also been linked to birthmarks, old scars and skin ulcers...immunosuppression caused by illness or chemotherapy ...human papilloma virus (the cause of warts) ...exposure to petroleum derivatives and other carcinogens.

Self-defense: Have birthmarks removed or checked annually...seek advice if a skin ulcer fails to heal or if a scar develops a growth or sore. If a wart doesn't respond to routine therapy, you may need a biopsy. A patient who is immunosuppressed or who has been exposed to carcinogens should seek advice if he/she develops a new growth or sore.

Rosacea Sufferers

Jonathan Weiss, MD, assistant clinical professor of dermatology, Emory University, Atlanta.

Ask your doctor about *MetroCream*. In a study of 128 patients, this prescription metronidazole *cream* resulted in a 58% reduction in redness and dry skin, compared with a 22% reduction with metronidazole *gel*. Improvements were noted within three weeks and continued throughout the study's 12 weeks. Rosacea, an acne-like condition that causes facial redness, usually appears after age 30.

Dandruff Shampoo Delay

John Reeves, MD, dermatologist, University Health Care System, Augusta, GA.

Dandruff shampoo can take up to a month to produce results—so don't give up too soon. The shampoos work by removing skin flakes...slowing production of flake-forming skin cells...minimizing scalp inflammation... and/or killing yeast that contributes to the problem. Various antidandruff shampoos appear to be equally effective, but which one is best varies from person to person.

The Big Mistake Shingles Sufferers Make

Michael N. Oxman, MD, professor of medicine and pathology at the University of California, and staff physician at the Veterans Administration Medical Center, both in San Diego. He is a member of the Scientific Advisory Board for the VZV Research Foundation, 603 W. 115 St., Ste. 371, New York 10025.

If you have ever had chicken pox—and 95% of Americans have—you are at risk for the blistering rash and severe pain of *shingles.*

People who get shingles are often tempted to wait for the problem to clear up on its own. But waiting is the worst thing you can do.

Without prompt treatment with antiviral medication, shingles pain may become chronic.

We asked University of California virologist Dr. Michael N. Oxman all about shingles...

● **What is shingles, and who gets it?** Shingles is a disease of skin and nerves caused by reactivation of the *varicella zoster virus* (VZV) —the same virus that causes chicken pox.

After a bout of chicken pox, the virus doesn't leave the body. It travels up sensory nerve fibers from the skin and establishes latent (dormant) infections in sensory ganglia that last for the rest of an individual's life.

We don't yet know what causes reactivation. We do know that shingles occurs most frequently in people with reduced immunity— individuals taking corticosteroids or immunosuppressant drugs...undergoing chemotherapy...or suffering from HIV infection.

In some cases, shingles may even be triggered by psychological stress.

Shingles is especially common among people over 50—presumably because immunity declines with age. Among people who live to 85, half will get the disease.

● **Is shingles contagious?** You can't get shingles unless you've had chicken pox—and you can't catch shingles from someone who has shingles. However, if you've never had chicken pox, you can catch *chicken pox* from a *shingles* sufferer.

The shingles virus is similar to *herpes simplex virus,* which causes genital herpes. Unlike herpes simplex virus, however, VZV is *not* transmitted through sexual contact.

● **What are the symptoms?** Shingles usually begins with pain on one side of the body —typically on the trunk or around the eye.

The pain—often quite intense—is caused by inflammation created as the virus reproduces within nerve tissue. Pain is generally followed by a rash in the same area one to three days later.

Until the telltale rash appears, shingles is notoriously hard to diagnose. Depending on where the pain is, shingles can resemble a heart attack...gall bladder attack...appendicitis ...kidney stone...or a ruptured spinal disk. Shingles can even be mistaken for glaucoma, if the eye is affected.

Once your doctor has ruled out these ailments, keep a close watch for the rash. It's essential to begin treatment as soon as the rash appears.

If treatment isn't started quickly, the virus may spread to other nerve cells. This can cause muscle weakness, hearing loss or other complications.

Most common complication: Chronic pain. Some patients with this disorder—called *post-herpetic neuralgia* (PHN)—are so sensitive that even the pressure of clothing on the skin can cause excruciating pain.

●**How is shingles treated?** Until a few years ago, there was no treatment. Then it was found that the antiviral drug *acyclovir* (Zovirax) was effective. But acyclovir must be taken in very high oral doses—or injected.

Some doctors used to prescribe steroids along with acyclovir. The thinking was that by reducing inflammation, steroids might prevent PHN.

Studies have shown that steroids do *not* prevent PHN. Moreover, they can lead to stomach ulcers and raise blood pressure.

Better: Two new antivirals, *famciclovir* (Famvir) and *valacyclovir* (Valtrex), are more easily absorbed than acyclovir...and these are far more effective.

●**What about controlling the pain?** Aspirin, ibuprofen or acetaminophen may be enough in some cases. For severe acute pain, doctors should prescribe codeine or another narcotic.

●**What if the pain becomes chronic?** Consult a doctor who specializes in pain management. Tricyclic antidepressants—prescribed at lower doses than for depression—are effective in 60% to 70% of patients with PHN.

Some patients appear to get relief from alternative treatments such as acupuncture or electrical stimulation.

An Itch May Be More than Skin Deep

Neal Schultz, MD, a dermatologist in private practice, 1130 Park Ave., New York 10128.

When troubled by itching, focus on the cause: *Trap:* Severe, prolonged itching can indicate disease of the thyroid, kidney or liver...lymphoma...or other problems, so consult a doctor.

To be more comfortable in the meantime: Cool the skin with compresses or nonprescription lotions like *Sarna Lotion.* Oral antihistamines help itching from allergic reactions—and can be used for sedation if itching keeps you awake. Topical cortisone cream helps inflamed skin. If those don't help, ask your doctor about prescriptions. Ultraviolet light helps eczema and itching that has no obvious cause.

How to Tell When the Sun Is Dangerous

Joseph P. Bark, MD, a dermatologist in private practice and a staff physician at St. Joseph Hospital in Lexington, KY. He is author of *Your Skin: An Owner's Guide.* Prentice Hall.

Here are some little-known facts about the summer sun and ways to protect yourself...

●**Shadow's length and sharpness.** If your shadow is shorter than you are—or there is no shadow—the sun is overhead and at its most powerful strength.

The same is true about the sun's intensity when your shadow—or the shade made by trees and other objects—is very sharp, deep and dark.

●**Altitude.** The higher you are in elevation, the thinner the ozone layer and atmosphere, and less protection against the sun's ultraviolet (UV) rays.

●**Sand/grass traps.** They reflect nearly 100% of the sun's rays. If you're at the beach or on a lawn when the sun is overhead, you get double the radiation.

• **Color.** The deeper the color blue of the sky, the less of a barrier there is between you and the sun's rays.

PROTECTING YOURSELF

• **Always wear the highest SPF sunscreen possible**—at least SPF 15—and be sure the sunscreen is waterproof.

Helpful: Men—use sunscreen in place of aftershave lotion. Women—use cosmetics that contain sunscreen.

• **Wear a hat with a wide brim** made from a tightly woven fabric that won't let much light pass through. Avoid baseball caps and sun visors…they don't protect the sides or back of the neck.

• **Wear large sunglasses** that fit close to your eyes and the bridge of your nose. Sunglasses stop you from squinting, protect against wrinkle formation and prevent cataracts and other eye disorders.

Caution: Avoid the small, John Lennon–style sunglasses. The dark lenses cause corneas to dilate, so they are exposed to light that slips in around the glasses. Instead, wear sunglasses at least as large as the eye's orbit—the hollow "cave" that houses the eyeball.

All-Year Sun Defense

Perry Robins, MD, chief, Mohs micrographic surgery, New York University Medical Center, and founding president of The Skin Cancer Foundation, 149 Madison Ave., Ste. 901, New York 10016. He is author of *Sun Sense*, which can be ordered through this foundation, 800-SKIN-490, *www.skincancer.org*.

Always use sunscreen if you will be in the sun for any amount of time. Also use sunscreen that blocks UVA rays when spending a lot of time near glass.

Reason: Glass does not effectively block damaging UVA rays.

Women should use moisturizers that contain a broad-spectrum sunscreen (which blocks out both UVA and UVB rays) under makeup.

Much…Much Younger Looking Skin in 15 Minutes a Day

Rachel Perry, founder and chief executive of Rachel Perry, Inc., a natural skin care and makeup company based in Van Nuys, CA. She is author of *Reverse the Aging Process of Your Face: A Simple Technique That Works.* Avery.

You can actually reverse the aging process of your face. How? By using good quality facial cleansers and scrubs along with a few simple isometric facial exercises and self-massage. It takes only 15 minutes a day—and those minutes can be in the shower. My regimen works for men and women.

The general idea is to speed up the process of removing and replacing dead facial skin tissue. It's the dead tissue that leaves the skin tired and muddy looking.

Men don't get those fine lines above the upper lip that many women get because most men shave daily, automatically epidermabrading or exfoliating—i.e., removing dead skin tissue.

CLEANSE AND SCRUB

Daily cleansing and scrubbing is the key to removing dead skin cells.

For a *cleanser*, use either a creamy cleanser or foaming facial cleansing gel. Look for a spreadable consistency. A cleanser should not soak into your skin too easily. The cleanser removes oil and dirt.

A *scrub**—which is used for an abrasive scrub-massage—should have as many natural ingredients as possible. The word "scrub" or "cleanser" should be clearly marked on the container you buy.

For a scrub, I find that two ingredients—sea kelp and sea salt—have the necessary abrasive action, are antibacterial and give a smooth, refined texture to the skin. If you can't find a product with these ingredients, buy them in bulk and add ¼ teaspoon each of sea salt and sea kelp for each ounce of purchased product.

*Facial scrubs made from natural ingredients are available in varying degrees of abrasiveness and can be found in your local health food store or the health food section of your supermarket.

When you use a scrub, dampen your fingers first with water—the additional moisture gives the scrub more spreadability. Always look for products that are pH-balanced.

Caution: Use the scrub gently at first, until you get used to its abrasive action. You don't want to overdo it and leave red patches, or worse, break blood vessels in your face.

You'll also want a supply of small, rough, white cotton terry-cloth towels. Hand towels are a good size. I have seven—enough to last a week.

NOW, THE EXERCISES

It's a good idea to do these exercises whenever you apply cleanser and facial scrub.

Women may also want to do them whenever they apply moisturizer, night cream or even makeup base. This allows your fingers to move smoothly over your face.

Men might find it easiest to do them in the shower. Once you learn the exercises, they will quickly become automatic. After all, you work out to keep your body in good shape. You exercise your arms, legs, abdomen—why not exercise your face?

THE ETERNAL "O"

This exercise firms up the mouth, cheeks, nose and eye area…

First, form a large oval "O" with your mouth, pulling your upper lip downward over your teeth. Smile slightly, but don't move your mouth from the O-shape.

At the same time, squeeze your eyelids shut. The purpose of this phase is to stretch the skin tightly across your face, so you can massage it without worrying about damaging the elasticity of your skin.

The massage: Holding the O position with your eyes closed, use the fingertips of each hand to trace a complete circle around each eye.

●**Starting from the corners**, move over the eyebrows, then under the eyes (including the upper cheeks), for a complete circle.

●**Do this quickly**, a minimum of 10 times. Eventually, you work up to 50 times or more.

Nose: Next, massage your nose with downward strokes, five times.

Mouth: Then massage in a full circle around your mouth, five times in one direction, five in the other.

Forehead: Finally, put your fingertips at the bridge of your nose, and massage upward and outward over your forehead to your hairline, using five to 10 long strokes.

THE FIRMING SMILE

Now, for the bottom half of your face, to help prevent jowls and a double chin…

●**Roll your lips inward over your upper and lower teeth**, leaving a space of about ½ inch between your lips.

●**Smile as widely as you can**—with your *lower* jaw only.

●**Holding the exercise position**, and using your fingertips, massage the entire lower part of your face in small outward circular motions.

●**Start at the tip of your chin**, move up to your ears and then back down again, to a slow count of 10. With practice, work up to 20.

THE NECK REJUVENATOR

To keep your neck muscles firm, and your neck tissue smooth and supple…

●**Place your thumb under your chin**, and curl your tongue back in your throat until you feel the muscle directly under your chin protrude.

●**Now you can take your thumb away**—but continue to keep your tongue curled back.

●**Next, with your chin pointing upward**, stretch your neck as far to the left as possible, to a slow count of 10.

●**Repeat, rotating to the right.** At the same time, massage upward from the base of the neck with the fingertips of both hands, in long, vigorous upward strokes, up to the jawbone.

THE UPPER-LIP SMOOTHER AND AROUND-THE-MOUTH STRENGTHENER

To prevent those upper-lip lines, smooth the furrows that run from the corners of the mouth to the chin, strengthen the muscles around the mouth and firm the lips…

●**Press your lips together in a straight line**, smiling slightly.

●**Using the index fingers of both hands**, massage in tiny outward circular motions around the mouth, to a slow count of 10.

•**Squeeze your lips together harder and harder**, until you feel a tingling sensation.

•**Then immediately make a small "O" with your mouth**, to a slow count of 10.

•**Pucker harder and harder while massaging** in tiny outward circular motions around the mouth, to a slow count of 10. Release.

Do this exercise with the massage at least twice a day. And also do it whenever you can without the massage—while driving, cooking, cleaning, reading. It's a truly portable exercise.

Acne Drug

Diane Berson, MD, adjunct assistant professor of dermatology, New York University School of Medicine, New York City.

The prescription lotion *sulfacetamide* (Klaron) clears blemishes by inhibiting the bacterial growth that causes acne—without drying the skin like other acne lotions.

In studies, acne sufferers who used sulfacetamide saw improvement within two weeks. It's effective in adults and adolescents.

UVB Rays Are Everywhere

Richard H. Grant, PhD, associate professor of agromicrometeorology, Purdue University, West Lafayette, IN.

Dangerous ultraviolet B (UVB) rays exist in shade as well as in direct sunlight. UVB exposure more closely correlates to how much *open sky* you can see than to whether you're in direct sunlight.

Example: If you're in a grove of trees with direct sunlight hitting you but with a limited view of the sky, you're probably getting *less* UVB exposure than you would get while standing in the shade of a lone tree where your view of the sky is less obstructed.

Helpful: Sunscreen, long sleeves, long pants and a broad-brimmed hat.

Skin Cancer Sufferer Risk

Morten Frisch, MD, PhD, senior epidemiologist, Danish Epidemiology Science Centre, Copenhagen. His study of 37,674 skin cancer patients was published in *Annals of Internal Medicine*, 190 N. Independence Mall West, Philadelphia 19106.

People with skin cancer face an increased risk of developing other kinds of cancer. Compared with the general population, patients who had at least one basal cell carcinoma before age 60 had a 37% higher risk of developing breast cancer and a two- to threefold higher risk of developing testicular cancer or non-Hodgkin's lymphoma.

Repairing Skin Damage

Joseph P. Bark, MD, a dermatologist in private practice and a staff physician at St. Joseph Hospital in Lexington, KY. He is author of *Your Skin: An Owner's Guide*. Prentice Hall.

Cosmetic surgery is the best option for repairing significant skin damage—deep wrinkles, severely sagging skin, pockmarks and surgical or wound scars (including the red, raised scars known as *keloids*). Consult two cosmetic or dermatologic surgeons to get a balanced picture of the potential benefits and risks of any recommended procedure (including chemical peels and dermabrasion). Ask to see before-and-after photos of previous patients. *Also:* Ask for the names and phone numbers of those patients, and contact them before proceeding.

Sunscreen Danger

Brian L. Diffey, PhD, professor of photobiology, Dryburn Hospital, Durham, England.

Applying sunscreen incorrectly can raise your risk of skin cancer. To get the full sun protection factor (SPF), adults of average size must use about 1.2 ounces per application to cover their bodies.

Problem: Most people apply far less. Though they're wearing too little sunscreen, sunbathers assume they're protected and therefore stay out in the sun too long.

Self-defense: Apply sunscreen liberally and uniformly. Let it dry before going into the sun.

Sun Protection

Vincent A. DeLeo, MD, clinical professor of dermatology, Columbia University, New York City.

When it comes to blocking sunlight, a fabric's *weave* is more important than its color, thickness or any special coating.

Test: Hold clothing up to a light. If you can see through it, it will not provide adequate protection.

What Keeps Skin Young... And What Doesn't

Gerald Imber, MD, clinical assistant professor of surgery at New York Hospital–Cornell Medical Center, and a plastic surgeon in private practice, both in New York City. He is author of *The Youth Corridor: A Renowned Plastic Surgeon's Revolutionary Program for Maintenance, Rejuvenation, and Timeless Beauty.* HarperPerennial.

Although I've been a cosmetic surgeon for more than 20 years, I'm quick to point out that surgery is *not* the only way to keep your face looking youthful.

Proper skin care is more effective than you might imagine at keeping wrinkles at bay. The earlier you start taking care of your skin, the better the results.

Begin in your 20s, and your skin should keep its youthful appearance into your 50s and beyond.

Even if you're over 60, you can undo much of the damage caused by the combined effects of time and environmental stress, such as extremes of temperature, dryness, pollution and sunlight. You can also slow the skin's aging process.

That does *not* mean you should stock up on costly lotions. Cosmetic counters and drugstore shelves sag under the weight of products that claim to work miracles. None do.

But here are five products that really will have a noticeable effect on your skin...

ALPHA HYDROXY ACID

Creams containing *alpha hydroxy acids* (AHAs) are the first over-the-counter antiaging preparations that really work.

Derived from natural sources including sugarcane, grapes and milk, AHAs act as exfoliants, encouraging new cell growth, fading discoloration and reducing or eliminating fine lines.

There are now dozens of AHA creams on the market, each with its own "special" acid (lactic, citric, glycolic, etc.). All work equally well. Just be sure the label specifies an AHA concentration of 10% or so. That's the minimum strength capable of really smoothing the skin.

AHA creams yield noticeable results only after several months of daily use—so you must be patient.

Caution: Since once-a-day application of AHA gets such good results, some people assume that they might as well slather it on morning and night. *Bad idea.* Overuse of AHA cream can cause severe skin irritation.

For faster results: Ask a plastic surgeon or dermatologist about getting a light chemical peel. Such peels use a solution containing 30% to 70% AHA. They're performed in the doctor's office with no anesthesia.

In most cases the only side effect is a slight tingling and redness for an hour afterwards.

SUNSCREEN

Used properly, virtually any sunscreen on the market filters out ultraviolet A (UVA) and ultraviolet B (UVB) light. Those are the rays that cause premature aging.

Best: A sun protection factor (SPF) of at least 15. Do not assume that sunscreen with an SPF 30 allows you to stay in the sun twice as long as a sunscreen with an SPF 15.

Sunscreen gets sweated off quickly. I recommend reapplying it liberally at least once an hour. If you go into the water, reapply it as soon as you come out. I also recommend wearing a hat when venturing outdoors in sunlight.

ANTIOXIDANT VITAMINS

Vitamins C and E are the only vitamins proven to be beneficial to the skin. These antioxidant vitamins work by preventing the breakdown of collagen. That's the structural protein that keeps skin strong, smooth and elastic.

There's even some evidence that C and E help the body build more collagen.

I recommend taking 1,000 milligrams (mg) of vitamin C and 800 international units (IU) of vitamin E daily.

Caution: Check with your doctor before you begin taking supplements.

These vitamins must be taken *internally* to have any effect. Though it's a popular practice, there's no evidence that rubbing vitamin E oil or lotion onto your skin does any good. The vitamin molecules are far too big to penetrate the skin.

TRETINOIN

This vitamin A derivative (sold as *Retin-A*) smooths skin and erases fine wrinkles. It does so by speeding cellular turnover and stimulating the skin to produce collagen.

It's effective, but Retin-A can cause red, scaly patches. Luckily, there's a moisturizer-like formulation of tretinoin called *Renova*. It's not quite as effective as Retin-A but is less likely to cause irritation.

For visible results, tretinoin must be used for at least four months. To minimize the risk of skin irritation, I tell my patients to stop treatment periodically to allow the skin to recover. When and for how long you use tretinoin should be discussed with your doctor.

Retin-A and Renova are available only by prescription. AHAs and tretinoin can be used at the same time.

MOISTURIZER

Moisturized skin isn't any healthier than dry skin, but it certainly looks and feels as if it is.

Moisturizer hydrates dead cells on the skin's surface, temporarily preventing them from flaking off.

Any water- or oil-based formula will do the job, as will Vaseline or even Crisco. There's no medical reason to pay extra for fancy brands—no matter what "special ingredients" they contain.

The Dangers of Ultraviolet Light

Johanna Adami, MD, MPH, department of medical epidemiology, Karolinska Institute, Stockholm, Sweden. Her study of medical records of 113,000 cancer patients was published in the *British Medical Journal*, Tavistock Square, London WCIH 9JR, England.

Skin cancer may not be the only malignancy caused by sunlight. In a study, the lymph system cancer *non-Hodgkin's lymphoma* was 1.4 times more common among malignant melanoma patients than among healthy people …and twice as common among patients with another common skin cancer, squamous cell carcinoma.

Theory: Ultraviolet light suppresses the immune system, crippling its ability to kill cancer cells.

 # Diabetic's Foot Ulcer Danger

Lawrence O. Kollenberg, DPM, a former podiatrist in private practice in Jacksonville, FL.

Diabetic foot ulcers that fail to heal sometimes necessitate the amputation of the toes, the foot or even the entire lower leg.

Now: Dressings containing freeze-dried bovine collagen help heal both infected and noninfected ulcers, helping to save the limb. In one study, all 24 diabetic foot ulcers treated with the collagen treatment healed within five months.

Also helpful: Don't walk barefoot…don't wear tight shoes…wash your feet every day with a mild, nondrying cleanser…and see a podiatrist on a regular basis.

Foot Pain Relief

Suzanne M. Levine, DPM, podiatrist and clinical instructor, New York Hospital–Cornell Medical Center, New York City.

People who suffer from chronic pain in the soles of the feet should avoid going barefoot.

Going barefoot—especially first thing in the morning—can rupture the scar tissue that forms overnight, forcing the healing process to begin anew the next night.

Self-defense: Until the foot has fully healed, always wear shoes or sandals.

Melanoma: What Your Doctor Isn't Telling You

Timothy McCall, MD, an internist, medical editor of *Yoga Journal* and author of *Examining Your Doctor: A Patient's Guide to Avoiding Harmful Medical Care.* Carol. *www.drmccall.com.*

The incidence of malignant melanoma, the deadliest form of skin cancer, has soared in recent years—probably because of the thinning of the ozone layer and our more active, outdoor lifestyles.

As you may know, your chance of surviving melanoma hinges almost entirely on how early it is detected. Found early, melanoma has a cure rate approaching 100%. Once the cancer has burrowed deep into the skin, however, the odds of long-term survival are slim.

Unfortunately, recent trends in the way doctors practice medicine may be making early detection of melanoma *less* likely. Because of their desire to reduce costs, health maintenance organizations (HMOs) are encouraging doctors to spend less time with patients. Yet the only effective way to check for skin cancer —and for precancerous conditions that might turn cancerous—is to examine the entire surface of your skin. That takes time.

Another factor interfering with early detection of skin cancer is that HMOs and other managed-care plans discourage primary-care doctors from referring patients to specialists. And *dermatologists* are the doctors most skilled at telling which moles are questionable.

Since you cannot count on your doctor to educate you about melanoma or do a careful screening of your skin, your best defense is to learn these things yourself. *Here are the basics...*

Fair-skinned people are at greatest risk. Blondes and redheads are two to four times more likely to develop melanoma than brunettes. Melanoma in blacks is uncommon, though it does occur. Melanoma tends to run in families. Be especially vigilant at checking your skin if a close relative had it. Any mole can become cancerous, but those present from birth are riskier.

The best way to prevent skin cancer is to avoid exposure to sunlight. That's especially important at midday, when ultraviolet (UV) radiation is peaking.

To reduce sun exposure, consider wearing a broad-brimmed hat, UV-blocking sunglasses and long pants and long sleeves. Cover all exposed areas with a sunscreen that has a sun protection factor (SPF) of 15 or greater. And don't assume cloudy days are safe. About 80% of UV rays make their way through the clouds. UV gets reflected into shady areas, too.

If you're at risk, examine your skin at least once every three months (or have a family member do it for you). *Look for the following warning signs...*

- **Diameter larger than a pencil eraser.**

- **Irregular color**, sometimes with areas of red, white, gray or purple mixed in.

- **Irregular borders**, sometimes notched, with the color "bleeding" outward.

Melanomas are most likely to develop on parts of the body that get lots of sun exposure —especially the back and legs. But they can pop up anywhere, including such unlikely areas as the soles of the feet.

If there is any doubt whether a mole could be a melanoma, have it checked. If your primary-care doctor cannot rule out melanoma, have the mole biopsied by a dermatologist.

The poster on the wall of my office says it best. In a takeoff on the old school readers, it proclaims: "See Spot. See Spot Change. See a Doctor."

Periodic self-exam:

1. Examine body front and back in mirror, then right and left sides, arms raised.

2. Bend elbows, look at forearms, back of upper arms and palms.

3. Look at backs of legs and feet, spaces between toes and soles.

4. Examine back of neck and scalp with a hand mirror. Part hair to lift.

5. Check back and buttocks with a hand mirror.

More Skin Cancer Facts

Hensin Tsao, MD, PhD, associate professor of dermatology, Massachusetts General Hospital, Boston.

Deadly skin cancer can lie dormant for more than a decade. Not too long ago, any patient who had a melanoma removed and then stayed cancer-free for 10 years was considered cured.

Finding: Melanoma can recur even after 15 years. Since treatments are now available for certain recurrences, melanoma survivors should have their skin and lymph nodes checked every year.

A Word About Surgery

Gerald Imber, MD, clinical assistant professor of surgery at New York Hospital–Cornell Medical Center, and a plastic surgeon in private practice, both in New York City. He is author of *The Youth Corridor: A Renowned Plastic Surgeon's Revolutionary Program for Maintenance, Rejuvenation, and Timeless Beauty.* Harper Perennial.

If you think you might decide to have cosmetic surgery, don't wait until you need a full face-lift.

Instead, start earlier and get several less invasive procedures (microsuction of the jowls, eyelift, etc.). That way, you'll look great all along.

What Causes Tiny Red Lines on the Cheeks?

Thomas N. Helm, MD, associate clinical professor of dermatology, State University of New York, Buffalo.

These tiny lines are usually nothing more than dilated blood vessels under the skin. Called *telangiectasia,* they're caused by sun exposure and by age-related thinning of the skin.

Good news: Dermatologists can remove them using an electric probe…or via laser therapy.

16

Health Alerts

All About Leg Cramps

Norman Marcus, MD
Norman Marcus Pain Institute

If you've been experiencing leg cramps but have neglected to do anything about them, you may be placing your life in jeopardy. *Reason:* While two of the three main types of leg cramps are benign, a walking-related cramp known as intermittent claudication can be a sign of heart disease.

●**Nighttime leg cramps** typically involve a spasm in the calf muscle that wakes you up.

To stop the pain: Gently massage the knot while alternately flexing and extending your toes.

Also helpful: Ask your doctor about taking the prescription medication quinine sulfate…and about taking a daily supplement that contains 500 to 1,000 milligrams (mg) of calcium…1,000 mg of magnesium…and 400 international units (IU) of vitamin D.

The minerals are critical to proper muscle contraction. Vitamin D assures proper absorption of the minerals.

●**Post-exercise leg cramps** are usually caused by electrolyte imbalances brought on by heavy perspiration. These imbalances cause muscle and nerve cells to malfunction.

Helpful: Rest…drink water or a sports drink like Gatorade before and during exercise …and massage after exercise.

●**Intermittent claudication.** If walking gives you a cramp in one of your calves, see a doctor right away. Unlike other types of leg cramps, intermittent claudication is caused by reduced blood flow in one of the legs. In most cases, this reduction in blood flow is caused by the buildup of fatty deposits in leg arteries (atherosclerosis).

Danger: People who have fatty deposits in their leg arteries often have similar deposits in

Norman Marcus, MD, director of the Norman Marcus Pain Institute, New York City. He is clinical associate professor in anesthesiology and psychiatry and director of Muscle Pain Research at New York University School of Medicine, and author of *Freedom from Pain.* Fireside.

their coronary arteries. In fact, if someone has claudication, there is a 50% chance that he/she also has heart disease.

Claudication causes bad cramps in one leg after walking even a short distance. Typically, the cramp disappears after a minute or two of rest…and recurs when you resume walking.

Other symptoms: Having one foot that has thicker toenails, is bluish in color, has less hair or is colder than the other foot.

Treatment for intermittent claudication is similar to that for coronary artery disease. In most cases, patients are urged to take long walks or get other regular aerobic exercise… quit smoking…and adopt a low-fat, low-cholesterol diet.

Some cases of intermittent claudication require leg surgery to clear away the blockages. In some cases, doctors are able to push aside the fatty deposits by snaking a balloon-tipped catheter through the skin and into the clogged artery. This procedure is called *balloon angioplasty*.

For severe cases, bypass surgery may be required. In this procedure the surgeon creates a "detour" around the blocked arteries by grafting a blood vessel from a large artery in the groin to an artery behind the knee.

In some cases, individuals who experience walking-related leg cramps are suffering not from claudication but from *pseudo*claudication.

This comparatively benign condition is caused by abnormal growth of bone tissue in the spine. As the bone grows, the bony sheath encasing the lower spinal nerves narrows. That compresses the nerves, causing them to register pain.

How can you tell pseudoclaudication from true claudication? Pain from claudication goes away within two minutes when you stop walking. Pain from pseudoclaudication persists for five to 10 minutes.

If pseudoclaudication is accompanied by leg weakness and loss of sensation, surgery may be needed. Injections of cortisone and local anesthetic into the spinal cord region may decrease the pain.

Diabetes Alert

John F. Amos, OD, dean, School of Optometry, University of Alabama at Birmingham.

Annual eye exams are essential for all diabetics. See an eye doctor *right away* if you experience vision changes—blurred, fluctuating or double vision.

Disinfectant Danger

David Lewis, PhD, adjunct senior research scientist, University of Georgia, Athens. His study was published in *Nature Medicine*, 310 Varick St., New York City 10013.

The disinfectant commonly used on medical and dental instruments does *not* kill the AIDS virus. Even when drill pieces and viewing scopes (endoscopes) used in the respiratory and gastrointestinal tracts spent two hours soaking in the disinfectant *glutaraldehyde*, the virus survived in blood-tainted lubricants used in these devices. While there's no evidence that contaminated lubricants have ever led to AIDS, occasional infections may go undetected.

Self-defense: Ask your doctor to sterilize endoscopes with ethylene oxide gas or peracetic acid, not simply disinfect them.

Rodent Danger

Bruno Chomel, DVM, PhD, assistant professor of population health and reproduction, School of Veterinary Medicine, University of California, Davis.

Hantavirus, which causes a respiratory illness that can be deadly, is thought to spread via inhalation of tiny particles of rodent droppings.

Self-defense: If you see signs of rodent infestation in storage rooms, cabins, etc., don't vacuum or sweep the floor. That can stir up feces-laden dust. *Better:* Don work gloves and a filter mask, then sprinkle or spray the floor with a mixture of bleach and water. Sweep the mess into a plastic bag, then dispose.

Another Danger In the Kitchen

Charles P. Gerba, PhD, professor of microbiology, University of Arizona, Tucson.

Dishcloths and kitchen sponges are often infected with *salmonella, staphylococcus* and other disease-causing germs.

Self-defense: Replace rags and sponges with paper towels. Or use a germ-resistant sponge such as Cell-O brand and wash it in hot water after each use. And be sure to wash your hands with soap after handling uncooked meat.

Good news: Adopting these simple strategies could prevent 90% of all food-borne illnesses.

The Scary Truth About Blood Transfusions

Edgar G. Engleman, MD, professor of pathology and medicine at Stanford University Medical School and director of the University's Blood Center, both in Palo Alto, CA. In 1983, under Dr. Engleman's direction, Stanford's blood center was the first in the world to test donated blood for the AIDS virus.

Although the nation's blood supply is safer today than ever before, many people remain fearful of catching AIDS or another disease from a transfusion.

For an update on transfusion safety, we spoke with Dr. Edgar G. Engleman, who pioneered the testing of donated blood for the AIDS virus in the early 1980s.

According to Dr. Engleman, the blood supply is now remarkably safe, especially when compared with 10 years ago. Risk of catching a serious infection is roughly one in 5,000. *There are several explanations for this increased level of safety...*

WIDESPREAD SCREENING

In the early 1980s, donated blood was screened only for hepatitis B and syphilis. Not until 1985 was testing for the AIDS virus (HIV) implemented on a nationwide basis.

Most blood banks did not launch efforts to screen for AIDS prior to the availability of a specific test, arguing that the risk of catching AIDS from a transfusion was tiny and the cost high. In fact, up to 2% of the units of blood transfused in some cities in the early 1980s harbored HIV. Thousands were needlessly infected, including Arthur Ashe and Ryan White.

Today, the Food and Drug Administration keeps close watch over blood banks. It doesn't hesitate to close down those that don't follow regulations.

MORE ACCURATE HIV TESTING

At one time, blood banks tested only for the presence of *antibodies* to HIV (not the virus itself). *Problem:* It can take a while after infection for antibodies to form. There is a window of time when a person's blood is infectious even though the virus isn't detectable via conventional antibody testing.

To offset this problem, more sensitive antibody tests have been developed.

Result: The window has shrunk from 24 weeks to about four weeks. In addition, the FDA has licensed a test for HIV itself. This test, which is mandated for use by all blood banks, shrinks the window even further.

And prospective blood donors are thoroughly questioned about possible risk factors for AIDS (homosexuality, intravenous drug abuse, etc.) before they are allowed to donate blood.

Bottom line: Roughly one in 400,000 transfusions now results in transmission of HIV. The new test should reduce the incidence to one in 700,000.

FEWER TRANSFUSIONS ARE GIVEN

A generation ago, doctors recommended transfusions even in cases that weren't life-threatening—to help people feel less tired after surgery, for example.

311

Today, doctors order transfusions only to save lives—not to make patients feel better.

BEYOND AIDS SCREENING

Blood banks now screen donated blood for the two strains of HIV, syphilis, hepatitis B and C, plus two other potentially deadly pathogens...

●**Human T-lymphotropic virus** (HTLV-1 and HTLV-2). Close relatives of HIV, these viruses cause cancer and other illnesses.

●**Cytomegalovirus** (CMV). It can cause a life-threatening infection in premature infants, chemotherapy patients, AIDS patients, transplant recipients taking immunosuppressant drugs and other individuals with poor immunity.

Diseases for which we are not yet testing, but which may be cause for concern, include...

●**Hepatitis G.** This newly discovered strain of hepatitis is less virulent than other strains—but more persistent.

●**Chagas.** This one-celled organism (protozoan) causes chronic infection, which can lead to heart failure.

As more people enter the US from areas where Chagas is endemic (chiefly Central and South America) the incidence of the disease in the US will increase. Even so, the number of cases spread by transfusion will probably remain low.

HOW TO AVOID BAD BLOOD

What can individuals do to protect themselves from tainted blood? First, it's important to remember that *blood transfusions save lives* ...and that people have died because they *refused* transfusions. *Having said that, there are ways to minimize your risk...*

●**Predeposit your own blood.** Autologous donation—banking your own blood—is the single most significant precaution you can take. Barring human error in the handling of your blood (extremely unlikely), your risk of contracting a transfusion-related illness is essentially zero.

●**Recycle your blood.** Many operating rooms are now equipped with "cell-saving" devices that collect blood draining from the surgical incision and reintroduce it into the body.

Called *intraoperative autologous transfusion* (IAT), this technique is often effective in emergency surgery—so it's definitely worth asking for. It cannot be used for intestinal surgery, tumor removal or any other operation in which blood could be contaminated with bacteria or cancer cells.

●**Know your options.** In California, surgeons are required to inform patients of their transfusion options. This is *not* the case in all states.

If your surgeon doesn't explain your options, ask him to do so. Alternatives should be discussed at least six weeks before surgery.

If significant blood loss is expected, a *series* of autologous donations may be required over several weeks. Blood cells can be stored for up to 42 days, frozen plasma for up to one year.

The surgeon isn't necessarily to blame if you should need a transfusion. However, you're likely to lose *less* blood under the hands of a good surgeon. Ask how many times he/she has done this procedure.

Some hospitals can provide plasma or platelets taken from one person. "Single donor" blood is generally less likely than "pooled" blood to carry disease. However, this isn't always practical. Given today's careful screening practices, the increase in safety is marginal at best.

Some patients scheduled for surgery ask friends and relatives to donate blood. The assumption is that blood from someone you know is safer than blood from anonymous donors.

In fact, friends and relatives are likely to be *first-time* donors (whereas the community supply consists mostly of blood from repeat donors), so their blood hasn't been subjected to repeated testing. Ironically, it may be less safe.

●**Ask about blood-boosting drugs.** Researchers have identified hormone-like substances that spur the production of red blood cells, white blood cells or platelets. In many instances, these factors can be synthesized using recombinant DNA technology—and used as drugs.

Erythropoietin (EPO), one of the first of these to become commercially available, helps the body make more red cells. It's helpful for some patients with kidney failure and other chronic conditions that used to require repeated transfusions.

However, since the body takes up to a few weeks to manufacture blood cells in response to the EPO, its value in surgery is limited.

Lead Danger

Charles V. Shorten, PhD, professor of health, West Chester University, West Chester, PA.

Salad dressing stored in a crystal cruet can quickly become contaminated with lead. It's long been known that crystal goblets can leach lead into beverages. But this hasn't been considered a threat to children because so few drink from crystal. *However:* A study found that lead rapidly leaches into salad dressing. After one hour in a crystal cruet, lead levels hit 162 micrograms per liter (mcg/L). After 42 days, levels hit 665 mcg/L, eight times the level in distilled water kept in crystal.

Drinking Danger

Nedra Wilson, PhD, assistant professor of anatomy and cell biology, Oklahoma State University, Tulsa.

Every glass of alcohol causes your body to lose water. If the water isn't replaced, you could become dehydrated.

Self-defense: Never use beer or any other alcoholic beverage as a thirst quencher. Remember to sip water whenever you're drinking beer, wine or any other alcoholic beverage.

Underwear Danger

Alan Matarasso, MD, a New York City–based plastic and reconstructive surgeon. His remarks were reported in *Archives of Internal Medicine*, 515 N. State St., Chicago 60610.

Tight garments may contribute to *deep vein thrombosis* (DVT), a potentially deadly ailment involving formation of a blood clot in the legs. Should the clot break away and travel to the lungs, this pulmonary embolism can kill within minutes.

Self-defense: Avoid restrictive clothing if you're at high risk for DVT. At-risk individuals include postsurgical patients, pregnant women and those who are bedridden.

Boating Danger

Neil B. Hampson, MD, medical director, hyperbaric department, Virginia Mason Medical Center, Seattle. His study of 27 poisonings was published in the *Journal of the American Medical Association*, 515 N. State St., Chicago 60610.

Pleasure boaters are vulnerable to carbon monoxide poisoning.

Danger: Air currents created behind a moving boat can draw carbon monoxide—colorless and odorless—from the engine exhaust into the boat. In a study of 27 onboard carbon monoxide poisonings, 21 involved engine exhaust...four involved emissions from onboard water heaters...and two involved emissions from gas generators. Many carbon monoxide poisoning cases go unreported because boaters blame their symptoms—headaches, nausea, dizziness and vomiting—on seasickness.

Self-defense: Install a carbon monoxide warning sensor with an alarm in all gasoline-fueled cabin cruisers.

Allergy Attacks And Food

Stephen F. Kemp, MD, associate professor of medicine, allergy and immunology, The University of Mississippi Medical Center, Jackson.

In a survey of 266 cases of the life-threatening allergic response *anaphylaxis*, 34% were caused by food, spices or food additives. *Usual culprits:* Shellfish and peanuts. Aspirin and non-steroidal anti-inflammatory drugs caused the most drug-related attacks. Anyone at risk for anaphylaxis should keep the drug *epinephrine* on hand.

Ear Thermometer Danger

Michael Yaron, MD, associate professor of surgery, University of Colorado Health Sciences Center, Denver. His study of 100 patients was published in the *American Journal of Emergency Medicine*, 360 Park Ave. S., New York City 10010.

In-the-ear thermometers are often unreliable. Only six of 10 adults with fever detected by an electronic rectal thermometer—considered the most accurate method for fever measurement—were found to have a fever with an ear thermometer. Oral thermometers are generally accurate.

Get a Tetanus Booster Shot Every 10 Years

Timothy McCall, MD, an internist, medical editor of *Yoga Journal* and author of *Examining Your Doctor: A Patient's Guide to Avoiding Harmful Medical Care*. Carol. *www.drmccall.com.*

The protection generated by a tetanus shot deteriorates over time. Older people, in particular, who have not had a booster shot in decades lose immunity to this completely preventable but potentially fatal disease.

Drinking Unfiltered Coffee May Raise Your Blood Cholesterol Level

Michael J. Klag, MD, dean, Johns Hopkins School of Public Health, Baltimore.

When Dutch researchers measured cholesterol levels of people who switched to unfiltered coffee brewed in French-press plunger coffee pots, they found that they rose by up to 20 points compared with those who stayed with filtered coffee. Scientists theorize that the jump was caused by two compounds that are trapped by coffee filters and have been shown to raise cholesterol levels and affect the function of the liver, which metabolizes cholesterol.

Another Secondhand-Smoke Danger

George Howard, DrPH, epidemiologist, Bowman Gray School of Medicine, Winston-Salem, NC, and leader of a seven-year study of 8,400 people.

Atherosclerosis—a thickening of the arteries that can lead to heart attack and stroke is another danger of inhaling second-hand smoke. Over time, the effects are cumulative. Regular inhalation significantly interferes with the ability of arteries to carry blood—increasing the risk of serious disease.

Yikes! Another Measles Shot?

Barbara Reynolds, Centers for Disease Control and Prevention, Atlanta.

If you were born after 1956 and received only one measles vaccination, a second may be needed to protect you. More than three million Americans are at risk of contracting measles despite inoculation. A single vaccination fails to provide immunity 5% of the time. That failure rate was only determined in 1989, and children up to age 12 then got second shots. You may not be protected if you were older than 12 in 1989.

Self-defense: Check your medical records. Have a second vaccination if necessary.

In-Line Skating Injuries On the Rise

Rodney M. Friedman, former editor and publisher, *University of California, Berkeley Wellness Letter*, Health Letter Associates, Box 420148, Palm Coast, FL 32142.

In-line skating injuries will send more than 100,000 Americans to hospital emergency rooms this year. About two-thirds of these injured skaters will not be wearing a helmet, elbow and knee pads or wrist guards when they fall.

Stroke Diagnosis Danger

Louis R. Caplan, MD, professor of neurology and medicine, Harvard Medical School, Boston.

Headaches, confusion, temporary blindness, seizures and other stroke-like symptoms are sometimes caused by a less serious neurological disorder called *reversible predominantly posterior leukoencephalopathy* (RPPL).

Danger: Some doctors begin treatment for stroke when the patient really needs adjustment of his/her blood pressure or immunosuppressant medication.

Good news: With proper treatment, patients with RPPL usually recover within days. RPPL is common among patients with high blood pressure and those taking immunosuppressant drugs after transplant surgery. It occurs when capillaries leak fluid into the brain.

Don't Cut Back on Caffeine Suddenly

Johanna Dwyer, RD, adjunct professor of society, human development, and health, Harvard School of Public Health, Boston.

You may suffer withdrawal symptoms if you cut back on caffeine suddenly. *Better:* Lower your intake gradually. Try cutting half a cup of coffee from your diet every few days… or mixing regular with decaffeinated and gradually increasing the proportion of decaf. Also ease up on consumption of other caffeine-containing beverages, like some teas and soft drinks.

Hidden Dangers in Household Products… In Everyday Foods, Too

Samuel S. Epstein, MD, professor emeritus of occupational and environmental medicine at the University of Illinois School of Public Health in Chicago, and chairman of the Cancer Prevention Coalition, at the University of Illinois at Chicago. He is coauthor of *The Safe Shopper's Bible: A Consumer's Guide to Nontoxic Household Products, Cosmetics and Food.* Wiley.

Everyone seems to worry about smog and other sources of pollution *outside* the home.

But many everyday foods are tainted with toxic chemicals…and an EPA study of air in six US cities found that certain airborne toxins can be up to 500 times more concentrated indoors than outdoors.

Where do these dangerous airborne toxins come from? From cleansers, paints, cosmetics and other household products.

Problem: Federal regulations that govern the labeling of consumer products are woefully inadequate. Consequently, it's difficult for consumers to find out precisely which products contain dangerous ingredients or contaminants —and which are safe.

To find out how consumers can protect themselves, we spoke with Dr. Samuel S. Epstein, a noted toxicologist and chairman of the Chicago-based Cancer Prevention Coalition…

DANGEROUS PRODUCT AND SAFER ALTERNATIVES

●**Beef frankfurters.** The nitrite preservatives in beef frankfurters interact with *amines*, which occur naturally in meat and fish, to form potent cancer-causing compounds called nitrosamines.

Franks also may be contaminated with the carcinogenic pesticides *benzene hexachloride, Dacthal, dieldrin, DDT* and *heptachlor*…and with residues of powerful hormones.

Safer: "Nitrite-free" franks or—better still—tofu franks.

●**Bug killer.** Many household pesticides contain *propoxur*, a compound that is both carcinogenic and neurotoxic.

Safer: Brands that substitute *pyrethrum* or another natural, herbal pesticide for propoxur.

●**Cat litter.** Many brands contain *crystalline silica*, an eye and lung irritant and suspected carcinogen.

Safer: Litter made of a natural ingredient such as pulverized paper.

●**Flea collar.** Many flea collars contain the pesticide propoxur.

Safer: Flea collars made with natural, herbal pesticides.

●**Air freshener.** Some aerosol brands contain *orthophenylphenol*, a skin irritant and carcinogen. This is particularly dangerous because tiny aerosol droplets are readily inhaled deep into the lungs.

Safer: Solid air fresheners made with plant-based scents. It's best to avoid all aerosol spray products, including air fresheners, cosmetics and household cleaners.

●**Hair conditioner.** Some brands contain *formaldehyde* and the carcinogenic dye *FD&C Red #4.*

Safer: Natural, plant-based conditioners.

●**Hair dye.** Black and dark brown hair dyes have been linked to several kinds of cancer, including non-Hodgkin's lymphoma, multiple myeloma and leukemia.

Safer: Hair dyes that substitute plant-based substances like *henna* for the synthetic dyes.

Warning: Never buy hair dye that contains *phenylenediamine.*

●**Laundry detergent.** Brands that contain washing soda are highly caustic. Some brands may also be contaminated with a carcinogen called *1,4 dioxane.*

Safer: Vegetable-based detergents or laundry soap.

●**Makeup.** Cosmetics often contain talc, *titanium dioxide* and/or the preservative *BHA*—all of which are carcinogenic. In addition, *lanolin* found in many brands is often tainted with DDT.

Safer: Natural, plant-based cosmetics.

●**Moth repellent.** These often contain *naphthalene*, a neurotoxin, or *dichlorobenzene*, a highly volatile compound that is a potent carcinogen.

Safer: Cedar blocks, chips and sachets.

●**Paint stripper.** Aerosol strippers often contain *methanol*, a neurotoxin that is also a potent skin and eye irritant…along with *methylene chloride*, a carcinogen.

Safer: Get rid of old paint by sanding or scraping it off. To avoid inhalation of dust, wear a respirator mask.

●**Shaving cream.** Some brands contain the carcinogenic preservative BHA…along with *triethanolamine* and/or *diethanolamine*, which are nitrosamine precursors.

Others contain *Blue #1* and other cancer-causing dyes.

Safer: Natural brands—especially those that are applied with a brush.

●**Talcum powder.** Talc irritates the lungs and has been linked to ovarian cancer.

Safer: Products made with cornstarch.

●**Toothpaste.** Many popular brands of toothpaste contain Blue #1, which is a carcinogen.

Fluoride is also a suspected carcinogen.

Safer: Natural toothpaste without fluoride.

●**Weed killer.** Some brands contain sodium 2,4-*dichlorophenoxyacetate* (2,4-D), a carcinogen and neurotoxin.

Safer: "Weed whackers" or other tools for cutting rather than poisoning weeds.

●**Whole milk**—including whole-milk products like cheese and milk chocolate.

Milk fat is often laced with the carcinogenic compounds DDT, dieldrin, heptachlor and/or *hexachlorobenzene.*

In addition, milk products are sometimes tainted with antibiotic residues. Some of these residues cause allergic reactions. Others are suspected of causing cancer.

Ingestion of these antibiotic residues also promotes growth of potentially dangerous antibiotic-resistant bacteria inside the body.

Safer: Organic skim milk, especially brands labeled "bovine hormone-free."

Meningitis Warning

Ronald Ruden, MD, internist in private practice in New York.

B*acterial* meningitis—the less common, *potentially deadly* type—is most prevalent in late winter/early spring. *Viral* meningitis is most prevalent in late summer/early autumn. Symptoms are the same—severe headache, fever, stiff neck. If you experience symptoms, see your doctor *immediately.* Bacterial meningitis requires antibiotics. Viral is treated simply with bed rest.

Prevention: Good hygiene—wash hands after using the bathroom…don't share food.

Even the Best Medical Labs Can Make Mistakes…

Charles B. Inlander, a consumer advocate and healthcare consultant based in Fogelsville, PA. He was founding president of the nonprofit People's Medical Society, a consumer health advocacy group in Allentown, PA. He is author of numerous books, including *Take This Book to the Hospital With You.* St. Martin's.

A nd these mistakes can be dangerous—even deadly. The biggest errors occur on routine tests—especially Pap smears and PSA tests (for prostate cancer). If a test comes back negative and you still think something could be wrong—*get retested.* Ask your doctor to send the test to a different lab…or to send it to the same lab but under a different name. *Never* use the doctor's *in-office* lab—their error rates are much higher than commercial lab rates.

Also: Always make sure the lab your doctor uses is certified by the College of American Pathologists. If you don't trust the lab that your doctor uses, ask him/her to use a properly accredited one.

Asthma Attacks Can Be Triggered by Thunderstorms

A. Craig Davidson, MD, consultant physician, Guy's and St. Thomas's Hospital, London.

T he culprit is grass pollen and other airborne allergens stirred up by wind and rain.

Nose Piercing Is Dangerous

William Castelli, MD, medical director, Framingham Cardiovascular Institute and former director, Framingham Heart Study, Boston.

B ecause the nose is designed to trap airborne bacteria, it is one of the dirtiest places in the body. Many virulent bacteria, such as *staphylococcus aureus,* are harmless as long as they stay in the nose. But should the piercing needle force them into the bloodstream, they can cause serious illness—even death.

Glucose Level Alert

Linda J. Rhodes, MD, assistant professor of psychiatry, University of Texas Health Science Center, San Antonio.

E levated glucose levels can trigger depression, fatigue, apathy and malaise. Diabetics should monitor feelings as well as glucose levels—and report problems to their doctor.

Cigar Dangers

Harlan Krumholz, MD, professor of cardiology at Yale University School of Medicine, New Haven, CT, and author of *No Ifs, Ands or Butts: The Smoker's Guide to Quitting.* Diane.

Cigars have all of the health risks of cigarettes—including lung cancer, heart disease and stroke.

Trap I: Thinking that smoking cigars is safe because you don't inhale.

Reality: Cigar smoke contains more tar, nicotine and carbon monoxide than filtered cigarettes. You may not inhale as you puff, but you still breathe in the "secondhand" smoke.

Trap II: Giving in to the "George Burns phenomenon."

Reality: Just because someone else lived a long life despite an unhealthy habit doesn't mean you will, too.

Reality: Any amount of smoking puts your health—and others'—at risk.

Even Moderately High Blood Pressure Can Damage Kidneys

Michael Klag, MD, MPH, dean of the Bloomberg School of Public Health, Johns Hopkins University, Baltimore. His 16-year study of 332,544 men was published in *The New England Journal of Medicine*, 10 Shattuck St., Boston 02115.

It has long been known that severely high blood pressure can cause kidney failure, but researchers have been unsure of what, if any, danger moderately high blood pressure poses to the kidneys.

In a study, men with blood pressure between 140/90 and 159/99 were three times as likely to suffer kidney failure as were men with blood pressure below 120/80. Those who had blood pressure readings of up to 179/109 had six times the kidney damage risk.

To the rescue: Your doctor will probably prescribe a pressure-lowering regimen.

Smokers' Sleep Trap

David Wetter, PhD, professor and chair, department of health disparities research, University of Texas, M.D. Anderson Cancer Center, Houston, and Terry Young, PhD, associate professor, preventive medicine, University of Wisconsin at Madison.

Smokers are more likely to have difficulty falling asleep, difficulty waking up, daytime sleepiness and nightmares. *Possible causes:* The stimulative effect of nicotine…nightly nicotine withdrawal…breathing difficulties associated with smoking. Over time, such sleep disturbances can result in fatigue, depression and impaired ability to think.

Shoveling Snow Stresses the Heart

Barry Franklin, PhD, director of cardiac rehabilitation, William Beaumont Hospital, Royal Oak, MI.

After two minutes of shoveling wet snow, heart rates of nine out of 10 men soared far above the zone recommended for aerobic exercise (70% to 85% of maximum heart rate). After 10 minutes of shoveling, heart rates reached 97% of maximum…and blood pressure was higher than when the men ran to the point of exhaustion.

Asthma Warning

Thomas Plaut, MD, asthma specialist and medical consultant to *Asthma Update*, 123 Monticello Ave., Annapolis, MD 21401.

Asthma patients cannot measure the ailment's severity by how they feel. A peak-flow meter is needed to determine lung function and ways to keep the disease under control. If you have asthma, make sure your doctor uses a peak-flow meter as the basis for determining therapy. And be sure the doctor teaches you how to use it at home between visits.

Lead Alert

Howard Hu, MD, ScD, chair, environmental health sciences, University of Michigan School of Public Health in Ann Arbor.

Very low levels of lead are dangerous to adults, too. Adults who pick up traces of lead from environmental sources—like food cans, water pipes and lead paint dust—can develop high blood pressure and reduced kidney function.

Self-defense: Take the same precautions for yourself that you would for a child. *Start here:* Have your water tested to ensure lead levels are safe. The danger posed by lead-based paint should be evaluated and possibly removed by professionals—don't do it yourself. Take extra care with hobbies that expose you to lead, such as staining glass and shooting.

Lead Poisoning Alert

Study of 23 types of pool cue chalk, led by Mary Beth Miller, DO, department of medical toxicology, Good Samaritan Regional Medical Center, Phoenix, reported in *Pediatrics*, 141 Northwest Point Blvd., Elk Grove Village, IL 60007.

Surprising source of lead danger: Pool cue chalk. Lead compounds are sometimes used to color chalk for pool cues. In one case, a 28-month-old girl who often put the chalk in her mouth developed elevated lead levels.

Self-defense: Buy pool cue chalk that does not contain lead. If unsure, take extra precautions to keep it away from children.

Toxic Chemicals Self-Defense

Robert G. Lewis, PhD, senior scientist, National Exposure Research Laboratory, Environmental Protection Agency, Research Triangle Park, NC.

To keep toxic chemicals out of your home, remove your shoes before coming inside, especially after working with insecticides or herbicides.

Also: Use a doormat...have carpets steam-cleaned...replace any carpet that is more than 20 years old. Traces of banned pesticides, such as DDT, can be found in some old carpets.

Who Should Be Vaccinated For Hepatitis B?

Mary Ann Littell, information specialist, American Liver Foundation, 75 Maiden Lane, Ste. 603, New York 10038.

The vaccine is a good idea for international travelers...infants and adolescents...doctors, nurses, paramedics, firefighters and police officers...people on hemodialysis... members of the military...morticians and embalmers...patients and staff members at institutions for the mentally handicapped... members of ethnic or racial groups with high rates of hepatitis B infection—African-American, Native American, Hispanic, Chinese, Korean, Indo-Chinese, Filipino, Alaskan Eskimo or Haitian...people with multiple sex partners...intravenous drug users...recipients of clotting factor and certain other blood products...people living with or having sex with a hepatitis B carrier.

Weight-Lifting Danger

John D. Cantwell, MD, team physician for the Atlanta Braves, and a cardiologist in private practice in Atlanta.

Intense weight-lifting can be dangerous for individuals with high blood pressure. Anyone with hypertension or another risk factor for heart disease (cigarette smoking, high cholesterol, diabetes, etc.) should do strenuous exercise only with a doctor's permission.

Drowning Fact

Centers for Disease Control and Prevention, 1600 Clifton Rd., Atlanta 30333. *www.cdc.gov.*

Avoid alcohol before swimming—or while boating. From 25% to 50% of all adult drowning victims were exposed to alcohol at time of death.

Plastic vs. Wood Cutting Boards

Don Schaffner, PhD, extension specialist, food science, Rutgers University, New Brunswick, NJ.

When it comes to preventing bacterial contamination, food safety experts now favor plastic. But the best solution may be to have a plastic board for meat and poultry *and* a wooden board for fruit, vegetables and bread. Keep the boards separate to avoid cross-contamination. Clean them after each use with a solution of two teaspoons bleach in a quart of water. Plastic boards can be put in a dishwasher.

Caution: Sanitizing a wooden board in the microwave can cause a fire.

To Beat the Heat...

Stuart R. Rose, MD, assistant clinical professor of emergency medicine, Tufts University School of Medicine, Boston, and president, Travel Medicine, Inc., Northampton, MA.

Drink two to three quarts of water a day, even if you do not feel thirsty.

● **Drink two glasses two hours before any exercise.** Keep drinking cool water—not cold—during exertion.

● **Review medications with your doctor**—some can restrict sweat or increase production of body heat.

● **If you take prescription diuretics,** ask your doctor if you should change the dosage while traveling.

● **Replace salt lost through sweating** by drinking a sports drink or eating salty foods. If you have salt restrictions, consult your doctor.

Milk and Diabetes Connection

Hans-Michael Dosch, MD, professor of pediatrics and immunology, Hospital for Sick Children, Toronto. His study of diabetes in 140 infants was published in *The New England Journal of Medicine*, 10 Shattuck St., Boston 02115.

Infants given cow's milk formula during their first three months face an increased risk of diabetes later in life.

Theory: A protein in cow's milk—*bovine serum albumin*—is similar to proteins found in insulin-producing cells in the pancreas. In infants genetically predisposed to diabetes, antibodies that form to attack bovine serum albumin wind up attacking the pancreas cells as well.

Lesson: If possible, mothers should breastfeed their infants for the first three months of life.

Have a Foot Problem?

John T. Langloh, MD, staff orthopedist, National Hospital Medical Center, Arlington, VA.

Diagnose foot problems by checking your footprints. Dip your feet in water, then walk along a piece of brown paper. If you have a "light" footprint—little or no link between the ball of your foot and the heel—you may have a high arch.

Helpful: "Stability" shoes with extra arch cushioning...high-top sneakers.

If you have a "heavy" footprint, you may have flat feet. This can lead to arch or knee pain.

Helpful: Molded arch supports...shoes with "control" features...orthotic inserts.

Who's Reading Your Medical Records?

Timothy McCall, MD, an internist, medical editor of *Yoga Journal* and author of *Examining Your Doctor: A Patient's Guide to Avoiding Harmful Medical Care.* Carol. *www.drmccall.com.*

Patients discuss private matters with their doctors with the implicit understanding that the information exchanged is private. In reality, more and more people are gaining access to these confidential medical records and using the information in ways you never intended.

These days, insurance companies, credit bureaus and the like have assembled sophisticated databases that contain loads of private information. Unbeknownst to you, this information may be shared with other insurers, potential employers, marketing firms—and sometimes sold to anyone who will pay for it.

Worst of all, information you divulged to help your doctor help you may be used with just the opposite result. *Here are four true horror stories...*

●**A company changes its insurance policy to limit coverage** for AIDS-related problems after learning that an employee has tested HIV-positive.

●**A man is denied life insurance** after telling his doctor he was feeling "down" because he feared his company might be the victim of a hostile takeover.

●**A woman is fired** after her employer learns she needs a kidney transplant.

●**A hospital employee uses a computer to access the phone numbers of teenage female patients**, then calls them up and sexually harasses them.

To provide top-notch medical care, doctors need complete access to the most sensitive matters—drug use, sexual habits, etc. We need our patients to trust that their secrets will remain secret. If a young man doesn't feel comfortable telling a doctor he's gay, for example, then the doctor may misjudge the significance of a symptom, order the wrong tests, miss diagnoses and the opportunity to treat.

Until legal loopholes that allow unauthorized dissemination of medical information are closed, how can you minimize your risk? I recommend several strategies:

●**Never sign a blanket disclosure form.** Before agreeing to the release of your medical records, make sure you know who will be allowed to see them, which information they'll be given access to and what they need the information for.

●**Remind your doctor that your information must not be shared with anyone without your consent.**

●**Consider asking your doctor not to include especially sensitive information in your record.** You might say, "If I tell you something very personal that may be relevant to my care but that I don't want to be written in my chart, would you respect my wishes?" If your doctor is unwilling to honor your request, you'll have to decide whether you still want to reveal the information.

Keep in mind that keeping important information out of your chart could compromise your care down the road—especially if you see another doctor or if your doctor fails to remember what you said. Keep information out of your record only if you feel doing so is absolutely essential.

●**Be wary of any medical information you give out**, no matter how innocent it seems. A TV ad once offered free information on pollen counts to anyone who called an 800 number. The names of those who called were then used by the drug company that had sponsored the ad to market an allergy medication.

●**Get a copy of your medical records** to make sure all information is factually correct. An error in your chart could lead to the loss of employment or future insurance coverage.

In most states, you have a legal right to your medical records. In the rest, you can ask your doctor for a copy of your chart. If your doctor won't provide it, you've got to wonder whether your doctor views health care as a democracy or a dictatorship.

Fibromyalgia... New Strategies for Controlling Mysterious Pain and Fatigue

Robert M. Bennett, MD, professor of medicine and chairman of the division of arthritis and rheumatic diseases at Oregon Health & Science University in Portland and a member of the medical advisory board of the National Fibromyalgia Research Association. For a free information packet on fibromyalgia, write the association at Box 500, Salem, OR 97308.

Fibromyalgia is a mysterious pain syndrome which afflicts four million Americans and is characterized by...

●**Chronic flu-like pain** in the muscles, tendons and/or ligaments.

●**"Tender points"**—areas of great sensitivity to touch.

●**Restlessness, numbness and/or tingling** in the arms and legs.

●**Sleep problems**—thought to be caused by pain and/or persistent leg twitching that makes deep, restful sleep impossible.

●**Chronic fatigue.** Many fibromyalgia sufferers feel tired even after a full night's sleep.

Some patients also report headaches, abdominal bloating and/or irritable bowel syndrome.

To learn more, we spoke with the nation's leading fibromyalgia researcher, Dr. Robert M. Bennett.

AN EMOTIONAL PROBLEM

For decades, doctors considered fibromyalgia an emotional problem. The consensus was that anxious or depressed individuals unwittingly "created" their symptoms.

Since the mid-1970s, several studies have proved this theory false. As it turns out, most fibromyalgia patients do *not* have emotional problems. In those who do, the problems are now believed to be the *result* of having to live with chronic pain—not the cause of the pain.

Fibromyalgia seems to be associated with chronic fatigue syndrome (CFS)—another disorder that has at least some connection with emotional problems. Up to 80% of CFS patients also have fibromyalgia.

Some researchers speculate that CFS and fibromyalgia are simply different terms for the same condition. Since neither syndrome is well understood, however, it's hard to know for sure.

HOW FIBROMYALGIA STARTS

While some cases begin with a flu-like infection, most start with lower back pain, whiplash or another localized pain. This pain then spreads to other parts of the body.

Why does the pain persist? What makes it spread? The culprit seems to be subtle changes in the central nervous system—possibly the result of abnormally high levels of certain neurotransmitters—that make people more sensitive to pain.

Because the disorder tends to run in families, researchers also suspect that there is a hereditary component.

THE GOOD NEWS...AND THE BAD

The good news is that fibromyalgia is neither crippling nor degenerative. It certainly isn't fatal.

Unfortunately, there is no cure. Most patients learn to manage their symptoms, but the pain may continue to flare up in response to injury, infection or stress.

Even worse, few doctors know much about the syndrome. That means it can be hard to get an accurate diagnosis.

If you think you have fibromyalgia, your best bet is probably a rheumatologist. To find one in your area, contact the Arthritis Foundation (800-568-4045, *www.arthritis.org*).

DRUG THERAPY

Conventional arthritis drugs, including aspirin, do *not* seem to be particularly effective against fibromyalgia. *Drugs that do seem effective include...*

●*Amitriptyline* (Elavil) and other tricyclic antidepressants. Taken at low doses (10 to 25 milligrams [mg] instead of the 100 to 200 mg prescribed for depression), tricyclics help to reduce pain and promote sleep.

●*Zolpidem* (Ambien). This short-acting sedative can help fibromyalgia sufferers get much-needed sleep. However, because of the danger of dependency, zolpidem should be taken no more than twice a week.

•**L-dopa and carbidopa** (Sinemet). Very low doses of this drug—used mainly to treat Parkinson's disease—relieve restless legs syndrome, a common problem for fibromyalgia patients.

•**Procaine or lidocaine.** These local anesthetics are injected into tender points. Injected properly, these drugs bring relief lasting several months.

•**Tramadol** (Ultram). A relatively new non-narcotic drug.

LIFESTYLE ISSUES

Since emotional stress can trigger pain, fibromyalgia patients must learn to pace themselves. Physical and occupational therapists can demonstrate less stressful ways to move... and suggest job modifications to make your work environment more comfortable.

It's particularly important to avoid long stretches of typing or other repetitive motions.

•**Exercise.** Although too much or too little exercise exacerbates fibromyalgia symptoms, gentle stretching or massage (including acupressure) and moderate exercise are essential. Shoot for 20 minutes of aerobic exercise three times a week.

•**Relaxation.** Since fibromyalgia pain isn't caused by muscle tension, deep breathing and other relaxation techniques aren't likely to reduce symptoms.

But learning to relax can keep tension from *exacerbating* the pain. Patients who know how to relax—via relaxation tapes, rhythmic breathing, hot baths, etc.—are better able to keep the problem in perspective.

•**Support groups.** As with many chronic diseases, fibromyalgia seems to be helped by active participation in a support group.

To find a group in your area—or to obtain more information on fibromyalgia—contact the Arthritis Foundation.

Aneurysm Alert

Harold Wilkinson, MD, professor and former chairman of neurosurgery at the University of Massachusetts, Worcester, MA.

When it comes to headaches, I consider myself lucky. I get them rarely, and I can always pinpoint the cause—most recently, giving up a three-cup-a-day coffee habit.

Though usually benign, headaches can be a sign of serious trouble—tumor, meningitis, etc. One cause that often gets overlooked is brain aneurysm—a weak, bulging portion of an artery—inside the skull. Left untreated, an aneurysm can rupture, causing a fatal "brain attack."

Each year, 25,000 Americans are stricken by ruptured aneurysms. Recently, a friend—just 36 years old—died after suffering a ruptured aneurysm.

What causes aneurysms? The risk factors include age (30 to 60 are the riskiest years), high blood pressure, atherosclerosis...and a family history of aneurysms.

The good news about brain aneurysms is that surgery is usually curative—if done within 24 hours of the rupture. Tragically, too many people shrug off their symptoms until it's too late.

If you suddenly get "the worst headache of your life"—especially if you have any of the risk factors—see a doctor right away.

Avoiding Drug Errors

David W. Freeman, former editorial director, *Bottom Line/Health*, 281 Tresser Blvd., Stamford, CT 06901.

Doctors are notorious for having bad handwriting. Making matters worse, many common medications have similar names—Accupril and Accutane, Lovastatin and Lotensin, Prilosec and Prozac...to name but a few.

Bad handwriting plus confusing drug names can cause big trouble. *Real-life example:* A doctor wrote an order for 2 milligrams (mg) of the blood pressure drug *Cardura* on a patient's hospital chart. But the pharmacist read the doctor's scrawl as 2 mg of the anticoagulant *Coumadin.*

Luckily for this patient, a nurse caught this potentially lethal error and called the doctor, who cleared things up. Of course, not every nurse is as vigilant.

How does one guard against such errors? I put that question to Diane D. Cousins, RPh, a prescribing error expert with the US Pharmacopeia, the nonprofit organization that sets national drug standards. *She said that each time a doctor writes a prescription for you, insist that he/she write legibly and...*

●**Avoid use of Latin words and abbreviations** for drug names and directions for use.

●**Include a brief notation of the drug's purpose.**

●**Include your age and weight.**

●**Specify dosages using metric values** (grams, milligrams, etc.) or international units (IU) instead of the old-fashioned apothecary terms (drams, minims, etc.).

●**Write a zero *before* a decimal point (for fractional doses)**...but not a zero *after* a decimal point. For example, 0.5 mg instead of .5 mg, but 3 mg instead of 3.0 mg.

Please take the time to see that your doctor complies. It just might save your life.

Gas Fumes Danger

Victoria Strand, MD, consulting physician, department of respiratory and allergic disease, Karolinska Institute, Huddinge University Hospital, Stockholm.

Fumes from gas appliances and heavy traffic can render the respiratory tract unusually sensitive to pollen.

Study: Adult asthmatics experienced an average 52% decrease in lung function when exposed to airborne pollen if they had breathed such fumes a few hours earlier.

Self-defense: Have gas appliances inspected annually...equip gas stoves with exhaust fans (or open a window when cooking)...open a window when operating a gas dryer...avoid jogging on busy streets.

Important: If sufficient household ventilation cannot be arranged, asthmatics should consider switching to electrical appliances.

Checking Up on Your Thyroid Could Save Your Life

Lawrence Wood, MD, a retired member of the thyroid unit at Massachusetts General Hospital in Boston, and co-author of *Your Thyroid: A Home Reference.* Random House. For more information, contact the Thyroid Foundation of America, One Longfellow Pl., Suite 1518, Boston 02114. 800-832-8321, *www.allthyroid.org.*

If you've been feeling run-down, the problem could be your thyroid gland. Research suggests that *hypothyroidism* (thyroid deficiency) is far more common than previously believed. One study found signs of the disorder in 8% of women and 3% of men.

Hypothyroidism is especially common among older people. Over age 60, up to 17% of women and 8% of men have it.

The thyroid gland, located just below the Adam's apple, is responsible for regulating body metabolism. Besides reducing your energy level, hypothyroidism can cause elevated cholesterol levels, weight gain, depression, constipation and/or brittle hair and nails.

CAUSES OF THYROID TROUBLE

The leading cause of hypothyroidism is scarring of the gland caused by inflammation. This condition is known as Hashimoto's disease.

Other causes include viral infection, certain drugs (including lithium and iodine) and radiation therapy delivered to the neck for cancer.

Mild cases of hypothyroidism often go undetected—because the symptoms are too subtle to be detected by the individual.

Doctors at Massachusetts General Hospital in Boston studied a group of patients with mild hypothyroidism. Most of these patients *thought* they were well. In a double-blind study, each was treated, in turn, with thyroid and placebo tablets.

Result: Most patients felt better when taking the thyroid tablets. Some felt more energy, others were less depressed or less constipated.

These findings suggest that low-dose thyroid treatment may be beneficial even for people who don't know they have thyroid trouble.

CHECKING THYROID LEVELS

The easiest way to detect hypothyroidism is via a blood test for a pituitary hormone called *thyroid-stimulating hormone* (TSH). Ordinarily, TSH stimulates the thyroid gland to make *triiodothyronine* (T3), *thyroxine* (T4) and other thyroid hormones.

If levels of these thyroid hormones fall too low, the pituitary automatically makes more TSH. So, abnormally *high* levels of TSH are a clear sign of hypothyroidism.

If your thyroid is producing too much hormone (a condition called *hyperthyroidism*), TSH levels in your blood will be abnormally low. If your TSH levels are abnormal, your doctor may order other tests.

The TSH test can be obtained by your primary-care physician during a routine checkup.

Cost: $40 to $80.

WHO SHOULD GET TESTED?

Everyone age 50 or older should have his/her TSH levels checked at least once every five years. *Start at age 35 if you have…*

● **A parent, sibling or child who has had thyroid trouble.**

● **A visibly swollen thyroid gland** (goiter). If you think you have a goiter, see a doctor. The condition can be the first sign of thyroid cancer.

● **Prematurely gray hair.** Even a single gray hair before age 30 is a sign that you may have an overactive or underactive thyroid.

● **Insulin-dependent (type 1) diabetes.**

● **A tendency toward left-handedness.** For unknown reasons, left-handed people seem to be predisposed to thyroid trouble.

● **Pernicious anemia.**

● **Spots on the skin lacking pigmentation known as vitiligo,** a thyroid-related immune disorder.

Important: A diagnosis of hypothyroidism should always be confirmed by a TSH test.

TREATING HYPOTHYROIDISM

Hypothyroidism is easily corrected by taking a daily tablet of T4 (from which the body can make T3). This treatment, taken indefinitely, can be prescribed by your regular doctor.

Most people with hypothyroidism feel well after two to three months of taking the pills.

Your doctor will probably start you on a low dose of thyroid hormone and check your TSH levels every few weeks until the proper dosage is found.

Dosing requirements can change, so have your TSH levels checked about once a year.

Caution: Thyroid pills should not be taken with iron supplements. Iron blocks the absorption of thyroid hormone.

OVERACTIVE THYROID

Low levels of TSH generally mean hyperthyroidism. This condition can occasionally be caused by inflammation of the gland or too much iodine in the diet. But the most common cause is a hereditary condition known as Graves' disease.

Graves' usually strikes between age 20 and 40. Signs include swelling of the thyroid, weight loss, anxiety, hair loss, muscle weakness and a rapid heartbeat.

If you're diagnosed with Graves', your doctor will probably refer you to an endocrinologist for additional testing and treatment.

THYROID LUMPS AND TUMORS

About one of every 25 people has one or more small nodules in their thyroid gland.

If a nodule is detected, your doctor should evaluate it further. Tests may include a TSH level, imaging studies (an ultrasound or a radioactive thyroid scan) and a thyroid biopsy.

Nodules that prove to be cancerous should be surgically removed. Surgery is often combined with radioactive iodine, thyroid supplements and X rays or chemotherapy. Most cases of thyroid cancer can be cured via these means.

Daytime Sleepiness And Narcolepsy

Michael Thorpy, MD, director of the Sleep–Wake Disorders Center at Montefiore Medical Center, Bronx, NY, and director of the National Narcolepsy Registry.

Do you find yourself nodding off several times a day? If so, you may be one of the hundreds of thousands of Americans who suffer from narcolepsy.

Narcolepsy usually starts around puberty. It's thought to be largely hereditary, although in many cases it shows up only after it's been triggered by a head injury, an intensely emotional experience or another event.

Narcolepsy symptoms start subtly and become more pronounced with time. The disorder is typically diagnosed about 10 years after symptoms first appear.

Telltale symptoms: Excessive daytime sleepiness and an uncontrollable urge to sleep.

Narcoleptics *know* they're about to fall asleep—they don't typically black out in mid-sentence—but can do nothing to keep from doing so.

THREE RELATED DISORDERS

Many people who suffer from narcolepsy also suffer from one or more related disorders...

●**Cataplexy.** This form of sudden muscle weakness is brought on by strong emotions. You might begin to argue with your spouse, for instance, only to have your head droop uncontrollably and your knees weaken.

●**Sleep paralysis.** This frightening phenomenon is marked by an inability to move the body after awakening in the morning.

Episodes of sleep paralysis can last anywhere from a few seconds to several minutes.

●**Hypnagogic hallucinations.** These unusually vivid dreams occur at the very onset of sleep.

Hypnagogic hallucinations come about when a person goes immediately from wakefulness to *rapid eye movement* (REM) sleep without first progressing through lighter stages of sleep.

GETTING HELP

If you think you have narcolepsy, organize your day so that you can take short, frequent naps (less than 20 minutes). To avoid accidents, always take a brief rest before driving or operating dangerous equipment.

Avoid alcohol and caffeine. Alcohol won't prevent sleepiness, and it can cause you to wake up late at night. Caffeine is simply not potent enough to keep you awake.

If these simple remedies don't help, consult a board-certified sleep specialist. He/she may ask that you spend a night in a sleep disorders center, where the type, depth and quality of your sleep can be measured.

For referral to sleep specialists in your area, contact the American Academy of Sleep Medicine at 708-492-0930, *www.aasmnet.org.*

HELPFUL MEDICATIONS

The newest medication for narcolepsy is *modafinil* (Provigil). It has been approved to treat people with sleep apnea and shift-work sleep disorders.

●**Stimulants.** *Pemoline* (Cylert), *methylphenidate* (Ritalin), *dextroamphetamine* (Dexedrine) and related drugs simply help you stay awake.

Although stimulants are quite effective at controlling drowsiness, they can have side effects, such as anxiety, headaches, insomnia and increases in heart rate and blood pressure.

●**Antidepressants.** Drugs like *protriptyline* (Vivactil) and *fluoxetine* (Prozac) fight cataplexy. Protriptyline can cause dizziness, dry mouth and sexual dysfunction. Fluoxetine can cause insomnia and sexual dysfunction.

●**Sleeping medications.** *Clonazepam* (Klonopin) and *zolpidem* (Ambien) improve nighttime sleep. However, clonazepam is addicting and can cause daytime drowsiness.

Zolpidem is nonaddicting, but it can cause daytime sleepiness, nausea and headache.

NATIONAL NARCOLEPSY REGISTRY

To learn more about narcolepsy and/or to add your name to the National Narcolepsy Registry, contact the National Sleep Foundation, 1522 K St. NW, Suite 500, Washington, DC 20005, 202-347-3471.

Web site: *www.sleepfoundation.org.*

E-mail: *nsf@sleepfoundation.org.*

17

Weight Success

The 10 Secrets of Successful Weight Loss

Anne M. Fletcher, MS, RD

If you're trying to lose weight, it's easy to be discouraged by the experts. Doctors and dietitians routinely cite pessimistic figures like the notorious "95% failure rate." According to this statistic, 95% of all dieters gain their weight back—and then some.

The truth about weight loss may not be nearly so dire. A survey by *Consumer Reports* found that one in four readers who used commercial diet programs had kept off at least two-thirds of the weight they had lost.

Twenty-five percent is still a lower success rate than most of us would like. But instead of focusing on dieting failures, I decided to look at what's different about people who *don't* gain weight back.

I consulted the experts who *really* matter—160 people, each of whom had lost at least 20 pounds (average weight loss for this group turned out to be 63 pounds) and who had kept the weight off for at least three years.

It turned out that there were 10 common threads among these "successful losers"…

1. They believed they could do it. Most of the people I surveyed had lost and regained their weight at least five times before successfully keeping it off. But they didn't give up.

The turning point for many of them came when they realized they were sick and tired of the weight-loss battle. Instead of using this feeling as an excuse to stop trying to lose weight, however, the successful dieters somehow felt empowered by it. The feeling made them resolve to take control.

2. They lost weight for themselves—not someone else. All her life, one young woman I interviewed had been told by her mother (and everyone else), "You have such a pretty face—if only you'd lose some weight!"

Anne M. Fletcher, MS, RD, author of *Eating Thin for Life: Food Secrets & Recipes from People Who Have Lost Weight & Kept It Off*. Houghton Mifflin.

327

She lost and gained weight repeatedly. Inside, she was angry that people didn't accept her the way she was. By the time she entered college, she weighed more than 200 pounds. But it was there that she met a man who loved her that way.

Ironically, because she finally felt accepted, she was able to lose weight once and for all—for her own sake.

3. They found out what worked for them. About half the people I talked to lost weight on their own. Others used a commercial diet center or a self-help group...or consulted privately with a dietitian.

In addition, successful people learned to accept a target weight that was realistic for them. This goal might be slightly above their ideal weight, but they knew they could go no lower without starving themselves.

4. They were willing to learn a new way of eating—for life. Many dieters go back to their old eating habits once they lose weight. That's why most dieters regain weight.

The weight-control masters accepted low-fat eating as a *way of life.* They learned to enjoy fruits, vegetables and grains. They found ways to add low-calorie flavor by using spices, lemon or lime juice and low-fat products. Gradually, they noticed that they didn't feel good when they ate high-fat foods.

5. They deal with slipups immediately. While they aren't obsessed with the scale, most weigh themselves once a week to once every few days. They have a narrow window of acceptable weight regain (typically five to 10 pounds). When their weight exceeds this "buffer zone," they do what's necessary to lose it.

Some people exercise more. Others cut back on sweets...pay closer attention to portion sizes...or keep a food diary to increase their awareness of what they eat. But each person I talked to had a plan of action—and used it before the weight gain could get out of hand.

6. They say nice things to themselves. Negative self-talk can be self-fulfilling. An example is the "now-I've-blown-it" phenomenon

that's familiar to many of us: *I ate one cookie. I'm a pig. I might as well eat the whole bag.*

The weight-loss masters give themselves positive and encouraging messages even when they make mistakes: *I resolved not to eat two helpings, but I slipped. I'll be more careful the rest of the day.*

7. They exercise. Nine out of 10 of the successful people I interviewed exercise regularly. They aren't fanatics, and few of them work out every day. But they've managed to find simple activities like walking that they can work into their daily routine.

8. They face their feelings. Back when they were overweight, many of the people I spoke to automatically turned to food whenever they felt upset, bored, lonely or anxious.

What they learned to do instead was get to the source of the negative emotion—by noticing the feeling, identifying the cause and figuring out a way to solve the problem.

Many of their solutions are quite simple. When bored, they leave the house and do something fun. When lonely, they call a friend. When angry, they confront the person who's mistreating them.

9. They enjoy life. A number of the now-successful people used to spend so much energy taking care of others that they neglected their own needs. Eating was their only reward.

Some people who kept weight off have developed what I call a "healthy selfishness." They're still considerate of others, but they take care of themselves, too.

As one woman put it, *I found that when my own needs were met, I was better at meeting the needs of others.*

They've also found ways to reward themselves without food—from pursuing a hobby to seeking more satisfying relationships.

10. They get support. They ask their families not to leave junk food laying around...call a buddy when they're tempted to overeat... and request encouragement and pep talks from friends and family.

Beer Drinkers Really Do Have Bigger Bellies

Bruce B. Duncan, MD, PhD, an epidemiologist at the Federal University of Rio Grande do Sul, Porto Alegre, Brazil. His study of the drinking habits of more than 12,000 adults was published in the *American Journal of Epidemiology*, 111 Market Pl., Suite 840, Baltimore 21202.

Compared with both nondrinkers and those who drink an equivalent amount of alcohol in wine, adults who drink six beers a week are rounder around the middle. *Danger:* Potbellies have been linked to increased risk of heart disease.

Why Diets Fail

Steven A. Lamm, MD, clinical assistant professor of medicine at New York University School of Medicine in New York. He is author of *Thinner at Last*. Fireside.

One out of three Americans is overweight, ranging from a few pounds to obese. Most of these people have been on numerous types of diets—many of which have failed.

Here's why dieting no longer makes sense—and new thinking about effective weight loss…

WHY DIETING FAILS

When you diet, your brain—in an act of self-defense against perceived starvation—signals your body that you need more food…and lowers your metabolism so you store more fat. Both actions make it harder to reach your dieting goals.

With each repeated cycle of dieting, it takes longer to lose weight and it comes back quicker. What's more, you are likely to accumulate extra pounds each time.

Important: Taking off weight isn't the main problem—keeping it off is. Despite the best nutrition, exercise regimens and diet plans in the world, 90% of dieters regain one- to two-thirds of lost weight within one year and almost all of it within five years.

Getting out of the diet mode requires that you accept that obesity is a complex medical problem that requires a multipronged solution, including possible drug intervention. Being very overweight is not a result of a lack of willpower or discipline, so stop blaming yourself for your size and deluding yourself that you won't wake up hungry tomorrow. You will, because your brain sabotages your best efforts at psychological control and makes it impossible to resist cravings.

Also recognize that constant dieting can perpetuate your weight problem by adversely affecting your metabolism.

Important: A chronic overweight problem can only be managed, never cured. To keep your weight in "remission," you must be constantly vigilant, eating healthfully and exercising regularly.

A HEALTHY EATING PLAN

Here's how to start on a healthy eating plan for life…

●**Stop obsessing over your weight and your appetite.** Rather than keeping you "in control," mental preoccupation with dieting is practically guaranteed to keep you overweight because you're constantly thinking of food.

●**Adhere to the following eating guidelines** developed by the Department of Agriculture…

●**Eat 20% of your calories from protein sources, 20% from fat and 60% from carbohydrates.** People with a weight problem should reduce their carbohydrate intake to about 40% and increase protein intake to 40%.

●**Cut back on foods that are high in saturated fats,** including potato chips, ice cream and red meat. They aren't good for you and seem to spark primitive hunger urges.

●**Decrease your intake of simple carbohydrates**—sugars. Instead, concentrate on eating more complex carbohydrates—breads, rice, pasta, potatoes, fruits and vegetables—which will give you energy and make you feel full.

●**Don't skip meals.** Not eating at regular intervals is a foolproof way to get fat—it convinces your body you're starving and need to conserve fat.

●**Don't eat less than 1,200 calories a day.**
When you go on such a low-calorie diet, your body starts to break down muscle tissue to use for energy so it doesn't have to dip into its fat stores. You lose weight, but you lose muscle as well as fat, which means that after your diet you'll end up with a higher percentage of body fat to muscle mass. That will make your metabolism work even slower.

●**Start or continue an exercise program.**
Ideal: Engage in aerobic activity—walking, running, swimming or bicycling—for an hour three times a week. *Second best:* Exercise moderately for 30 minutes five times a week.

To build muscle and offset muscle loss brought on by dieting, also engage in resistance training—using free weights or weight machines—twice a week. Weight training can speed your loss of fat, help you ward off osteoporosis as you age and enhance your endurance.

Important: Unless you are willing to exercise regularly, you will not succeed in keeping weight off.

FINDING A PHYSICIAN

Discuss drug treatment for obesity with your primary care doctor. If your doctor won't prescribe drugs for you, ask for a referral to an obesity specialist. Or contact the American Society of Bariatric Physicians (877-266-6834), *www.asbp.org* for the name of a doctor who prescribes medication as part of a comprehensive weight-control program. Approximately 60% of physicians today offer such a program.

Wonderful Ways to Keep Weight Off Once You've Lost It

Joyce D. Nash, PhD, a clinical psychologist in Menlo Park, CA. She is author of several books on behavioral medicine, including *Now That You've Lost It.* iUniverse.

It's a lot easier to lose weight than it is to keep off the excess pounds. When you are trying to lose weight, you're singularly focused on the task at hand. But once you're down to your target weight, you have to balance weight maintenance with other factors in your life.

On a daily basis, that requires you to continually correct yourself and bring yourself back on course.

Weight management is a journey rather than a destination.

PSYCHOLOGY OF WEIGHT MAINTENANCE

Positive thinking patterns are crucial to successful, long-term weight management. *People who are not successful at managing their weight tend to...*

●**Make excuses** that let them overeat or not exercise.

●**Focus narrowly on the pleasure of eating** and forget their weight-management goals.

●**Doubt their ability to change.**

●**Set unrealistic expectations** for themselves or others.

●**Judge themselves—and other people—harshly.**

In contrast, those people who are successful tend to...

●**Remind themselves of their long-range goals.**

●**Notice even small successes** in weight management.

●**Use positive self-talk** to keep themselves on the right track.

STRATEGIES FOR WEIGHT MAINTENANCE

●**Make exercise a regular part of your life.** Without regular exercise, weight maintenance is exceedingly difficult.

Of course, making exercise a part of your daily routine is easier said than done. I recommend you choose a range of activities that you enjoy and can turn to when you're in different moods—or confronted by bad weather.

Example: I walk outside for an hour a day. On days when it rains, I cycle on a stationary bicycle indoors.

●**Reduce fat calories to 30% of your daily intake.** Most Americans eat more fat than they need. We're exposed to a lot of fatty, highly palatable foods, so we develop a taste for foods that are readily available. However, you can change your taste buds and actually learn to prefer low-fat foods.

Strategy: Start small. Eat bread without butter, salad with little or no dressing and chicken without its skin.

Bonus: After consuming low-fat foods for a while, you'll find that eating fatty foods makes you feel physically and psychologically uncomfortable…bloated, sluggish, even nauseous.

• **Control binges.** Between 25% and 50% of all people who attend weight-management programs are bingers. The biggest trigger for binges is negative emotions—anger…depression…anxiety.

Strategy: Keep a two-week journal to record your eating behaviors—meals, snacks, binges. Also record the circumstances—how you feel, what you are doing and your thoughts when you are eating. This will help you identify triggers for eating and develop strategies to avoid them.

Example: I recently treated a female patient who often felt angry and responded to her negative emotions by bingeing. Once she identified her anger as a trigger for excessive eating, she was able to examine her anger cycle and pick and choose which battles to fight and when to let the anger pass away. She also learned to express her anger—by confronting the person who had precipitated the anger in her, for instance—in ways other than eating.

• **Eat moderately.** To successfully maintain a low weight level, you must keep your caloric intake under control.

Strategy: Eat anything you want, but keep your calories in a moderate range. The government recommends between 1,600 and 2,800 calories each day to maintain weight for most adult men and women. However, your best range for maintaining weight will depend on your age, sex, lifestyle, activity level and other factors. Experiment with adding on and taking off calories to find the range that's best for you.

• **Think smart.** Focus on your long-term goal of weight maintenance, give yourself instructional thoughts and pat yourself on the back for positive behaviors.

Mistake: At the office, a coworker is passing around slices of cake. As a slice comes your way, you see only the cake, not your goal. You rationalize, telling yourself that you've been good for weeks and you shouldn't be deprived when everyone else is eating it.

Better: As a slice comes your way, remind yourself that you've worked hard to lose weight, you feel great and you want to keep the weight off. You tell yourself that the momentary pleasure of the cake isn't in your best interest. You decline the cake. As your coworker moves on to someone else, you feel good about yourself and congratulate yourself for forgoing temptation.

• **Handle lapses.** Everyone backslides on occasion.

Strategy: Avoid turning a lapse into a relapse. Instead of having a second donut, go to the gym to burn off the calories or cut back on calorie intake tomorrow.

• **Create a lifestyle that is satisfying to you.** The last thing you want to say at the end of your life is that you devoted the majority of your life to watching your weight. While weight maintenance is important to health and psychological well-being, your life should be about something more meaningful.

Create a mission that makes you feel your life is worth living. Find a way to be creative, contribute to society or do something that's important to you.

Maximize Your Gardening "Workout"

Jeffrey Restuccio, author of *Fitness the Dynamic Gardening Way*. Balance of Nature Publishing.

Heavy digging, raking, laying sod, turning compost and other garden chores burn 300 to 400 calories an hour.

To burn even more: Use hand tools, such as an old-fashioned push mower instead of a power mower, a rake instead of a leaf blower …wear wrist and ankle weights to increase calories burned…split tasks into 30-minute segments so you'll get a good workout each day.

Caution: Don't overdo it.

Metabolism Slows With Age

Johanna Dwyer, DSc, RD, director, Frances Stern Nutrition Center, New England Medical Center, Boston.

Metabolism slows with age—beginning as early as age 35.

Result: Weight gain simply from continuing to eat as you did when you were younger.

Self-defense: Weight training and regular aerobic exercise to increase muscle mass and keep your metabolism running more quickly. *Also:* Consume foods that are full of nutrients but low in calories—drink vegetable juice instead of soda, eat multigrain bread instead of white. You can continue eating most of your favorite foods—just reduce the portion sizes.

Dieting for People Who Have Trouble Dieting

Louis J. Aronne, MD, director of New York Hospital's Comprehensive Weight Control Center. He is author of Weigh Less, Live Longer. *Wiley.*

If you're like most people, you have probably tried all the weight-control approaches—but haven't been successful in losing all the weight you want...or keeping it off.

WHY WE OVEREAT

One of the major reasons you're overweight may be that you can't control your urge to eat. Food cravings are a result of a chemical imbalance in the brain. They start in the hypothalamus, the brain's hunger center, which sends out chemical messengers—*neurotransmitters*—to tell you when, how much and what to eat.

Although it sounds very simple—some neurotransmitters say eat...others say stop eating—the delicate balance between messengers can easily be disturbed.

Add to that the unlimited amounts of food available everywhere today and the fact that you don't have to physically exert yourself to get food, and you've got a setup for out-of-control eating.

HOW TO CONTROL FOOD URGES

To fight your cravings, you must learn how to curb the levels of neurotransmitters the brain sends out. The only way to stifle your urge to eat now is to change your exercise and eating patterns. *Here's how...*

•**Keep a weight-control journal for one month.** Research has shown we don't know how much we really eat in a day—sometimes we underestimate by as much as 75%.

Helpful: Buy a small notebook that you can carry with you everywhere. Each time you eat or drink something, write down what it was, how much you consumed, when and where, what you were doing before and how you felt while eating.

Reason: If you use the journal every day—all day—you'll identify hidden food traps in your routine...determine if stress prompts you to eat...discover the types of foods that trigger you to overeat...learn how exercise affects your appetite.

•**Start an exercise program.** You've heard it over and over again, but exercise is truly the key to weight-control success.

Build exercise into your everyday life—climb the stairs instead of taking the escalator...walk to the corner store instead of taking the car...park far away from the mall so you'll have farther to walk.

Engage in up to an hour of aerobic exercise—walking, running, biking—and resistance exercise—calisthenics or weight training—at least three times a week.

Example: Do 10 minutes of aerobic activity mixed in with resistance training three times a day...or 30 minutes once a day. Studies show that both ways are equally beneficial for people who are just starting to exercise.

If you're already someone who works out regularly but wants to burn more calories, vary the intensity of your workout.

Example: Set the treadmill so that you walk up hills of different heights, followed by flat surfaces.

- **Learn about the components of a nutritionally balanced diet.** *The government recommends that adults eat the following daily…*

  - **Six to 11 servings of pasta, cereal, rice and bread.** *Example:* One serving equals a half cup of pasta.

  - **Three to five servings of vegetables.** *Example:* One serving equals a half cup.

  - **Two to four servings of fruits.** *Example:* One serving equals one banana.

  - **Two to three servings of dairy products.** *Example:* One serving equals eight ounces of milk.

  - **Two to three servings of meat, poultry, fish and eggs.** *Example:* One serving equals two to three ounces.

  - **Sparing amounts of fats, oils and sweets.**

Exception: If you suffer from *insulin resistance*—a condition where the body must produce increasingly large amounts of insulin to maintain blood-sugar levels—moderate your intake of cereal, bread, pasta and other carbohydrates. Instead, follow a slightly higher-protein, lower-carbohydrate diet than the government recommends.

Reason: You actually crave carbohydrates, but carbohydrates make you eat more because they quickly raise and then lower your insulin levels. Your body thinks your blood-sugar level will drop too much and sends out a signal requesting more food.

You can find out if you are insulin-resistant—a quarter of the population is—by keeping your weight journal and tracking your response to carbohydrates. Or you can talk to your doctor about it.

- **Don't skip meals or severely limit your food intake.** This prompts your brain to produce more *neuropeptides*, which trigger a gnawing desire for carbohydrates.

If you ignore the urge, your brain dispatches another chemical, called *galanin*, which instructs your body to eat and store fat. Together, the two produce irresistible cravings.

- **Be prepared for cravings as you change to a healthier diet.** The good news is that the cravings will fade.

Helpful: Satisfy cravings for carbohydrates by eating small amounts of food—a small piece of fruit, a pretzel.

Manage your cravings for sweets by eating a small portion of a nonfat product, such as a graham cracker or a hard candy. Large portions may have lots of calories, so beware. If you must have chocolate, eat a few chocolate kisses.

- **Control stress.** When you are under pressure, your body produces *cortisol*—a hormone that tells your body to put out more neuropeptides and galanin. As a result, you crave carbohydrates and fats.

Helpful: While you can't eliminate stress entirely, you can learn to control it. Find the best stress-buster for you—exercise…practice deep-breathing or meditation…perform muscle relax-and-release exercises…take a warm bath…read a book…or listen to music.

For some people, stress reduction actually suppresses the appetite by decreasing levels of certain compounds in the body that can spur weight gain.

Surprising Calorie-Burner

Harold Bloomfield, MD, a leading psychological educator, and coauthor of *The Power of 5.* Rodale.

Sipping ice water burns calories. Whenever you drink something cold, your body raises your metabolism to keep your body temperature from falling. That process burns calories—eight 16-ounce glasses of ice water will burn an extra 200 calories per day.

The Fat Bank

50 Essential Things to Do When the Doctor Says It's Heart Disease by Fredric Pashkow, MD, medical director of the Queens Medical Center Heart Institute in Honolulu. Hyperion.

Use "fat banking" to maintain a healthful diet without feeling as if you can never have fatty foods. Look at calorie and fat allotments as balances in a bank account. You can draw on them as you would from a bank. If you know you will want a high-fat food on a certain day, you can "build up your bank balance" by cutting your fat intake for some days before…or reducing fat intake afterward to bring your account back into balance.

Also helpful: When eating a meal containing high-fat food, eat a small amount of that food and balance it with low-fat choices—lots of vegetables, or fruit for dessert.

Simple Secrets of Permanent Weight Loss

Kathleen Thompson, coauthor of *Feeding on Dreams: Why America's Diet Industry Doesn't Work & What Will Work for You.* HarperCollins.

Each year, Americans spend $33 billion on commercial diet programs—and much of that sum is essentially wasted.

Reason: The premise on which these programs are based—cut calories and lose weight—is at least 20 years out-of-date. In study after study, it has been thoroughly discredited.

Weight loss isn't that simple. The hard part isn't losing weight, but keeping it off. Unless you're willing to eat frozen dinners and drink low-cal shakes for the rest of your life, that is almost impossible on most of the commercial weight-loss programs.

Not surprising, then, that many dieters shuffle unsuccessfully from one diet plan to the next—losing weight on one program, putting it back on and then moving on to another plan.

In fact, counselors working for the leading commercial diet plans freely admit that perhaps nine of 10 people who try one commercial diet program wind up trying two or three…or more.

WEIGHT-LOSS PRINCIPLES

How do you take weight off and keep it off—once and for all? *There are three fundamental principles for effective and lasting weight loss…*

Principle #1: Take control of your life and your weight. Turning responsibility for what you eat and what you do over to anyone else is deadly. You must design a program for yourself. You also must open your life to self-inspection.

Often, eating is a survival skill. It's a way of coping with frustrations and disappointments. Life can be very difficult. Eating can get you through it.

Overeating becomes a way to maintain emotional health—although physical health is jeopardized as a result.

To overcome this self-destructive approach to food, you must learn to separate food itself from its emotional symbolism. You may need the help of a psychologist specializing in weight problems.

For referrals to a psychologist in your area, contact the National Association of Anorexia Nervosa and Associated Disorders, Box 7, Highland Park, IL 60035, 847-831-3438, *www.anad.org.*

Principle #2: Accept your body. Focus not on how your body looks, but on what it enables you to do. Don't compare yourself with the ideal body put forth in sexy movies or magazine ads. After all, body shape is determined largely by heredity. We tend to look like our mothers and fathers—and that persists even if we're successful at losing weight.

Principle #3: Make food a pleasure. Avoid thinking of food as a moral issue. "Good" foods are those you think you should be eating—fruits, vegetables, beans, pasta, etc. "Bad" foods taste good but are fattening—cakes, candy, sugary soft drinks, etc.

Substituting good foods for bad *sounds* like a good idea, but odds are it's just setting you up for failure. *Problem:* Even if you could steer clear of "bad" foods for several months, you'd give in to temptation—possibly by going on an eating binge.

Better way: If you like cheesecake, allow yourself the freedom to eat it on occasion. By removing this cheesecake "taboo," you reduce your obsession with it.

DIETING VS. YOUR SET POINT

The only way to ensure lasting weight loss is to lower your set point—the weight your body "thinks" it should weigh. When people overeat, they generally gain weight only temporarily, returning to their usual weight, or "set point" when they resume their previous eating habits.

Similarly, when you go on a low-calorie diet, your body wants to keep you from starving. As a result, your metabolism slows to maintain your set point. *Result:* Weight loss occurs very slowly. When you resume your normal eating patterns, your weight quickly rises to its former level.

To lower your set point, reduce your intake of dietary fat and increase your lean muscle mass. In other words, lighten up your eating habits and exercise enough to build muscle.

CUTTING OUT DIETARY FAT

●**Start small.** You're not going on a diet, you're changing the way you eat for the rest of your life. So there's no need to cut out dietary fat all at once.

You might start by switching to milk instead of cream in your coffee, then switching to low-fat mayonnaise on your sandwiches, etc.

●**Eat what you like.** If you already enjoy certain low-fat foods, make them staples of your diet. Make a list of your favorite high-fat foods, and find a way to substitute low-fat versions for some of them.

●**Keep track of your fat intake.** Buy a nutritional guide that lists the fat content of each food. Use it to calculate how many grams of fat you consume each day.

The maximum number of grams of fat you can eat each day and still lose weight is determined by your age, sex and medical condition, among other things.

A woman over 30 should probably consume no more than 20% of her calories in the form of fat. A man over 30 can probably get away with up to 25%. (One gram of fat equals about nine calories.)

●**Make sure the whole family adopts healthful eating habits.** If your spouse has an ice cream sundae for dessert, you probably won't feel satisfied with a pear. But if everyone in the family starts eating healthfully, there's less temptation.

THE IMPORTANCE OF EXERCISE

The more you exercise, the more muscle you build. And because muscle cells burn dietary fat more efficiently than fat cells do, gaining muscle mass speeds your metabolism. *Payoff:* A thin person can eat much more fat than a fat person without gaining weight.

If you've been inactive for a long time, begin by exercising just five or 10 minutes a day. Gradually build until you're exercising at least 20 minutes a day, three to four days a week.

The point is to do what you like. Otherwise, you'll quickly give up exercising. If you used to play a lot of volleyball or softball, for example, try to work these activities back into your schedule. If you're joining a gym, look for one where you feel comfortable. One reason people stop going to the gym is that they feel they don't measure up. If you feel intimidated by a fancy club, try the local "Y" instead.

Consider hiring a personal trainer. If you can't afford one, pool your money with a few friends and hire a trainer to come to one of your homes. Invest in headphones and a few good exercise tapes.

Free Yourself from Food Cravings

Elizabeth Somer, MA, RD, author of *Food and Mood.* Holt. She is editor-in-chief of *Nutrition Alert*, Nutrition Communications, 4742 Liberty Rd. S, Suite 148, Salem, OR 97302.

Here are some simple ways to rid yourself of food cravings...

●**If you crave something sweet,** eat a bagel with low-sugar jam instead of candy.

●**Make gradual changes in your diet**—not abrupt ones, which can upset mood-altering brain chemicals.

●**Eat regularly**—not skipping breakfast. *Helpful:* Eat smaller amounts more often.

●**Take a daily multivitamin** containing minerals, too.

●**Drink at least six glasses of water** every day.

Body Shape and Health Risk

Stephen P. Gullo, PhD, president, Institute for Health and Weight Sciences, New York City, and author of *Thin Tastes Better*. Dell.

Extra weight at your waist increases risk of heart attack, high blood pressure, stroke and diabetes—but extra weight centered on the hips and thighs may not.

To check out your "body shape risk," measure your waist at its narrowest point, and your hips (over your buttocks) at their widest point. Divide the inches measured at your waist by those measured at your hips.

An increase in health risks are related to a ratio that's greater than 1.0 for men, and 0.8 for women.

A Diet for Life

James Merker, MPA, CAE, executive director, American Society of Bariatric Physicians, Englewood, CO.

Don't start a diet simply to meet some short-term weight goal.

Example: Trying to drop a few dress sizes in time for a special party.

Problem: Pounds that are shed quickly are likely to return just as fast—if not faster.

Better: Focus on long-term, permanent weight control, which requires a similar long-term, permanent change in lifestyle.

Vegetarian Diets: Results Last Longer

Neal D. Barnard, MD, president, Physician's Committee for Responsible Medicine, 5100 Wisconsin Ave. NW, Suite 40, Washington, DC 20016. A physician and psychiatrist, he is also author of *Eat Right, Live Longer*. Three Rivers.

Totally vegetarian diets are best at successfully modifying eating habits in a way that produces lasting results.

Mistake: Many doctors recommend moderate diets because they believe patients will cheat on strict diets or give up on them entirely. But research shows dieters are *more* likely to follow strict diets than moderate ones.

Reasons: The diet regime is clear-cut, so cheating can't be rationalized. And...strict diets bring faster results—and with them the vital positive reinforcement of visible success.

Do Your Feet Hurt?

Carol Frey, MD, orthopedic surgeon, University of Southern California Foot & Ankle Clinic, Los Angeles, and author of a five-year study of 580 women.

As weight increases, feet grow larger and a person is more likely to have foot and ankle trouble.

Example: Overweight women were three times as likely to have ankle pain as women of normal weight.

Lose Weight—Even While You're Sleeping

Keli Roberts, a personal trainer in Los Angeles and author of *Keli Roberts' Fitness Hollywood*. Summit Publishing Group.

To lose weight...lift weights. The number of calories burned in any one weight-lifting workout is not very high—but a person with more muscle mass uses up more calories *all the time*, even while sleeping.

In one study, one group of people exercised aerobically three times a week for 30 minutes, while another split the sessions between aerobics and strength training. The aerobics group members lost four pounds during the study, but people who added strength training lost 10 pounds...*and* gained muscle mass.

Diet Doctors' Weight-Loss Secrets...and How They Keep Weight Off

Mary Dan Eades, MD, an internist specializing in weight loss and metabolic medicine. She is in private practice, with her husband, Michael Eades, MD, in Little Rock, AR...Stephen Gullo, PhD, president of the Institute for Health and Weight Sciences in New York City, and author of *Thin Tastes Better*. Dell...John McDougall, MD, founder and director of The McDougall Program in Santa Rosa, CA.

The secret to looking and feeling younger than your years is following a nutritious diet and exercising regularly. But there are many different strategies for battling everyday temptation and staying slim. *We asked three top diet doctors how they do it...*

MARY DAN EADES, MD

My diet is focused on getting the correct balance of foods so that metabolic hormones, particularly insulin, help the body use nutrients as they should. As a result, I consume moderate amounts of protein and fat, and I'm selective about the carbohydrates I eat.

Today I weigh 135 pounds and stand five feet, five inches tall—with less than 24% body fat.

●**I eat adequate amounts of protein.** Protein is the most essential food that the body needs to survive. I eat at least 10 to 12 ounces of protein each day when I am trying to lose or maintain my weight.

I get the protein in the form of lean red meat, fish, poultry, low-fat cheese, eggs and tofu. By eating protein in correct proportion to other dietary components, I am able to burn the incoming fat as fuel for energy rather than store it—as would be the case if I were eating a lot of protein-rich foods and not enough of the other types.

●**I select my carbohydrates carefully.** I keep my carbohydrate intake to a minimum—about 60 to 80 grams daily because of their adverse impact on insulin—especially starchier sources and refined carbohydrates. I primarily get those carbohydrates from a wide variety of fruits and vegetables that pack a big vitamin punch.

●**I take a daily multivitamin supplement** to ensure I'm getting all of the nutrients I might otherwise miss.

●**I exercise regularly.** I practice kung fu—a high-impact aerobic and resistance training regimen—four times a week for one hour. Or, if I can't get to kung fu class, I run and work out with weights.

STEPHEN GULLO, PhD

Living a very busy lifestyle surrounded by fine foods, I frequently find myself tempted to overeat. Obesity runs in my family, and I have the same weight-control problems as my patients. If I'm not careful about what I eat, I can easily add eight to 10 pounds to my 5'11", 168-pound frame. I'm especially prone to weight gain around the abdomen. And that is particularly unhealthful.

Pizza is my downfall. Just one slice can cause me to experience continuing cravings for more pizza, bread and other flour products for weeks. *To cap my craving for pizza, I try to minimize my trigger-food problem by "boxing it in"...*

●**Limiting** the quantity I eat.

●**Controlling** how often I eat it.

●**Avoiding** all the locations at which I usually am inclined to eat this particular food.

If self-control doesn't work, I "box it out"—temporarily banish pizza from my diet. It's hard at first, but eventually I stop craving the food. If I find myself thinking about it, I use diversion. Some activity that diverts the mind usually turns off the craving almost instantly.

To avoid temptation, I follow a few basic guidelines...

●**Shop carefully at the supermarket,** since that's where most weight problems begin. I avoid shopping in the late afternoon or right after work, when blood sugar plummets and we're prone to impulsive food purchases. Before I put any product in my shopping cart, I ask myself, *Is this a food I have* *a history of abusing?* If it is, I put it back on the shelf.

•When traveling, I don't accept hotel mini-bar keys. I also ask the maid not to leave cookies or candy on my pillow. Availability creates craving.

•Never show up at a restaurant hungry. It is easy to attack the bread basket. Instead, I eat sugar-free Jell-O, nonfat yogurt, nonfat soup or fruit before dining out. Sometimes before a meal I have cold tomato juice, which is a natural appetite suppressant.

•Exercise regularly. I jog or put in time on the "strength trainer" NordicTrack for 45 minutes two to three times a week and do additional strength training. This helps me burn 10% to 15% more calories than I would normally.

•Take supplements. I believe in the importance of vitamins and antioxidants. Every day, I take vitamin E (400 international units [IU]), vitamin C (500 milligrams [mg] in the morning and 500 mg at night), folate (400 mg), selenium (100 mg) and a baby aspirin.*

•Use cognitive-switching techniques. This involves replacing negative food thoughts with healthy ones.

Example: Instead of saying, *I'll have just one slice of pizza* (which is not true to my history with this particular food), I tell myself that the craving I'm feeling is only temporary...the desire will pass...and that as much as I want a slice of pizza at that instant, I want to be healthy and in control of my life.

JOHN McDOUGALL, MD

At age 22, I weighed 220 pounds and stood six feet, one inch tall. Today, I'm 49 and I weigh 175 pounds. I'm a vegetarian who relies on the starch-based diet followed by the people from China, Japan and the Middle East.

In these cultures, people have lower levels of obesity, heart disease, breast cancer and other health problems than do those who follow the typical high-fat American diet. *Here's what I do...*

*Consult your doctor for the amounts that are appropriate for you.

•I eat minimal amounts of protein and fat. As a vegetarian, I don't eat meat, fish, poultry or dairy products. I believe they lead to medical problems. I get all the protein I need from vegetable sources. I also avoid vegetable oils, margarine and shortenings as well as refined and simple sugars.

•I eat mostly carbohydrates. My diet consists largely of whole grains (such as breads, pasta and rice)...root vegetables (potatoes, sweet potatoes, yams, turnips, parsnips)...beans, peas and lentils...and green and yellow vegetables. I can eat these foods until I've satisfied my hunger. I eat limited amounts of fruits (because they can be high in sugar and calories) and limited amounts of low-fat dressings and sauces.

•I don't take vitamin supplements because I get all the nutrients I need from my diet. While I don't eat dairy products, I get sufficient calcium from potatoes, rice, corn and other vegetables that contain the mineral.

•I exercise moderately. Luckily, my low-fat diet doesn't call for intensive activity to maintain my weight. I try to be physically active in my routine. I downhill ski in winter and swim, windsurf and walk in summer. I also work out with weights with a personal trainer one hour each week year-round...although I wish I had time to do more.

Calorie Buster

Pietro Tonino, MD, director, division of sports medicine, Loyola University Medical Center, Maywood, IL.

Running on a treadmill burns more calories than using any of five other common exercise machines. Exercisers who ran on a treadmill burned about 700 calories per hour, compared with those who used a stair machine (627 calories per hour)...rower (606)...cross-country ski machine (595)...stationary bike with arm motion (509)...and standard stationary bike (498).

The Real Reason It's So Hard to Lose Weight

The late Albert Ellis, PhD, creator of rational emotive behavior therapy and author or coauthor of more than 700 papers and books, including *The Art & Science of Rational Eating*. Barricade. He was the president emeritus of the Albert Ellis Institute, 45 E. 65 St., New York 10065.

W hy is it so hard to lose weight? It is not because we don't know which foods to eat (and which to avoid).

In most cases, persistent obesity is the result of *irrational beliefs.*

These are the things we tell ourselves—consciously or unconsciously—about the events in our lives and our reactions to them.

They're why so many of us wind up using food to satisfy *emotional,* not physical, hunger.

By replacing these beliefs with sound self-statements, it's possible to change your eating behavior—and your weight.

START WITH SELF-ACCEPTANCE

Few people recognize the incredible irony that underlies most cases of obesity—that is, if you're serious about losing weight, you must first learn to accept yourself. You must do so *unconditionally,* with all your eating and weight problems.

Putting yourself down—for being fat, for falling short of your eating goals or for any other reason—may *feel* like a powerful motivational tool. In fact, it hampers your efforts to change your eating habits.

Trap: If you habitually put yourself down, you'll eventually come to view yourself as weak and unable to change—and, perhaps, not *worth changing.*

Self-flagellation also makes you feel bad. And people regularly use overeating to soothe bad feelings.

How does one move toward greater self-acceptance? *There are two key strategies…*

●**Focus on behavior.** Don't confuse what you *do* with who you *are.* Just because you overeat (behavior) does not mean you're a bad person (character).

Each of us does millions of things during a lifetime. Some are good. Some are bad. Learn

to say, "*Overeating* is bad" rather than, "*I* am bad."

●**Change "shoulds" and "musts" to preferences.** Shoulds and musts are among the most common—and most destructive—irrational beliefs. *If you think that…*

●**Life *should* be less stressful…**

●**You *should* be able to eat whatever you want…**

●**You *must* become thinner…**

●**Other people *must* treat you fairly…**

…then you'll feel angry and miserable when these demands aren't met.

Let's face it. Life *isn't* fair, and others don't always treat us the way we'd like them to. Yet insisting that things be otherwise doesn't change things. It just wastes time and energy—and makes us chronically upset.

When we recast these demands as *preferences,* they lose their power to make us miserable.

Example: Don't tell yourself, "I *must* be thin." Tell yourself, "I *prefer* to be thin."

THE ABCD METHOD

Each time you catch yourself overeating, analyze the situation using the following simple technique. Some people find it helpful to do this in writing. *Pause for a moment, and…*

●**Identify the *Activating* event.** This is the situation that preceded your distress.

Examples: Your boss gave you a poor performance evaluation…you had an argument with your spouse…you stepped on the scale only to see that you'd gained five pounds.

●**Notice your irrational *Beliefs* about the negative event.** In addition to using *should* and *must* and putting yourself down, irrational beliefs can stem from *awfulizing* (blowing events out of proportion)…and *low frustration tolerance* (viewing frustration and discomfort as *intolerable* rather than *inconvenient*).

Examples: "My boss *should* appreciate me more, and it's *awful* that he/she doesn't"…"My spouse *must* always be supportive and good-natured"…"Dieting is *too hard* and I cannot *stand* it."

There's nothing wrong with feeling frustrated, depressed or angry occasionally. But when you convince yourself that these feelings are to be avoided at all costs, you subject yourself to needless pain.

●**Consider the *Consequences* of your irrational thinking.** The greater your awareness of your irrational beliefs, the easier it will be to see that they lead to undesirable consequences—emotional *and* behavioral.

Example: If you believe life should not include problems and challenges, you're likely to spend much of your time feeling resentful and discouraged. You're also likely to avoid taking responsibility for choosing what to eat.

When you accept that restricting your eating may be difficult but not *horrible* or *impossible*, you can focus on pleasures other than eating.

●*Dispute* **your irrational beliefs.** Simply identifying problematic events, beliefs and their consequences isn't enough. You must vigorously *challenge* your ineffective self-statements. *Ways to dispute irrational beliefs...*

●**Evidence.** Is it *proven* that fat people are worthless? That you should always get what you want?

●**Logic.** How does it follow that going off your diet once or twice means you'll never lose weight?

●**Pragmatism.** Is this belief really helping you to reach your goal? Would a different belief be more helpful?

●**Role-playing.** Have a friend repeat your own irrational beliefs one at a time—while you forcefully argue against them.

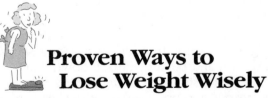

Proven Ways to Lose Weight Wisely

Anne M. Fletcher, MS, RD, author of *Eating Thin for Life: Food Secrets & Recipes from People Who Have Lost Weight & Kept It Off.* Houghton Mifflin.

Based on interviews with more than 200 people—each of whom successfully lost an average of 64 pounds and kept off the excess weight for at least three years—I've found that it isn't necessary to spend a lot of money to lose weight.

Most of these people accomplished their goals without spending thousands on a gym membership or spa vacation. They didn't buy a $3,000 treadmill...have surgery to reduce their stomachs' capacity to hold food...or go on an expensive diet-drug regimen.

Instead, they made reasonable changes to both their eating and exercise habits—changes that last a lifetime.

Lessons from the people I interviewed who lost weight without going broke...

●**Write down what you eat.** Some of us underestimate by up to half what we eat when we don't record each morsel. It's the little snacks—the handful of peanuts or the bite of your spouse's dessert—that can trip you up.

Helpful: Many people find it helpful to keep track—in a notebook—of everything they eat while they are losing weight. And—most of those I surveyed continued to record what they ate on a weekly or occasional basis to maintain weight loss. Just the act of keeping track of what is consumed helps many people to cut back.

●**Buy a digital food scale, measuring cups and spoons and a fat and calorie counter.** Many people are unaware of what constitutes an accurate food portion. We're all used to "supersizing" our meals, so our servings often are much larger than those listed on food labels.

Example: Some calorie counters list a bagel as weighing two ounces. Yet the plump, fresh bagels we get at the bakery typically weigh four ounces—doubling their calorie count to more than 300.

Total cost: Less than $100.

Once you get a handle on *real* portion sizes, you will be able to put away the scale and books. But don't discard them.

Reason: It's a good idea to periodically check to make sure you are still eyeballing portions correctly and that your calorie and fat counts are on target.

●**If you need help losing weight, shop around for a value-conscious program.** Half of the people I studied lost weight on their own. The other half needed help from professionals or programs. There's nothing wrong with signing up for commercial programs, but they don't have to cost an arm and a leg.

Nonprofit support groups like TOPS (Take Off Pounds Sensibly, 800-932-8677, *www.tops.org*) and Overeaters Anonymous (505-891-2664, *www.oa.org*) cost just a few dollars a week. Some programs don't charge at all.

Weight Watchers (800-651-6000, *www.weightwatchers.com*) is affordable, costing about $20 to join and approximately $10 a week to attend meetings.

●**Walk it off.** By far, walking was the top exercise choice of the people whom I surveyed.

Reasons: It doesn't cost anything…you can do it outdoors or indoors at a mall…with a dog or friends…near your home or at a local university or school…at a low, moderate or high intensity—whatever you are comfortable with.

Important: More than half of the people I surveyed did more than one kind of exercise to break the monotony of a daily workout.

●**Take advantage of community adult education exercise programs.** At night, many local schools open their doors to adults for physical education classes such as aerobics, calisthenics, swimming or country line dancing. These classes are typically inexpensive (less than $50), last for several weeks and are taught by experts.

●**Borrow low-fat cookbooks from the library.** Test the recipes, and if you like one book especially well, buy it…and use it.

Or, since most of us tend to eat the same 10 dinners over and over again, select five to 10 low-fat recipes and copy them from the book onto recipe cards.

●**See a registered dietitian (RD) at the local hospital.** Not only can RDs assess where your eating habits are falling short, they can devise a personalized plan for you that will help you to control your food intake and get the nutrition you need.

Cost: A visit to an RD costs about $40. If you have a weight-related medical illness, such as diabetes or high blood pressure, the cost may be covered by your health insurance.

●**Spend your snack money on fruits and vegetables.** The people I interviewed told me that this was their biggest secret of weight loss and weight maintenance.

More on How to Control Food Cravings

Leslie Bonci, RD, director of sports medicine nutrition, University of Pittsburgh Medical Center.

Distract yourself by taking a short walk or doing something else for five minutes, until the craving passes…set limits on your consumption—two cookies instead of half the bag…find a healthful substitute for what you're craving—an apple instead of a brownie, for example.

Scent Therapy Can Help You Lose Weight

Alan R. Hirsch, MD, assistant professor of neurology and psychiatry at Rush–Presbyterian–St. Luke's Medical Center in Chicago. He is also founder and neurological director of The Smell & Taste Treatment and Research Foundation, Water Tower Place, Suite 990W, 845 N. Michigan Ave., Chicago 60611. He is author of *Dr. Hirsch's Guide to Scentsational Weight Loss.* Element.

Physicians have long been aware that people who lose their sense of smell (a condition known as *anosmia*) often wind up gaining weight.

My research shows that overweight people who sniff food aromas do just the opposite—they *lose* weight.

Study: More than 3,000 overweight people were given a pen-like inhaler containing the scent of apple, peppermint or banana. They were asked to sniff the scent whenever they felt hungry.

Over the course of the six-month investigation, participants took from 18 to 288 whiffs a day…and lost an average of 30 pounds apiece.

The more frequently the subjects sniffed, the less hungry they felt—and the more weight they lost. Some people wound up losing even more weight than they intended to lose.

It's not yet clear whether these individuals will be able to keep the weight off. My hunch, however, is that scent-induced weight loss will prove to be no easier or harder to maintain than weight loss brought about via more conventional means—special diets, exercise regimens, appetite suppressants, etc. Follow-up studies may provide an answer to this important question.

WHY SNIFFING WORKS

What explains the connection between sniffing food and losing weight?

One likely possibility is that *sniffing* food somehow tricks the brain into *thinking* that the body is actually consuming food.

Another theory: Inhaling a pleasant food aroma helps eliminate the subtle anxiety that often causes people to overeat.

Whatever the explanation, it's clear that food scents do help curb overeating.

PRACTICING SCENT THERAPY

If you'd like to lose weight via "scent therapy," try these simple strategies...

●**Take time to sniff your food before eating.** Inhale as deeply as possible to make sure the aroma-causing molecules reach the olfactory bulb. That's the part of the body responsible for the sense of smell.

●**Chew your food thoroughly.** The more thoroughly you chew, the more scent is liberated. If you're eating alone—or can do so without offending your dining partner—you might even try "blowing bubbles" into each mouthful of food before swallowing.

By doing so, you maximize the mixing of food molecules with air molecules.

●**Opt for fresh foods whenever possible** ...and eat them hot. Fresh, unprocessed foods tend to have stronger scents than packaged or canned foods. Hot food is more aromatic than cold food.

●**Add a pungent herb, spice or condiment to bland foods.** If you're eating rice, for example, you might top it with steak sauce. You might sprinkle chopped garlic on your salad ...or add a splash of ketchup on cottage cheese.

USING AN INHALER

If you prefer, you can use a scent inhaler. For information on where to purchase one, contact The Smell & Taste Treatment and Research Foundation at 312-938-1047, *www. smellandtaste.org*.

Keep the inhaler with you at all times. When you find yourself feeling hungry, inhale the scent three times into each nostril.

Vary scents you inhale, and stick to food odors you like. If you don't find an odor pleasant, it *won't* help you lose weight.

Caution: Do not use an odor inhaler if you suffer from asthma or migraine headaches. These conditions may worsen if you do.

How the Weight-Loss Scientists Lost Their Weight

Richard Heller, PhD, and Rachael Heller, PhD. He is adjunct professor of pathology at Mount Sinai Medical School in New York and professor emeritus of biomedical sciences at City University of New York (CUNY). She is clinical professor of pathology at Mount Sinai and professor of biomedical sciences at CUNY. They are coauthors of several books, including *The Carbohydrate Addict's Lifespan Program*. Signet.

As scientists who have been overweight, we know firsthand that food cravings and weight gain don't always result from lack of willpower.

Instead, they may be caused by biological addiction to carbohydrates and an overabundant production of the hormone insulin.

CARBOHYDRATES AND INSULIN

Our research shows that as many as 75% of overweight people—and 40% of normal-weight people—suffer from a biological imbalance involving insulin.

Insulin is a hormone that helps your body use and conserve food energy in three ways...

●**Insulin *tells* your body when to eat.**

●**Insulin *delivers* food energy** to wherever the body needs it.

●**Insulin *commands* the body to save food energy** stored in fat cells for a time when no food is available.

Many people produce so much insulin that their bodies are unable to absorb it all. As a result, they wind up with an excess of insulin in their bloodstreams. This imbalance leads to a cycle in which they experience overpowering cravings for carbohydrates, such as breads, pastas, snack foods and cakes. When they eat carbohydrates, the body releases even more insulin.

The result is constant hunger pangs, intense and recurrent cravings for carbohydrates, easy weight gain and difficulty losing weight.

Fortunately, carbohydrate addiction and insulin imbalance can be corrected so that you can lose weight and be healthy for the rest of your life—without feeling deprived or struggling to manage your eating patterns and your weight.

ARE YOU A CARBOHYDRATE ADDICT?

Ask yourself the following six questions. *They will help you find out if your body has trouble managing carbohydrates...*

• **After eating a full breakfast, do you get hungrier** before it is time for lunch than you would if you had skipped breakfast altogether?

• **Do you get tired after eating a large meal** or find that you get sluggish and/or hungry in the afternoon?

• **Have you been on diet after diet,** only to regain all the weight that you lost and more?

• **Does stress, boredom or tiredness make you want to eat?**

• **Do you sometimes feel that you aren't satisfied,** even though you have just finished a meal?

• **Do you find it harder to take off weight** —and keep it off—than when you were younger?

If you answered "yes" to *two* of these six questions, you are probably mildly carbohydrate-addicted.

If you answered "yes" to *three* or *four* questions, you are likely to be moderately carbohydrate-addicted.

If you answered "yes" to *five* or *six* questions, you probably have a severe carbohydrate addiction that may be greatly affecting your life.

MANAGING YOUR CARBO INTAKE

We have created a simple plan to help restore the carbohydrate addict's body to its natural balance.

This regimen has worked for both of us— Rachael lost 165 pounds and Richard lost 45 pounds, and we have maintained that weight loss for more than 12 years. It has also worked for 80% of the 1,000 carbohydrate-addicted patients we counseled at Mount Sinai Hospital in New York.

The plan does not require you to deprive yourself of carbohydrates, only that you limit them to one meal a day to prevent the release of excessive amounts of insulin.

TWO CATEGORIES OF FOOD

• **Carbohydrate-rich foods,** including breads ...grains...cereals...ice cream...milk...yogurt... fruit and juices...luncheon meats...pasta...noodles...rice...snack foods...sweets...and starchy vegetables—beets, squash, carrots, zucchini, corn, tomatoes, peas and potatoes.

• **Craving-reducing foods,** including red meat...poultry...fish...cheese...tofu...oils...fats ...dressings...nonstarchy vegetables—brussels sprouts, green beans, peppers, lettuce, asparagus, broccoli and mushrooms.

OUR BASIC PLAN

• **Eat one balanced Reward Meal® every day for breakfast, lunch or dinner.** This is a balanced wholesome meal—not a binge— that includes all of the foods you need for good nutrition and health. Start with two cups of fresh salad. *The rest of the meal should consist of...*

• **One-third craving-reducing protein,** such as meat, poultry, fish, cheese, eggs or tofu.

• **One-third nonstarchy vegetables.**

• **One-third carbohydrate-rich foods** such as starches, starchy vegetables and snack foods, fruits, juices or sweets.

We don't believe that you need to weigh your food or count calories or fat grams when following the plan. Simply use good sense and listen to your body when sizing up portions.

• **Complete your Reward Meal® within one hour.** If the meal lasts longer, your body will continue to release insulin in response to the carbohydrate-rich foods, and you'll be hungry all over again.

• **Eat only craving-reducing foods at all other meals and snacks.**

We're not saying our plan will work for everyone. All programs must be individualized to suit particular lifestyles and needs. But we believe that carbohydrate addiction is so pervasive that, for most people, our plan is worth trying.

Working with your physician, follow the program for two weeks. You should immediately notice a lessening of your cravings.

If you don't, try adjusting the program until you notice a difference—for example, you may need to eat between-meal snacks...adjust the proportions of your meals...or adjust your intake of nutritional and other dietary supplements.

Another Benefit of Losing Weight

Gary Zammit, PhD, director, Sleep Disorder Institute, New York.

It is possible to cure snoring by losing weight.

Study: Males who snore heavily were placed on a six-month weight loss program. *Result:* Among the men who lost six pounds, the amount of snoring dropped 50%. Among those who lost 13 pounds or more, snoring was virtually eliminated.

How to Tell How Many Calories to Eat Each Day

Ellen Coleman, MPH, nutrition consultant, The SPORT Clinic, Riverside, CA.

Use the *Harris-Benedict equations* to determine your *basal energy expenditure (BEE)*.

For men: BEE = 66 + 13.7W + 5H − 6.8A.

For women: BEE = 665 + 9.6W + 1.7H − 4.7A.

In each equation, W equals weight in kilograms (kg), H equals height in centimeters (cm) and A equals age.

To make metric conversions, multiply your height in inches by 2.54 and divide your weight in pounds by 2.2.

Example: A 40-year-old man who is 5 feet 10 inches (178 cm) tall and who weighs 195 pounds (88.6 kg) needs 1,897 calories a day. 66 + (13.7 x 88.6) + (5 x 178) − (6.8 x 40).

Note: The BEE is based upon how many calories are needed each day by people who are *sedentary*.

Add *another* 100 calories for every 15 to 20 minutes of light exercise (walking, gardening, etc.). Add 150 to 200 calories per 15 to 20 minutes of vigorous exercise (running, swimming, etc.).

18

Healthy Attitudes for Your Work and Home Environment

Carpal Tunnel Syndrome: New Preventive Steps

George Piligian, MD
Irving J. Selikoff Center for Occupational and Environmental Medicine

The medical condition that is known as *carpal tunnel syndrome* (CTS)—and related disorders belonging to the category of *cumulative trauma disorders* (CTD)—are among the most widespread and most frequently discussed workplace disorders.

BACKGROUND TO THE PROBLEM

CTS results from the entrapment of one of three main nerves supplying the hand as it goes through the wrist. It can be diagnosed by a physical exam and an objective diagnostic test called nerve conduction velocity and EMG. Related ailments or CTDs as a group may be harder to diagnose because objective diagnostic tests are not yet available for all of them.

Common symptoms to train employees to watch for: An early sign of CTS is a change in the sensations in your hand—such as tingling—or just being aware that the hand doesn't feel right. Later on, pain, numbness or weakness may occur.

If ignored, CTS can progress to the loss of hand-muscle control and crippling.

COST THREAT

As if difficulty in diagnosing CTDs weren't bad enough, once a person has gotten to the advanced stages of a CTD, the symptoms are often impossible to reverse completely.

Implication for businesses: Prevention of such ailments is a company's best—and virtually only—defense. The next best defense is trying to help workers who do become affected as soon as the very first symptoms appear.

Risk of ignoring early signs: Once symptoms become severe, the employee will probably

George Piligian, MD, occupational medicine physician at the Irving J. Selikoff Center for Occupational and Environmental Medicine, Mount Sinai Medical Center, New York.

face disability leave and prolonged medical treatment—with surgery the most likely treatment for very severe cases.

Result: The cost of coping with an employee suffering from a CTD very often falls most heavily on the business through its health insurance and disability insurance policies. Difficulty of diagnosis notwithstanding, CTS and related conditions are a real and growing problem for business.

REDUCING THE RISK

Employees are most at risk when they do repetitive tasks, especially when they must work in an awkward manner, using poorly designed tools and equipment.

Increased use of computers is believed to be a leading cause—because of several factors involving work style and use of the body while at the computer.

Assume that complaints of CTS are real and justified. In fact, since symptoms are progressive, the more you can encourage workers to come forward at the first hint of possible trouble, the better for the worker and for the business.

Milder cases, caught early, may be stopped from progressing by making minor changes in the work function, coupled with physical therapy to ease the symptoms. Some people may be able to continue working at a fairly high level while getting treatment. But often, significant changes in work pace and work style are needed to arrest progression of the symptoms.

ADDITIONAL PREVENTIVE MEASURES

•**Listen to employee complaints** that certain jobs, especially repetitive jobs, are causing discomfort or pain. Worker complaints of headaches, neck or back pain, persisting fatigue of hand and arm muscles, and changes in sensation from these parts can all be early warning signs of CTDs.

•**Adjust workstations.** Watch out for employees who look uncomfortable at their tasks. Watch for jobs that seem to force workers into awkward postures. Are work desks and tables adjustable for the workers using them? Are there tools that workers seem to be having trouble using? Listen for complaints that certain tools "just don't feel right." Don't assume that "one size fits all" when it comes to office equipment. Some equipment may have to be redesigned to accommodate individual workers.

•**Redesign jobs to minimize repetitive motions.** Try to rotate jobs among several employees so no one worker must perform the same task over and over again. If repetitive work can't be reduced, at least provide frequent breaks and rest periods.

•**Reduce stress.** Since stress or workplace organizational factors are apparently contributing factors to some CTDs, do whatever is possible to reduce the stress level in the workplace. If frequent absences and irritability levels are increasing, it is likely that stress is too great.

•**Consider using outside expertise.** Seek the nearest university hospital center that has an occupational health clinic with experience in research in this relatively new field. Consult with people on the staff who have experience in spotting and eliminating workplace hazards.

Caution: Many entrepreneurs have begun to do business in ergonomics—claiming expertise in preventing CTDs. The quality of many of these so-called experts is hard to evaluate.

Stand Up Straight

Susanne Callan-Harris, MS, PT, physical therapist, department of sports medicine, University of Rochester, NY.

Surprising cause of carpal tunnel syndrome: Slouching. Poor posture while working at a computer weakens the shoulders and upper back due to lack of use. When the upper body is weak, the forearms and wrists have to do more work when typing. Repetitive-motion strain, such as carpal tunnel syndrome, may result.

Healthier Computer Use I

Study by Alan Hedge, PhD, director, Human Factors Laboratory, Cornell University, quoted in *Office Systems 97*, 1111 Bethlehem Pike, Box 908, Springhouse, PA 19477.

Avoid computer eyestrain by occasionally shifting your focus to distant objects to relax eye muscles. Also, keep the monitor at or below your horizontal line of sight and 18 to 30 inches from your eyes. Symptoms of eye strain include blurred vision, dizziness and headaches.

Healthier Computer Use II

Steelcase Corp., office furniture and design specialists, Grand Rapids, MI.

Antiglare filters on computer screens reduce health and vision problems while increasing productivity among full-time computer users. In a study of optical glass antiglare filters, 80% of users said the filters made it easier for them to read computer screens, and 89% said filters increased the quality of the screen image. The percentage of computer users complaining of tired eyes dropped from 86% to 40%...lethargy from 78% to 36%...itching or watery eyes from 60% to 28%...focusing trouble from 60% to 33%...dry eyes from 52% to 24%...headaches from 53% to 32%.

What HMOs Won't Tell You

Alan Mittermaier, president, HealthMetrix Research, Inc., a company that assists employers in evaluating HMOs and other managed-care providers, Box 30041, Columbus, OH 43230.

When a company contracts for any outside services, the customary procedure is to monitor the supplier to ensure that it consistently delivers what it committed itself to deliver. When it comes to health maintenance organizations (HMOs), however, many companies ignore that basic business practice.

The lapse could be especially expensive today. *Reason:* No matter what happens in Congress in regard to health insurance, health care costs are still expected to rise in the coming years.

CRUCIAL COMPARISON

The good news: It is easier to monitor the performance of an HMO than those at most companies might think.

Essential: At least once a year, compare the company's current HMO with nationwide HMO performance measures.

Advantages: By giving the HMO an annual checkup, the company can pick up early warning signals of potential trouble. Even if it remains in good shape, knowing how the HMO stacks up against competitors puts the company in a better bargaining position when the contract comes up for renewal.

How to do it: Use the *Healthcare Effectiveness Data and Information Set* (HEDIS), available from the National Committee for Quality Assurance (NCQA) in Washington, DC. The database establishes guidelines for comparing HMOs in approximately 71 key areas of performance.

Nearly all HMOs—especially those with superior performance—provide the HEDIS data to companies that request them.

When a company first compares its HMO against industry norms, it often hires a consultant. For $5,000 to $10,000, most health care consultants will steer a company through the initial procedure and also teach managers how to do it themselves in the future. *Several important performance criteria include...*

● **The medical-loss ratio.** The term refers to the ratio of an HMO's medical expenses to the revenue it collects in premiums. Most managed care industry observers agree that a medical-loss ratio of less than .80—where less than 80% of premium income is spent on medical coverage—is inappropriate.

On the other hand, a ratio of .80 to .85 is a reliable sign that the HMO is financially stable and not spending an excessive portion of its income on marketing or administrative overhead.

Caution: Be careful about renewing a contract with an HMO whose ratio fluctuates

347

significantly from year to year. A severe downward dip might indicate that the organization has suddenly found a need to market itself more aggressively. That can occur if an HMO suddenly loses a large number of members.

An upward surge can be a bad omen, too. It could indicate, for instance, that an HMO has incurred unexpected medical expenses which could spell financial difficulty. This can result if the HMO finds itself with a large number of unexpectedly costly medical cases.

If trouble does occur, an HMO may try to cut corners on service or concentrate on attracting new members instead of servicing current ones.

Exceptions: New HMOs may have more fluctuations in their medical-loss ratio than HMOs that have been in business for many years.

● **Disenrollment rates.** This term refers to the percentage of employees who have dropped out of the HMO.

The statistics aren't as obvious as you might think, since meaningful figures can't include employees who drop out because they change employers or move away. The statistics to look at are those of workers who opt out of the plan and go into another.

Rule of thumb: Be leery of an HMO with a disenrollment rate of more than 10% a year or one with a steadily rising disenrollment rate.

● **Preventive care.** While there's no guarantee, companies can usually hold down health care premiums by using an HMO that stresses preventive care. For that reason, periodically check HEDIS statistics for the HMO's performance, compared with industry norms, in children's immunization, mammography and prenatal care.

A reduction of these services can point to higher costs in the future.

EVALUATING A NEW HMO

If the company decides to change HMOs, or if it is considering using one, the first step is, again, to get the HEDIS data for organizations the company is considering.

Next, check with current and past clients as you would with any other supplier. *But also take a hard look at...*

● **Prices.** The best HMO isn't necessarily the one with the lowest premium, but the one whose services match up closest with the company's benefits policy.

Example: If a company's current policy requires no employee copayment for office visits, it might look for a less expensive HMO than a business that currently recoups part of its health care outlay by requiring a $25 copayment.

● **Quality.** As a rule, try to contract with an HMO that's accredited by either the NCQA in Washington or the Joint Commission in Oak Brook Terrace, Illinois.

Both organizations set rigorous standards. Information supplied by the NCQA is generally supplied in layman's terms and is therefore easier to understand. Nevertheless, it is prudent for companies that use managed care for the first time to hire a consultant to evaluate the data.

● **Access to primary-care physicians.** The key here is the number of physicians that an HMO lists that are actually accepting new patients. Often, an HMO's provider directory lists an impressive array of family physicians, internists and pediatricians, but many of them don't accept new patients. HEDIS tracks the percentage that do.

Rule of thumb: Select HMOs where at least 75% of the listed physicians accept new patients.

● **Patient satisfaction.** That's easy to overlook but critically important. *Reason:* The best health care plan in the country won't do a company much good if employees don't like it.

Recommended: In addition to talking with past and current clients, ask a prospective HMO for results of its latest patient satisfaction survey, preferably one conducted by an independent organization. If the HMO conducts its own survey, ask to see the questionnaire in order to spot any question-bias.

Rule of thumb: There's usually a trade-off between employee satisfaction and limiting choice of providers, a big factor in lowering costs.

Example: An HMO that limits employees to a small network of physicians may save a company money, but it is also likely to create dissatisfaction, especially if employees cannot continue to use their own personal physicians.

Are You Taking Advantage Of the Family and Medical Leave Act?

US Department of Labor Research, cited in *Benefits and Compensation Solutions*, 10 Valley Dr., Greenwich, CT 06831.

Only 2% to 4% of eligible employees are taking advantage of the Family and Medical Leave Act, despite fears that the Act would put a strain on business. Under the law, businesses with 50 or more employees must allow employees to take as much as 12 weeks a year of *unpaid* leave to handle family illnesses, births or adoptions.

Everyone Has Anxiety— More...or Less

Jerilyn Ross, MA, LICSW, director, The Ross Center for Anxiety & Related Disorders, 5225 Wisconsin Ave. NW, Suite 400, Washington, DC 20015. Ross is author of *Triumph Over Fear: A Book of Help and Hope for People with Anxiety, Panic Attacks, and Phobias.* Bantam.

You're suffering from anxiety when, stuck in traffic and late for an appointment, your heart starts pounding and your hands start sweating.

Or—an argument with your spouse makes your muscles tense up, and your knees feel weak.

An occasional bout of some anxiety is not only unavoidable, it's healthy. This emotion serves a constructive function—to prepare you to deal with stressful situations...to motivate you to avoid adversity and to solve problems.

But *frequent*, intense anxiety is not a healthy condition...

WHEN ANXIETY ITSELF IS THE PROBLEM

There is reason to be concerned about anxiety when the symptoms are out of proportion to the triggering event or situation...or the anxiety interferes with your ability to attend to everyday activities and responsibilities.

High-performing managers who live and work in a stressful environment of challenge and change usually can tell the difference between normal anxiety and anxiety that is out of control. *Typical...*

● **An executive has been a polished speaker for years**, experiencing a normal case of jitters before he/she begins each presentation but never afraid of the experience. Then during a particular presentation, for no apparent reason, he has a panic attack—his heart begins to race, he experiences shortness of breath and lightheadedness—and is sure he is going to pass out. As a result, the manager begins to be fearful that those jitters will overwhelm him in the *next* presentation—and so starts to make excuses and refuses invitations to speak.

● **A manager has made many business trips by plane**, experiencing the usual anxieties when planes hit turbulent air or landings are delayed because of bad weather. Then, for some reason, the anticipation of those fears becomes overwhelming. The manager begins to balk at taking business trips and declines a promotion that would require even more travel.

Problem: Fears caused by the anticipation of a panic attack can interfere with normal everyday living. These are fears of the actual feelings themselves.

These are not fears of flying or fears of talking before groups of people. They are fears that the feelings themselves will be overwhelming...turning talks and presentations into total disasters. A person fears he may lose control or make a fool of himself—that the racing heart and shortness of breath will kill him or that he may be losing his mind.

Caution: Competent managers very often self-diagnose these symptoms as "all in their heads"—to be conquered by self-discipline.

They often work in a business culture and environment that encourages people to be strong and tough it out.

They are embarrassed to reveal their fears. And even though many of these symptoms are overwhelming to the person experiencing them, their peers and subordinates may not see any outward signs of the terrors within.

Anxiety disorders are the most common mental health problem in America today. Between 13% and 25% of Americans suffer from these problems—which can manifest themselves as panic attacks, phobias or obsessive-compulsive disorder.

Fortunately, anxiety disorders are also among the most easily treatable mental disorders.

Like hypertension and diabetes, the symptoms generally respond favorably to medication and training in behavior modification by qualified psychotherapists.

Trap: While anxiety sufferers have no reason to be embarrassed about their feelings, or to believe that there is no remedy, fewer than 25% of the people who suffer these irrational fears actually receive treatment.

THE RIGHT MEDICINE

Anyone who went to a doctor over 10 years ago in search of relief from an anxiety problem and had a disappointing experience with prescribed medication should not be reluctant—if necessary—to try again now. Prior to the mid-1980s, doctors usually treated panic symptoms with drugs that were potentially habit-forming and not always very helpful. More effective treatments are now available.

No one pill will make all the symptoms of an anxiety disorder magically disappear. Even though many people do recover completely from their distressing symptoms, anxiety disorders are generally a chronic condition that can be greatly relieved, though rarely eradicated by, the right medication and behavior therapy.

A psychiatrist trained in managing anxiety disorders may prescribe *Xanax* (alprazolam) or *Klonopin* (clonazepam), although these might be habit-forming...or *Prozac* (fluoxetine hydrochloride)...or *Paxil* (paroxetine)...or *Tofranil* (imipramine).

Many more medications specifically designed to treat panic disorders are undergoing Food and Drug Administration testing.

A psychotherapist who specializes in anxiety disorders can generally train patients in ways to modify their thoughts and behavior effectively and efficiently, and at far less cost than for other mental conditions. Consult your doctor for referrals to experienced psychotherapists in your area.

"OUTS"

In addition to using medication it is often possible to learn to manage irrational anxieties on your own.

Key: Use your creativity to give yourself an "out"—either actual or imaginary—from anxiety-provoking places or situations.

Example: If you start sweating due to anxiety related to a luncheon meeting to discuss renewal of a contract with a major customer, take note of the location of the restaurant's phone and restrooms—places you can easily retreat to for a needed emotional break—and then make a graceful retreat if you need to.

Important: An out—something that helps you to face the scary situation—is not a crutch. A crutch is something you use to keep yourself away from the activity. A crutch is having someone else do the shopping because you are afraid of stores...sticking to side streets while driving instead of using highways...walking up steps instead of using elevators. An out, on the other hand, is anything that gets you *in*.

Workaholism Self-Defense

Joyce Kilmartin, former president, Equilibrium, Inc., a company that provides seminars and workshops to help people balance their lives.

A major problem with workaholism is that today many businesspeople wear it almost as a badge of honor. In their minds, being overworked is tantamount to success.

Reality: Truly successful people know how to keep their lives in balance. They know the importance of work but also of family and physical and emotional health. In the end, managers with balance in their lives are more creative, more productive...and more likable.

By contrast, a person who pursues work to the exclusion of all other activities is headed for trouble.

Example: Late in life, you begin to think back on your accomplishments and the first thing that comes to mind is a set of Italian luggage or a condo on Maui. Then you start wishing that you'd been closer to your children.

HOW MUCH IS TOO MUCH

The question, of course, is how to tell when commitment to work changes from a healthy drive to succeed—into a prescription for despair. *There's no clear answer that applies to everyone, but there are some very reliable warning signs...*

●**It's dark when you leave for work and dark when you return from the office**, even in summer.

●**No matter how hard you work**, it never seems to be enough.

●**You have no fun in your life**, but you do have fantasies of escaping.

●**You don't really know what's going on in the lives of your loved ones.**

●**You're plagued by aches and pains** and are too tired for sex.

LESS OBVIOUS SIGNALS OF WORKAHOLISM

●**Forgetting things that you've known for years**—such as your ATM password or a close relative's birthday. That kind of forgetfulness is a sign that professional concerns are monopolizing your mind.

●**Inability to get into the car without turning on the radio**—or getting on the phone. The habit is often a sign that you feel obliged to juggle facets of your life instead of focusing on the real task—in this case, driving.

●**Buying exercise equipment**—or a health club membership—but never using it. Successful people are purposeful. They understand the importance of following through, whether it's finishing a marketing report or losing five more pounds. Burnout candidates have good intentions, but can't get off the track toward exhaustion.

REGAINING BALANCE

It's rarely easy to change your behavior. *How to facilitate change...*

●**Take active steps to remain focused on the goal of leading a life that's balanced among work, family and your emotional well-being.** One of the most effective ways is to isolate yourself for an hour or two. A setting close to nature is especially helpful.

Ideal: By the ocean. In this environment, list the 10 people and things that are most important in your life. Almost always, family appears ahead of work.

●**Enlist the help of a friend.** Choose a person who has known you for a long time, both professionally and personally.

Be honest with this confidant about your desire to be successful and to enjoy life more fully. Listen to his/her feedback, and ask him to recommend specific actions you can take.

If you're married, bring your spouse into the change process. Nearly always, you'll discover that your spouse has been hoping that you'd achieve more balance.

●**Avoid major shifts in lifestyle.** Instead, make small, incremental changes, such as delegating someone to attend an unimportant meeting.

Monumental changes are nearly always impossible, but small ones are self-reinforcing. If your productivity rises once you start delegating, for instance, it's unlikely that you'll go back to the days of slavish attendance at every meeting.

Ask your confidant to encourage you to take a chance on small lifestyle changes. Surprisingly, many small changes will become part of your permanent regimen.

●**Learn something new that you've always wanted to know.** New knowledge isn't just satisfying for its own sake. It makes you a more interesting and creative person. And it serves the purpose of adding variety to your life, refreshing your spirit and thereby reducing the chances of filling all of your time with work.

But again, take it in small steps. Start lessons on a musical instrument you like, but don't bite off more than you can chew.

●**Improve your health.** Eat more healthfully, get more sleep, exercise more frequently and spend more time outdoors. *Also helpful:* Yoga and meditation.

Almost always, better health brings a higher level of confidence, and that too is self-reinforcing.

Highly confident people don't have to prove themselves by working 14 hours a day.

Most top achievers, consciously or otherwise, follow these steps. They know what their priorities are in life and never stop learning. They take care of their health. And with the help of a confidant, they work toward incremental improvements in the overall balance of life.

Hostility, Stress And Disease

Redford B. Williams, MD, professor of psychiatry, Duke University Medical Center, Durham, NC. He is also coauthor of *Anger Kills*. HarperTorch.

Intense anger is nearly as likely as strenuous activity to cause a heart attack. People with stressful jobs also have a higher incidence of high blood pressure. After a heart attack, an optimistic outlook and supportive social ties can play a major role in successful recovery.

Simple Stress-Reducing Office Routine

Chicago Institute of Neurosurgery and Neuroresearch.

Millions of Americans who suffer from back and neck pain are unable to identify a specific incident as the root of their discomfort.

Surprisingly, it doesn't take bungee jumping or moving a piano to bring on a backache. In fact, one of the most common causes of back and neck problems is simply doing too much of nothing at all.

Sedentary jobs that necessitate sitting at a desk or computer terminal for extended lengths of time can be hard on your body. Maintaining the same position for hours on end can lead to constant muscle tension, joint strains, permanent muscle shortening, decreased circulation and other damaging conditions that contribute to back and neck pain.

Are those of us who make a living glued to an office chair hour after hour, day after day, destined for bad backs? Absolutely not. You can counteract the negative effects of prolonged sitting by breaking up your day with brief, frequent periods of activity.

Perform the following five-minute series of stretches twice a day and supplement this quick routine with hourly strolls around the office. Stretching, coupled with a minute or two of upright movement each hour, helps reduce stress, ease muscle tension and strain, improve circulation and relieve pain.

If you're experiencing severe or persistent pain, consult a doctor.

1. Reaching behind your back, clasp your fingers together with your palms facing in. Slowly raise and straighten your arms. Hold this position for several seconds, then slowly release. Repeat three times.

2. Raise your elbows while keeping your hips stationary. Twist your upper body at your waist to the right. Hold this position for several seconds, then repeat on your left side. Repeat this stretch on each side three times.

3. Place your fingers behind your head. Squeeze your shoulder blades together until you feel tension through your upper back, then slowly release. Repeat three times.

4. Stretch your right arm across your upper body. With your left arm, pull your right elbow toward your left shoulder. Hold this position for several seconds, then reverse arms. Repeat three times.

5. Clasp both your hands together above your head. While stretching your hands upward, slowly lean to the right side, then left. Do not arch your back. Keep your knees slightly bent. Repeat three times.

6. Lean against a support with your left leg forward and your right leg back. Your left leg should be bent and your right leg should be straight. With your right heel on the floor, slowly move your hips forward until you feel a stretch in your right calf. Hold for 30 seconds before releasing, then reverse legs. Repeat three times.

7. Extend and separate your fingers until you feel the stretch. Hold this position for five seconds. Relax, then gently bend your fingers.

8. Bring your left hand to your upper back from above while bringing your right hand to your upper back from below. Slowly move your hands as close together as possible and hold. Release after several seconds, then reverse arms. Repeat three times.

9. Tuck in your chin slowly. Hold this position for two seconds, then release. This exercise counteracts the effects of leaning forward to stare at a computer monitor.

10. Sit up straight and extend both of your legs out from your body. Hold this position for several seconds, then release. Repeat three times.

How to Reduce Job Stress

Valerie O'Hara, PhD, founder of the La Jolla Institute for Stress Management, a psychotherapist in private practice in California and author of *The Fitness Option: Five Weeks to Healing Stress*. La Jolla Institute for Stress Management.

It has gotten to the point where you can't sleep. Your body aches. You snap at your spouse...your kids...and your dog. These symptoms are common. So is the cause—*job stress*.

How can you get relief *without* quitting? Regular exercise, sound nutrition and some form of daily meditation are effective stress-busters. *But there are some lesser-known antidotes to try...*

TAKE A SICK DAY

Do so *before* you feel you can't stand the stress any longer. Temporarily removing yourself from the work environment gives you the time and the distance you need to reflect on the precise causes of your stress...and how to eliminate them.

If you don't call in sick now, your body may soon force you to. Epidemiologists say that more than 80% of all visits to primary-care physicians are for stress-related illnesses.

KEEP A JOURNAL

Use your time off to experiment with keeping a journal. The idea behind "journaling" is to create a stress diary, in which you detail the sources of your work stress...and list what you like about your job.

When it comes to psychological stress, the way you *perceive* your circumstances plays a big part in determining your response to them. Often, we exaggerate work problems in our own minds. Writing them down helps us recognize this exaggeration.

Example: Jenny, a registered nurse, came to me complaining bitterly about "never-ending paperwork." She insisted that she hated her job.

Journaling helped her realize that she spent only one-quarter of her time dealing with paperwork. The rest was devoted to caring for patients—something she truly loved.

By changing the way she perceived her job, Jenny learned to contain her stress—not exaggerate it.

MAKE A CHART

A thought-replacement chart is a tool that helps retrain your immediate responses to stressful situations.

What to do: Take a piece of paper, and divide it into three columns. Label the first column "Trigger Situations," the middle column "Negative Self-Talk" and the third column "Positive Thought Replacement."

In the first column, jot down the regular sources of your job stress. In the center column, describe your usual responses to these situations. In the third, write what a friend would say to make you feel better...or what you would tell yourself if you were in a good mood.

Next time you find yourself in one of these situations, use those statements from the third column to talk back to yourself. Doing so will change your perception and defuse your stress.

Example: Larry felt overwhelmed by the increased workload associated with his recent promotion. Whenever his boss gave him a new project, he thought, "I'll never get this done on time. I might as well give up. I don't deserve this promotion."

Larry's thought-replacement chart helped him change this self-talk to: "I can take it one step at a time. I can prioritize and delegate. I can do this job."

Larry still has just as much work. But his new, more positive perspective on the situation has helped him better deal with it.

SCHEDULE WORRY TIME

Sometimes talking to yourself about a problem isn't enough to solve it. In such cases, you must take action.

If you find yourself spending too much time agonizing over what action to take, schedule regular "worry focus" sessions.

Allot 30 minutes a day to focus on what's stressing you out. Brainstorm possible solutions on your own...or with the help of a coworker. When your time is up, banish any worries by telling yourself, "No, those thoughts are for the next worry focus."

DON'T FORGET TO RELAX

Balance your worry focus sessions with one or more daily "worry breaks"—predetermined times when you simply refuse to dwell on anything stressful.

If the idea of having to remember to take your break makes you anxious, tie it to a regular activity—a shower, jog, commute, meal or something else that's already been incorporated into your routine.

Many people would like to try deep breathing or another relaxation exercise—but they get so caught up in the workday that they forget to take a break.

In such cases, the solution is to set up a visual reminder.

Example: Vicki, a personnel manager, found that a few moments of deep breathing and visualizing herself sitting by a waterfall did much to calm her nerves. But she kept forgetting to take advantage of this technique—until she hung a picture of a waterfall in her office to prompt her.

THINK TWICE ABOUT CAFFEINE

The coffee, tea, soda, etc., that you depend on to get through a stressful morning may *cause* additional stress later in the day.

Two cups of coffee a day contribute to anxiety. More than two cups *creates* anxiety.

Find out how much caffeine is contained in the beverage you drink. To encourage yourself to have noncaffeinated alternatives, tape a note

on your mug reminding you to have herbal tea instead.

Better still, keep a half-gallon bottle of water on your desk. Try to finish it by the end of the work day. It will keep hunger at bay, discouraging stress-related snacking. When your body is properly hydrated, it works better and produces more energy—energy you need to do your job well and fight stress.

Indoor Pollutants... Easy Avoidance Strategies

Leo Galland, MD, director of the Foundation for Integrated Medicine in New York City. His latest book is *The Fat Resistance Diet*. Broadway. *www.fatresistancediet.com*. Dr. Galland is a recipient of the Linus Pauling award.

Environmental pollution can cause all sorts of ailments, including asthma, allergies, immune system suppression and even cancer.

Smog, toxic-waste dumps, chemical-laden streams and other examples of *outdoor* pollution get lots of media attention. But for most of us, pollutants *inside the home* pose much bigger threats to our health.

Here's how to create an environmentally safe home...

PROHIBIT SMOKING

Establish a firm no-smoking policy. That goes for pipe and cigar smoking as well as for cigarette smoking.

If someone in the family smokes and is unable or unwilling to quit, make sure he/she smokes outside. To discourage smoking by guests, get rid of ashtrays...and consider posting a sign that reads NO SMOKING PLEASE.

In addition to raising your risk for cancer and heart disease, secondhand smoke aggravates asthma and raises children's susceptibility to sore throats and ear infections.

Cancer-causing tars in tobacco smoke cling to curtains and upholstered furniture long after cigarettes have been extinguished.

DON'T WEAR SHOES

If you wear shoes in your home, you track in pesticides, lead and other toxins each time you come home. These chemicals can be difficult to clean up—especially if they're deposited on carpets.

In Japan and many other countries, it's customary for house guests and occupants to leave their shoes at the door. Follow their example. Go barefoot…or wear slippers, if you prefer.

CONTROL MOLD

Household mold can cause everything from eczema and asthma to joint pain, fatigue and headaches. Some molds excrete *tricothecenes*, toxic compounds that suppress the immune system and cause leukemia.

Molds flourish in moist air. Use a dehumidifier to keep relative humidity indoors below 50%. Simple models are available for about $100 at hardware stores.

Make sure your basement and attic are well-ventilated. Install exhaust fans in your kitchen and bathrooms—to get rid of moisture that builds up during cooking and showering.

Do not install carpeting in bathrooms, basements or other areas where dampness or high humidity is a problem.

Check your refrigerator daily. Remove food with any signs of mold. Once a week, clean showers, tubs, cabinets under the sink and other mold-prone spots. Using gloves, apply an antiseptic solution made of 50% hydrogen peroxide and 50% water.

CHECK GAS APPLIANCES

Gas stoves, heaters and clothes dryers must be properly vented to avoid exposure to carbon monoxide (CO), nitrogen dioxide (NO2), formaldehyde and other toxic emissions.

Especially hazardous: Gas appliances with a pilot light. If your home has any such appliances, replace them with electric appliances…or with pilotless gas appliances, which have an electrical ignition system.

Even low-level exposure to CO—if prolonged—can cause memory impairment and hearing loss. Nitrogen dioxide can cause persistent cough and sore throat.

Self-defense: Install a CO monitor in your kitchen. *Cost:* About $30 and up. For more information, call the US Consumer Product Safety Commission at 800-638-2772, *www.cpsc.gov.*

WATCH OUT FOR FORMALDEHYDE

Formaldehyde is commonly found in particle board, plywood and other building materials. It can leach out of these materials into the air.

Breathing formaldehyde-laden air can cause dizziness, shortness of breath and a burning sensation in the eyes, nose and/or throat. Prolonged exposure has been linked to chronic headache, memory loss and cancer.

If you're planning to remodel your house, use formaldehyde-free building materials.

If your home already contains materials made with formaldehyde, give them a coat of *Safe Seal* varnish or another hard lacquer.

Since new clothing, carpets and furniture can give off formaldehyde, too, it's a good idea to air them out for several days before using them. Put them in an unoccupied room with open windows.

GET AN AIR FILTER

Every home should have an air-filtration system. *There are three major types of filters available…*

•**Negative ion generator.** By giving particles of smoke and dust a small electrical charge, it makes them adhere to floors, walls and furniture, where they can be removed by sweeping or dusting.

•**HEPA (high-efficiency particulate arrestor) filter.** This is a folded paper element that filters out dust, pollen and smoke.

•**Activated charcoal filter.** It filters out formaldehyde and *volatile organic compounds* (VOCs), which can irritate the lungs and cause cancer.

…AND A WATER FILTER

In most parts of the country, tap water has been treated with chlorine to kill bacteria.

Unfortunately, chlorine reacts with organic matter (typically leaves that fall into the water system) to form *chloroform* and other *trihalomethanes.* These compounds are known to cause bladder and rectal cancer.

Self-defense: Use an activated carbon water filter (such as those made by Brita and Water Pik) for any water used for drinking or food preparation. Such filters, which also remove lead, are inexpensive and widely available. *Cost:* About $20.

Since trihalomethanes can evaporate into the air while you shower, it's also a good idea to install a charcoal filter on your shower head. *Cost:* About $70 and up.

What about bottled spring water? It's generally chlorine-free, but some brands are contaminated with bacteria. Call the manufacturer to make sure it comes from a protected spring, and request an analysis.

CONTROL DUST

House dust can contain lead (from lead paint and lead-tainted soil), as well as VOCs from paint, adhesives, carpeting and cleaning solutions.

Self-defense: Damp-mop all floors and other horizontal surfaces (windowsills, furniture, etc.) once a week. Vacuum carpets three times weekly.

CHOOSE PRODUCTS CAREFULLY

Paints, solvents, cleansers, furniture polishes, air fresheners and other common products can contain a wide range of toxins. To limit your exposure to these noxious chemicals, use nontoxic alternatives.

Helpful resource: Dr. Samuel Epstein's *The Safe Shopper's Bible* (Wiley).

Caution: Never mix products containing ammonia and chlorine. These compounds react to form *chloramine*, a toxin that can cause severe lung damage.

MAKE YOUR HOME OFFICE SAFE

Computers, copiers, fax machines and especially laser printers often emit VOCs. Keep all such devices in one room—not a bedroom. Make sure the room is well-ventilated, and install an air filter.

If possible, leave the room each time you print out a document.

Environmental Control of Allergies

Harold Nelson, MD, professor of medicine, allergy and immunology, National Jewish Medical and Research Center for Immunology and Respiratory Medicine, Denver.

Often, the best defense against airborne allergens that trigger hay fever and other allergies is to control your environment. This means avoiding situations in which allergies are likely to strike and taking steps to minimize allergic reactions when avoidance isn't possible. *General strategies...*

●**Do not plan outdoor activities for the middle of the day or afternoon.** Ragweed pollen peaks between 11 a.m. and 1 p.m. Grass is the "safest" in the late afternoon and early morning.

●**Take "safe" vacations during the height of allergy season.** *Best destinations:* The mountains or the beach, which are often pollen free.

●**Avoid alcohol.** In some people with nasal allergies, alcohol swells blood vessels in nasal passages, causing increased nasal stuffiness.

●**Don't hang clothes and sheets outdoors to dry.** They'll catch windblown pollen and molds.

●**Stay away from smokers.** Cigarette, pipe and cigar smoke—as well as cooking smoke from grills and campfires—can trigger sinusitis.

ALLERGY-PROOF YOUR HOME

●**Rent an air-filtration system before buying one.** This will let you try it out first to see if it works. A filtration system is not all that useful for house dust mite allergy, but may help those allergic to animal dander.

●**Cover your mattress with plastic.** *Also:* Pillows need to be covered or washed...replace feather pillows with polyester—foam pillows can get moldy. *Helpful:* Wash bedding in hot water at least once every two weeks.

●**Consider removing carpeting from your bedroom.** Even when cleaned regularly, carpets and rugs can harbor mites. To limit animal dander problems, keep pets away from those areas that are carpeted.

19

Taking Care of Your Eyes, Ears and Teeth

The Simple Secrets of Avoiding Serious Eye Troubles

James F. Collins, MD, FACS
Center for Eye Care

Everyone over 40—not just those who wear glasses or contact lenses—should see an ophthalmologist once every year or two…and then *annually* after age 65. Most eye problems develop slowly, but the major diseases increase sharply after age 65.

Tests for eye health cost approximately $50 to $125. A visual field test for peripheral vision costs another $75.

Downside: Medicare may not pay for preventive care, especially if the doctor doesn't find a problem.

The three most common eye diseases are cataracts, glaucoma and a disease that is less familiar to most…macular degeneration. A cataract is a human eye lens that has lost some of its clarity and become cloudy or opaque. Age-related cataracts, the most common type, can start as early as age 40.

Rarer causes: Eye injuries…certain drugs, including steroids (such as prednisone or cortisone)…diabetes. Many people have some degree of cataract formation by their 60s or 70s.

The extent of impairment depends on the location and extent of haziness in the lens—as well as to what the individual person is accustomed. A person who does crossword puzzles or fine sewing might be more bothered by cataracts than someone who doesn't do close work or much reading.

The most common types of cataracts progress slowly and symptoms can be treated as they develop. In early stages, cataracts are treated with new eyeglass prescriptions and the use of sunglasses. Relatively few people with cataracts

James F. Collins, MD, FACS, a practicing ophthalmologist and medical director of the Center for Eye Care in West Islip, NY. Dr. Collins is author of *Your Eyes…An Owner's Guide.* Prentice Hall.

require surgery. When surgery is necessary, however, it's nice to know that cataract surgery is one of the most consistently successful operations performed today. Unless an additional eye disease has intruded, the chance of restoring vision to its former level is more than 95%.

The surgeon removes the cloudy inner part of the human lens (cataract) and replaces it with an artificial lens. The outer part of the human lens (the capsule) is left in place. About one-third of the time, the capsule grows hazy and an opening must be cleared with painless laser treatment months or years later.

Previously, treatment techniques required waiting until a cataract was "mature" before it could be frozen and removed. Now the timing is based on individual need, such as a person's inability to drive a car or play golf. Cataract surgery enables many people to drive for the first time in many years.

GLAUCOMA

Glaucoma is a group of disorders that involves excessive pressure within the eye. Damage to the optic nerve causes partial vision loss. The degree of severity varies greatly.

Only an ophthalmologist can interpret the subtle tests required to make a diagnosis. Most cases of glaucoma can be controlled before loss of vision is significant.

Keys to success: Early detection...proper treatment...compliance with doctor's orders.

The most common type—*primary open angle glaucoma*—is an insidious disease that's treatable in early stages but can progress to permanent blindness.

The "angle," formed by the cornea and iris, contains the meshwork of the eye that permits fluid to drain out.

The incidence increases dramatically after age 40 (striking about 2% of people in that age group), and increases steadily after that.

Symptoms usually don't appear until loss of peripheral vision becomes noticeable. Only regular eye exams will catch this type of glaucoma early.

The slow loss of peripheral vision can creep up on you. *Tip-offs:* You trip over furniture... drive up on curbs...turn your head more broadly to see around you.

Treatment: Eye drops, pills, laser surgery and possibly conventional incisional surgery.

Much rarer: Narrow angle and acute angle closure glaucoma. Drainage from the eye shuts down. This may cause sudden, severe pain (usually in one eye), blurred vision, redness and swelling in the eye, headache and nausea.

MACULAR DEGENERATION

A frequent cause of the loss of sharp vision is macular degeneration. The macula is the central portion of the retina, which is a thin, transparent tissue that serves as the nerve cell layer of the eye.

The most common type by far is dry (*atrophic*) macular degeneration, which often causes no symptoms. Only an ophthalmologist can properly diagnose it.

Rarer: Wet (*exudative*) macular degeneration, a hemorrhage into the macula, accounts for about one-tenth of cases but more than 90% of severe visual loss caused by age-related macular degeneration.

Main symptom: A gradual loss of central vision or, in the case of "wet" macular degeneration, a sudden drop-off of vision.

Other causes of sudden vision loss include acute glaucoma, blood clots and hemorrhages. Migraines can also cause sudden, temporary loss of vision, usually off to one side.

Photodynamic therapy, which uses a low-powered laser in concert with the drug *verteporfin*, has shown great promise in arresting the downward course of the "wet" variety.

RETINAL BREAKS...AND DETACHMENT

A retinal break is a round hole or horseshoe-shaped tear in the retina. Fluid can pass through and accumulate under the retina, pulling it away from the layers of the eye underneath—leading to a retinal detachment. A tiny detachment may not be noticed but larger detachments can lead to profound vision loss and even blindness.

At risk: Anyone who has had an eye injury or blow on the head...is very nearsighted ...has a family history of retinal breaks or detachment...has severe diabetes. Some diabetics develop abnormal scar tissue in the vitreous gel (a thick, clear, jelly-like substance that fills the eyeball, cushioning and protecting it from within) that can contract, causing retinal tears and detachments.

Modern advances have made retinal tears and detachment much less common after cataract surgery than they used to be.

More rarely, a retinal tear can also cause a torn retinal blood vessel, resulting in bleeding into the vitreous gel. This in turn can cause sudden loss of vision.

Symptoms of a retinal break: You may see "flashers" or "floaters" or suddenly notice that a specific part of your vision is "missing," suggesting that a large section of the retina has become detached. Some retinal detachment can also cause few or no symptoms and only be discovered during a thorough eye examination.

Treatment for a retinal break: An ophthalmologist carefully tracks any retinal break for the development of retinal detachment. Laser treatment is often used as a preventive measure.

Treatment for retinal detachment: Surgical reattachment, sometimes involving multiple procedures. The prognosis for recovery is best when treatment is prompt.

PROTECT YOURSELF

- **Wear sunglasses** with ultraviolet-blocking lenses.
- **Keep your blood pressure normal.**
- **Take supplements of vitamins A, C and E and minerals zinc and selenium.** The compounds made specifically for eyes are generally better than multivitamins because they contain larger amounts of zinc and selenium.
- **Eat a healthy diet.** A proper diet is better for your eyes than vitamin supplements. Favor dark green, leafy vegetables such as spinach and collard greens.

In one impressive study of people with early macular degeneration, those who ate a diet heavy in dark green vegetables were three to four times more likely to preserve good vision than those who did not.

- **Don't smoke.** Smoking robs the eyes of important nutrients and aggravates cataracts.

Follow the above recommendations even more closely if you have either of two risk factors that can't be controlled: A genetic predisposition—the condition tends to cluster in families—and eye color.

People with light-colored eyes, especially those with blue irises, have a much higher incidence of macular degeneration.

To be sure all's well, take a simple test with your glasses on. Cover one eye at a time. Do you see equally well through both?

A Sign of Diabetes?

The late Michael Yablonski, MD, former chairman of ophthalmology, University of Nebraska, Omaha.

Bloodshot eyes can be a sign of diabetes. If your eyes are often red, consult a doctor.

Other causes: Allergies, eyelid infections, sickle-cell anemia.

Solutions for Bloodshot Eyes

Anne Sumers, MD, ophthalmologist in private practice, Ridgewood, NJ.

Eyes become red and irritated when the blood vessels on the surface of the eyeball dilate, often due to too little sleep, too much alcohol, allergies or excessive rubbing.

Self-defense: Although bloodshot eyes will improve on their own in one or two days, applying a cold compress may help because cold causes *vasospasm* (shrinkage of blood vessels).

Important: Bloodshot eyes can be a sign of *conjunctivitis* (pink eye), a disorder in which the tissue that lines the inside of the eyelid is inflamed. It can be caused by a viral or bacterial infection, allergy or irritating substances (such as shampoo, dirt, smoke, pool chlorine, etc.).

If you suspect you have an eye infection: Consult your doctor. Vasoconstrictor drops, such as *olopatadine* (Patanol) or *epinastine* (Elestat), may be recommended to reduce redness and itching. You also may need antibiotic drops, such as *ofloxacin* (Ocuflox) or *ortobramycin* (Tobrex), to clear up the infection.

Cataract Self-Defense... Sunglasses... Supplements... Surgery

Julius Shulman, MD, assistant clinical professor of ophthalmology at Mount Sinai Medical Center, New York City. He is the author of *Cataracts: The Complete Guide From Diagnosis to Recovery for Patients and Families*. St. Martin's.

Like gray hair and wrinkles, a gradual clouding of the eye's crystalline lens—the transparent light-focusing structure just behind the iris—represents a normal part of aging.*

While removal of the cloudy lens remains the only cure for cataracts, modern surgical techniques make this operation far simpler and safer than it used to be.

We've also learned a great deal about the role that environmental factors play in cataract formation—and how to slow the process...

PREVENTING CATARACTS

Scientists now know that sunlight and other sources of ultraviolet (UV) light may hasten formation of cataracts—not to mention macular degeneration and other potentially blinding eye disorders.

Self-defense: Just as you use sunscreen to protect your skin from sunlight, you should use UV-blocking eyeglasses to limit your eyes' exposure.

Whenever you venture outdoors in bright sun, wear sunglasses that block UVA and UVB light. Both glass and plastic lenses are okay. There is no advantage to polarized lenses.

If you wear corrective lenses, be sure to choose lenses that screen UV. Other strategies for forestalling development of cataracts include avoiding smoking and limiting your exposure to air pollution.

Inside the body, toxins found in cigarette smoke and air pollution have an oxidizing effect, causing formation of highly corrosive

*Some people develop cataracts at 50, some at 90. Past age 65, about 30% have them, and by 75, more than 50%. Cataracts can also be caused by eye trauma— a ball or fist striking the eye, for instance.

compounds called *free radicals*. These compounds attack cells, including those in the crystalline lens.

Antioxidants—especially vitamins E and C —will help limit production of free radicals.

Diabetics are at special risk for cataracts, apparently because of fluctuations in blood sugar levels. These fluctuations cause the lens to swell, which disturbs its delicate metabolism and causes clouding.

If you have diabetes, check your blood glucose levels often and take other measures to keep your blood sugar tightly controlled.

Long-term use of *prednisone* or another oral corticosteroid—prescribed for rheumatoid arthritis, ulcerative colitis, asthma, lupus, etc.— causes a steep increase in cataract risk. Ask your doctor about nonsteroidal anti-inflammatory drugs (NSAIDs) and other alternatives.

Self-defense: Have your eyes examined every two years if you are under 60...every year if you are older or have diabetes...twice a year if you are taking corticosteroids.

WHEN TO TREAT CATARACTS

The first symptoms of cataracts are often unusual sensitivity to bright light (photophobia) and blurred vision—a problem that's especially noticeable while you're driving at night.

As lens transparency declines, you may develop nearsightedness (myopia), which makes reading glasses unnecessary. If you're already myopic, you may need a stronger prescription.

Anyone who experiences symptoms suggestive of cataracts should see an ophthalmologist right away. He/she can give you a stronger eyeglass prescription, if necessary...and conduct tests to rule out other causes of vision loss, such as glaucoma and macular degeneration. Without prompt treatment, these eye conditions can lead to blindness.

Good news: As long as eyeglasses can correct your vision to 20/50 or better—that's the point at which vision trouble begins to affect daily activities—cataract surgery is generally unnecessary.

Exceptions: Prompt surgery for cataracts is necessary if...

● **You drive and your corrected vision falls below 20/40**—the legal standard in most states.

- **You have chronic eye inflammation.**
- **Your cataracts threaten to cause glaucoma.**

Ultimately, when to have surgery is a *personal* decision. A passionate reader or stamp collector may want his cataracts removed sooner than someone whose leisure pursuits are hiking or movies.

If a doctor recommends cataract surgery, ask why. Do not agree to surgery unless you are having significant problems with your daily activities...or your symptoms are reducing your quality of life.

SURGICAL OPTIONS

The treatment of choice for most cataracts is an outpatient procedure known as *phacoemulsification*. In "phaco," the surgeon pulverizes the lens with sound waves from a tiny ultrasound probe inserted into the eye.

Phaco requires only one tiny ⅛-inch incision —and no or very few stitches. Healing takes two to three weeks.

An older technique—*extracapsular cataract extraction* (ECCE)—requires a ½-inch incision that must be closed with up to 10 sutures.

ECCE is also performed on an outpatient basis, but it's almost always less desirable than phaco because healing can take up to eight weeks.

Exception: ECCE is better than phaco for advanced cataracts, which are too hard to break up with sound waves.

Since phaco is usually preferable, be suspicious of any doctor who recommends ECCE.

Both phacoemulsification and ECCE are performed under local anesthesia (injected into the eyelids). Some surgeons now use *topical* anesthesia, in which anesthetic is delivered to the eye via eyedrops.

Cost of surgery: $1,500 to $2,000.

REPLACING THE LENS

Until the 1970s, people who underwent cataract surgery had to wear thick "Coke bottle" lenses afterward—to make up for the lost lens.

With modern surgery, thick eyeglasses are unnecessary. The surgeon simply replaces the lens with a plastic or silicone intraocular lens prosthesis.

Unlike a natural lens, the prosthesis has a fixed focal length—that is, it cannot change shape to accommodate both near and far vision.

In most cases, you must make a choice—do you want the lens primarily for reading and other close work...or for distance vision?

If you pick near vision, you'll need ordinary looking (not Coke-bottle) eyeglasses for distance vision—and vice versa.

If cataract surgery is to be performed on both eyes, ask the surgeon about placing a near-vision lens in one eye and a distance-vision lens in the other. That way, you may avoid the need for eyeglasses entirely.

Obesity and Cataracts

Robert J. Glynn, PhD, ScD, professor of medicine, Harvard Medical School, Boston. His five-year study of 17,764 male physicians 40 to 84 years of age was published in *Archives of Ophthalmology*, 515 N. State St., Chicago 60610.

The fatter you are, the greater your risk of cataracts. In a study, the leanest men had the lowest risk. Smokers also face an increased risk of cataracts.

Protect Your Eyes with Good Nutrition

Studies quoted in *Health*, Box 56863, Boulder, CO 80322.

People who eat at least five servings of vegetables a week cut in half their risk of suffering *macular degeneration*—the most common cause of blindness in older Americans. Researchers believe that antioxidants in vegetables tie up oxygen molecules known as "free radicals," which otherwise damage the eyes over time. Also, the vitamin A in vegetables prevents loss of night vision.

Asthma Danger

Samy Suissa, PhD, director, division of clinical epidemiology, Royal Victoria Hospital, Montreal. His review of medical records of 48,118 asthma patients was published in the *Journal of the American Medical Association*, 515 N. State St., Chicago 60610.

Long-term use of high-dose steroid inhalers can cause glaucoma. Steroid inhaler use has increased sharply over the last 10 years. But in a study, asthmatics who used high-dose steroid inhalers eight times a day for three months or more were 44% more likely to develop glaucoma than were similar asthmatics who did not use inhaled steroids.

Self-defense: Asthmatics who use high-dose steroid inhalers should have their eyes checked by an ophthalmologist.

Glaucoma Busters

Sally Mellgren, MD, an ophthalmologist in private practice in Oceanside, CA. Her study was presented at a meeting of the American Academy of Ophthalmology.

Fight glaucoma with a low-fat diet and regular exercise. A common age-related eye disorder, glaucoma is caused by the buildup of pressure inside the eyeball. *Study:* Doctors put their glaucoma patients on a primarily vegetarian diet and a program of moderate exercise. After two weeks, fluid pressure in their eyes fell an average of 11.3%.

Glaucoma Treatment Without Side Effects

Joel S. Schuman, MD, professor of ophthalmology, Tufts University School of Medicine, and director of the glaucoma service, New England Eye Center, both in Boston.

The glaucoma eyedrops *brimonidine* (Alphagan) seem less likely than other glaucoma drugs to cause troublesome side effects. *Brimonidine* works by reducing production of *aqueous humor* (the clear, watery fluid in the eye). It's unlikely to cause heart rate and blood pressure disturbances, which prevent glaucoma patients with asthma and heart conditions from using other glaucoma drugs. Everyone age 40 or older should be checked for glaucoma every two years.

Better Glaucoma Testing

Richard Mills, MD, clinical professor of ophthalmology, University of Washington in Seattle.

The standard glaucoma test, which measures pressure inside the eye, may not be the most effective way to diagnose the disease.

Reasons: Eye pressure fluctuates, so any single measurement may be normal...and some people with glaucoma never develop above-normal eye pressure. *Better:* An inspection of the back of the eye to find damage to the optic nerve and measure any loss of peripheral vision.

Eye Exam Timetable

John Shoemaker, assistant vice president, Prevent Blindness America, 211 W. Wacker Dr., Ste. 1700, Chicago 60606.

Healthy adults 20 to 39 years of age should see an optometrist or ophthalmologist once every three to five years (every two to four years for African-Americans). Between ages 40 and 64, it's every two to four years for both Caucasians and African-Americans. For

Caucasians and African-Americans age 65 or older, it's every year or two.

Important: People with a family history of glaucoma or another eye ailment should have their eyes examined more frequently. Consult an eye doctor right away if you experience any vision problems.

Eye Exercise

Paul Planer, OD, an optometrist and author of *The Sports Vision Manual.* International Academy of Sports Vision.

Exercise your eyes while working at your computer by hanging a newspaper page on the wall about eight feet from where you sit …every 15 minutes, look away from the computer screen and focus on the newspaper…bring the headlines into focus and then shift your gaze back to the computer screen…repeat five times before returning to work.

Itchy Eyes?

George Fulk, OD, PhD, professor emeritus of optometry, Northeastern State University College of Optometry, Tahlequah, OK.

Your eyelashes might be infested with mites. These microscopic bugs are usually harmless—unless they become too numerous.

Self-defense: Ask your doctor or optometrist about using the topical gel *pilocarpine* (Pilopine) to treat the problem.

"Red Eye" Danger

The late Michael Yablonski, MD, former chairman of ophthalmology, University of Nebraska, Omaha.

Though usually a minor condition caused by a bacterial or viral infection, red eye is sometimes symptomatic of *iritis*—a potentially blinding inflammation of the iris.

Other symptoms: Excessive tearing…pain in reaction to light…cloudy vision…headaches.

Good news: The problem usually clears up following a few days or weeks of treatment.

Treatment: Cortisone-like eyedrops to control inflammation. They are sometimes used in conjunction with a drug to dilate the pupils… and pain medication.

Does My 10-Year-Old Need Bifocals?

George Fulk, OD, PhD, professor emeritus of optometry, Northeastern State University College of Optometry, Tahlequah, OK.

Bifocals help keep certain children from becoming extremely nearsighted. They work by relieving eye stress when kids do "close work." Mildly nearsighted kids fitted with bifocals may be 50% less likely to become extremely nearsighted than kids fitted with regular eyeglasses.

Eyedrop Danger I

Douglas D. Koch, MD, professor of ophthalmology, Baylor College of Medicine, Houston. His study of 70 people was published in *Archives of Ophthalmology*, 515 N. State St., Chicago 60610.

Decongestant eyedrops used to clear redness can cause eyes to become even redder. In 70% of patients studied, increased redness was caused by the "rebound" effect. That is, patients using the nonprescription eyedrops developed even greater redness when the effects of the drops wore off. The other 30% were allergic or had a toxic reaction to *tetrahydrozoline* or another ingredient.

Good news: Rebound redness and inflammation usually clear up when sufferers stop using the drops.

Self-defense: Use nonprescription eyedrops for no longer than four days. Or try artificial tears—they contain no irritating ingredients. If redness persists, see an ophthalmologist.

Eyedrop Danger II

Douglas D. Koch, MD, professor of ophthalmology, Baylor College of Medicine, Houston. His study of 70 people was published in *Archives of Ophthalmology*, 515 N. State St., Chicago 60610.

Vasoconstrictor eyedrops—widely available without a prescription—can hurt eyes if used too frequently, by causing conjunctivitis (pinkeye).

Self-defense: If you develop inflammation, redness, discomfort or discharge while using drops, stop using them immediately. Be especially cautious about using drops containing *naphazoline* or *tetrahydrozoline hydrochloride.*

Examples: Clear Eyes, Murine Plus and Visine.

Sunglasses Update

Stephen Miller, executive director, College of Optometrists in Vision Development, St. Louis.

Cheaper sunglasses may protect eyes as well as the more expensive ones. As long as the label promises UVA and UVB blockage of at least 99%, a $15 generic pair of sunglasses will give just as good protection from ultraviolet radiation as a $200 pair. With higher-priced sunglasses, you are paying for the frame design and a brand name.

Eye Injury Reduction

Paul F. Vinger, MD, clinical professor of ophthalmology, Tufts University School of Medicine, Boston.

To reduce the risk of eye injury, ask for *poly-carbonate* lenses whenever you purchase eyeglasses. They resist shattering far better than glass or other plastics. *Test:* Lenses made of *high-index plastic* shattered when hit by a tennis ball going 40 miles per hour. Lenses of *allyl resin* shattered when struck by a tennis ball moving at 55 mph. Glass withstood impacts of up to 89 mph. *Polycarbonate* lenses did not shatter even when bombarded at speeds of up to 130 mph.

Wraparound Sunglasses Offer Best Protection

Safe in the Sun by Mary-Ellen Siegel, MSW, clinical instructor and therapist, department of community medicine, Mount Sinai School of Medicine, New York. Walker & Co.

Any sunglasses that fit closely are also good. If sunglasses do not fit closely, almost three times as much UV radiation reaches eyes. Make sure sunglasses fit comfortably and snugly.

Ideal: Frame distributes weight evenly on your nose...hinges are sturdy...and ear pieces don't have too much play.

Food for Your Eyes

Johanna M. Seddon, MD, associate professor of ophthalmology, Harvard Medical School, Boston.

In a study, those who ate spinach or other dark, leafy green vegetables, such as collard and mustard greens, two to four times a week had healthier maculas (central part of the retinal layer) and better vision than those who did not. Eating greens five or six times a week resulted in greater benefits. Results combined vegetables of all types, canned or fresh, cooked or raw.

Possible explanation: These greens are rich in lutein and zeaxanthin, pigments that are vital to the visual process but that can become damaged or destroyed by light and with age.

Surprise: Carrots—usually considered good for vision—contain very little lutein and zeaxanthin.

Better Hearing

George A. Gates, MD, professor of otolaryngology–head and neck surgery, University of Washington, Seattle.

Profoundly deaf adults may benefit from a cochlear implant. This device—long recommended primarily for deaf *children*—is surgically implanted behind the ear. It transforms sounds into electrical impulses that the wearer can "hear."

The implants improved lip-reading ability in 90% of those who got them...and 10% to 20% of people who got them were able to communicate without lip-reading.

Free Hearing Test

George Biddle, executive director, DAHST (Dial A Hearing Screening Test), 300 S. Chester Rd., Ste. 301, Swarthmore, PA 19081.

Free hearing test by phone can reassure you about a feared loss of hearing—or warn you of the need for medical attention. The call involves listening to four tones in each ear. Failure to hear a tone warns of a problem. Call 800-222-EARS between 9 a.m. and 5 p.m. Eastern time to obtain the phone number of a local hearing clinic through which the test will be administered.

Exercise May Improve Hearing

Study of 26 people by Helaine Alessio, PhD, professor of exercise physiology, Miami University, Oxford, OH.

Subjects were able to hear faint sounds twice as well after they had worked out for one-half hour two or three times a week for two months. *Possible explanation:* Improved circulation to the inner ear may improve hearing ability.

How to Prevent Hearing Loss

Christopher Linstrom, MD, chief of otology at New York Eye and Ear Infirmary in New York City, and professor of otolaryngology at New York Medical College, Valhalla.

We tend to take our hearing for granted—until we start to lose it. And once hearing loss occurs, it's usually *irreversible*.

The gradual loss of hearing that occurs as we age is called *presbycusis*. It's very common. By age 60, most people have a slight weakness in their ability to hear sounds above 4,000 hertz (cycles a second). Unfortunately, that's the range in which speech falls.

The first sign of presbycusis is usually an inability to make out consonants—to distinguish between "sit" and "spit," for example, or "pants" and "dance."

Irreversible hearing loss can also be the result of high fever, measles, scarlet fever and certain other diseases...or, rarely, a side effect of surgical anesthesia.

A third form of hearing loss occurs when a small bone in the middle ear called the *stapes* loses its ability to transmit sound to the auditory nerve.

This hereditary condition, *otosclerosis*, afflicts 3% of the population, mostly women. It may start at puberty, but typically comes on in the 20s, 30s or 40s.

PROTECTING YOUR HEARING

You can't do much about your genes or your age, but you can protect yourself against the major enemy of hearing—exposure to loud noise.

Sustained noise above 85 decibels (the loudness of a shout or a crying infant) damages the nerve endings that transmit sound signals to the brain. Similar to presbycusis, the speech frequencies around 4,000 hertz are the first to go. Then higher and lower frequencies are affected.

A 30-year-old who has spent years using a jackhammer without hearing protection may have the hearing of someone 50 years older.

You run a similar risk if your nights are spent at a disco, club or bar where the music is deafening. Or if you keep the volume of your Walkman too high.

Self-defense: Do everything necessary to avoid prolonged exposure to loud noise. If the noise level at a club causes pain or ringing in the ears, *leave*.

If sustained noise is unavoidable—at work, for example—use a noise-blocking headset… or foam rubber or molded wax earplugs. For maximum protection, wear a headset *in addition* to earplugs.

When buying ear protection, look for a noise-reduction rating (NRR) of 15 or higher. Putting cotton in your ears is *not* very effective. Cotton has an NRR of only five to 10.

What about brief exposures to loud noise? You probably won't suffer any hearing loss from the occasional fire engine roaring past (though it is a good idea to plug your ears with your fingers). But even one *very* loud burst—a gunshot, for example—can cause permanent trouble.

If you experience ringing in the ears and your hearing seems less acute after a loud noise, *and it's not back to normal in a day or two*, consult a hearing specialist. To find a good one, call a local hospital's ear, nose and throat department…or contact the American Academy of Otolaryngology–Head and Neck Surgery at 703-836-4444, *www.aaohns.org*.

CHRONIC EAR INFECTIONS

A bad cold or flu often causes fluid to build up in the ear. If fluid accumulation becomes chronic, delicate structures in the middle ear can be permanently damaged.

If your stuffiness persists for longer than a month, or if ear infections recur frequently, your doctor may prescribe a powerful decongestant or insert a ventilation tube through your eardrum.

To prevent injury to your eardrum, avoid flying when you have fluid in your ears. If

your trip can't be postponed, ask your doctor for a good decongestant. During the flight, gently pop your ears by swallowing hard.

COPING WITH HEARING LOSS

Your doctor will probably recommend a hearing test to pinpoint the extent and cause of your problem. It's rare, but hearing loss can stem from a tumor of the brain or cranial nerve. It's especially important to rule out a tumor if your hearing loss is more pronounced on one side.

A hearing test is conducted in a noiseless, insulated testing booth. It tests both the *level* (speech-reception threshold) and the *clarity* (word discrimination score) of hearing.

Some hospitals and hearing aid makers offer a "telephone hearing test," but such tests aren't very accurate.

Does your hearing loss stem from a problem in the transmission of sound through the inner ear? From damage to the auditory nerve? What frequencies are affected? The hearing test should answer these questions.

Some conditions can be corrected surgically. If you have otosclerosis, for example, a simple outpatient procedure to insert a tiny "piston" in the inner ear restores normal hearing 90% of the time.

If you need a hearing aid, get an audiologist's help in choosing the most appropriate model.

Today's devices—which must be painstakingly calibrated—are different from those of decades past. Most are small enough to fit inside or behind the ears or on eyeglass frames. And most have electronic filters and precise volume controls that let you amplify just the frequencies that give you trouble.

Some state-of-the-art devices are programmable. You can preset them for listening comfortably to conversation or music, indoors or outdoors. *Cost:* $400 to $2,000.

Caution: Never buy a hearing aid via mail-order or telephone.

COCHLEAR IMPLANTS

The latest treatment for hearing loss is the *cochlear implant*. Implanted in a bone next to the ear, this miniature computer turns sound into electromagnetic energy, which is fed into the inner ear to stimulate the auditory nerve.

Cochlear implants are appropriate only for individuals with profound hearing loss in both ears that cannot be helped by a hearing aid.

Though cochlear implants can boost the hearing of otherwise deaf people, they cannot provide the same sound quality of a good hearing aid.

Earlobes...What They Can Tell You

William J. Elliott, MD, PhD, professor of preventive medicine and pharmacology, Rush-Presbyterian–St. Luke's Medical Center, Chicago. His study of 264 heart patients was published in *The American Journal of Medicine*, 360 Park Ave. S., New York City 10010.

Creased earlobes are a better predictor of future heart trouble than diabetes, high blood pressure, smoking, high cholesterol, family history of coronary disease or obesity. In a study, having one creased earlobe raised the risk by 33%. Having both earlobes creased raised the risk by 77%. The link between earlobe creases and heart disease is not yet understood.

Self-defense: If your lobes are creased, ask your doctor about strategies to lower your risk.

No More Earaches When Flying

Jeffrey S. Jones, MD, research director, department of emergency medicine, Butterworth Hospital, Grand Rapids, MI. His study of 190 fliers with recurrent ear pain was reported in *Annals of Emergency Medicine,* 360 Park Ave. S., New York City 10010.

Take one decongestant tablet containing *pseudoephedrine* at least 30 minutes before your flight leaves. A study found that following this regimen relieved discomfort in 68% of travelers with recurrent ear pain, compared with only 38% of those who took a placebo. One pill works all day, so there's no need to take more if your flight is delayed.

Important: Check with your doctor before trying this regimen to ensure that the pseudoephedrine does not conflict with other medications or health conditions.

Getting Help for Ringing in the Ears From Tinnitus Sufferer Dr. Stephen Nagler

Stephen M. Nagler, MD, director of the Southeastern Comprehensive Tinnitus Clinic in Atlanta. A tinnitus sufferer himself, he is a member of the board of directors of the American Tinnitus Association, Box 5, Portland, OR 97207.

Forty-four million Americans experience the hearing disorder *tinnitus*—ringing in the ears—on an occasional basis. Six million have chronic tinnitus.

Tinnitus makes it hard to concentrate and can disrupt sleep. It can lead to depression—or even suicide.

WHAT CAUSES THE NOISE?

Tinnitus is *not* a normal consequence of aging. It's usually caused by damage to the delicate "hair cells" lining the *cochlea*, a snail shell-shaped structure of the inner ear.

The most common causes of hair cell damage are...

•**Loud noise.** A single loud noise (such as an explosion) can permanently damage the hair cells. More often, tinnitus stems from years of exposure to loud music, factory noise, etc.

Self-defense: Avoid loud music. Wear sound-absorbing earplugs whenever you spend time around a noisy machine.

Inexpensive earplugs are available at hardware stores. If you anticipate repeated or prolonged exposure, custom-molded earplugs from an audiologist—or sound-absorbing earmuffs—offer better protection.

Ineffective: Stuffing your ears with cotton.

•**Drugs.** Transient tinnitus can be caused by many common drugs, including aspirin. Among the drugs that can cause *permanent* tinnitus are *cisplatin* and certain other chemotherapeutic agents…and aminoglycoside antibiotics like *streptomycin* or *gentamicin.*

Self-defense: Anytime your doctor prescribes a drug, ask about the risks—including the risk of tinnitus. Make sure the benefits outweigh the risk.

●**Diseases.** Tinnitus can be symptomatic of high blood pressure, arteriosclerosis, thyroid disorders, diabetes and certain other diseases.

Tinnitus can also stem from head and neck injuries…or from disorders of the middle or inner ear, including otosclerosis and Ménière's disease. In rare instances, tinnitus is caused by a tumor of the auditory nerve.

Self-defense: If you suffer from any of these ailments, be sure to get adequate treatment. If you develop tinnitus, consult a doctor right away.

SOUND MASKING

Most tinnitus sufferers crave silence. Ironically, the most effective treatment is often to "bathe" yourself in sound.

●**Music.** Try listening to different kinds of music. Notice if any helps mask the tinnitus or simply distracts your attention.

●**White noise generators.** These tabletop devices produce static noise or nature sounds (wind, surf, etc.). They're available from electronics stores. *Cost:* $100 or less.

●**Tinnitus maskers.** These are white noise generators worn in or behind the ear, like a hearing aid. Certain maskers function as both a white noise generator *and* a hearing aid.

Tinnitus maskers must be custom-fitted by an audiologist. *Cost:* $1,000 or more.

AUDITORY HABITUATION

Auditory habituation combines use of a tinnitus masker or hearing aid with educational sessions that help the tinnitus sufferer change the way he/she perceives the sound.

This technique—administered by an audiologist or physician—can be quite effective. Eighty percent of those who try it get significant relief. However, the process can take two years.

Ultimately, the person with tinnitus comes to have a *neutral* rather than a *negative* perception of the sound. It's like wearing pants—you can feel the cloth against your skin if you think about it. Most of the time, however, you're unaware of the sensation.

MIND/BODY TECHNIQUES

●**Cognitive-behavioral therapy.** It helps tinnitus sufferers avoid the distorted thinking that aggravates their suffering.

Example: "The noise is driving me crazy. I cannot get any work done."

For referral to a cognitive-behavioral therapist, call the American Psychological Association at 800-374-2721, *www.apa.org.* Make sure the therapist has experience treating tinnitus.

●**Self-hypnosis.** Some unscrupulous hypnotherapists claim that tinnitus sufferers can be hypnotized to no longer hear the sound. Not true. But self-hypnosis can help them come to terms with their ailment.

More information: Contact the American Society of Clinical Hypnosis, 140 N. Bloomingdale Rd., Bloomingdale, IL 60108, 630-980-4740, *www.asch.net.*

●**Biofeedback.** This technique employs electronic gear that lets you monitor your brain waves and muscular contractions. Using this gear, tinnitus sufferers learn to control their own physiological reactions to the noise.

For a list of biofeedback practitioners in your area, send a self-addressed, stamped, business-sized envelope to the Association for Applied Psychophysiology and Biofeedback, 10200 W. 44 Ave., Suite 304, Wheat Ridge, CO 80033, 800-477-8892, *www.aapb.org.*

●**Guided imagery.** Simply imagining yourself in a tranquil setting can help eliminate the frustration caused by tinnitus.

What to do: A few times a day, close your eyes and spend a few minutes picturing yourself aboard a sailboat. Imagine the smell of the sea, the feel of the sun on your skin, the sound of spray, etc.

You're headed for an imaginary island where your tinnitus magically disappears.

TINNITUS MEDICATION

Some patients get relief from *alprazolam* (Xanax). If congestion or allergies seem to be compounding the problem, an antihistamine may be helpful.

The herb *ginkgo biloba* has been used with some success.

Caution: Ginkgo can interfere with blood clotting. If you take it on a regular basis, make sure your doctor checks your bleeding and clotting time at least twice a year.

Help for Teeth and Gums

Walter J. Loesche, DMD, PhD, Marcus Ward Professor of Dentistry Emeritus, University of Michigan School of Dentistry, Ann Arbor, and leader of a study of 90 patients with periodontal disease, published in *The Journal of the American Dental Association,* 211 E. Chicago Ave., Chicago 60611.

Nonsurgical treatment for periodontal disease can save teeth and make extractions unnecessary.

Recent study: Aggressive cleaning, known as root planing and scaling, plus antibiotic treatment for two weeks made 87% of surgeries and extractions unnecessary. Benefits lasted five years. If you have periodontal disease, ask your dentist about alternatives to surgery.

Cleaner Kids' Teeth

Eli Grossman, DDS, consultant, New Institutional Service Company, Northfield, NJ. His study of 32 children eight to 12 years of age was published in *The Journal of the American Dental Association*, 211 E. Chicago Ave., Chicago 60611.

Electric toothbrushes help children keep their teeth cleaner.

Study: Kids who used an electric toothbrush with a small head designed especially for children (Braun Oral B Plaque Remover for Kids) removed 65% of dental plaque.

Kids who used a regular manual toothbrush removed 42% of plaque.

Best Dental Floss

Peter L. Jacobsen, DDS, PhD, professor of diagnostic sciences, University of the Pacific Dental School, San Francisco.

If your teeth are tightly spaced, use Glide, Colgate Total or another low-friction floss. For widely spaced teeth (if you can see between your teeth at gum level), use a woven floss like Oral-B Ultra Floss or Super Floss. If you tend to shred floss, use dental tape instead.

Better Brushing

Academy of General Dentistry, 211 E. Chicago Ave., Suite 900, Chicago 60611. Send for the Academy's free pamphlet *Brush Up on Your Dental Facts for Adults and Seniors.*

Three to four minutes of brushing are needed to get teeth really clean. The average person brushes for less than one minute.

Helpful: Listen to the radio or stereo while you brush. Most popular songs last three to four minutes.

Vegetarians Are at Higher Risk for Periodontal Disease

Holly Lucart, Academy of General Dentistry, 211 E. Chicago Ave., Suite 900, Chicago 60611.

The diets of strict vegetarians may lack sufficient calcium, vitamins D, B2 and B12, and complete proteins.

Self-defense: Replace the calcium by eating green vegetables, grains and nuts. Replace other missing vitamins by taking a daily multivitamin. Vegans—who eat no animal products at all—are at greatest risk.

Brushing and Flossing Are Not Enough

Tom McGuire, DDS, president of the Dental Wellness Institute in Sebastopol, CA. He is author of *Tooth Fitness, Your Guide to Healthy Teeth*. Diane.

We all know the importance of brushing and flossing. But when it comes to other aspects of tooth care, there remains a great deal of confusion. *Here are the answers to the most common questions patients have about teeth...*

● **How often should I have my teeth professionally cleaned?** The usual advice—once every six months—is rather arbitrary. Go as often as your dentist or dental hygienist says is necessary. If you have advanced gum disease, or if you're bad about brushing, that might be as often as once a month.

● **My gums bleed when I brush. Should I be worried?** Many people think a little bleeding is normal. *Not true.* Bleeding gums are an early sign of gum disease (*gingivitis*). Untreated, it can lead to serious bacterial infection.

Gingivitis can usually be reversed in one to three weeks by daily flossing and by brushing after meals.

Helpful: After brushing, rinse with a mixture of one-quarter teaspoon salt and four ounces of water, to get rid of bacteria.

If bleeding persists for more than three weeks, see your dentist. You might have *periodontal* disease. An advanced form of gum disease, it won't respond to self-treatment.

Other danger signs: Sensitivity to heat or cold, sugar or acidic foods...sudden pain in the affected area...bleeding...the sensation that something is pressing on the root of a tooth.

Over time, periodontal disease can cause bone loss in the jaw. Left untreated, it may result in tooth loss.

Warning: Periodontal disease can increase the risk of heart disease. If you suspect you have gum disease, see your dentist at once—especially if you are predisposed to heart disease.

● **What causes gums to recede?** The likeliest cause is gum disease, although after age 50, gums naturally begin to pull away from the teeth. Though severe recession can lead to tooth decay, most cases of receding gums are a *cosmetic* problem.

● **What can I do to prevent gum disease?** Supplements of vitamins C, A and B-complex have been shown to help. So has eating less sugar. Sugar speeds formation of plaque (film made of food particles, bacteria and saliva), which causes decay and gum disease.

● **What kind of toothbrush is best?** A teardrop-shaped model with soft bristles about one inch long. If your mouth is small, choose a "junior-size" brush.

The brush should have no more than four rows of clear (not colored) bristles. They make it easier to detect signs of bleeding from brushing.

Brushes with clear plastic handles stay cleaner longer—they allow bacteria-killing ultraviolet light to penetrate to the bristles.

After brushing, rinse your toothbrush in warm water. Stand it up to dry. Allowing a brush to lie flat permits the water to pool...and bacteria to grow. To help control bacteria, soak brushes once a week in mouthwash.

● **How often should I replace my toothbrush?** Every three months—sooner if the bristles become flattened or frayed.

It's also a good idea to replace your brush after each professional dental cleaning—to prevent exposing clean teeth to bacteria from the old brush.

● **Do electric toothbrushes do a better job?** Electric and ultrasonic brushes provide more brush strokes per second, but they're often less effective than manual brushes at reaching the back teeth and the inner surfaces of the lower front teeth.

Instead of an electric toothbrush, you might consider buying an *oral irrigating device*. Such devices send a jet of water deep below the gumline, where brushes and floss can't reach. They should be used *in addition to* brushing and flossing.

Best model: The Water Pik, with the Pik Pocket subgingival irrigation tip attachment.

When using an irrigator, keep the pressure low. For maximum benefit, fill the reservoir with antibacterial mouthwash or saline solution, instead of water.

●**What brand of toothpaste is best?** They are are all pretty much alike. It's the *brushing* action that cleans the teeth and keeps the gums healthy.

For adults, use the toothpaste that tastes best to you. If you hate the taste of your toothpaste, you're apt to avoid brushing.

People who have gum problems should avoid "whitening" toothpastes, which tend to be abrasive.

Important: Don't swallow toothpaste. Most brands contain artificial coloring, flavoring, sweeteners, etc., whose health risks aren't fully known.

Since children tend to swallow toothpaste when they brush, I recommend a natural toothpaste like Tom's of Maine for them. It's free of additives.

●**What about special flosses?** Unwaxed floss, which has a rough surface, is better than waxed, thin or "friction-free" floss at removing plaque and dislodging food.

Exception: If your teeth are closely spaced, or if unwaxed floss causes pain or becomes frayed, try a coated or ultrathin floss. Otherwise, you're likely to forgo flossing altogether.

Avoid *colored* flosses. They make it hard to detect bleeding.

Flossing technique is more important than what type of floss you use.

Proper way: After inserting a 12- to 18-inch piece of floss between two teeth, press it to one side, and guide it down using a back-and-forth, shimmying motion.

Caution: Pulling floss "up and out" can dislodge a filling. Instead, let go of one end of the floss and slide it through the space between the teeth.

Floss at least every night—after brushing but *before* spitting out all the toothpaste. If you have an area in which food gets trapped, floss every time you brush.

●**Should I be using a fluoride or anti-plaque rinse?** Yes. I recommend using these before brushing (or when you cannot brush following a meal). Fluoride is very good at fighting decay.

If your water isn't fluoridated, children should be given fluoride drops, from age one-and-a-half until age 16. Fluoride taken during that time is the best way to prevent tooth decay in adulthood.

●**What's the best way to whiten teeth?** For superficial stains caused by cola, coffee or cigarettes, try a whitening toothpaste. Follow instructions carefully. Overuse can strip protective enamel from your teeth.

For severe stains, ask your dentist about tooth-bleaching. Dentist-administered bleaches are faster, more effective and less likely to irritate your gums than do-it-yourself bleaches. *Cost:* $100 to $300 per bleaching.

●**How often should I have dental X rays?** When starting with a new dentist, have a set of *full-mouth, bitewing and periapical* (root) X rays. After that, have bitewing X rays annually (every six months if you're prone to decay). Depending on your checkups and your dentist's recommendations, you can go up to five years between full-mouth and periapical X rays.

●**Are amalgam (silver) fillings really dangerous?** Amalgam fillings, which contain the toxic metal mercury, can cause nausea, memory loss and neurological problems. If you're concerned about mercury toxicity, consider replacing them. Look for a dentist who advertises mercury-free or cosmetic dentistry.

For Sweeter Breath

Alan A. Winter, DDS, associate clinical professor of dentistry, New York University School of Dentistry and partner, Park Avenue Periodontal Associates, 532 Park Ave., New York 10021.

Rinse your mouth after eating. Rinse carefully after eating starchy or sugary foods.

●**Scrape the back of your tongue every day** with a toothbrush to remove bacteria. (The tendency to gag will decrease.)

●**Avoid coffee**, alcohol, tobacco and sulfur-containing foods like garlic and onions.

●**Drink water or chew sugarless gum** when your mouth is dry to produce more saliva.

●**Eat parsley**—a natural breath freshener.

●**Avoid over-the-counter mouthwashes.** Most just disguise bad breath briefly.

Important: Sucking on candy mints and cough drops is not a solution because they cause decay.

If the problem persists, see your dentist and doctor to see if you have an underlying dental or digestive problem.

Laser Whitening Procedure

Gary F. Alder, DDS, director, dental residency program, Rush–Presbyterian–St. Luke's Medical Center, Chicago.

Discolored teeth can now be whitened quickly and painlessly with a laser. In this procedure, teeth are painted with peroxide bleach, then zapped with a blue argon laser.

The 90-minute treatment—performed in a dentist's office—works on coffee and tobacco stains as well as on the discoloration caused by the antibiotic tetracycline. Teeth are noticeably brighter immediately after treatment...and continue to whiten for several days. Laser whitening is better and faster than home bleaching.

What Causes a Burning, Itching Sensation Inside the Mouth?

Trey Petty, DDS, associate professor of medicine, University of Calgary Medical School, Calgary, Canada.

Several serious ailments can cause this sensation, so those experiencing the problem should be examined thoroughly by a dentist or doctor. However, you may be suffering from *burning mouth syndrome* (BMS), a mild but mysterious ailment that affects mostly postmenopausal women.

Helpful: Lozenges containing *capsaicin*—the substance that puts the kick in cayenne pepper. Capsaicin lozenges are not available commercially, but they can be made by a pharmacy—or even at home.

Recipe: Dissolve two cups of brown sugar, ¼ cup molasses, ½ cup butter, two tablespoons water and two tablespoons white vinegar in a heavy pan over low heat. Boil gently, stirring frequently until the mixture reaches 300°F. Stir in ½ teaspoon cayenne pepper. Drop by teaspoonfuls onto wax paper and let harden. Start with three lozenges per day. Taper back as pain subsides.

20

Keeping Fit Pays Off

Jack LaLanne's Fitness Magic

Jack LaLanne

Life is survival of the fittest. You have to be in shape for that! Run a personal fitness check. Do you get enough rest? Eat the right foods? Have a hobby that relieves stress? Exercise to accumulate reserves of energy that will be like money in the bank for the day you need it?

The only way to increase your strength, energy and vitality is to stress your body beyond what it's accustomed to doing.

People up to 95 years old have *doubled* their strength and endurance in a short time with weight-training programs.

A 90-year-old person can't lift a weight as heavy as a 21-year-old person can. But each can work to his own capacity…and get results.

People rationalize about not exercising. Their main excuse—*I don't have the time.*

Would you sell your arm for $100 or your leg for $1 million? No, because your most priceless possession is your body. Shouldn't you spend a little time keeping it in good shape?

How you look is a billboard of the way you regard yourself. As you become fitter, and look and feel better, your self-esteem will rise…a good first step for improving your sex life as well.

If you're afraid you'll have a heart attack—be aware that the people who have heart attacks are the ones who *don't* exercise.

MAKE GOOD USE OF COMMERCIALS

When a commercial interrupts a TV show, don't get a snack—exercise instead. *Here's an easy one…*

●**Get up/get down.** Lower yourself gently to the floor and lie on your back. Stand up.

Jack LaLanne, fitness expert who opened his first gym in 1936 and has promoted physical culture for 65 years. Mr. LaLanne is author of several books, including *Revitalize Your Life After 50: Improve Your Looks, Your Health and Your Sex Life.* Hastings House.

Repeat slowly...then quickly. Practice until you can do it fast 15 times in a row. Invite your children or grandchildren to join in.

MAGIC FIVES

I devised these five simple exercises to trim and firm every part of the body. You can do Magic Fives almost anywhere. Your only gym equipment is a straight-backed chair and one or two books.

Start by doing each exercise slowly to a count of 10. Build stamina by exercising a little more vigorously each time, four or five times a week. Consider watching yourself in a mirror to see how well you're doing. Visualize yourself as you want to look. Breathe deeply to bring oxygen to your bloodstream and burn fat.

1. Swings. These work many muscles simultaneously. Hold a light book between your hands. Place your feet shoulder width apart. Bend your knees slightly.

Bend over at the waist. Breathing out, slowly swing the book down between your legs, trying to touch an imaginary wall behind you. Breathing in, swing the book back up again over your head. Keep your arms straight and try to touch the imaginary wall immediately behind you with the book.

2. Knees to chest. Excellent for the waistline, hip flexibility, abdominal muscles and lower back.

Sit at the very edge of a straight, hard chair. Holding both sides of the seat to keep your balance, lean back until your shoulders touch the back of the chair. Draw both knees as close to your chest as you can (or lift one knee at a time until you can lift both at once). When you become advanced, hold a book between your knees.

Lower your legs. Then make pedaling motions, pretending you're riding a bicycle. Progress from short movements to large ones. With each rotation, extend your leg down close to the floor before continuing.

For variation, do these exercises while lying on your back on the floor or on your bed.

3. Leg lunges. For sagging hips and flabby thighs.

Stand to one side of a chair. Hold on to the back of it. With your right leg, lunge forward as if you were fencing. Bring it back. Repeat with your left leg. As you get stronger, bend your knee more and step farther out. Keep your upper body erect throughout.

4. Leg extensions to the back. Tremendous for your back muscles all the way down from your neck to the bottoms of your feet. Firms the buttocks.

Facing a chair, bend at the waist and hold both sides of the seat. Keep your arms straight and back away from the chair until you feel comfortable.

Slowly lift your right leg backward as high as possible while pointing your toes, looking up, breathing in and tensing your hips tightly. You can bend your left knee a bit. As you lower your leg, breathe out...put your chin on your chest...and round your back, tensing your abdominal muscles. Repeat with your other leg.

5. Two-way punches. These cardiovascular exercises work most of the upper body muscles. They'll burn calories and trim your waistline.

• **Forward punches**. Helpful for your arms, shoulders, upper back and chest. Stand with your feet shoulder-width apart. Bend your knees a bit. Visualize a punching bag in front of you and punch it hard with one hand at a time. Imagine that your elbow is hitting a wall behind you as it comes back. Increase the pace.

• **Overhead punches.** Works the backs of your arms, the sides of your waist and your calves. Improves your posture.

Clench your fists, stand erect and punch your right arm overhead, pretending you're trying to hit the ceiling. Rise up on your toes as you go. Drop the opposite elbow down as low as you can. Alternate arms. Do this exercise rapidly.

• **Combination punches.** Assume the position for forward punches. Pull your waist in and punch forward rapidly, hitting your elbows against an imaginary wall behind you. Quickly switch to an overhead punch. As each arm comes down, push your elbow down as low as you can. The faster you punch, the more calories you'll burn. When you become more advanced, hold a book in each hand for extra resistance.

TRIM UPPER-ARM MUSCLES

The muscle on the back of the upper arm typically gets flabby as people age. That is because the triceps are not used very often. *To tone that muscle...*

• **Do overhead punches** (described above).

• **Push a weight**, such as a small barbell, above your head.

• **Stand with your back to the wall and your arms down**, with your palms against the wall. Push yourself away from the wall and back again. *Bonus:* You'll exercise the backs of your shoulders and improve your posture.

TAKE RESPONSIBILITY

I spend at least one hour a day lifting weights...and another hour swimming. Can't you find 20 minutes a few times a week to keep yourself in shape?

Caution: Always check with your doctor before starting an exercise regimen.

The Dangers Of Too Much Exercise

Kenneth H. Cooper, MD, MPH, president and founder of the Cooper Aerobics Center, 12200 Preston Rd., Dallas 75230. He is author of numerous books on health and fitness, including *Dr. Kenneth H. Cooper's Antioxidant Revolution*. Bookman.

When I was writing my first fitness book, *Aerobics*, back in 1968, I believed that a regimen of sustained, strenuous exercise was necessary for health and longevity...and more was better.

In the decades since then, countless studies have helped to radically refine this basic "exercise prescription."

It has become increasingly clear that the health benefits of less exercise—less strenuous *and* less time-consuming—are almost as great as a very demanding workout program.

We've also learned that *excessive* exercise exacts a toll on our bodies—in the form of everything from musculoskeletal injuries to increased risk of cancer.

Finally, we've come to recognize the vital role that *antioxidants* can play in protecting exercisers against cancer, heart attack, arthritis and other diseases.

HOW MUCH EXERCISE IS BEST?

In 1989, Steven Blair, PED, a researcher here at the Cooper Institute, shook the scientific world.

In measuring the fitness of more than 13,000 American men and women, Blair found that the 20% who were fittest were 75% less likely to die over the next eight years than the 20% who were least fit. No surprise there.

The shock was that the biggest reduction in mortality came from only a *slight* increase in exercise. Those who were just a tad fitter than their most sedentary peers enjoyed a 55% lower death rate.

Implication: Very moderate physical activity gives the biggest health return on your investment of time and energy.

A modest exercise regimen confers increased energy and endurance and a stronger, more resilient cardiovascular system. This "aerobic training effect" lowers your risk of disease...and raises your life expectancy by up to two-and-one-half years.

I now believe that there's no *health-related* reason to do anything more strenuous than take a brisk walk for 30 minutes five times a week.

I walk or run two to three miles, four or five times a week. I want to stay at a higher level of fitness so I can safely engage in more strenuous activities like mountain climbing, skiing and an occasional five-kilometer running race.

WHY MORE ISN'T BETTER

People who exercise harder than this may be doing themselves more harm than good. I'm talking especially about individuals who run 30 miles a week or more.

For starters, the risk of muscle injury rises *steeply* once you run much more than 15 miles a week.

Most people I know who used to work out at this level have had to cut back sharply—because of chronic injuries. Many of those who kept running long distances eventually had to quit altogether. Some required hip or knee replacements.

But muscle and joint problems are just the beginning. It turns out that serious exercisers may be unusually vulnerable to life-threatening illnesses.

One of my friends, a 50-mile-a-week runner, died of a brain tumor at age 50. Another friend who loved to run marathons succumbed to cancer at age 60.

In my practice, I've seen many cases of cancer and heart disease among elite athletes.

Studies examining the relationship between exercise and health, like Dr. Blair's, indicate that the death rate goes up slightly for those at the peak of the fitness pyramid.

What's to blame? I'm now convinced that the most likely culprit is a class of highly unstable oxygen molecules.

HOW TO PROTECT YOURSELF

Oxygen is essential for life, as we all know. But when chemical reactions strip an oxygen molecule of one or more electrons, it becomes highly reactive. This so-called *free radical* launches an attack on the body's cells.

Result: Arteriosclerosis, cancer, immunity problems—even an increased risk of cataracts.

Free radicals are plentiful in polluted air (including air tainted with automobile exhaust and cigarette smoke). They're also generated during the normal energy-burning process of metabolism.

Fortunately, the body is equipped with special enzymes that neutralize free radicals. But while moderate exercise helps this self-defense system "gear up" for battle, *excessive* exercise floods the body with free radicals. This may overwhelm this system.

At special risk: People who run outdoors in an urban setting. They get an extra dose of free radicals from car exhaust, smog and other airborne toxins.

To protect yourself—especially if you exercise regularly—you need *antioxidants* to help the body neutralize free radicals. These include vitamins C and E and beta-carotene (a precursor of vitamin A).

Like many health experts, I think it's best to get these antioxidants by eating five to seven servings of fruits and vegetables each day.

Dark-green and yellow vegetables are rich in beta-carotene.

One-and-a-half medium-sized carrots or one sweet potato a day provides enough to give you protection. Citrus fruits are good sources of vitamin C. Seeds, nuts and vegetable oils have vitamin E.

For an extra margin of protection, take supplements every day. *Here's what I've found to be best for regular exercisers...*

- **1,000 milligrams (mg) of vitamin C** (2,000 mg if you run over 30 miles per week).

- **400 international units** (IU) of vitamin E (1,200 IU if you run over 30 miles per week).*

- **5,000 IU of beta-carotene** (10,000 IU if you run over 30 miles per week).

- **400 micrograms** (mcg) of folic acid. (800 mcg if you run over 30 miles per week).

- **400 mcg of vitamin B-12.**

To keep vitamin costs under $5 a month, buy generic supplements in bulk (500 tablets at a time).

Just be sure the vitamin E is in its natural form (d-alpha tocopherol). It gets into cells and body fluids more efficiently than the synthetic form.

*Due to the possible interactions between vitamin E and various drugs and supplements, as well as other safety considerations, consult your doctor before starting a vitamin E regimen.

Walking Your Way to Better Health

Mort Malkin, DDS, attending surgeon emeritus at Brooklyn Hospital Center, New York. A noted authority on fitness and walking, he is author of *Aerobic Walking—The Weight-Loss Exercise*. Wiley.

Walking may be *the* ultimate form of exercise. It can provide just as much of a workout as running—even cross-country skiing—without the inconvenience, expense or risk of injury associated with those activities.

With a few simple alterations to your stride, walking is also a great way to melt away pounds and strengthen muscles. And, of course, walking is a weight-bearing exercise (good for bone-building)...and it can be done anywhere. All you need is a decent pair of shoes.

OPTIMIZING YOUR STRIDE

Conventional walking is too easy to be much of a workout. That's because it uses only a small part of the body's muscle mass.

According to a Columbia University study, conventional walking is mostly momentum. Only in the final third of the stride do the muscles produce power for forward movement... and even then the power comes from only the modestly sized calf muscles—the *soleus* and *gastrocnemius*.

To boost the fitness value of walking, you must put more muscle to work. The larger the muscle mass you involve with each stride, the greater the health benefits, including weight loss.

Here are three ways to optimize your stride...

●**Make the muscles work earlier.** Most walkers apply power only to the *end* of each stride, as they push off with the ball of the foot and the toes.

Instead: Start extending a backward force against the ground the instant your heel touches down. Think of pulling the ground under your body with your leg. This action involves the back of the thigh (hamstrings) and the buttocks (*gluteals*). Together, these muscles are up to five times bigger than your calf muscles. End each stride with a push-off as you normally would.

●**Swing your hips.** Most people use only the legs to carry their feet forward.

Better: Reach forward with the hip of the leg that is coming forward for the new stride.

Picture a line through your hips, running from left to right. If you're strolling, this line stays perpendicular to the direction of travel. In aerobic walking, the line should be at a 45 degree angle to the direction you're headed.

Result: You work your abdominals, lower back muscles and even more of the gluteals.

●**Boost your speed.** Focus on acceleration as soon as your heel strikes the ground. Imagine your eyes on a level plane. As you walk, keep them level, with no bouncing.

Look at a lamppost, tree or another object that is relatively close to you. Walk so smoothly that the object does not jiggle.

BODY BENEFITS

Put more muscle mass to work, and you will more quickly derive the benefits of walking—better fat metabolism, improved glucose tolerance, a lower resting heart rate, reduced stress, etc.

The difference between plain walking and aerobic walking is dramatic.

Example: A woman with type 2 diabetes who is taking insulin joined one of my walking classes. For several years, she had been walking five miles six days a week. She needed 20 units of insulin a day. Her blood sugar level averaged 135.

After trying the proper technique for one month, she found she needed less insulin—12 units daily. Her blood sugar level had declined to a more normal 99.

GETTING STARTED

To reduce your risk of injury, start your walking program gradually. You can begin by taking a 10- to 20-minute stroll, three or four days a week, even if you're already fit.

Add five minutes a week, working up to an average of 40 to 50 minutes a session. This is the ideal workout length for weight loss and health benefits.

As you increase workout time, also increase your speed. *You'll know you've reached the proper intensity if...*

- **You're *slightly* out of breath** throughout the workout.
- **You're a bit above the comfort zone** but are able to finish the workout. On a scale of 5 (resting) to 20 (all-out effort), your level of exertion should be about 14.
- **You're able to talk in phrases only,** not complete sentences. In fact, you won't feel like talking at all.

PICKING THE RIGHT SHOES

Try on a wide variety of walking and running shoes to find the pair that best fits your feet.

Look for: Moderate cushioning...a low, beveled heel...roominess in the toe box...flexibility...an "Achilles notch" at the back of the collar (to allow space for your Achilles tendon).

Have a salesperson check the wear pattern on your old shoes before he/she recommends a new pair.

Inexpensive Ways To Shape Up

Patrick Netter, home fitness expert and consultant, Netter Marketing Group, 333 N. Bonhill Rd., Los Angeles 90049.

Rent—or buy—workout videos from your local video store...contact an area high school about evening exercise classes for adults ...create your own home gym by buying a single well-made exercise machine—the cost will be less than joining a health club...exercise with friends to make it more difficult to put off working out.

Health Clubs Can Be Unhealthy

Rodney Basler, MD, dermatologist and past chairman of the American Academy of Dermatology's task force on sports medicine, Lincoln, NE.

Even the cleanest-looking health club can, in actuality, be full of hidden germs.

Self-defense: Grab a towel when you walk in and keep it between your body and the equipment...instead of wearing skin-baring tank tops and short shorts, exercise in T-shirts and thigh-length shorts...wear flip-flops in the shower. Pooled water on shower floors and damp carpeting can lead to athlete's foot...before using a hot tub, make sure the water is clear—cloudy water and deposits along the sides of the tub are signs of bacterial growth.

Beware of Health Club Scams

Stephen Isaacs, a lawyer and coauthor of *The Consumer's Legal Guide to Today's Health Care.* Houghton Mifflin.

The costly lifetime memberships that health clubs advertise are a bad deal. *Reason:* They last for the club's lifetime, *not yours.* When you do join a health club, read the fine print in contracts *very carefully.* Some contracts contain a comprehensive liability waiver that relieves the health club of responsibility for all accidents...even those that are caused by its own negligence.

Exercise Beats Dieting

John P. Foreyt, PhD, professor of medicine and psychiatry at Baylor College of Medicine in Houston and director of its Nutrition Research Clinic.

Exercise is more important than dieting for weight loss. In a study, researchers followed three groups of people who wanted to lose weight. One group exercised and dieted, the second dieted without exercising, the third exercised without dieting. After two years, only the group that exercised without seriously dieting maintained their weight losses.

Reason: These people said that, after working out, they didn't want to fill up on high-calorie, high-fat foods and instead ate sensibly and lost weight.

The Right Time To Exercise

Tom Thomas, PhD, professor of nutritional sciences, University of Missouri, Columbia, quoted in *Runner's World,* 33 E. Minor St., Emmaus, PA 18098.

Exercise *before* a fatty meal to minimize the artery-clogging effects of the food. A one-hour exercise session about 12 hours before a high-fat meal significantly cuts the amount of fat circulating in the blood after the meal. Exercising after the meal has little effect. *Bottom line:* If you expect to eat a high-fat dinner at night, do a one-hour run, for example, first thing in the morning.

Smarter, More Effective Exercising

Mort Malkin, DDS, attending surgeon emeritus at Brooklyn Hospital Center, New York. A noted authority on fitness and walking, he is author of *Aerobic Walking—The Weight-Loss Exercise.* Wiley.

Unless you take the proper precautions, you should avoid using weights when walking for fitness.

Why: Hand weights can cause shoulder and back pain...ankle weights can strain knees and throw you off balance.

More effective than weights: Increase your walking pace.

Exercise and Longevity

Urho Kujala, MD, PhD, unit for sports and exercise medicine, University of Helsinki, Finland.

Exercise prolongs life regardless of heredity. A study of 16,000 adult twins who were tracked for 19 years found that the active twin had a substantially lower chance of dying prematurely.

General finding: Persons who jogged, walked briskly or performed equivalent exercise for 30 minutes at least six times a month had a 43% lower death rate than persons who were sedentary.

Dr. Kenneth Cooper's Exercise Plan

Kenneth H. Cooper, MD, MPH, president and founder of the Cooper Aerobics Center, 12200 Preston Rd., Dallas 75230. He is author of numerous books on health and fitness, including *Dr. Kenneth H. Cooper's Antioxidant Revolution.* Bookman.

I've been a fitness enthusiast for several decades. But my ideas about exercise and health have changed with the times, as new medical data have emerged.

EXERCISING WISELY

For the average American, it is clear that moderate exercise is best. Moderate exercise minimizes the risk of musculoskeletal injury... it's a realistic level of exercise for most people...it's easy...and it doesn't take a lot of time.

At the Cooper Aerobics Center, we have shown that moderate activity reduces deaths from heart attack, stroke, diabetes and cancer by 55%—and increases longevity significantly.

The best exercises to perform to obtain health and longevity benefits, in no particular order, are cross-country skiing...swimming... running...cycling...and walking.

You can perform indoor or outdoor versions of these activities—and mix and match among them to keep up your interest.

A WEEKLY WORKOUT PLAN

Before you start an exercise program, consult a physician for a checkup and an exercise stress test if you're a healthy male over age 40 —or a healthy female over age 50.

Here's a great moderate-level weekly workout plan almost anyone can do...

Aerobic exercise: Perform an aerobic activity at least three times a week. *Make sure each session includes...*

- **A three- to four-minute stretching session.** Stretch your legs—hamstrings, quadriceps and Achilles tendons—and your back before and after exercising. Also stretch out your shoulders if you're preparing to do an activity with intensive arm movements, such as swimming or cross-country skiing.

Stretches should be gentle and continuous, not pulsing. Breathe evenly while stretching and stretch to the point of resistance, not to the point of pain.

- **A five- to 10-minute warm-up.** Do your chosen exercise at a slower pace to ready your musculoskeletal system for more intense activity.

Example: Walk at 75% of your usual speed until you break out in a light sweat.

- **A 20-minute aerobic segment** performed at a sustained low speed. After six to 10 weeks, gradually increase your speed and distance, and add arm movements to intensify the workout.

To become aerobically fit, walk up to 45 minutes, five times a week…or 60 minutes, two to three times a week.

- **Five-minute cool-down.** Exercise slowly again to bring your heart rate back down to normal.

- **Integrate muscle-toning exercises into your regimen.** Use weight machines or hand-held weights, or perform push-ups or stomach crunches at least twice a week for 20 minutes.

Reason: Toning exercises keep your muscles in shape—including your heart—improve strength, stamina and flexibility, and reduce the potential for injury.

You can perform muscle-toning exercises on the same days you perform aerobic activities or on alternate days.

KEEP IN MIND

- **Aging increases the risk of injury.** Therefore, the intensity of exercise becomes less important than the duration of exercise. You get as much cardiovascular aerobic benefit from walking a 12-minute mile as you do from running a nine-minute mile.

Important: Shoot for a 12- to 15-minute-per-mile pace when walking.

- **Stretching becomes more important.** It can reduce stiffness and risk of injury and improve athletic performance.

Important: If you feel pain, immediately stop what you're doing. If pain persists, have it evaluated by a physician.

- **You may gain some weight as you age**—but that's not unhealthy if you continue to exercise. Don't worry about extra pounds if you're within 20% of your ideal weight.

Better Weight-Lifting Workouts

Patrick Netter, exercise/fitness equipment consultant, 333 N. Bonhill Rd., Los Angeles 90049.

You'll develop better muscle tone and strength if you increase the weight rather than the number of repetitions. As soon as you can do three sets of 12 reps with moderate effort, add five to 10 pounds to the weight. *Also:* When doing reps, do them slowly. Fast and jerky repetitions build up momentum. That can cause strain or injury to your muscles and joints.

Short Exercise Sessions May Be Better

John Jakicic, PhD, assistant professor of behavioral medicine, Brown Medical School, Providence, RI, and leader of an exercise study of 56 women.

In a study, overweight women who exercised in three 10-minute sessions lost more weight than women who exercised in one 30-minute session.

Possible reason: The shorter-duration workouts seemed easier for the women to do—so they did them more diligently, and ended up doing more total exercise than the women who did longer workouts.

Do-It-Yourself Sports Drink

Nancy Clark, MS, RD, author of *Nancy Clark's Sports Nutrition Guidebook*. Human Kinetics.

During strenuous workouts lasting an hour or more, sports drinks such as Gatorade and Powerade are better than water for replacing carbohydrates depleted during exercise. But athletes can save money by making their own sports drinks.

Recipe: Dissolve one tablespoon sugar and a pinch of salt in a glass with one tablespoon of hot water. Add one tablespoon orange juice (or two tablespoons of lemon juice) and seven ounces of ice water.

Exercise Is Good for Asthmatics

Francois Haas, PhD, pulmonary physiologist and director, Pulmonary Function Lab, New York University Medical Center, Rusk Institute, 400 E. 34 St., New York 10016.

Aerobic conditioning helps increase lung capacity and strengthens the heart, making it easier to draw oxygen into the lungs and easier for the heart to pump oxygen-rich blood.

Helpful: Any exercise that raises the heart rate above normal limits...even walking.

Self-defense: Take medication to open the bronchial tubes at least 20 minutes before exercising. Warm up for 10 minutes before strenuous exercise. Avoid asthma-provoking situations like exercising in cold, dry weather or when the air is filled with pollution or allergens.

How to Fight Arthritis With Exercise

Marian Minor, PhD, PT, an associate professor at the University of Missouri School of Medicine, Columbia.

Walking and cycling—dynamic exercise—are good for people with arthritis.

A study found that dynamic exercise produced greater improvement in muscle strength, physical conditioning and joint mobility than the isometric or range-of-motion exercises usually recommended for people with rheumatoid arthritis.

Improved joint mobility makes it easier to move around and perform everyday bending and stretching activities.

The best way to get into a suitable noncompetitive exercise program that does not overstress your capabilities—join a group with other people who know about arthritis.

Local chapters of the Arthritis Foundation may be able to direct you, or visit their Web site at *www.arthritis.org*.

How to Stick With Your Exercise Regimen

Charles Roy Schroeder, PhD, professor of exercise physiology at the University of Memphis. He is author of *Taking the Work Out of Working Out*. Chronimed.

Have you ever committed yourself to an exercise routine—only to quickly abandon it?

If so, your commitment was probably based on the prospect of *future* goals—weight loss, lower cholesterol, firmer muscles, etc.

There's nothing wrong with these goals, but they are rarely enough to keep you motivated.

To stick with a routine, you must find ways to enjoy exercise itself. How do you do *that*? *Dr. Charles Roy Schroeder, one of the country's leading exercise physiologists, recommends these strategies...*

●**Consider your personality and lifestyle when picking an exercise routine.** If you have a demanding, people-oriented job, you might enjoy a repetitive, solitary workout like swimming or jogging.

If you thrive on competition, pick a competitive sport like tennis, basketball, etc....or pepper your workouts with goal-oriented elements, such as timed sprints.

●**Be aware of bodily sensations.** It's easy to overlook the pleasurable feelings that accompany exercise. Make it a point to be aware of these *kinesthetic* sensations—the rhythm of your breathing...the motion of your joints...the ebb and flow of tension as your muscles contract and release.

●**Add music.** The right music can make your movements more graceful and rhythmic. It can also set a pace for you.

Avoid loud or insistent music—the kind favored by many aerobics instructors. Blaring music directs your attention away from the pleasurable kinesthetic sensations.

If you're running, bicycling or skating, it's best not to wear earphones. They can make it hard for you to hear traffic or other potential hazards.

●**Work out with a mirror.** Mirrors enable you to see your muscles at work at the same time you *feel* them working—and that helps focus your mind.

Mirrors also let you check for correct form...and let you enjoy the gradual improvement in your appearance as you get into shape. That helps keep you motivated.

●**Vary your exercise routine.** *Make your workout interesting by varying...*

●**Speed and intensity.** Alternate between light and heavy weights. Experiment with different resistance settings on the exercise bike. Vary your running pace.

●**Range of motion.** Instead of lifting a weight all the way up on each repetition, lift it one-quarter of the way and then lower it. Then lift it halfway and lower it...and then lift it three-quarters of the way.

Also: Add motions that spread the work over additional muscles.

In the arm curl, for example, standard form is to hold dumbbells with hands down at sides, then bend at the elbows to bring forearms up in front of chest.

As you raise your forearms, try moving your elbows forward at the same time. That works the shoulder muscles.

●**Form.** On a bicycle, move your hips from side to side as you pedal...or push harder on alternate sides (LEFT right left, RIGHT left right).

●**Get a workout partner**—someone who is open to the idea of exploring pleasure in movement. Motivate and inspire each other.

●**Be playful.** Throw in some skipping steps as you jog. In the pool, pretend you are a dolphin or a submarine. No one has to know what you're thinking.

Giving free rein to your imagination will make exercise more enjoyable.

Better Stationary Biking

Hold It! You're Exercising Wrong by Edward Jackowski, founder of Exude, a one-on-one motivational and fitness company based in New York. Fireside.

Unless you want to add bulk to your lower body, don't bike with much tension on the wheels. The more tension, or resistance, you ride with, the bigger your leg muscles will become. *To improve muscle tone without building size:* Pedal with little or no tension at a high speed—80 to 120 rotations per minute (RPM).

 # Exercise vs. Insomnia

Peter Tanzer, MD, in private practice in Pittsburgh and author of *The Doctor's Guide for Sleep Without Pills.* Tresco.

Exercise can help beat insomnia. Exercise *well before* bedtime. Later, as you cool down, you will begin to relax and be ready for sleep.

Exercise too near bedtime is stimulating, causing increased alertness that can interfere with falling asleep.

Caution: If an exercise routine helps you sleep better, keep it up. If you stop, insomnia may return in a few days.

Exercise Surprise

Kenneth H. Cooper, MD, MPH, president and founder of the Cooper Aerobics Center, 12200 Preston Rd., Dallas 75230. He is author of numerous books on health and fitness, including *Dr. Kenneth H. Cooper's Antioxidant Revolution.* Bookman.

Shorter exercise sessions held more frequently may be better for weight loss than fewer, longer sessions.

Reason: The body burns additional calories for several minutes after exercise ends.

In theory, the calories burned during one 30-minute session equal the ones burned in three 10-minute sessions of the same intensity. But the three-session approach means the body has three post-exercise calorie burns instead of one.

"Tubing" Your Way to Strong Muscles

Brian B. Cook, senior kinesiologist (exercise specialist) at Total Physio, a physiotherapy and rehabilitation clinic in Hamilton, Ontario. He is coauthor of *Strength Basics: Your Guide to Resistance Training for Health and Optimal Performance.* Human Kinetics.

If you'd like to boost your strength and muscular endurance but weight lifting isn't right for you, "tubing" is a safe, effective alternative.

Tubing—stretching a length of rubber hose—is perfect for older individuals and for anyone just beginning or resuming an exercise program after a sedentary period. It's also good for those who lack access to weights...who want a break from conventional weight training...or who wish to stay toned while traveling. (Rubber tubing takes up little room in a suitcase.)

Tubing is very inexpensive. The recommended 12-foot length of ⅜- to ½-inch diameter tubing costs about $20. It's available from sports/fitness stores and medical supply houses.

You can make handles on the tubing simply by tying a loop on each end. If you prefer, look for tubing made just for exercise—it comes with built-in handles.

Caution: Check the tubing before each use. If you find nicks and/or tears, replace the tubing.

TUBING SCHEDULE

Do at least three 30-minute tubing workouts each week. First, stretch for five to 10 minutes. Then do two sets of 10 repetitions of each of the following exercises. After three weeks, progress to three sets of 10 reps each.

Important: Unless otherwise indicated, the tubing should be lightly stretched when you are in the starting position.

CHEST PRESS

Lie on your back with your legs bent and feet flat on the floor. Anchor the tubing under your shoulders. Place your elbows on the floor at chest height and your hands above your elbows.

Exhale and stretch the tubing to arm's length. Inhale as you slowly return to the starting position.

HALF SQUAT

Stand on the tubing at its midpoint, with feet shoulder-width apart. Holding the tubing handles, extend your arms straight down at your sides. The tubing should be fully stretched. Look straight ahead, with your abdominals tight and chest up.

Inhale as you slowly squat until your knees are bent at a 90-degree angle. Exhale as you slowly return to the starting position.

BENT-OVER ONE-ARM ROW

Lean on a chair with your left hand. Slightly bend your knees and hips, keeping your back parallel to the floor. Stand on the tubing with your right foot. Place the left foot behind you to stabilize your body.

Hold the slightly stretched tubing in your right hand, letting your arm hang straight down from the shoulder. Inhale as you pull your hand up toward your shoulder, keeping your elbow snug against your body. Exhale as you lower your hand to the starting position. Repeat, then switch arms.

BICEP CURLS

Stand on the tubing with your feet shoulder-width apart, knees slightly bent. Keep your arms against your sides and palms pointed slightly forward, with the handles in your hands.

Exhale as you slowly curl your hands up to your shoulders, keeping your elbows next to your body. Inhale as you lower your hands to the starting position.

SEATED CALF PRESS

Sit on the floor. Straighten your right leg and loop the tubing around the arch of the right foot. Keep the left leg bent, with the foot flat on the floor.

Hold the handles in both hands at chest level. Exhale as you point the toes of the right leg. Inhale as you return to the starting position.

Repeat. Then switch sides and do the exercise using the left leg.

How to Get the Most Out of Your Workouts

Miriam E. Nelson, PhD, chief of the Human Physiology Laboratory at the Jean Mayer US Department of Agriculture Human Nutrition Research Center on Aging at Tufts University in Boston. She is author of *Strong Women Stay Young*. Bantam.

Working out at a health club can be a great way to build strength and endurance. But only a fraction of the estimated 19 million Americans who now belong to health clubs are getting their money's worth.

Here's how to make sure *your* money—as well as your time and sweat—are well spent.

ASK FOR GUIDANCE

You may *think* you're exercising under the watchful eyes of the fitness trainers who are on duty at your health club.

But most trainers adopt a hands-off approach to interacting with club patrons. To avoid seeming rude, they'll correct your technique *only* if you're about to injure yourself.

Unless you take the initiative and ask for help, you may never know that you're leaning too heavily on the handrails of the stair climber...or that the short jerks you use to move the weight on the "lat pull-down" are less effective than slow, smooth movements.

Next time you work out at the gym, ask an instructor, "Am I using this piece of equipment correctly? Is there a way I could get more out of it?"

DO STRENGTH TRAINING FIRST

If you're just beginning an exercise program, don't start with aerobics classes or another cardiovascular workout. If you do, you'll probably find it hard to keep up. That's because your muscles, ligaments and bones aren't yet strong enough to take the punishment.

Instead, get a couple of weeks of strength training under your belt. Aerobic activity will then be more enjoyable.

CHALLENGE YOURSELF

It's definitely not true that you must experience pain to make fitness gains. But if you want to see noticeable improvements in strength, you must be willing to push yourself a little.

How much weight should you lift? In general, you should be able to lift a given weight only eight to 10 times before your muscles become so fatigued that you must rest.

Sharp pain is a signal to stop exercising immediately, since it could indicate a joint problem.

If you have any medical concerns, consult a doctor before beginning an exercise regimen.

BUILD BOTH SIDES OF YOUR BODY

Even if their bodies look perfectly symmetrical, most people are stronger on one side. They tend to favor that side when working out with leg-extension machines and other weight machines that involve use of both arms or legs at the same time. As a result, the stronger side always stays stronger.

When exercising both legs or arms at the same time, be conscious of challenging the weaker limb. Do not depend on the stronger one to lift the weight.

DON'T HOLD YOUR BREATH

Most people instinctively hold their breath while lifting heavy weights. But breath-holding during exertion is hazardous—especially for individuals suffering from heart disease, high blood pressure, diabetes or glaucoma. It causes excessive pressure in the chest and abdomen.

Safer: Exhale as you lift the weight…and inhale as you lower the weight. If you have trouble getting the rhythm right, count out loud as you lift.

PREVENT DEHYDRATION

You already know that it's important to drink water while working out. But it's just as important to down at least eight ounces of water *after* a workout—even if you're not thirsty.

Sports drinks such as Gatorade are appropriate only for long-distance runners and other endurance athletes.

MAKE YOUR WORKOUTS SOCIAL

Exercise with a friend. Good conversation makes those minutes on the treadmill zip by… and just being near someone you like can keep you going through a series of weight lifts.

Your workouts are also a good way to keep up with people you might otherwise be too busy to see. Finally, knowing that your workout buddy will be waiting for you at the gym makes it more likely that you'll stick to your exercise schedule.

RECORD YOUR PROGRESS

Motivate yourself by keeping an exercise log that charts your growing fitness. Such a log makes it easy to remember the proper seat adjustment, the resistance and the other settings for each machine.

Overrated Exercise Machines

Research led by William Whiting, biomechanics specialist, Los Angeles, reported in *Women's Health Letter*, Box 467939, Atlanta 31146.

Abdominal muscle exercise machines are highly overrated. They are no more effective than old-fashioned crunch exercises. Claims like losing 10 pounds in 10 days are based on using them with nutrition and aerobic exercise programs. Crunches—done with or without a device—do not burn enough calories to achieve significant weight loss. And—they

do not provide enough resistance to help users get a rippling, washboard-type abdomen.

Dance for Health and Fun

David Nieman, DrPH, professor of health and exercise science, Appalachian State University, Boone, NC 28608.

Dancing is better exercise than walking. Ballroom dancing burns 210 to 385 calories per hour. More vigorous Western or swing dancing burns up to 400 calories per hour. Walking 2.5 to 4.5 miles per hour burns about 210 to 315 calories per hour. In addition, dance classes are an excellent way to meet people— since you usually rotate partners throughout the lesson.

Better Sleeping

Donald Bliwise, PhD, former director of the Sleep Disorders Clinic at Emory University School of Medicine, Atlanta.

Exercise during the day can help you sleep better at night. Researchers set up a program of moderate exercise four times a week for a group of people between age 50 and age 76 who had difficulty sleeping at night and they found that they were able to sleep more soundly. Experts say that to help sleep, exercise should be done earlier in the day, well before supper time. *Best:* Bike riding, brisk walking or other moderate aerobic exercise.

Finding the Fountain Of Youth

Research conducted by Gary Hunter, PhD, professor of exercise physiology, School of Education, University of Alabama, Birmingham.

Strength training is the closest thing to a "fountain of youth."

Study: Women as old as age 77 who began training on weight machines increased their physical strength more than 50% within four months. Such strength is vital in preventing debilitating injuries often associated with aging—from gradual weakening and lessening of mobility, to osteoporosis and injuries from falls. The women in the study also increased their walking speed by 18% even though walking was not part of their training.

Important: Aerobic exercises such as walking and swimming, while excellent for general health, do not provide strength benefits. Resistance training with weights or machines is necessary to accomplish this.

Sore Muscle Relief

Patrice Morency, MS, director, Innerweave Clinic, Portland, OR.

Soothe sore muscles with a hot/cold shower. Start with two minutes of hot water, then change to cold water for two minutes. Repeat this hot/cold cycle five times.

Why it works: The temperature changes cause alternating constriction and dilation of blood vessels. That helps flush lactic acid—the chemical that underlies soreness—from the muscles.

Hot Weather Jogging

Jeff Galloway, former Olympic runner who conducts fitness clinics in the US, writing in *Runner's World*, 33 E. Minor St., Emmaus, PA 18098.

Keep your head wet by pouring water over yourself at the start of your run and every 10 to 20 minutes…wear light, synthetic clothing so sweat will evaporate faster…after the run, cool down by pouring water over yourself or taking a cool swim or shower.

Best Swimming Exercise

Men's Fitness, 21100 Erwin St., Woodland Hills, CA 91367.

When swimming for exercise, use a basic crawl stroke. Cover as much water as possible with each stroke. Measure progress by how many strokes it takes to swim the length of the pool. Breathe every other stroke. Avoid holding your breath for several strokes. Keep power coming from your arms—two or three relaxed, shallow kicks per stroke are plenty. To sharpen strokes, swim as fast as possible with clenched fists.

Exercising to Lose Weight

Robert McMurray, PhD, professor of sports science and nutrition, University of North Carolina, Chapel Hill.

Exercising to lose weight works if you can do at least 45 minutes of aerobic and strength training five days a week. *Regimen:* Change your routine on a daily or weekly basis to lower the risk of muscle strain and reduce monotony.

Example: Switch between swimming and walking. Performing a variety of exercises will keep more muscles toned and may burn more calories.

Easy Rheumatoid Arthritis Relief

Mary J. Bell, MD, staff rheumatologist, Sunnybrook Health Science Center, University of Toronto. Her six-week study of 150 rheumatoid arthritis patients was presented at a meeting of the American College of Rheumatology.

Exercise helps ease joint stiffness caused by rheumatoid arthritis. Patients who did light exercise—walking and stretching—for as little as three hours over a six-week period reported a significant reduction in stiffness. Exercise is also effective against osteoarthritis.

Walking with Weights Works!

David Nieman, DrPH, professor of health and exercise science, Appalachian State University, Boone, NC.

Walking with weights burns more calories than walking without weights.

To avoid injury: Start with a one-pound weight in each hand. Gradually increase to five pounds. Keep stride length normal and consistent...and walk slowly until you've adjusted to the weights.

Caution: Swinging your arms excessively while carrying hand weights can cause elbow or shoulder injuries. If possible, alternate use of hand weights with ankle weights and weight vests.

How to Develop the Exercise Habit

Adele Pace, MD, an Ashland, KY, psychiatrist with a special interest in fitness. She is author of *The Busy Executive's Guide to Total Fitness.* Prentice Hall.

Everyone knows that exercise is good for you. That it reduces your risk for heart disease, diabetes and cancer. That it lowers your weight while raising your spirits. But for too many of us, the gap between couch and gym is just too great.

Many people embark on an ambitious exercise program only to lapse back into inactivity after a few workouts. These people fail to develop the *exercise habit* that keeps some people up and active through all kinds of moods and weather.

A POSITIVE ADDICTION

As with food and sex, we have an innate appetite for physical activity. Working out triggers production of *dopamine* and other pleasure-giving neurotransmitters, and the brain comes to crave this rewarding "bath" of neurotransmitters.

Consequently, people who work out regularly develop a sort of addiction to exercise.

For them, exercise is no longer a chore or obligation. It's a pleasurable habit.

How do you reach that point? The key is finding a way to *enjoy* your workouts. If you dread exercise—if you expect it to be painful and/or boring—it will be. Anticipate pleasure, and you'll find that instead.

SELF-EDUCATION IS KEY

Having a vague notion that exercise is beneficial does nothing for your attitude. You must read up on the specific, concrete rewards of exercise.

Good sources of information: *The American College of Sports Medicine Fitness Book* (IBS)...and Dr. Robert Cooper's *Health and Fitness Excellence* (Houghton Mifflin).

Find out exactly how exercise strengthens the muscles and boosts endurance. Learn how regular workouts cut your risk for heart disease as effectively as quitting smoking.

Talk to enthusiastic exercisers. Get them to tell you how they feel during and after working out. Ask them why they do it. Catch their excitement.

When I was a medical resident, I knew I should exercise. But I had no time—or so I thought. I asked a student—a 25-mile-a-week runner—why he wasted the time when his schedule was already jammed.

He explained vividly how running gave him extra energy and honed his concentration. He claimed that the 30 minutes a day he spent running actually made him a better student.

Guess what? He graduated first in his class.

REWARD YOURSELF

One good way to train yourself to become a habitual exerciser is to bolster your brain's natural reinforcement system with external rewards.

During your workouts, envision the cold drink you'll treat yourself to after it's over...or promise yourself a bagel or low-fat muffin.

Set up a system of short-term rewards for meeting your goals. If you've faithfully walked 30 minutes a day all week, indulge yourself with a good book or movie...a new article of clothing...or an afternoon off from work. Enjoy this special treat with a clear conscience.

To maintain your interest—and boost your fitness—continually revise your goals upward.

As your conditioning improves, shoot for a 20-minute-a-mile pace, then a 15-minute-a-mile pace (or whatever pace seems reasonable for you).

Record your progress in an exercise journal. Review it periodically to remind yourself of just how far you have come.

SECRETS OF EXERCISE SUCCESS

•**Exercise with a buddy.** Running, walking or weight-training with a like-minded individual is far more pleasurable than working out alone.

When you have an exercise buddy, each exercise period becomes a social occasion as well as a workout. You look forward to getting together. You can compare notes and encourage each other, too.

•**Help others with their exercise programs.** In addition to *seeking* help in forming an exercise habit, *give* help to a friend or family member who wants to get into shape. Doing so makes it harder to accept your own excuses for not working out.

If you have kids, exercising together certainly qualifies as "quality time." By encouraging your kids to exercise, you help them cultivate a life-long, life-giving habit.

Helping others works even if the other "person" is a dog. I became a committed runner as a result of taking my overweight Collie-Shepherd mix, Sam, on a daily two-mile run. No matter how tired I feel, I refuse to let the pup miss his exercise.

•**Combine exercise with another activity.** I exercise outdoors as much as possible, resorting to the gym only when bad weather hits (or for weight-lifting).

Like many people, I find stair-climbers and stationary bicycles boring. To make working out on them more palatable, I read magazines and medical journals as I step or pedal.

When I run on a treadmill, I listen to self-help audio tapes. One of my favorites is Dr. Denis Waitley's six-tape set *The Psychology of Winning* (Nightingale Conant).

•**Include several different kinds of exercise in your repertoire.** You might run one day, bike the next, swim the next, etc. "Cross-training" helps you achieve full-body fitness while staving off boredom.

EXERCISING ON THE ROAD

Before departing, call ahead to find out if health club facilities are available at your hotel (or nearby). If you return to the same city frequently, scout out the best exercise opportunities.

If you've been cross-training, you'll have no trouble getting in a good workout—whether the available facilities are geared to running, bicycling, swimming, etc.

Exercise vs. The Blues

Kathleen Moore, PhD, research associate, department of psychiatry, Duke University Medical Center, Durham, NC. Her study of 57 depressed people 50 years of age or older was presented at a meeting of the Society of Behavioral Medicine.

Even short workouts—as brief as eight minutes—are enough to enhance mood.

Earlier studies showed the psychological benefits of *sustained* exercise. But this is the first to suggest that brief workouts reduce feelings of sadness, tension, fatigue, anger and confusion.

21

The Whole You— The Mind/Body Connection

Deepak Chopra's Secrets of Having Boundless Energy

Deepak Chopra, MD
Chopra Center

Fatigue is one of the most common problems doctors are asked to treat. Complaints about exhaustion are likely to continue, given our busy schedules and many demands on our lives.

Yet despite the large number of people who feel tired day after day, fatigue is an unnatural state. Such fatigue does not occur in animals or children. When children and animals are tired, they rest and awaken renewed.

But adults have the ability to maneuver around their biological needs. They drive themselves...resist the natural, biological cycle of alternating rest and activity...and become depleted.

To banish common fatigue, we need to rediscover our basic harmony with nature. The secret of recovering our harmony can be found in a mind/body system of health, which is based on the understanding that your own mind/body system is inseparably connected to the systems of nature.

WATCH WHAT YOU EAT

You can increase your energy by eating fresh, pure foods. By contrast, foods that lack freshness and are highly processed deplete the body of energy. *Foods especially rich in natural energy include...*

- **Fresh fruits and lightly cooked vegetables.**

- **Wheat, rice, barley and other whole grains.**

- **Nonmeat sources of protein**, such as dried beans. For those who balk at a vegetarian diet, fish and poultry are acceptable substitutes.

Deepak Chopra, MD, founder of the Chopra Center in Carlsbad, CA. He is author of numerous books, including *Boundless Energy* (Rider) and *The Seven Spiritual Laws of Success* (Amber-Allen).

●**Honey as a substitute for refined sugar.**
Foods that deplete energy and should be avoided include red meat, aged cheese, alcohol, coffee and smoked and canned foods. This does not mean you must completely avoid anything but energy-boosting foods.

Any system that is too rigid will create further imbalance. Instead, experiment with these suggestions and notice what proportion makes a significant difference in your own energy level.

STRENGTHEN YOUR DIGESTION

Poor digestion can sometimes lead to fatigue in two ways…

●**Energy for the body is lost when food is not adequately metabolized.**

●**When food residue lingers undigested**, impurities and toxins may accumulate, placing stress on the body.

How to strengthen your digestion and boost your energy level…

●**Create a calm atmosphere for dining.**
Instead of always working through lunch and watching TV during dinner, enjoy yourself and pay attention to your meal. Conversation is fine —but avoid controversial subjects.

When the body is accustomed to a routine, digestion will be automatic. So stick to regular mealtimes.

●**Eat your biggest meal at lunch.** Research indicates that this is the time when metabolism is most efficient.

●**Sip warm water or herbal tea throughout the day** to normalize the metabolic rate and eliminate toxins.

Helpful: Fill a thermos with warm water, which enhances digestion. Keep it nearby and take a few sips every half-hour.

REDUCE STRESS

Tension drains the body of energy, causing it to function less effectively.

Better: Make it a priority to spend time on relaxing activities. Everyone has favorite pastimes, and some of these can even take place during the work day.

Classic stress-relievers: Meditation, a massage, sex, a warm shower or bath, playing or listening to music…and a change of scenery.

EXERCISE IN MODERATION

Americans' obsession with strenuous exercise is creating an epidemic of exhaustion. Pushing ourselves past what our bodies are naturally designed to handle results in long-lasting fatigue.

Solution: For maximum energy, exercise seven days a week for 15 to 20 minutes at a time. Some fitness experts recommend taking a day off between workouts—but that's because our average workouts are too strenuous. Instead, exercise daily, but to only 50% of your capacity.

Example: If you are able to swim 20 laps, only swim 10. You'll feel energetic—and over time, your capacity will increase.

KEEPING NATURAL RHYTHMS

The body is most responsive to certain activities when they are performed at specific times of the day.

Before electric light was invented, our schedules were more in keeping with these natural rhythms under which our bodies evolved. Rediscovering them will help you feel energetic every day.

●**Awaken between 6 a.m. and 7 a.m.**

●**Exercise in the morning**—or, if this isn't possible, no later than three hours before bedtime.

●**Eat lunch between 12 p.m. and 1 p.m.**

●**Eat dinner between 6 p.m. and 7 p.m.**
…and wind down with restful activities afterward, such as going for a walk, reading, playing games with your family or listening to music.

●**Go to bed between 10 p.m. and 11 p.m. each night.**

Helpful: If you try going to bed at 10 p.m. but find you have trouble falling asleep, don't worry about it. Just rest quietly with your eyes closed. Clear your mind, and avoid dwelling on anything that is troubling you. Your body will get the rest it needs. Over time, you'll gradually notice an increase in energy in the morning, and you'll be able to fall asleep at the earlier hour.

TAKE PLEASURE IN LIFE

Joy is a natural energizer. If you're having a good time, you'll never be fatigued. In fact, studies have found that 80% of people suffering from chronic fatigue score higher than normal on measures of depression and anxiety.

Solution: Practice shifting your awareness to the positive. We can't avoid negative events, but we don't have to dwell on them.

Treat others with kindness, tolerance and love...refuse to entertain negativity...and pay attention to the joy and playfulness that can be found all around you. Learn to meditate to help you get in touch with nature and enable you to see these simple joys.

EXCEPTION TO THE RULE

If you are bothered by persistent fatigue, have a thorough medical checkup to rule out a treatable physical cause—such as anemia, thyroid problems or mononucleosis.

Mind/Body Techniques for Enhanced Wellness

David S. Sobel, MD, director, regional health education, Kaiser Permanente Northern California, Oakland. He is coauthor of *The Healthy Mind, Healthy Body Handbook.* Time-Life.

What's the most powerful healing tool you can find? Your brain. While drugs are usually used to treat an existing medical condition, mind/body techniques may be more effective than medication in *preventing* some medical problems. They are also less expensive, safer and have longer lasting benefits than medication.

POSITIVE THINKING

People with an optimistic, confident attitude are healthier than others. Optimism boosts the immune system...increases longevity...reduces symptoms of illness...and improves the outcome of surgery.

To think more positively: Track your thoughts in different situations by writing down what is bothering you, what physical symptoms you feel and what negative thoughts are passing through your mind.

Think about how realistic your pessimistic reactions are...and write down some alternative, more positive responses.

Focus on what you have, not what you lack. Think of the good things in your life—family, friends, enjoyable pastimes.

Inventory your talents, skills, achievements and positive qualities—big and small. When something goes wrong, put your disappointment in perspective by consulting your list of "positives."

LAUGHTER IS KEY

A hearty laugh gives a good "workout" to your face, shoulders, diaphragm and abdomen ...and sometimes even your arms and legs. This "inner jogging" burns calories at the same rate as brisk walking. It reduces your susceptibility to pain, curbs stress and boosts the immune system.

Harness the health benefits of humor: Seek out funny movies, books and comedians...look at the cartoons in books and magazines—cut out those that particularly amuse you and post them where you can see them...tell your favorite jokes to other people—and listen to theirs.

When something happens that inconveniences you, don't get mad—get funny.

SENSORY STIMULATION

Sensory pleasures reduce stress, anxiety and depression...lower blood pressure...decrease pain...and enhance immune function. *To increase your sensory enjoyment...*

•**Touch.** Warm your hands by rubbing them together rapidly, then cup them over your eyes.

•**Sight.** Get a small aquarium with tropical fish. Watching fish for 20 minutes has been shown to reduce blood pressure.

•**Hearing.** Learn to play a musical instrument...join a singing group...or exercise in time to music.

•**Taste.** Pay close attention to the flavors and aromas of your food. If you savor each bite, you will eat less and enjoy it more.

BETTER COMMUNICATION

Communicating poorly can make you feel defensive, hostile and/or frustrated. Effective communication makes you feel in control of events and connected to other people. *Communication secrets...*

●**Listen well.** If what someone tells you is unclear, ask friendly questions to clarify it. Paraphrase—but don't parrot—his/her statements back to him.

Listen attentively to understand the feelings that underlie his words. Let him know that you understand his feelings.

●**Watch your body language.** Make sure that it matches your words.

●**Be assertive, not passive or aggressive.** Passivity implies that you feel weak and inferior, leading you to bottle up anger, resentment and hurt. Aggressive responses imply that you feel superior and may produce retaliatory and defensive reactions.

Assertive responses convey the attitude that while you and the other person may differ, you are equally entitled to express yourselves. This makes it easier to resolve problems.

To be assertive: Explain how you see the situation as objectively as you can...state *your* opinions and *your* feelings about the subject, without blaming the other person for making you feel that way. State requests clearly and specifically. Look for win–win outcomes.

HELPING OTHERS

Doing good not only makes you feel better—it also keeps you healthier. Excessive concern with your own comfort leads to depression, poor health and a life with little meaning. People involved in helping others form stronger social ties. That has a positive effect on health.

A recent study of 3,300 volunteers found that 95% of them felt that personally helping other people provided an immediately pleasurable sensation—the so-called "helper's high." This is a sudden warmth, a surge of energy and a feeling of euphoria immediately after helping.

Ninety percent said they were healthier than other people their own age. Many reported fewer colds, headaches and backaches...and improved eating and sleeping habits.

20 Minutes a Day To a Much Happier, Much Healthier Life

Herbert Benson, MD, associate professor of medicine at Harvard Medical School, and director emeritus of the Benson Henry Institute for Mind/Body Medicine, Chestnut Hill, MA, and coauthor of Timeless Healing: The Power and Biology of Belief. Scribner.

In more than 30 years of practicing medicine, I have found that the most impressive healing force—one that is universally accessible—is the power of the individual to cure himself/herself.

REMEMBERED WELLNESS

Doctors have long known that many patients will show improvement if they are given a placebo—a "dummy" pill—simply because they believe that the pill prescribed by the doctor will be effective. Most of the success physicians had before the modern era of scientific medicine probably came from this effect, because most of the medicines they used back then had little or no pharmaceutical value.

Example: During my college years, I spent one summer working as a seaman on a merchant ship. Knowing I was a premed student, my fellow sailors came to me after shore-leave carousing to cure their hangovers. I gave them vitamin tablets, the only pills I had to dispense, and was amazed to see how effectively they cured my shipmates' symptoms.

Most researchers dismiss this "placebo effect" as an unwanted complication that makes it difficult to carry out objective research into the effect of medical treatments. But, the placebo effect shows how powerful belief can be in enlisting the body's own curative powers.

When patients trust a physician, a treatment he recommends can be remarkably effective even though scientific medicine says it should not work. I think we should recognize the remarkable ability of the human mind to direct the body away from illness and toward health by dropping the expression "placebo effect" in favor of a positive term such as "remembered wellness."

Examples: In 1979, Harvard's Dr. David P. McCallie, Jr., and I studied a variety of treatments that had been used to relieve angina in the past—but that were revealed to have no physiological effect. We found that as long as the medical profession still believed in them, they worked 70% to 90% of the time. Later, when better-informed physicians began to doubt them, the effectiveness of these treatments dropped by more than half.

More recent studies have shown that remembered wellness helps patients obtain relief more than 70% of the time from chest pain, fatigue, dizziness, back pain and congestive heart failure.

MIND AND BODY

Remembered wellness is a powerful tool for restoring health. You can use it purposefully by training your body to enlist the mind's power of belief.

Brain researchers have found that thinking about a particular event produces the same pattern of activity in the brain as actually experiencing the event. The brain sends signals to the body that make it react the same way to the mental image as it would to the actual experience.

Example: When the old blockbuster movie *Lawrence of Arabia* was playing, movie theater concession stands experienced record demand for drinks. Moviegoers who had been watching desert action for two hours emerged during the intermission as thirsty as they would have been had they actually spent that time in the Arabian desert.

Our brains continuously produce images with powerful bodily effects. In particular, most of us today are continually exposed to stressful situations of one type or another, from heavy traffic...to work deadlines...to family problems.

The brain's natural response to stress, known as the fight-or-flight response, is to pump out adrenaline and other stress hormones. These substances increase blood pressure and produce harmful effects on the body, including blockage of blood vessels, disturbances in heart rhythm, anxiety, depression, anger and hostility.

Medications are not effective in the long run in dealing with the symptoms of stress.

A better way is to enlist the body's own recuperative power of remembered wellness.

One particularly effective method is to practice the *relaxation response*.

LET HEALING BEGIN

The *relaxation response* is the result of practicing mental focusing techniques that prevent an agitated mind from jumping from one stress-producing thought to another. When the mind calms down, the body follows suit. The relaxation response slows the body's metabolism and produces slow brain waves that are associated with pleasurable feelings.

To produce the relaxation response: Sit in a comfortable position, close your eyes, relax and breathe slowly and naturally while silently repeating a particular phrase you have chosen.

The focus phrase can be a religious word, phrase or prayer of particular significance to you, or a secular term that has a calming effect. *Examples:* "God, grant me the serenity"... "Peace"..."Relax."

If your mind wanders, passively disregard the disturbing thoughts and return to your focus phrase.

Continue for 10 to 20 minutes, then allow other thoughts to return to your mind, open your eyes and sit for another minute before getting up.

Free of distraction, the body will be encouraged to use its own recuperative powers.

THE LIFESAVING POWER OF BELIEF

When people believe that life is meaningful and that they have a mission to accomplish, they are strongly motivated to commit all their inner mind/body resources to help them fight illness. That combination sometimes produces medical miracles.

Example: My patient, a deeply religious 71-year-old widow, having overcome diabetes and several heart attacks, was suffering from an advanced case of throat cancer. When her doctor recommended surgery to remove half her jaw, she refused, insisting that she would be able to survive with radiation therapy, another proven but less aggressive therapy.

As she suffered the devastating side effects of radiation, she never lost the belief that she would survive so she could continue helping other people. She bolstered her powers of resistance by practicing the relaxation response, and her many friends and relatives across the country complemented her fervent prayers with prayers of their own.

Five years later, the tumor has vanished, and my patient is fitter than she has been for a long time.

BOTTOM LINE

Modern medicine has many effective medications and procedures that target specific diseases. Both physicians and patients need to recognize that these techniques work best when they are used in combination with the patient's own inner beliefs.

How to Use Guided Imagery for Wellness

Mitchell L. Gaynor, MD, clinical assistant professor of medicine at Weill Cornell Medical College, New York City. He is author of *Healing Essence: A Cancer Doctor's Practical Program for Hope and Recovery.* Kodansha.

Can your imagination protect you from cancer and other serious ailments? Can it cure disease? Extend life? Can it make you less anxious and more fulfilled?

Although more research needs to be done, preliminary studies suggest that the answer to each of these questions is *yes*.

To harness the power of your imagination, you must practice guided imagery on a daily basis.

This easy mental exercise involves creating and then focusing on a tranquil mental picture —basking in the warm sun on a sandy, windswept beach, for instance. Psychologist Jeanne Achterberg has called *guided imagery* "thinking without words."

HOW THE MIND HEALS THE BODY

Over the last eight years, I've taught thousands of cancer patients to use guided imagery for healing and recovery...and the same technique can be used by *healthy* individuals to become happier, more relaxed—and less vulnerable to illness.

My imagery regimen, which I call *Essence*, is not a substitute for medical care. It's an adjunct to conventional cancer therapies like chemotherapy, radiation and bone marrow transplantation.

A scientific field called *psychoneuroimmunology* (PNI) has demonstrated clearly that the mind plays a key role in health and illness.

Specifically, negative psychological factors like stress, depression and pessimism impair the immune system...while joy, optimism and other positive emotions enhance it.

In one landmark study, breast cancer patients who practiced meditation and guided imagery in addition to receiving conventional medical care lived *twice* as long as a control group who got only conventional medical care.

In another study, conducted at Yale University, patients suffering from depression began to feel much better when they visualized scenes in which they were praised by people they admired.

By using my Essence program, you can cultivate positive, health-promoting emotions— and assist in your own healing.

ESSENCE AT WORK

One of my patients, a 28-year-old man, had experienced a complete remission from cancer after receiving a bone marrow transplant. But he hadn't slept in three months. He was afraid he would never wake up.

Guided imagery gave him a sense of peace that enabled him to release the fear. Soon, he was able to get the restorative sleep he needed to stay well.

Another patient was benefiting from chemotherapy, but the nausea caused her so much suffering that she was thinking about discontinuing it.

With my program, her anxiety and nausea dissipated. She was able to get on with her lifesaving treatment.

When another of my patients discovered that cancer had spread to his liver, he was sure that the disease was too advanced for chemotherapy to help.

My program helped him realize that he was a person, not a statistic...and that the outcome *in his case* was uncertain. He had a partial remission, and is back at work a year after his diagnosis.

Even if your illness cannot be cured—and not all can—my program can help eliminate *emotional* suffering.

THE ESSENCE OF ESSENCE

Most of us were brought up with a clear picture of how our lives were supposed to turn out. We suffer because our lives fall short of our expectations.

We struggle against the reality of disease. *It's not supposed to be this way*, we think…or *Life's not fair.*

But deep within each of us lies the true self —our "essence." It's the part of you that doesn't judge your life, but accepts it. It doesn't smother unpleasant feelings. It doesn't turn physical pain into emotional pain with thoughts such as, *I just can't stand this* and *Why must this happen to me?*

You experience your essence only when your mind becomes quiet and your thoughts recede. Meditation helps, but I've found that my program works faster.

I ask my patients to do this for 20 minutes, twice daily…

Sit in a quiet setting, breathing slowly. Let the breath come through your nose, into your upper abdomen and out through your mouth.

Focus on a positive thought, preceded by the word "infinite." *Examples:* Infinite peace… infinite love…infinite healing. *Next…*

• **Experience whatever negative emotion is troubling you.** Try to envision the emotion as a physical thing, endowed with shape, temperature, color, etc.

• **See your essence as a white light just above your head.**

• **Surrender your pain**, suffering or sadness. Imagine the negative emotion being swallowed by the white light.

• **Empower your healing.** Breathe deeply, and as you inhale, visualize white light going into the region of your body once occupied by suffering or pain.

• **Nurture the idea of a positive outcome.** Imagine a life free of pain, fear and suffering.

• **Create an imaginary channel** that lets the white light of your essence continuously flow into the place where you experience negative emotions.

• **Embody your own healing power.** Imagine each cell of your body being suffused with the white light.

While I developed this technique for cancer patients, it can also heal the suffering caused by any illness, including heart disease, arthritis, etc. It can even help people who are healthy.

We all suffer fears, painful memories and disappointments. We forget who we truly are as we struggle to meet unrealistic expectations …and condemn those around us who fail to meet our expectations of them. We push these feelings aside, but they take their toll.

Simply focus on whatever is bothering you —job stress, marital strife, etc. At the same time, visualize your essence. Let its healing power flow through your mind and body.

How to Use Your Mind to Improve Your Health

Steven Locke, MD, former chief of behavioral medicine, Harvard Pilgrim Health Care, New England's largest health maintenance organization. He is now in private practice in Wayland, MD. Dr. Locke is coauthor of *The Healer Within*. HarperOne.

While some doctors still caution against using creative visualization and other "mind–body" techniques to the exclusion of conventional medicine, studies make it increasingly clear that one's attitude and emotional state play key roles in the prevention of—and recovery from—illness.

We asked Harvard Medical School scientist Steven Locke, MD, about the relationship between the mind and the immune system…

• **What effects do positive emotions have on immunity?** Close relationships with friends and family members seem to have significant and highly beneficial effects on the immune system. Several studies have shown, for example, that married people live longer than those who are single or divorced. Other studies have linked happiness and positive emotions to longer survival among cancer patients.

Study I: Eighty-six women with advanced breast cancer were divided into two groups.

One group received standard medical care... the other received medical care *and* weekly group therapy sessions.

Result: The women who received group therapy lived nearly twice as long as those who received only medical care.

Study II: Melanoma patients were divided into two groups. The first group received medical care only...the second group received medical care as well as stress-management training.

Result: Those in the second group suffered far less distress over their cancer diagnoses than those in the first group...their immune functions were much stronger...and their rate of survival was greater. *Also:* There was a greater trend—though not statistically significant—for melanoma to recur in the first group.

●**How do negative emotions affect the immune system?** Stressful events, such as the death of a family member, marital separation, the loss of a job—even taking a college exam—cause marked deficits in the immune function, as measured by changes in the number and function of specialized blood cells.

Unknown: Whether or not these events increased susceptibility to illness. Also unknown is whether depression and other emotional problems cause cancer. While they can lead to self-destructive habits that cause cancer, there is no clear evidence that they themselves result in the illness.

●**Is there a cancer personality?** Some researchers suggest that there are behavior patterns—including suppression of hostility or a helpless/hopeless attitude—that place some people at greater risk for cancer.

In my opinion, the notion that your personality determines your cancer risk is simplistic and emotionally destructive. Cancer is bad enough without believing your illness is your fault.

Reality: People develop cancer not because of personality defects but because of hereditary predispositions to the disease...exposure to tobacco smoke or other carcinogens...a high-fat, low-fiber diet...or excessive alcohol use.

●**Is there any value in guided imagery, deep relaxation and other "alternative" techniques?** Such techniques certainly give those who are ill a psychological boost by engendering a sense of empowerment.

Less certain: Whether these techniques do what they are intended to do—marshal the immune defenses against pathogens.

In a study at Ohio State University, elderly people received training in progressive muscle relaxation.

Result: The subjects had significantly more natural killer-cells—a type of immunity that protects against viral illness and cancer—in their bloodstreams after the training than they did before.

Caution: These techniques are unproven for cancer or other life-threatening illnesses. Patients who wish to use them should not abandon their conventional treatments in the belief that these techniques will cure them.

●**Does laughter play a role in the battle against illness?** Norman Cousins, the late editor and essayist who wrote about his personal health battle in *Anatomy of an Illness*, was among the first to argue that laughter does *not* play a role. He felt misunderstood about the power of laughter. He believed what made the difference for him was the sense of empowerment from being an active participant in his treatment. Although he used comedies to induce positive emotions, he emphasized hope, a sense of control and loving support as critical factors in healing. Research, however, suggests laughter may affect immunity.

Study: Watching a humorous video (in this case a comedian) reduced levels of adrenaline and cortisol in the bloodstream—according to scientists at Loma Linda University in California. These and other substances that suppress immunity are produced by the body in great quantities during times of stress.

●**Is it true that hostile, angry people die younger?** Dr. Redford Williams and his associates at Duke University found that certain forms of hostility—cynicism and mistrust—are associated with higher mortality. Other studies suggest that people who are either too angry or who never express their anger may be at higher risk. At Harvard, my colleagues and I did a study of various psychosocial factors and immunity.

Among our findings: People who were deemed most hostile had lower natural killer-cell activity.

Possible explanation: Hostile and mistrustful individuals may have poor social networks. Many studies suggest that the support of friends and family plays a protective role in health.

● **Can mind power combat a common cold?** Stress increases the likelihood of developing colds. Since relaxation techniques have increased immune responses in other studies, deep breathing and meditation might be helpful in strengthening resistance to the cold virus. Although this hasn't been well researched, it seems worth a try.

Your Mind And Your Health

Elliott S. Dacher, MD, practices internal medicine and conducts healing and wellness seminars nationwide. He is author of *Whole Healing: A Step-by-Step Program to Reclaim Your Power to Heal.* Plume.

When left unexpressed and unresolved, emotions such as anger, hostility and feelings of loss and stress are dangerous to your health. So are feelings of powerlessness.

Example: A study in *The Journal of the American Medical Association* showed that people who had little or no control over their jobs reported feeling "helpless and powerless"—and were more likely to develop heart problems and elevated blood pressure levels.

Though feelings of anxiety will arise, they can be managed so that your health is not compromised by them.

WHY PALMS SWEAT

Our minds have greater influence over our well-being than most of us realize. The human brain produces chemicals called *neuropeptides* —messengers that deliver information to various parts of the body. The medical world recently discovered that neuropeptides are also produced outside the brain—in tissues, organs and even in the immune system's white blood cells. Neuropeptides, nerves and other neurotransmitters link every part of the body, creating a kind of inner conversation. What happens in one area or organ can affect numerous other organs.

Example: If you are about to give a speech and are feeling nervous, your brain may send neuropeptides carrying an anxiety-provoking message to your stomach (creating butterflies). In turn, your stomach may send similar messages to the back of your neck (triggering stiffness), your heart (causing palpitations) and your hands (resulting in sweaty palms).

Medical researchers now recognize that it is impossible to separate the mind's health from the body's health. What you believe, think or feel will affect your body in the short and long term, and a growing number of experts strongly suspect that you can use your mind not only to ward off illness but also to heal yourself when you get sick.

USING YOUR MIND

● **Tap into your power of choice.** To combat feelings of helplessness and powerlessness— in the workplace, in personal relationships or in your health care—make informed, intelligent choices.

Example: In the area of health care, it's crucial to realize you can't allow yourself to be helpless, relying on practitioners or institutions to make the best choices for you or to ensure your long-term health. You need to take charge.

When you see your doctor, make sure you're armed with information about your condition. Visit your public or hospital library …read medical journal articles…check out online sources, such as HealthWorld *(www. healthy.net)*, which provides access to articles on medical conditions.

By making informed choices in every area of your life—and by acting rather than being acted upon—you will gain that important sense of control.

● **Listen to and trust your body.** Each day, I see patients who complain of sore throats or colds that just won't go away. When I ask them, *Have you taken time off work to get well?* the answer is almost always, *No.*

My message to them: *If you were any animal other than a human, you would listen and respond to your body telling you to rest. You would find a resting place somewhere, curl up and go to sleep until you felt better.*

Too often our "intelligent" mind tells us we absolutely must finish a project at work or we must devote a Saturday afternoon to coaching our child's soccer team, even though we're exhausted. We ignore the signals sent by our bodies and our more intuitive and wiser minds.

Symptoms of illness may be more than signs of a physical problem. Often, they are a signal that something is out of sync in your life, that some aspect of your approach to life needs changing.

If you're chronically tired or sluggish, your body may be telling you to exercise more or change your diet—or simply unplug your phone and crawl into bed for a healing rest.

When you learn to listen to and trust the messages your body sends, you will be taking an important step toward achieving optimal health.

●**Give your mind a rest.** Just as your body needs sleep for renewal and optimal health, your mind needs periods of quiet and solitude.

A quiet mind reveals important things about your life, changes you may need to make to create a healthier and richer lifestyle. Inner information such as this cannot break through constant mental chatter. A period of solitude "recharges" the brain and the body.

Helpful: I often tell people, especially working parents, to take a half day off from work …or spend a Saturday alone…or go to a retreat or spa for a weekend and reflect, read, walk or listen to music.

●**Confide in a friend and/or keep a journal.** When you think only about your problems, it's likely that you'll end up obsessing about them—and feeling even more stressed.

Helpful: Spend time with a trusted friend, sharing your innermost fears, your sadness over the loss of a loved one or your feelings of anger or bitterness about a problem at work. Research shows that something as simple as social support greatly enhances one's health.

Or spend 15 to 20 minutes every evening writing in a journal. Research shows that talking with a close friend about your feelings or writing them down greatly relieves stress. Writing also imposes order on a particular situation, so you are more able to resolve problems.

I've kept a journal for 20 years and when I look back on what I've written, I discover thought and behavior patterns—good ones and bad ones. I see decisions I've made and directions I've taken. Often I realize that I need to change certain patterns in order to achieve a more truly healthful life.

●**Look for meaning in every part of your life.** Finding meaning in one's life, studies show, is an essential part of good health. While it's easy to discover meaning in the positive aspects of your life, such as your loving relationship with your children and joy in your work, it is difficult to find meaning and purpose in life's difficulties and crises.

When you face a difficult situation at work or in a personal relationship, rather than feeling powerless or angry or resentful, ask, *Is there something I can learn from this situation?*

When you find positive meaning in every aspect of your life and start to realize that there is a greater force operating, you begin to develop the spirituality essential for true health.

●**View health as a lifelong process.** Most of us think of "health" as the absence of disease. But health is much more than being symptom-free and more than fixing what's broken. Everything we do, feel or experience plays a role—good or bad—in our health.

I like to think of health as an art—a lifelong process of developing, shaping and composing our lives.

How to Make Your Mind Very Sharp

Harry Lorayne can memorize every person's name in a room of 500 people and recite from memory random pages of the latest issue of *Time* magazine. He is author of several books on memory, including the *Memory Power* package (book, audio and video cassettes).

I am over 70 years old. I can remember 500 names at a time or numerals consisting of an almost infinite number of digits. When I'm not applying my memory systems, then my memory isn't as good as when I was young. But, when I am using my memory systems, I remember better than anyone alive today!

You can use my systems to *regain* memory. Bob Norland did. He wrote to me when he was 75. Bob had had a stroke, and doctors told him he would never be able to remember again. His daughter brought him my systems. Now 80, Bob still works, but can't write with his right hand. So when he takes orders on the phone, he must rely on his memory for names, order numbers, prices and phone numbers.

When I was just starting out back in the 1950s, the big memory guru was David Roth. I first met him when he was 91. A few years later, he told me the Rotary Club was throwing him a party for his 94th birthday. He said, "I won't do much, just get everyone's name and telephone number...and repeat it back...person by person."

He died at age 96, with his full mental capacity. Applying these ideas keeps you young.

ONE-A-DAY MENTAL EXERCISES

Mental exercises are the key to keeping your memory sharp. I do crossword puzzles regularly. I also do "one-a-day" mental exercises. They force me to think. *Here are three examples (answers at end of article)...*

1. Take a pad and pencil. Draw a line, from left to right, about one inch long. How can you make it shorter without erasing, cutting or folding the paper?

2. Chickens are 50 cents each, ducks are three dollars each and turkeys are 10 dollars each. You want to spend exactly 100 dollars, but also take home 100 birds. How many of each bird should you buy?

3. Look at the Roman numeral IX. How can you add one symbol, and make the number 6?

WORKING THE "SYSTEMS"

All you need to do to use my systems effectively is stay alert and aware. They're based on ancient memory systems going back to Aristotle, with a few twists of my own. I use these systems constantly, whether walking down the street, driving or waiting in line. *Here's how to start...*

- **Original awareness.** You can't forget something if you never remembered it in the first place. *Turn that around, and you've got the solution to remembering:* If you remember something originally, how can you forget it?

- **Observation.** Essential to *original awareness*—anything you wish to remember must first be observed.

- **Association.** This is the best way to sharpen your observation, and thus your *original awareness.*

In order to remember any new piece of information, it must be associated to something you know or remember in a ridiculous way.

- **Linkage.** Once you *associate* an item by picturing it in a *ridiculous* way, you can *link* it to anything else. That's how you can remember long sequences.

Let's say you want to remember the following six words, in sequence—airplane, tree, envelope, earring, bucket, sing. *Here's how...*

Airplane: Picture an airplane. Now you want to link "airplane" to "tree." Think of a ridiculous image that connects, or associates, those two things in your mind's eye.

Examples: A gigantic tree flying instead of a plane...an airplane growing up out of the earth like a tree...airplanes growing on trees...millions of trees as passengers boarding an airplane. These are crazy, impossible pictures.

Envelope: Picture millions of envelopes growing on a tree. See it clearly, just for a second.

Earring: You open an envelope and millions of earrings fly out and hit you in the face. Or you're wearing envelopes on your ears instead of earrings.

Bucket: A gigantic bucket is wearing earrings.

Sing: The gigantic bucket is singing.

Putting it all together: Your first image is of an airplane. Then a gigantic tree is flying out of an airplane. When you think of tree, your next "link" is of millions of envelopes growing on a tree. You open an envelope and millions of earrings fly out. A gigantic bucket is wearing earrings. The gigantic bucket is singing. Practice thinking of those images, and you'll have the sequence. Using the same method, you can remember 10, 15, 20 or 30 or more items in sequence.

MAKING THE CONNECTION

Making your pictures ridiculous is key. *Four ways to do that are...*

•**Substitution.** Picture one item instead of the other. *For example,* imagine a tree flying instead of an airplane.

•**Change proportion.** Try to see items larger than life. That's why many of my suggestions are "gigantic."

•**Exaggeration.** That's why I often suggest you see "millions" of an item.

•**Action.** Action is always easy to remember. The *link*, tying ridiculous images to each item, can work with *anything.*

You can even do it with numbers. It's easy, once you learn how to associate each number with a specific image.

For names, even foreign words, you make your image by substitution.

Example: Let's say you want to remember the states in alphabetical order. After "Minnesota" comes "Mississippi." How to link them? Well, you can't picture Minnesota, but you can picture a "mini soda." Now, imagine a "Mrs. Sipping" a "mini soda." So, when you think of mini soda (Minnesota) you will automatically think of a Mrs. Sipping (Mississippi).

We all forget mundane things. It's the unusual, the obscene, the violent that we remember.

That's what makes the systems work.

The use of images in memory systems isn't new. Aristotle wrote, "We must speculate with images."

I added the ridiculous aspect. For kids it's not a problem. I asked some kids to visualize a piano coming out of their ears. Adults sometimes have a problem with that. But kids don't. One said, "I saw a piano coming out of my ear and a platypus was playing it!"

Society dulls your imagination. Don't let it!

Answers to one-a-day exercises: 1) Draw a line above it that is two inches long. The first line is shorter. 2) 94 chickens, one duck, five turkeys. 3) Add a capital S. Now you have: SIX.

How to Stimulate Your Cerebellum

Arthur Winter, MD, FICS, a neurosurgeon at the New Jersey Neurological Institute, Livingston, NJ. He is coauthor of *Build Your Brain Power—The Latest Techniques to Preserve, Restore and Improve Your Brain's Potential.* St. Martin's.

The cerebellum lies at the back of the skull, beneath the cerebrum. It is responsible for coordinating body movements, and is particularly vulnerable to age.

Helpful: Practice new motor skills to stimulate the region.

Cerebellum test: Stand with your hands at your sides and close your eyes. Touch your nose with one index finger, then the other. Repeat four times.

Do this exercise and at least some of the ones listed below daily...

•**Charades** (which substitutes body control for speech).

•**Pat your head with one hand and rub your stomach with the other** for a count of 20—then reverse hands and repeat.

•**Use a pair of scissors to cut out a picture** from a newspaper or magazine, sticking as closely to the outline as possible.

•**Try to stack 100 pennies** or dimes as high as you can before they tumble.

•**Play tennis or go bowling**—both sports require coordinating body movements and vision.

•**Listen to dance music** (this actually stimulates the "dancing" areas of the brain).

Mind/Body Made Easy

David W. Freeman, former editorial director, *Bottom Line/Health*, 281 Tresser Blvd., Stamford, CT 06901.

We've all heard about the health benefits of meditation and other mind/body techniques. But who has time to practice these techniques?

We all do, says Gloria Keeling, president of the Mind/Body Fitness Training Institute in Maui, Hawaii. *Even if you can't always find time to meditate, the following strategies can easily be incorporated into your daily routine...*

●**Start each day with a positive thought.** Don't get out of bed until you've had one. *Example:* "I am a healthy, loving person." If you can do so without disturbing your bedmate, say the affirmation out loud.

●**When brushing your teeth, *only* brush your teeth.** Focus on the taste of the toothpaste, the feel of the foam, etc. Practice this type of "mindfulness" whenever you wash the dishes, make the bed, etc.

●**Practice "eating meditation."** Eat slowly. Savor the taste and texture of each bite. You'll enjoy food more...and make more healthful food choices.

●**When someone talks to you, focus all your attention on what he/she says.** Do not think about how you'll respond. Good listeners are good thinkers—and have better relationships.

●**Do "mini-checkups."** While driving or doing chores, notice how you feel. If you feel anxious or tired, spend a few minutes doing deep breathing.

●**Get outside.** Stargaze. Walk barefoot. Listen to birds singing, water flowing, etc. Affirm your connection to nature.

Empower Yourself

Jane Shuman, motivational speaker, Shuman & Associates, 1425 Ashford Ln., Aurora, IL 60504.

Empower yourself by visualizing and affirming what you want to have happen—*as though it has happened already.* Pick a situation in which you want to have more control. Relax. Breathe deeply and quietly. Visualize the situation in as much detail as possible. Imagine yourself having a powerful, positive response to it. Focus on the image of your success daily until you actually meet the challenge.

The Healing Power of Friendship

Jacqueline Olds, MD, associate clinical professor of psychiatry at Harvard Medical School in Boston, and a psychiatrist in private practice in Cambridge, MA. She is coauthor of *Overcoming Loneliness in Everyday Life.* Carol.

America is in the midst of a loneliness epidemic—and the isolation is undermining our health. Yet because our culture esteems self-reliance and abhors dependency, many of us are ashamed to admit we're lonely...and too proud to reach out.

In American society, saying you're lonely suggests that you're weak—or unable to attract friends. Yet total self-reliance is a myth, and loneliness is *not* a sign of weakness. It's an alarm system—a signal that we need to bring people into our lives.

A HIDDEN PROBLEM

Because of the stigma of admitting to loneliness, many people don't even *know* they're lonely—much less what to do about it.

They may call the problem "low self-esteem" and look to the past for solutions. What they really need to do is get more involved with the people around them. Of course, those who are too depressed to do so need to have their depression treated first.

Our seeming obsession with the most intimate details of strangers' lives—as evidenced by the rise of "tell-all" television talk shows—is another manifestation of our isolation.

When you lack a circle of people you know well, gossiping about strangers is a way to fill the gap. But it isn't very satisfying.

HEALTH RISKS OF LONELINESS

Evidence is growing that loneliness has serious health consequences...

James House, PhD, a University of Michigan sociologist, reviewed studies of 37,000 people in the US, Sweden and Finland.

What he found: People who had no serious medical problems but who lived alone and/or had few friends were twice as likely to die over a decade as people who had more social connections.

●**A Duke University study found** that heart attack survivors who were married or had confidants had an 82% five-year survival rate. Those who had neither had a 50% five-year survival rate.

●**Ohio State University researchers have shown** that having a close circle of friends helps block stress-related declines in immune function, as measured by natural-killer cell activity.

INCREASING ISOLATION

Harvard's Robert Putnam has reported a serious decline in the number of Americans involved in church groups, political clubs, the Red Cross and similar community organizations.

A 1992 survey bolsters Putnam's contention. It found that 39% of Americans said they socialized with neighbors no more than once a year ...compared with 28% in 1974. It doesn't look as though this trend is going to change anytime soon.

Several college students have told me that having a significant relationship will only hinder their careers. Their priorities are so skewed that they see such a relationship as a burden that will make it hard to reach their "real" goals.

CULTIVATING FRIENDSHIPS

No matter how busy our lives, it's essential that we make room for others. Even if you're married, you need close friends *other* than your spouse. It's unreasonable to expect one relationship to meet all your emotional needs.

Even if your spouse *could* meet all your needs, it's risky to depend solely on him/her. What would happen to you if something happened to him?

Many people assume that a friendship forms naturally when we meet people we like and invite them to get together once in a while.

But liking someone and intending to get to know that person aren't enough. To grow, friendships need a context—a shared endeavor that provides regular contact.

INTEREST GROUPS

Interest groups can provide this environment—but only if they have a long-term focus. Helping out on a one-time political campaign doesn't give you the same sense of connection that you would get from helping on the park cleanup crew every week.

If you're shy about approaching new groups, consider inviting someone you already know to go *with* you to a meeting.

In addition to a context, friendships need some degree of mutual dependency and mutual obligation.

Examples: Watering each other's plants when one of you is out of town...holding a joint garage sale...looking after each other's kids for the afternoon...sharing a vegetable garden that joins two yards.

One obvious way to start this kind of exchange is to *offer* your help. Ask if you can bring some groceries by for a coworker who's sick, or collect mail for a neighbor who's out of town.

Even better approach: Ask for a favor. For many of us, this goes against the grain. We worry that people will stop liking us if we impose. This is one of the first cultural values we acquire in America.

More often than not, though, people are delighted to be asked for their assistance. Because you were willing to go out on a limb by asking them for help, they'll be more likely to turn to you when they need a hand.

STRENGTHENING FAMILY TIES

Asking for help is also a terrific way to strengthen bonds *within* families.

Example: My husband's 98-year-old grandmother seemed depressed at family gatherings.

She's still an excellent seamstress, so on one of these occasions we asked if she'd mind trying her hand at a pile of mending that had stacked up. Suddenly, she felt happy and useful. She left the gathering more cheerful than we'd seen her in months.

Even if your family is spread out across the country, working on shared projects will bring you closer together.

Example I: Geographically dispersed siblings can help each other catalog old family photos or compile oral histories.

Example II: Families can take on charitable causes that hold particular meaning for them—such as contributing to the American Liver Foundation if a relative needed a liver transplant.

Once we acknowledge our need for other people, we open the door to a life that is healthier, more connected and more satisfying.

How the Great Self-Help Experts Help Themselves

Joan Borysenko, PhD, cofounder of the Mind/Body Clinic at New England Deaconess Hospital in Boston and president of Mind/Body Health Sciences in Boulder, CO. She is author of *Minding the Body, Mending the Mind* (Da Capo) and *A Woman's Book of Life* (Riverhead)...Wayne Dyer, PhD, a renowned motivational speaker and author of numerous books, including *Your Erroneous Zones* (Time Warner) and *A Promise Is a Promise* (Hay House)...Bernie Siegel, MD, founder of Exceptional Cancer Patients in Middletown, CT, which provides information and therapeutic support to people with life-threatening and chronic illnesses. He is author of several books, including *How to Live Between Office Visits.* Harper.

The stress and tension that accompany the demands of work and family affect everyone today. Yet some of us handle the pressure better than others, by calmly dealing with the struggles we face.

To uncover the secrets of people who keep cool while pursuing excellence, three of the country's leading self-improvement experts share the techniques they use when tension strikes...

JOAN BORYSENKO, PhD

A demanding schedule that keeps me on the road about 200 days a year is a source of great pleasure and potential stress. Lectures and workshops for hospitals, corporations, churches and civic groups on topics ranging from medicine and psychology to spirituality, stress and women's health require constant research. There's a never-ending series of book-writing deadlines and production schedules for audiotapes, all of which make a busy life. And until five years ago, when my younger son left for college, I was also balancing family and career.

Research on stress hardiness reveals that when work is deeply meaningful—when we are committed and passionate about what we do—there is less stress. That is certainly true for me.

Self-defense: While attitude helps me manage stress, so do family, friends and health habits. Medical research shows that meaningful relationships are critical to health and well-being. Being in touch with friends and family is a priority for me—even if it means enormous phone bills when I call from abroad.

Health habits are important, too. But the busier and more stressed our lives become, the easier it is to make excuses for being couch potatoes.

Example: I live high in the Rocky Mountains, where I love to hike in the stark beauty and crystal-clear air. For me, hiking and yoga are priorities when I'm home. When I'm traveling, I have to be more creative. I specifically request hotel accommodations near hiking trails rather than in downtown areas...I take the stairs rather than the elevator...and I order take-out lunches and use the spare time to take walks.

Eating well is another challenge when life is hectic. I eat oatmeal and fruit for breakfast and adhere to a largely vegetarian, whole-foods diet to cut down on fat and junk.

Since I teach meditation and extol the benefits of prayer, I am fortunate that my work reinforces this great source of comfort and creativity.

Most mornings and evenings, I meditate, which reinforces my gratitude. During the day, I try to become aware of my breathing. Is it shallow stress breathing...or deep, energizing, relaxing breathing?

A few minutes of the latter makes a big physiological and psychological difference. And when I shift my breathing, it makes me more aware of what's on my mind. Am I complaining...or am I aware that life is the most precious gift?

When I remember to be grateful, it shifts me into the now. Stress is replaced by peace, and I realize that life—with all its joys and sorrows—is an incredible and awesome adventure.

WAYNE DYER, PhD

My life is full of stressful things—demanding writing deadlines, complex travel schedules and the special stress of canceled or delayed flights.

And...I'm a parent of eight children, ages six to 22—seven of whom live at home, which is where I work.

With a crush of obligations, it's important to realize that it is not *things* that make us upset. The events themselves are meaningless. It's how we react that counts. How we choose to process any event is entirely up to us. If we choose inner peace, we'll have peace.

Self-defense: To help change my thoughts and stress levels, meditation is the most important thing I do. Every day, I meditate for at least 20 minutes in the morning and again at night.

I also avoid a sedentary lifestyle, which can make me more susceptible to stress. To be in the natural flow of health, healing and love, we must move about.

Examples: Instead of driving to the store to buy milk, I walk. And when I went away for two months to write my latest book and my office was on the eighth floor, I made a commitment to use the steps, not the elevator. I also get up most days at 4:45 a.m. and run 12 to 15 miles.

When annoying things happen, I remind myself that the universe has a purpose and things happen for a reason.

If tensions or stress levels rise in a group situation, I excuse myself and find a quiet place to meditate for 10 minutes. By the time I come back, peace has usually returned.

And—I make sure to be inspired at all times. The word inspired comes from *in-spirit*. When you're inspired by what you do, you're removed from the stress of the physical realm

and deep into what is called the *zone*. You have an overriding objective...and you are on track.

BERNIE SIEGEL, MD

As a doctor, I see many heartbreaking situations each day. To help me better understand and cope with them, I started keeping a journal years ago.

At first, I made notes to myself during the day. But after I got home, I did not always remember the details of the day. So I learned to write more elaborate notes to help my recollections. Despite my efforts, I was still unable to resolve my emotions. I knew the events were affecting me because I knew how my mind and body felt each evening.

To the rescue: Instead of viewing difficult events as stressful, I remembered what my mother had taught me—that difficulties are part of life...that they can be viewed as redirections...and that something good can come of them.

I began to realize that I have only one real problem—*me*. I found that I could refocus my thoughts by reminding myself that everything in life is fragile...that we are mortal and are here for just a limited period of time. By refocusing my thoughts, I am able to concentrate on what I truly love rather than be distracted by the details of everyday life. This is not about selfishness but about how we contribute our love to the world.

Another lesson that I have learned is that whatever happens in life will happen, regardless of what I think. I do not judge events as good or bad. Situations I might have short-changed as "problems" or "failures" have redirected my life and led to things for which I am now grateful.

Helpful: Every morning, I go running for at least one hour and listen to my inner voice and any other voices that want to speak to me. I also leaf through inspirational books that I keep on a shelf in my office, reading a paragraph or two to keep refocusing on what is truly important. The *Hazelden Meditation Series* (Hazelden) is particularly helpful.

Throughout the day, I meditate. My goal is to turn my entire day into a meditation. Once I can love enough and have enough faith, that will occur.

Several times a day, I stop to think about my behavior and how I am acting. I find that I'm never entirely happy with how I have behaved. But I forgive myself and continue to rehearse and practice—just as any athlete would do—to stay in touch with myself.

To stay in touch with my feelings, I keep a journal, and at least once a week, I write poetry or prose, paint pictures or construct something with my hands. These activities help me integrate what I'm experiencing rather than shut off events from my emotions.

Exceptional Cancer Patients Live Longer And Happier

Bernie Siegel, MD, founder of Exceptional Cancer Patients in Middletown, CT, which provides information and therapeutic support to people with life-threatening and chronic illnesses. He is author of several books, including *How to Live Between Office Visits*. Harper.

In more than 30 years as a surgeon, I treated thousands of cancer patients. Over the years, I noticed that while some of my patients denied their true feelings about their illnesses, others remained upbeat and insisted on taking responsibility for their lives.

These "exceptional" cancer patients managed to thrive emotionally despite being sick. In many cases, they fared better *physically* as well—outliving their less optimistic counterparts by months or years.

What's the secret of being an exceptional patient? Two factors are involved—*inspiration* and *information. Even if you do not have cancer, pondering these eight questions—developed by George Solomon, MD—should inspire you and provide you with helpful information...*

•**Do I get a sense of meaning from my work, daily activities and relationships?** People who dislike what they do often get sick as a result of the inevitable psychological stress

...or because sickness offers a convenient way out of an unpleasant situation. Each of us should work at something we see as contributing to the world.

I've seen many cancer patients suddenly quit their jobs and start doing what they always wanted to do. Many of these individuals lived longer, healthier lives.

Each of us must realize that despite the apparent constraints on our lives, we are free to do what we want to do.

•**Am I able to express anger appropriately?** When an infant isn't given what he/she wants, he bellows—for food, affection, a dry diaper, etc.

Like babies, adults deserve to be treated with respect and love. If we don't get treated that way, we must express our displeasure. We must tell others that we do not intend to let ourselves be stepped upon.

Sadly, most of us have been taught that expressing anger is wrong. We block our negative feelings instead, inhibiting our own healing powers and building up a reservoir of rage.

•**Am I capable of asking friends and family (and my doctor) for help?** You have an absolute right to ask for help whenever you need it. This goes for practical day-to-day items like food and transportation, as well as for emotional support when you're feeling sad or lonely.

Asking for help isn't a matter of selfishness. It's a matter of survival.

•**Am I able to say "no" when asked for a favor I can't do—or do not feel like doing?** Just as you have the right to ask others for favors, you have the right to decline requests from others.

Doing so doesn't mean you don't love the person asking the favor. It means you recognize that it's you alone who gets to choose how to spend your time.

Of course, your family and friends have every right to say no to your requests.

•**Do I engage in health-promoting behaviors based on *my* needs?** Others have no right to decide what you should or shouldn't do regarding exercise, diet, the treatments you seek (or don't seek), etc. You alone do.

Listen to others, but don't be afraid to follow your own path.

●**Do I spend enough time playing?** By play, I mean any activity so enjoyable that it causes you to lose track of time. If you can lose track of time, you won't feel as if you're ill for the duration of the play—no matter how dire your prognosis.

●**Do I frequently feel depressed and/or hopeless?** Many cancer patients fall into the trap of getting depressed *about* being depressed. Instead, you must confront your depression and learn from it.

You may need antidepressants and/or psychotherapy. No matter what, *learn* from the darkness—and accept that having cancer actually gives you a sense of freedom.

●**Am I dutifully playing a role while neglecting my own needs?** Many people identify themselves only by the roles they play —husband or wife, mother or father, valued employee, etc.

When these individuals are no longer able to play that role because of cancer, they lose all sense of identity.

I often ask cancer patients, "How would you introduce yourself to God?" If you introduced yourself as a lawyer or a teacher, I think God would say, "Come back when you've learned who you really are." Each of us is a unique creation. We are much more than the obvious roles we play.

Intentional Healing: The Do-It-Yourself Way to Perfect Health

Elliott S. Dacher, MD, practices internal medicine and conducts healing and wellness seminars nationwide. He is author of *Whole Healing: A Step-by-Step Program to Reclaim Your Power to Heal.* Plume.

To most people the word "healing" means doctors and drugs—regaining health with the help of others.

But the most powerful kind of healing is what we do for ourselves, by our own thoughts and actions, by the way we live.

This *Intentional Healing* is based on a conscious decision to maximize well-being. *Instead of passively enduring the physical ravages of stress, suffering the consequences of bad health habits and allowing negative emotions to plague our days and nights, we...*

●**Tap into the powers** that are naturally within us.

●**Take control of our minds and bodies** to use these powers to the maximum.

If you're in good health, Intentional Healing will help you stay that way. If you're ill, it can combine with medical care (if needed) to make you well.

KEYS TO HEALING

The twin pillars of Intentional Healing are *mindfulness* and *self-regulation*.

Mindfulness is becoming aware of what your mind is doing.

Self-regulation is harnessing the mind's power to ease your body into a healthier state.

Most people go through life barely conscious of the thoughts and feelings that course through their minds. But many of these thoughts and feelings are destructive.

Examples: Worry, anger and fear all tighten muscles, tax the circulation and trigger the release of stress hormones that in time take their toll on every system of the body.

MEDITATION

Mindfulness involves *waking up* to what's going on in your mind, observing patterns of thought and patterns of feeling in order to change and control them.

The first step to mindfulness is a daily meditation exercise...setting time aside to stop, be still and listen to what's going on within your mind. *For 30 minutes each day...*

●**Sit in a quiet place, eyes closed,** hands comfortably on your thighs. Take a deep breath and then breathe normally, counting each cycle of inhalation and exhalation up to 10. Do this three times.

●**Now focus your attention on your abdomen,** how it rises and falls with each inhalation and exhalation.

• **When thoughts enter your mind, simply observe them** without getting caught up in them. Let them pass. Then turn your attention back to your breathing.

• **If you feel restless, bored or uncomfortable, observe these feelings, too.** Then, when your mind quiets, focus again on your breathing.

You may feel extremely relaxed and peaceful after a few minutes...or you may not. There's no right or wrong way to feel...the point of the exercise is simply learning *to experience the present.*

IN THE MOMENT

Everyday life offers constant opportunities to practice mindfulness. *Examples...*

• **When you eat,** slow down. Eat slowly and mindfully, to keep your digestive system in a relaxed condition. Be aware of the color and aroma of the food. Note the feeling of each mouthful, the changing subtleties of flavor and texture, the movement of your jaws, the sensation of swallowing.

• **When you wash the dishes,** be conscious of the way each plate and utensil feels, the sensation of water on your skin. Be aware of your thoughts in a detached way, then return your full attention to the task at hand.

• **When talking with others,** pay complete attention. Erase judgments and reactions from your mind...instead of planning your response, be silent and listen fully to what the other person has to say.

LEARNING TO REGULATE YOUR BODY

Health is a natural result when your body functions in a balanced way, neither too revved up nor too fatigued. We run into trouble when external pressures and events—or our own feelings (particularly anxiety) disrupt the balance. That creates stress...widely recognized as a villain in a host of illnesses, from eczema to backache to heart attack.

By learning to regulate your own body, you cease to be at the mercy of health-destroying stress. Whenever you wish, you can ease your body into a healthy balance.

• **Relaxation** is a critical skill. Many people find that regular practice of mindfulness makes them more relaxed and eases stress. *Practice an exercise called complete breathing...*

Sit in a straight-backed chair. Close your eyes and place both hands on your abdomen. Feel your hands rise as you inhale deep down into your abdomen, making it expand as if it were a balloon. Continue breathing in to fill your chest with air—feel your chest muscles expand. Draw in more air so your shoulders rise slightly.

Release the breath, allowing it to flow smoothly out of the chest, then slowly contract your abdomen to expel the rest of the air.

Repeat the cycle 10 times. Do three groups of 10 complete breaths.

• **Healthy lifestyle.** This is another important way to take control of your body. By exercising regularly, you reduce stress, strengthen your heart and circulatory system and enhance the activity of your immune system.

Brisk walking, at least 20 minutes, four times a week, is a sensible, healthy exercise schedule.

The foods you eat have a significant effect on how your body functions. Choose a diet that will promote the health of your heart, arteries and digestive system...

Build your diet around fresh fruits and vegetables, and unprocessed foods rich in carbohydrates and fiber.

• **Keep animal fats to a minimum.**
• **Reduce your intake of salt.**
• **Drink lots of water.**
• **Have modest-sized meals.**

CREATE A HEALTHY LIFE

Our *attitudes* have a constant impact on our bodies.

Greed, selfishness and contentiousness generate relentless stress. But when we resolve to live at peace with the world and other people, we create for ourselves an environment that promotes healing. *Strive for...*

• **Contentment.** This mental attitude finds satisfaction in what life gives you. This doesn't mean abandoning your goals, but being patient with the pace of progress, enjoying each day.

• **Simplicity.** This requires you to know the difference between what you want and what you need. The simpler you make your life, the less turmoil you will cause yourself.

- **Honesty.** Be honest with yourself and all around you.

- **Harmlessness.** Abstain from actions and words that injure others. Make a conscious choice to nurture feelings of goodwill toward everyone.

- **Solitude.** Only when outside noise quiets down can you listen to your mind and body. Spend a half hour a day alone in a quiet room or out in nature. Give yourself space for reflection…it's as necessary for healing as food or sleep.

For Deep Relaxation: Yoga Made Very Simple

Alice Christensen, founder and executive director of the American Yoga Association, PO Box 19986, Sarasota, FL 34276. She is author of *20-Minute Yoga Workouts.* Wellspring/Ballantine.

If you're chronically anxious or simply feel "stressed out," consider giving yoga a try. This 5,000-year-old system of exercise, breathing and meditation is wonderfully effective at clearing the mind and easing muscular tension.

It also fosters a profound sense of self-confidence—a feeling that you can handle whatever comes your way.

BASIC YOGA PROGRAM

A basic program takes about 20 minutes each day. Some people prefer doing yoga in the morning. Others prefer early evening. Either way is okay. Just make sure you do it at the same time of day—every day.

The only "equipment" you'll need is a quiet room…loose, comfortable clothing…and a blanket, large towel or another pad on which to sit comfortably.*

YOGA BREATHING

To help focus your attention inward, start with two minutes of "complete breath" exercises.

Sit cross-legged on a firm cushion on the floor, or find another seated position in which your back is straight but relaxed.

*For more information on yoga, contact the American Yoga Association at 941-927-4977, *www.americanyoga association.org.*

Begin inhaling slowly and deeply through the nose. Relax your belly so that it expands with each incoming breath, and let your chest and rib cage expand. At the very "top" of each inhalation, your shoulders will lift slightly. At this point, exhale by relaxing your shoulders and then your ribs. Then tighten your belly to squeeze the air out. Relax and repeat.

Important: When we breathe ordinarily, each inhalation lasts longer than each exhalation. With yoga breathing, inhalation and exhalation should take the same amount of time.

Breathe *in* for a count of five…then *out* for a count of five until you've established a rhythm. Then focus on the sound of your breath.

ARM AND SHOULDER STRETCHES

These three stretches—each done while standing—loosen the joints and ease muscular tension.

- **Arm roll.** Hold your arms out to the side, elbows straight, hands held up as if stopping traffic. Rotate your arms forward in three large circles, then backward in three large circles. Then do three *small* circles in each direction.

- **Head roll.** With arms at your sides, bend your head forward while relaxing the muscles in the back of your neck. Slowly tilt your head to one side, then back, then to the other side, then to the front.

Do this head rotation three times clockwise, then three times counterclockwise.

- **Side stretch.** Keep your feet slightly more than shoulder-width apart, with arms held out to the side. Inhale deeply. Then exhale as you bend to the right. Slide your right hand down your right thigh toward the knee, and bring your left arm overhead. Breathe in, and return to an upright position.

Do the same stretch on your left side. Repeat three times on each side.

SPINE STRETCHES

These poses are especially beneficial if you work at a desk.

- **Sun pose.** Stand with feet together. As you inhale, raise your arms from the side until they're overhead. Look upward. Exhale as you bend from the waist. Reach as far forward as you comfortably can, and grasp your ankles, calves or knees.

Hold for a moment, then inhale as you return to an upright position, raising arms to the side until they're overhead. Lower arms in a circle as you exhale. Repeat twice.

•**Baby pose.** Sit on your feet. Slowly bend forward until your head approaches the floor. Let your arms rest at your sides with elbows bent. Hold for at least one minute.

•**Corpse pose.** Lie on your back with feet slightly apart and arms at sides, palms up. Close your eyes. Relax your entire body, paying particular attention to the face and stomach. Rest for at least one minute.

YOGA MEDITATION

Meditation teaches us to *observe*—rather than worry about or act upon—the thoughts that constantly flit through our minds.

This lets us withdraw from the never-ending bombardment of desires, fears, regrets, etc.... and find peace by turning our attention solely to the present moment. Start by lying face up on your pad, with arms at sides, palms up. Remain as still as possible.

For the next two minutes or so, focus on each part of your body in turn. Envision each part separately...and relax it.

Start with your forehead, then your eyes, face, neck and shoulders. Move down your body, relaxing each in turn—arms and hands...chest and abdomen...hips, legs and feet...then back up the spine to the neck and head.

Gently bring your attention to your forehead. Silently repeat "om" several times.

Your aim is to think of nothing. If thoughts intrude, don't worry—and don't try to *force* them to stop. Gently return your attention to the experience of silence.

Trap: The more you fight to *control* your thoughts, the harder your thoughts will resist you. Instead, just observe the thoughts as if they were passing by in the distance.

After meditating for 10 minutes or so, open your eyes. Wiggle your fingers and toes, open and close your fists. Take a deep breath. Stretch your arms and legs. Your yoga session is over.

As you become more skilled at meditation, you should be able to *remember* and *reproduce* the feeling at will—to achieve instant relaxation anytime, anywhere.

Midlife Wisdom

Kathryn Cramer, PhD, psychologist and founder of the Cramer Institute, which helps individuals and organizations master transition and change, 231 S. Remiston, Ste. 102, St. Louis, MO 63105. She is author of Roads Home: Seven Pathways to Midlife Wisdom. Quill.

Restlessness, boredom, physical and emotional changes, a lack of creativity and/or a sense of something looming on the horizon are often signs of a midlife crisis.

I call them the *readiness signals* that tell you to begin a journey to midlife wisdom—which happens by traveling seven important pathways.

MENTAL MASTERY

Mastery is your ability to capitalize on your accumulated knowledge and experience to solve problems.

Conscious attention to the details of your life will lead to better judgment in problem-solving. However, experts say that today we are bombarded with information at 1,000 times the rate our grandparents were.

We decide which of these bits of information to notice or ignore in the first place—but most of us don't realize that we've overdeveloped this skill because we've done a lot of selective *not noticing* by midlife.

Helpful: To become more aware of the details in your life, ask yourself these questions at the end of each day...

•**What did I learn today?** Be specific. Write down what you accomplished, what you thought and said. Recall any new skill or understanding you acquired.

•**How did I learn what I learned?** This will help you pinpoint how you learn best and most naturally.

•**How can I increase the use of this type of learning in my everyday life?** If you find yourself learning through reading, consider expanding your reading to other areas.

PHYSICAL VIGOR

There are two reasons that people who are between the ages of 35 and 65 must tune in to how they feel about their bodies...

•**The physical component of your journey** is intricately tied to all the other components. Your mind, emotions and relationships cannot be at their peak if your body is not functioning at least near its best.

●**Much of what upsets midlifers can be fixed or improved upon.**

These simple habits can have a powerful impact on your physical and mental well-being…

- ●**Eat breakfast daily.**
- ●**Avoid snacking.**
- ●**Maintain your ideal weight.**
- ●**Exercise regularly.**
- ●**Sleep seven to eight hours a night.**
- ●**Don't smoke.**
- ●**If you drink, drink moderately.**

EMOTIONAL VITALITY

To remain emotionally healthy, you must be able to recover from past and present disturbing situations and enrich your connections to people and events.

I've found that during the first half of life, experiences of joy usually emanate from events that go your way.

During the second half of life, however, emotionally healthy adults are capable of experiencing true joy despite the bad things that might happen to them. We lose the grandiosity of youth that says we can and must be the force at the center of life.

Unfortunately, most of us have little emotional training before midlife, so we have trouble responding competently to anger, pain and fear.

Helpful: Write down what disturbs you about an experience for which you would like to have a different emotional response. Recall childhood experiences that triggered similar negative feelings. How did you react? Feel the pain of not expressing your feelings as a child. Feel compassion for the child you were.

INTERPERSONAL EFFECTIVENESS

Interacting well with others requires that we be able to establish caring relationships and unify the strong and sensitive aspects of our personalities.

Example: Are you happy when you give someone a gift? For mature adults, the satisfaction of giving a gift far outweighs the thrill of receiving one. In fact, experts call this altruism the hallmark of maturity and the foundation of satisfying relationships.

Many midlifers have problems stemming from a lack of this altruistic development. Some couples have lost their ability to reach out to each other in truly compassionate ways. Or parents don't know how to be compassionate toward their teenage children.

Helpful: Select a person you feel is an adversary. Write down traits you admire and traits you loathe. Then write a few sentences about your adversary as though you have no feelings toward him/her. Be objective and detached.

Reflect on the admirable, negative and neutral traits you assigned to your adversary. Pretend you're getting to know this person for the first time.

Watch for insights as a result of your more balanced view. Once you have achieved emotional distance from this person, try approaching him anew, emphasizing the attractive and neutral traits over the negative. You'll see your former opponent's viewpoint more clearly.

EXCEPTIONAL COMPETENCE

We need to perform complex tasks, assume leadership and mentor roles and contribute significantly to the world based upon our talents and desires.

By the time we hit midlife, we've become good at tasks we have performed for years. Use this competence to free your time and attention and get focused on the important goals of the second half of your life. It is a time to confirm or readjust priorities and develop a vision, as you did when you were young.

Important: Do not compare your successes and failures with those of others. This will deflate or inflate your view of yourself unnecessarily. You will underestimate the value of what you have done, or you may end up with a false sense of superiority that will squelch your motivation.

SPIRITUAL SERENITY

Midlife spiritual anxiety is exceedingly normal. If we don't struggle to find more satisfying answers to age-old questions about life and our mortality, we risk facing old age with fear and anger as our main companions. *Helpful…*

●**Come to terms with life.** Our mortality is less frightening when we feel we have made the most of our lives.

●**Give in to feelings about your mortality.** Crystallizing your feelings can lead to a clearer sense of life purpose and a greater degree of life satisfaction.

PERSONAL INTEGRITY

Being happy with yourself and your work requires personal integrity, an integration of the many parts of your personality working together as one cohesive whole. People with personal integrity don't act one way at work and another way at home. They have the same standards of honesty, behavior and emotional response wherever they are.

Strive to bring out the best in yourself and others. Remind yourself to help others who need help, and be generous with your time and energy. Your reputation and enthusiasm will soar.

Four-Step Plan for Beating Obsessions and Compulsions

Jeffrey M. Schwartz, MD, research professor of psychiatry at UCLA School of Medicine. He is author of Brain Lock: Free Yourself from Obsessive-Compulsive Behavior. Harper Perennial.

You're not sure you turned off the stove, so you go home to check. After you leave again, you're *still* unsure. What if the house burned down? So you check *again*. And *again*. This is classic *obsessive-compulsive* behavior. Dread arising from intrusive thoughts (obsessions) leads to repetitive behavior (compulsions).

One of my patients washed his hands 100 times a day. He knew they were clean but he could not shake the feeling that they were dirty...and scrubbed until his hands were cracked and raw.

Five million Americans suffer from *obsessive-compulsive disorder* (OCD), whose symptoms make daily life exceedingly difficult. Countless more have minor obsessions and compulsions they would like to get rid of.

Examples: Getting up at night to check and recheck a lock...rereading the same passage to make sure you got every word...having unspeakable thoughts of violence that you can't get out of your mind.

We've made great strides in pinpointing the cause of the maddening symptoms...and developing a therapy that really helps.

A GLITCH IN THE BRAIN

OCD is caused by a biochemical imbalance in the *caudate nucleus*, a region of the brain whose function is to control another part of the brain called the *orbital cortex*.

Ordinarily, the orbital cortex serves as a sort of "error-detection system." When the caudate nucleus malfunctions, the orbital cortex is left stuck in the "on" position. This "brain-lock" condition creates a "something-is-amiss" feeling that won't go away.

To the rescue: My four-step program can control OCD within a matter of weeks.

STEP 1: RELABEL

Since obsessions and compulsions won't go away of their own accord, your first step is to *relabel* them by making mental notes.

If you feel compelled to count all the blue cars you pass on the highway, for example, tell yourself, "I don't *need* to count the blue cars. I'm having a *compulsive* urge to do so."

This inner dialogue brings you back to reality. By *observing* your brain—neither giving in to the compulsion nor pretending it doesn't exist—you bolster your "Impartial Spectator." That's the innermost part of your personality...and what will allow you to conquer OCD.

STEP 2: REATTRIBUTE

The next step answers the question, "Why won't these terrifying thoughts, urges and behaviors go away?" *Reattribute* these symptoms to their true cause—a biochemical imbalance in the brain.

Think of OCD anxiety as a mental alarm system—with a hair-trigger. The siren may wail incessantly, but that *doesn't* mean you must pay attention to it.

Helpful: Silently reflect on the phrase, "It's not me, it's OCD." Doing so stresses the distinction between your thoughts and fears… and your real self.

Once you learn to separate yourself from your urges and anxieties, you can *choose* not to act on them.

STEP 3: REFOCUS

Each time your obsession or compulsion resurfaces, *refocus* your attention on a pleasurable, constructive activity—taking a walk… gardening…doing needlepoint…listening to music…playing a computer game.

Your goal is to pursue the activity for at least 15 minutes. At first, however, you may be able to go no longer than five minutes.

The longer you refrain from acting on a compulsive urge, the weaker it becomes. Even if you ultimately give in, you still come out ahead. You're learning to tolerate psychological discomfort…and building up your power to say "no." This is profoundly empowering.

STEP 4: REVALUE

The more diligently you practice relabeling, reattributing and refocusing, the more fully you'll recognize your obsessions and compulsions for what they are—worthless distractions having no value whatsoever.

This process will gradually become automatic. Without even thinking, you'll be able to devalue the thoughts and urges and fend them off until they fade.

BENEFITS OF THIS METHOD

Some people experience a profound sense of relief after using my four-step technique for only a single day. For most people, however, it takes about eight to 10 weeks.

Do *not* expect your urges to go away completely. Each incremental improvement—you put off checking the lock for five minutes—brings you closer to full control. Praise yourself for each step forward!

The four-step method is more than a behavioral technique—it has physiological effects. Studies using *positron emission tomography* (PET) show that in individuals who practice the four-step method, brain function returns to normal.

WHAT ABOUT MEDICATION?

Some recently developed drugs—including the antidepressants *fluoxetine* (Prozac) and *fluvoxamine* (Luvox) and the antianxiety drug *buspirone* (BuSpar)—greatly weaken the fear that makes OCD urges so hard to resist.

I think of these drugs as "training wheels"— a useful aid when you're just getting acquainted with the four-step method.

Once you master my program and your brain biology begins to change, you'll be able to reduce the dosage…or give up the drugs completely.

22

Natural Ways and Herbal Solutions

Herbal Teas...
How to Grow Them and Brew Them, Too

Marietta Marshall Marcin

Many herbs can be used for tea. Although they won't reach the fullness or height they would outdoors, you can grow them indoors. Simply choose a spot where the plants will get plenty of sun—ideally a south-facing window that gets light all day.

HERBS THAT MAKE GREAT TEAS

Your gardening store likely stocks the seeds or will know a mail-order source. *Here are some of my favorites...*

- **Fennel seeds, leaves and root** are excellent stomach and intestinal remedies. When brewed, they also arouse appetite and expel mucus accumulations. The tea tastes like anise, peppermint and licorice.

- **Lemon balm tea** has been used for colic, cramps, bronchial catarrh, dyspepsia, some forms of asthma and headaches.

- **Mint tea** can be made from 30 different varieties. Mint teas relieve cramps, coughs, poor digestion, nausea, heartburn, abdominal pains, headaches and other ailments attributed to nerves.

- **Thyme tea** is ideal for calming nerves, alleviating indigestion and clearing the mucous membranes.

DRYING AND STORING

- **Using scissors**, cut leaves just before the flower forms for the fullest flavor and best leaf color when dried.

- **Wash leaves or branches quickly in cool water**...and lightly towel dry. Then spread on a mesh rack and place in a slow oven set at 100°F to 125°F. Leave the oven door open, and stand nearby, as the leaves dry in just a few minutes.

Marietta Marshall Marcin, a gardener in Winnetka, IL, grows 34 herbs in her garden. She is author of several books, including *The Herbal Tea Garden: Planning, Planting, Harvesting & Brewing*. Storey.

413

Or dry them in a microwave on a very low setting for one minute or less.

BREWING

Cover one teaspoon dried leaves—or three teaspoons fresh crushed herb—with one cup boiling water. Steep for 10 minutes and strain.

Spices and Self-Healing

James A. Duke, PhD, a botanist in Fulton, MD. He is now retired after spending 30 years at the US Department of Agriculture in Beltsville, MD. He is author of numerous books, including *The Green Pharmacy*. Rodale.

Did you know that celery seed fights gout? That bay leaves stop headache pain? *We didn't know either—until noted botanist James A. Duke, PhD, shared with us his picks for the most useful medicinal spices*...*

BAY LEAF

Good for: Migraines, diabetes.

Healing properties: Bay leaves are rich in pain-killing compounds called *parthenolides*.

They also contain a compound that boosts insulin's ability to control blood glucose.

Eating food seasoned with bay leaves helps prevent diabetes...and helps keep adult-onset (Type 2) diabetics from worsening to the point that they need daily insulin shots.

How to use: Make a tea by steeping several bay leaves in hot water. Or add bay leaves to chicken or bean soup.

Caution: Bay leaves themselves should not be eaten.

CAYENNE

Good for: Chronic pain, arthritis, ulcers, bronchitis, colds, influenza.

Healing properties: Cayenne contains *capsaicin*, a compound proven to block *Substance P*. That's the brain chemical involved in transmission of pain impulses.

*Check with your doctor before using spices for medicinal purposes. Do *not* substitute "spice therapy" for medication prescribed by your physician.

Capsaicin also boosts the body's production of natural painkillers called *endorphins*...and destroys the ulcer-causing stomach bacterium *Helicobacter pylori*.

How to use: For pain relief, soak gauze in a hot pepper sauce containing cayenne, and apply it to the painful area. My wife has found this very effective for her back pain.

For ulcers or for blocked air passages, add one-half teaspoon hot pepper sauce or cayenne to hot lemonade, and drink.

CELERY SEED

Good for: Arthritis, gout.

Healing properties: Celery seed contains more than a dozen distinct anti-inflammatory compounds. The same compounds are found in celery stalks.

How to use: Take two capsules of celery seed extract (available in health-food stores). You can also eat four stalks of celery.

GARLIC

Good for: Heart disease, high blood pressure, impaired immunity.

Healing properties: One of nature's most potent antibiotics, garlic inhibits growth of fungi, yeast and bacteria—including strains that are becoming resistant to synthetic antibiotics.

Garlic also contains *allicin*, a compound that works like aspirin to thin the blood. Because of this blood-thinning effect—plus its proven cholesterol- and blood-pressure-lowering powers—garlic is effective at preventing atherosclerosis.

How to use: I add garlic cloves to almost every dish I cook. I also cook with chives, leeks and onions. All have properties similar to those of garlic.

Each time my grandchildren visit, I take garlic pills to ward off any infections they might have brought along with them.

Fearing bad breath, some people prefer "deodorized" garlic pills. But I'm convinced that the more a garlic pill stinks, the better it is for you.

Beware: If you take aspirin to prevent a heart attack, garlic may thin your blood too much. Discuss this with your doctor.

LICORICE

Good for: Enlarged prostate, ulcers.

Healing properties: *Glycyrrhizic acid*, the major active ingredient in licorice, prevents conversion of testosterone to dydrotestosterone. This reduces swelling of the prostate, thereby putting an end to frequent urination, the most common symptom of prostate enlargement.

Licorice also contains numerous antibacterial compounds, including some that kill ulcer-causing bacteria.

How to use: Munching on licorice candy will *not* work. That's because most licorice candy sold in the US is made with anise, not licorice.

Instead, use a piece of licorice root to stir your tea. The active ingredients will steep into the tea—and act as a natural sweetener, too.

You can also add licorice root extract to hot drinks. Licorice root and licorice root extract are available at health-food stores.

Caution: Too much licorice can raise blood pressure...and cause heart problems. If you have high blood pressure, consult a doctor before using licorice.

ROSEMARY

Good for: Alzheimer's disease.

Healing properties: Sometimes called the "herb of remembrance," rosemary contains five compounds that seem to prevent the breakdown of *acetylcholine*, a neurotransmitter that's deficient in patients with Alzheimer's.

I believe that rosemary works just as well as the Alzheimer's drug *tacrine* (Cognex). Tacrine works in only 25% of patients...and it can cause liver damage.

I also believe that eating rosemary can reduce one's risk of *developing* Alzheimer's.

How to use: Rosemary can be added to all sorts of recipes, including fish and chicken dishes.

Since there's evidence that rosemary can be absorbed through the skin, you might try tossing rosemary sprigs into your bath...using rosemary shampoo...and rubbing rosemary lotion into your skin.

Ginger for Upset Stomach...and More

Stephen Fulder, PhD, a biochemist and private research consultant in Galilee, Israel, and a former lecturer at London University. He is author of numerous books, including *The Ginger Book: The Ultimate Home Remedy*. Avery.

If you're like most Americans, the closest you get to ginger is an occasional glass of ginger ale.

But in many parts of Asia, ginger is highly valued as a medicine. It's part of daily life for billions of people—as a safe, effective home remedy for a variety of ailments, including stomach upset, the common cold and poor circulation.

Powdered ginger—the kind you find in the spice section at the supermarket—is potent enough. But fresh ginger is even more potent ...and organic fresh ginger more potent still. *Here's how to use ginger...*

•**Stomach upset.** A ginger "tea" made with one-third teaspoon of powdered ginger (or one teaspoon of grated ginger) in a cup of hot water with a squeeze of lemon provides fast relief for motion sickness, nausea, vomiting or simple indigestion.

You can also buy ginger capsules or tablets at health food stores. In that case, you'll want to take two 500-milligram (mg) capsules.

Ginger calms the stomach, stopping the sensation of nausea, and speeds the digestive process.

•**Common cold.** Take two cups of ginger tea (or two 500-mg capsules) three times a day.

•**Poor circulation.** For cold hands and/or feet, take one cup of ginger tea (or a 500-mg ginger capsule) once a day, preferably in the morning. You won't see results quickly—it's more of a preventive measure than a cure.

But don't wait for an illness to come along. I love to add a slice of fresh ginger to ordinary tea...or grate it into stir-fried vegetables. I take some every day. So should you.

Medicinal Herbs: Growing Your Own to Improve Physical and Emotional Health

Miranda Smith, horticultural writer and teacher at the New England Small Farm Institute, 275 Jackson St., Belchertown, MA 01007. She is author of *Your Backyard Herb Garden*. Rodale.

In recent years, we've come to appreciate anew the medicinal value of herbs. Used properly, herbs offer a safe, natural alternative to many drugs—to energize, relax, help wounds heal, etc.

Most people buy their herbs at a health food store. But many herbs are easy to grow, whether you've got a big backyard or just a few pots on a porch.

GARDENING IS GOOD FOR YOU

Gardening is a wonderful antidote for psychological stress...a source of solitude...a respite from everyday problems. And with all the digging, hoeing, etc., it gives a pretty good workout.

You might even discover that gardening is good for the spirit. It's one thing to *read* "all things are connected," quite another to *experience* it in your garden.

Tending your herbs every day, you see in concrete terms how sun, rain, soil and your own care affect your plants. You begin to feel as if you were an integral part of the rhythms of nature.

Herbs can be grown from seedlings or seeds. You can get them from a local nursery...or a mail-order company, such as Richters, 357 Hwy. 47, Goodwood, Ontario L0C 1A0. 905-640-6677, *www.richters.com.*

CHAMOMILE

This plant produces daisy-like flowers on stalks that grow up to three feet tall. Full sunlight is best, but it tolerates partial shade.

German chamomile grows erect and can be planted six to eight inches apart. *Roman* chamomile is low, with creeping stems. Allow 18 inches between plants.

Uses: Chamomile tea, prepared from freshly picked or dried chamomile flowers, is quite relaxing. Taken 15 minutes before bedtime, it induces sleep. Chamomile tea also calms cranky toddlers and eases teething pain.

Caution: If you're allergic to ragweed, avoid chamomile tea.

COMFREY

This bushy plant grows three to five feet high, with drooping tubular flowers that range in color from blue to yellow and cream. Comfrey prefers full sun but will grow in partial shade. Give each plant at least three square feet.

Uses: Comfrey is for *external* use only. A strong comfrey *decoction*—a tea-like solution used on the skin—promotes healing of cuts, burns and bruises.

FENNEL

This herb grows up to five feet tall, with tiny yellow flowers that appear at midsummer. Plant six inches apart, preferably in full sunlight.

Uses: Fennel tea aids digestion. It also reduces colic in infants...and flatulence in children and adults.

FEVERFEW

This hardy two-foot perennial bears white daisy-like flowers. Plant seedlings in full sun or partial shade, spacing them 12 inches apart. Feverfew thrives even indoors in a pot, as long as it gets direct sunlight.

Uses: A tea of feverfew leaves has been shown to reduce the severity *and* intensity of migraine headaches. It can be drunk up to three times a day, between meals. Or simply chew one to four fresh leaves a day.

Caution: Stop using if you develop mouth sores.

LAVENDER

This plant grows up to two feet tall. Its lovely flowers yield a sweet, clean fragrance. Plant in full sun or partial shade, one to three feet apart. It will grow in containers, too.

Uses: Lavender tea calms jangled nerves. A cold lavender tea compress relieves headaches.

LOVAGE

One lovage plant, which grows up to six feet tall, can supply your needs for a full year. It prefers partial shade.

Uses: Use lovage as you would use celery, in cheese and egg dishes, soups, stews, salads, etc. You can apply lovage tea to wounds as an antiseptic. Or—drink it to stimulate digestion.

MARJORAM

This plant grows one foot tall, with tiny white or pink blossoms. Space seedlings six to eight inches apart, in full sun if possible. It will grow in containers.

Uses: Marjoram tea helps settle an upset stomach. Use it lukewarm as a gargle for throat inflammation.

PENNYROYAL

This perennial grows up to one foot high, with bluish flowers. Set plants in full sun or partial shade, six to 10 inches apart.

Uses: Pennyroyal is a natural insect repellent. Rub the leaves on your skin…or put a bouquet of pennyroyal sprigs on your picnic table. Occasionally crush the leaves to release their bug-unfriendly fragrance.

Caution: Do not take pennyroyal internally. It is poisonous.

THYME

Thyme grows up to 15 inches high. Set groups of plants one foot apart, in full sun or partial shade.

Uses: Thyme tea settles the stomach. Also, add to bath water. Thyme's antiseptic qualities help raw, rough skin.

MAKING HERBAL TEA

Steep fresh or dried herbs for 20 minutes in a tightly stoppered container. Immediately refrigerate any unused portion.

Some herbs can cause stomach irritation, headache and other side effects. To start out, make an extremely weak tea. See how it affects you. Once you're confident that you can tolerate weak tea, increase the strength a bit to find what works best for you.

Flower Remedies

Jamison Starbuck, ND, a naturopathic physician in family practice and a lecturer at the University of Montana, both in Missoula. She is past president of the American Association of Naturopathic Physicians and a contributing editor to *The Alternative Advisor: The Complete Guide to Natural Therapies and Alternative Treatments.* Time-Life.

Dried flowers of *calendula officinalis* are good for burns, cuts, scrapes, acne, tonsillitis and canker sores, vaginitis, rashes, athlete's foot and sunburn.

During the Civil War, these bright orange and yellow flowers provided the major line of defense against infection. Today you can buy dried calendula flowers, ointment, tincture or spray at most health food stores…or grow your own.

Calendula flourishes in almost any climate, whether it's planted in a pot or in the ground.

Most nurseries sell bedding plants in the springtime. Be sure to ask for *calendula officinalis*—not marigolds.

Flowers harvested between June and September are most potent. Dry them out of direct sun on a mesh screen for one to two weeks. Store in an airtight container.

Hot calendula tea helps soothe ulcers. Gargle with cool tea for inflamed tonsils or canker sores.

To make tea: Pour 10 ounces of boiling water over ⅔ cup of the flowers. Let it steep for 15 minutes. Or add five to 10 drops of calendula tincture to a cup of hot water.

Apply tincture or spray to rashes, cuts, scrapes or acne with a cotton ball. Spraying is good for sunburn, vaginitis and pinworms. Use ointment on scabs, eczema and psoriasis.

To make ointment: Melt ½ cup of petroleum jelly over low heat in a double boiler. Add a handful of dried calendula flowers. Heat on low for an hour. Strain out the herb and pour into a glass jar.

When to Consider Alternative Therapies

Timothy McCall, MD, an internist, medical editor of *Yoga Journal* and author of *Examining Your Doctor: A Patient's Guide to Avoiding Harmful Medical Care.* Carol. *www.drmccall.com.*

Consider alternative therapies if your ailments do not respond adequately to conventional medicine…and for stress-related problems like anxiety and insomnia. But do not abandon conventional medicine for unproven approaches marketed as homeopathic or natural. And—remember that even natural treatments have side effects. Some herbs and vitamins can cause problems if taken in large doses…in combination with certain other herbs and vitamins…or with conventional medicines.

Treat Stress and Depression the Natural Way

Michael J. Norden, MD, clinical associate professor of psychiatry at the University of Washington, Seattle. He was among the first to publish medical accounts of the varied uses of Prozac and has been a pioneer in the integration of psychopharmacology and alternative treatments. Dr. Norden is author of *Beyond Prozac*. Collins.

The stress of modern life has given rise to a worldwide epidemic of depression. Mood disorders are more prevalent now than ever before, and they're occurring at younger ages.

What's causing this epidemic? Much of the blame may well rest with technology, and the sweeping lifestyle changes it has encouraged.

Our bodies and brains evolved for a Stone Age existence, when daily life was governed by the rising and setting of the sun and the changing of the seasons. Today, people seem to live at a breakneck pace, 24 hours a day, all year long.

Problem: Fast-paced living brings reduced levels of the neurotransmitter *serotonin*, a key buffer against depression.

On the advice of their doctors, many people have turned to antidepressants to relieve their malaise. For serious depression, that's prudent. *However, it often makes more sense to find natural, nondrug ways to boost serotonin levels…*

GET MORE LIGHT

Exposure to bright light has been shown to raise serotonin levels. Unfortunately, indoor lighting averages only 200 to 500 lux. That's too weak to do the trick. Outdoors, sunlight can climb above 100,000 lux.

Being exposed to artificial light *at night* (when our ancestors would have been asleep) throws off the production cycle of *melatonin*. This key neurochemical affects a variety of bodily functions, including serotonin synthesis, making it another important buffer against depression.

Antidote: Get outdoors as much as possible during the day. If you live in a "gray" climate, consider buying a light box (10,000 lux). This device—available for $200 and up—can be used while reading, exercising or watching TV.

Caution: Light boxes should not be used by people with retinal disease.

Best brands: Apollo Health (800-545-9667, *www.apollolight.com*) and The SunBox Company (800-548-3968, *www.sunboxco.com*).

Also helpful: Dawn simulators. These devices use light to awaken you naturally on dark winter mornings.

SEEK OUT NEGATIVE IONS

Air with high concentrations of negative ions—molecules with an extra electron—is clearly linked to positive moods. Unfortunately, city air contains 10 times fewer negative ions than air in the country or by the seashore. Ion concentrations are even lower inside air-conditioned offices.

Antidote: If you can't live in the country or near the ocean, buy a negative-ion generator. These devices boost serotonin levels, improving mood and promoting sleep.

Be sure the machine you buy generates *small* negative ions. That's the kind shown to yield psychological benefits.

Best brand: The Happy Machine (866-466-4937).

GET MORE SLEEP

Adults today get 20% less sleep than before the invention of the electric light. Most of us need at least eight hours of sleep a night. Nearly 50% of Americans get less.

Sleep deprivation produces a sharp decrease in serotonin levels. It is strongly linked to depression.

Antidote: Make sleep a priority. If you feel sleepy during the day, or if you need an alarm clock to wake up, you probably need more shut-eye.

Strategies: Keep the bedroom cool and dark…avoid work or stimulating TV for at least one hour before bedtime…cut down on caffeine and alcohol…exercise late in the day (but at least five hours before bedtime)…rise at the same time each day. On days when you can't get the sleep you need, nap.

GET REGULAR EXERCISE

Exercise—an excellent serotonin booster—is linked not only with better moods, but also with better overall health. Yet despite the so-called "fitness revolution," Americans get less exercise today than even 10 years ago. We get far less exercise than our hunter-gatherer ancestors.

Antidote: Find an exercise you enjoy, and do it regularly. Aerobic exercise several times a week is ideal, but any kind of exercise is better than none.

RETHINK YOUR DIET

Our ancestors survived mostly on green plants and small game animals, which were low in fat but high in cholesterol.

Lesson: While some middle-aged men and others at high risk for heart attack should take steps to lower high cholesterol levels, cholesterol levels below 160 confer a heightened risk of depression, accidents and suicide. Apparently, low cholesterol levels interfere with the regulation of serotonin.

That doesn't mean we should binge on saturated fat. It does suggest that we should be wary of cholesterol levels that are too high *or* too low.

What about carbohydrates? They do appear to improve serotonin function *temporarily.* Over the long term, however, a high-carbohydrate diet diminishes your sense of well-being.

Reason: Carbohydrates quickly raise blood sugar and insulin levels. Elevated insulin signals the body to store food as fat—making it less available for energy. Insulin also boosts production of certain prostaglandins linked to depression.

Antidote: Eat a diet that's more in line with that of our hunter-gatherer ancestors…

•**Emphasize fruits and vegetables** while limiting consumption of grains and sweets. When you do eat grain, stick to whole grains. They have a less drastic effect on blood sugar than white bread or processed cereal.

•**At every meal, maintain a protein-fat-carbohydrate** calorie ratio of 30%-30%-40%.

•**Keep meals under 500 calories.** Don't let more than five hours pass between meals (except when you're asleep). Frequent, small meals keep insulin levels lower than a few large meals.

•**Do not eat red meat or egg yolks more than once a week.** These foods contain a chemical precursor to a brain chemical that is associated with depression.

WHAT ABOUT ANTIDEPRESSANTS?

Anyone who is so depressed that he/she has trouble functioning at work or at home should seek a medical diagnosis.

•**Fluoxetine** (Prozac) is the best known of a group of antidepressants called *selective serotonin reuptake inhibitors* (SSRIs). These drugs avoid many of the serious medical risks of older drugs.

But Prozac can cause decreased libido, delayed orgasm, insomnia and agitation…and may suppress melatonin levels.

Over the short term, this is probably not a concern. For patients who take the drug for a year or more, however, the effect on melatonin might have negative implications for long-term mood and health.

•**Sertraline** (Zoloft) and *paroxetine* (Paxil) are similar to Prozac but may be better or worse in a given individual.

•**Fluvoxamine** (Luvox) is another SSRI that appears to have fewer side effects than Prozac. Unlike Prozac, it raises melatonin levels.

•**Nefazodone** affects serotonin more subtly and seems free of Prozac's most objectionable side effects. It may be particularly helpful in treating depression accompanied by anxiety or insomnia.

•**Venlafaxine** (Effexor) acts on serotonin and boosts levels of *norepinephrine* (the neurochemical affected by earlier antidepressants called tricyclics). It has a good track record in treating cases that fail to respond to other medication.

•**Bupropion** (Wellbutrin) does *not* act on serotonin. In fact, we're not quite sure *how* it works. In a tiny percentage of cases, it has been associated with seizures. This risk can be minimized by lowering the dosage.

Effective Remedies from Your Kitchen Cabinet

Jamison Starbuck, ND, a naturopathic physician in family practice and a lecturer at the University of Montana, both in Missoula. She is past president of the American Association of Naturopathic Physicians and a contributing editor to *The Alternative Advisor: The Complete Guide to Natural Therapies and Alternative Treatments*. Time-Life.

Next time you're searching for relief from an acute ailment, look in your kitchen. Chances are you'll find as many remedies there as in your medicine chest.

● **Cold.** Try ginger tea. Both an antiviral and anti-inflammatory remedy, it helps prevent chills and reduces the buildup of phlegm. *What to do:* Peel and thinly slice a two-inch piece of fresh gingerroot. Put it in a saucepan and cover with 12 ounces of water. Bring to a boil, then gently simmer for seven minutes. Strain, add honey and the juice of one-half fresh lemon. Sip six ounces every three hours.

● **Sinus congestion.** To clear your nasal and sinus passages, try a *steam inhalation with dried thyme leaves.* Thyme is a good antiseptic and decongestant. *What to do:* Pour a quart of boiling water into a bowl. Add a heaping teaspoon of dried thyme leaves. Drape a large, dry cotton towel over your head and hold your face about 12 inches above the bowl. Breathe in the thyme-laced steam for eight minutes. Then gently blow your nose.

● **Bladder infection.** If you experience early symptoms of a bladder infection—such as pain when urinating or increased frequency—try *parsley tea.* Parsley is a mild natural diuretic that contains virtually no calories and also flushes the bladder of pesky organisms that can cause infection. *What to do:* Bring one quart of water to a boil, turn off the heat and add one cup of fresh parsley, stems and leaves. Cover and steep

for 15 minutes. Strain and drink one cup of cool tea over a two-hour period. Repeat the process four hours later. If your symptoms worsen or persist for more than 24 hours, see your health-care provider.

All About Herbal Remedies

Daniel B. Mowrey, PhD, president of the American Phytotherapy Research Laboratory, a nonprofit research facility in Lehi, UT. He is author of several books on herbal medicine, including *Herbal Tonic Therapies*. Keats Publishing.

Even if you eat right, exercise regularly and get plenty of sleep, herbal supplements can raise your health to a whole new level.

As explained here by one of the country's leading herbalists, Dr. Daniel B. Mowrey, so-called "tonic" herbs confer an impressive array of health benefits, including increased energy and stamina…heightened immunity…reduced risk of heart disease…improved liver function …reduced joint inflammation.

If you'd like to add herbal remedies to *your* medicine chest, start with the following eight tonic herbs.* All are available at health food stores.

Unlike drugs, herbal preparations are not regulated by the FDA. Ask the store clerk to recommend a reputable brand.

The doses listed are based on capsules containing 850 milligrams (mg) to 900 mg of the herb.

Caution: Consult a doctor before starting any herbal regimen—especially if you have a heart ailment or another chronic illness and/or you are using prescription or over-the-counter medications. Herbal remedies can dangerously interact with certain drugs.

*Editor's note: Certain remedies are inherently unsafe. *Comfrey, borage, chaparral* and *coltsfoot* can cause liver disease…*ma huang* can cause a rise in blood pressure that is particularly unsafe for those with heart or thyroid disease or diabetes…*yohimbe* can cause tremors, anxiety, high blood pressure and rapid heart rate.

If you develop a rash, nausea, hives, headaches or hay fever-like symptoms while taking an herb, stop using it immediately.

CAYENNE

Cayenne is good for the cardiovascular system. A mild stimulant, the herb also helps maintain muscle tone in the stomach and intestinal walls and enhances digestion. Cayenne is also an excellent "activator herb," amplifying the benefits of other herbs you take.

Daily dose: Two capsules. Or use ground cayenne as a spice.

ECHINACEA

Echinacea fights illness on two levels. First, it boosts levels of white blood cells, *B*- and *T-lymphocytes* and *phagocytes*—the key components of a healthy immune system. Second, it neutralizes invading microorganisms.

German researchers have shown that echinacea stops staph, strep and fungal infections, along with a variety of viruses.

Daily dose: Two capsules. Be sure the capsules contain the *whole* root in powdered form, not extract.

Used intermittently, liquid extract of echinacea makes a soothing balm for sore throats. Using an eyedropper, let a few drops fall against the back of your throat.

GARLIC

This spice helps prevent heart disease by lowering cholesterol levels and blocking formation of fatty deposits in the coronary arteries. It also boosts levels of T-cells, a critical component of the immune system.

Animal and human studies have shown that garlic also relieves arthritis. It contains sulfur compounds, which are known to have significant anti-inflammatory properties.

Daily dose: Two pills. Or use a garlic clove or garlic powder in your cooking.

GINGERROOT

Gingerroot is an excellent remedy for indigestion, constipation, diarrhea and nausea (including morning sickness). There's no good explanation for why it works. But my research suggests that ginger is even more effective than Dramamine at preventing motion sickness. It is also effective against the flu.

Be sure to buy capsules made from the *whole* gingerroot—not extract.

Daily dose: For mild motion sickness, two capsules 15 minutes before you depart (and two to four more every hour or whenever symptoms return). For serious gastrointestinal upset, take six to 12 capsules an hour.

LAPACHO

A South American herb, lapacho contains *napthoquinones* (N-factors), unique compounds that have antiviral and antibiotic properties. It's effective at preventing colds, flu and bacterial and fungal infections.

Taken in capsule or tea form, lapacho soothes painful joints...and boosts energy levels. Lapacho also stimulates activity of enzymes in the liver, enhancing its ability to remove toxins from the blood.

In Brazil, lapacho is used to treat leukemia and cervical cancer, and lapacho salve is used to treat skin cancer.

Studies suggest that the herb may also be effective against breast cancer.

Make tea by simmering the purplish paper-thin inner lining of the bark in hot water for 20 minutes, then strain and let cool. Leftover tea can be refrigerated.

Daily dose: To prevent illness, four capsules or two cups of tea. To treat an infection, six capsules or one to two quarts of tea.

MILK THISTLE

One of the world's most studied plants, milk thistle is very good for the liver. By stimulating protein synthesis, it boosts levels of key liver enzymes, speeding regeneration of damaged liver tissue. It also inhibits *lypoxygenase*, an enzyme that destroys liver cells.

Studies show that milk thistle can help reverse the effects of hepatitis and cirrhosis.

Daily dose: Two capsules.

PYGEUM EXTRACT

Derived from the bark of an African tree, pygeum has been shown to prevent—and even relieve—benign enlargement of the prostate. It contains *phytosterols*, which are potent anti-inflammatory compounds. Pygeum also contains *triterpenoids*, compounds that have an antiswelling effect.

Daily dose: To prevent prostate enlargement, two capsules. To shrink an enlarged prostate, four capsules.

YERBA MATE

This South American herb boosts energy and stamina without causing the jitters that caffeine can cause. Anecdotal reports suggest that yerba mate is also effective against asthma and allergies, though the mechanism is unknown.

Yerba mate is best taken as a daily tea. Pour boiling water over yerba mate leaves, let sit for 10 minutes, then strain and serve.

Daily dose: Two to four cups.

Fight Allergies with Stinging Nettle

Nancy L. Snyderman, MD, associate clinical professor of otolaryngology at University of Pennsylvania Health System. A medical correspondent for ABC-TV's "Good Morning America," she is also author of *Dr. Nancy Snyderman's Guide to Good Health.* William Morrow.

As an ear, nose and throat doctor, I prescribe lots of allergy and cold preparations. I used to rely on conventional antihistamines and decongestants. Unfortunately, these drugs can cause drowsiness, dry mouth, nervousness and other side effects. They often do more harm than good.

While preparing an interview with an alternative medicine advocate, he told me about *stinging nettle* (Urtica dioica). This herb is great for stuffy noses caused by allergies. It takes a little longer to work—up to 48 hours—but *doesn't* cause side effects.

Since then everyone in my family has used the herb. I recommend it to my patients, too, particularly those with seasonal allergies like hay fever.

Nettle is safe even when taken over an extended period. In fact, you can use it throughout allergy season. Or take it as soon as you feel a cold coming on. Be sure to follow the dosage directions listed on the bottle.

It's unclear how nettle works. It may constrict small blood vessels in the nose...or it may block the body's production of *histamines*, chemicals that stimulate production of mucus.

Stinging nettle is available in capsules or in tincture form. I prefer Eclectic Institute's freeze-dried nettle capsules because I believe they're especially potent. They are available at health-food stores or from the manufacturer at 800-332-4372, *www.eclecticherb.com.*

Alternative Remedies for Hay Fever

Freeze-dried preparations of the herb *stinging nettle* (Urtica dioica) are often helpful... and unlike antihistamines and decongestants, they do *not* cause troublesome side effects.

Caution: *Nettle tea* and capsules containing air-dried stinging nettle are less effective.

Also helpful: *Quercetin,* a compound derived from citrus fruits and buckwheat. Quercetin supplements should be taken as a preventive measure starting several weeks before allergy season. Consult a doctor before taking stinging nettle or quercetin.

Healing Secrets From a Mayan Medicine Man

Rosita Arvigo, DN (doctor of naprapathy, a branch of chiropractic), founder of the Ix Chel Tropical Research Foundation, Belize. She is coauthor of *Rain Forest Remedies: One Hundred Healing Herbs of Belize.* Lotus Press.

In the past decade, the National Cancer Institute has tested nearly 2,000 rain forest plants for anticancer and anti-AIDS activity. Hundreds of drugs have been developed this way, including *vincristine* (Oncovin) for leukemia and *paclitaxel* (Taxol) for ovarian cancer.

For the past several decades, Dr. Rosita Arvigo of Chicago has lived in the rain forest of the tiny Central American nation of Belize.

There, she and Michael Balick, PhD, associate director of the New York Botanical Garden, have studied medicinal plants, including those used by the late Don Elijio Panti, a 103-year-old "medicine man," who was legendary among the Maya of Belize.

Unlike modern drugs, these plants have been proven over thousands of years of use to be effective and safe. They are available at grocery stores, health food stores and garden centers.

Caution: Plant remedies should not be used by people who are allergic to that plant. Anyone who experiences heart palpitations or a skin rash from a medicinal plant should discontinue its use.

Recently, we asked Dr. Arvigo about these plants—and how we can put them to work in our own lives...

●**Basil.** Basil tea relieves fever, indigestion, anxiety and insomnia. Lab tests have found that basil oil has antibacterial and antifungal properties.

Boil a handful of fresh leaves (or two tablespoons of dried leaves) in two cups of water for five minutes, then strain. Drink hot before meals or at bedtime.

●**Lemon grass.** Among the Maya, lemon grass tea is widely used to reduce fever. It is also effective against coughs and colds.

Lemon grass causes perspiration and promotes the excretion of phlegm.

For treating fever in an adult, boil one mashed root and 10 leaves of the plant in three cups of water for 10 minutes. Drink hot, go to bed and wrap up warmly.

For fever in children, boil 10 leaves in three cups of water for 10 minutes. Give the child one-half cup of tea six times daily.

●**Marigold.** Taken as a hot tea, the larger, yellow varieties of marigold are great for treating colic. Marigold tea also relieves fever, stomach pain, flatulence and headaches.

To make tea, boil two or three flower heads in one cup of water for five minutes. Let the tea steep for 10 minutes. Give a baby spoonfuls of the warm tea.

Herbal bath: Boil a double handful of marigold flowers and leaves in a large pot of water for 20 minutes. Let the water cool, then pour it into a plastic baby tub. Bathe the infant for 10 minutes, then wrap him/her warmly and put him to bed.

●**Oregano.** This herb is widely used in Belize as a remedy for upper respiratory tract infections. It also relieves indigestion.

Oregano can be taken in tea form...or fresh or dried oregano leaves can be added to soups, stews and sauces.

To make tea, pour three cups of boiling water over one-half cup of fresh-picked leaves or three tablespoons of dried leaves. Let steep for 15 minutes, then strain. Drink one cup before each meal.

●**Periwinkle.** Although periwinkle contains potent anticancer compounds, it's best used as a remedy for sore throats.

Place nine pink flowers in a pint of water, and soak in sunlight for three hours. Sip the resulting tea all day long when you have a sore throat or cold.

●**Red rose.** This garden favorite makes a cooling tonic for hot, humid days. It also helps cool fevers and prevent diarrhea. *For children:* Boil one red rose and nine leaves in one cup of water for five minutes, then steep for 15 minutes. Strain and drink. *For adults:* Boil three roses and nine leaves per cup of water.

Safe, Simple Fix for Minor Injuries

William Pawluk, MD, MSc, assistant professor, Johns Hopkins Medical School, Baltimore.

From sprains and bruises to toothache, bone fracture and postsurgical discomfort, the homeopathic remedy *arnica* is good for just about any pain caused by physical trauma. Unlike aspirin and other over-the-counter painkillers, arnica pills have no side effects.

In a 1991 English study on patients hospitalized for acute injuries, arnica relieved stiffness and improved psychological well-being in 98% of patients, compared with 57% of patients given a placebo.

Arnica works *fast*. One of my coworkers fell and pulled a muscle. Ordinarily, it would take a week or two for pain from such an injury to subside. Yet within three days after he started taking arnica, his pain was gone.

It may even be beneficial to take arnica *before* sustaining an injury. Many marathoners use it before they race. In Canada, horse trainers have begun to use arnica to coax a little more speed out of their thoroughbreds.

Arnica is derived from a mountain plant called *leopard's bane*. It's sold in "potencies" ranging from 6x or 6c (low potency) to 200c (high potency).

In general, higher potencies are best for chronic conditions, low potencies for acute conditions. But speak with your doctor before taking a dose.

Arnica is safe in a wide range of dosages—from one pill every eight hours to four pills an hour. If pain persists, see a doctor.

Arnica is available in health-food stores, pharmacies and mail-order homeopathic pharmacies.

Two Herbs that Calm the Colon

David Edelberg, MD, instructor at the University of Chicago and assistant professor of medicine at Rush Medical College, both in Chicago. He is also chairman and medical director of American WholeHealth centers, a group of clinics offering physician-supervised alternative medical care.

If you're plagued by diarrhea, cramping and intestinal gas, you may have *irritable bowel syndrome* (IBS).

What causes IBS? Emotional stress is often involved.

Whatever its cause, IBS can be controlled with two herbs…

•**Peppermint** relaxes smooth muscle surrounding the large intestine, curbing spasms.

During flare-ups of IBS, I tell my patients to take *enteric-coated* peppermint oil—one or two capsules three times a day between meals.

If this dosage causes a burning sensation during bowel movements, lower the dose.

•**St. John's wort** eases anxiety by acting as a mild tranquilizer and antidepressant. It lowers levels of the brain chemical *monoamine oxidase* (MAO). High levels of MAO have been linked to depression.

The usual approach to reducing MAO levels is to take an MAO inhibitor such as Marplan, Nardil or Parnate. But foods that contain *tyramine*, including aged cheese, bananas and pepperoni, can interact with MAO inhibitors—*perhaps lethally*.

There are no dietary restrictions with St. John's wort (though it can make fair-skinned individuals sensitive to sunlight). Take one capsule twice a day with meals.

Both herbs are available at health-food stores.

Mail-order source: Arrowroot Natural Foods Direct (800-456-7818, *www.arrowroot.com*).

Food and Healing

Annemarie Colbin, founder of the Natural Gourmet Institute for Food and Health, 48 W. 21 St., New York 10010. A certified health education specialist and certified culinary professional, she is author of several books, including *Food and Healing*. Ballantine.

You are probably well aware that a low-fat, high-fiber diet can help prevent disease. But is there such a thing as food that heals?

The answer is *yes*.

For more than 30 years, I've been studying the effects of food on health. I have also tried out many remedies based on centuries-old folk wisdom.

Based on my observations and those of my students, I'm convinced that certain foods *do* help the body heal more quickly from a number of minor ailments…

COLDS AND FLU

The best natural remedy is garlic. By boosting the immune system and killing bacteria, it helps keep a mild viral illness from turning into a serious bacterial infection.

Swallow one small clove or several small pieces every four to six hours until symptoms subside. Wash this garlic "pill" down with a glass of orange juice or water.

Don't worry about bad breath. If you don't chew the garlic, no one will be able to smell it on your breath.

CONSTIPATION

You probably know that whole grains and fresh fruits and vegetables—especially prunes —help "normalize" colon function.

But these natural remedies won't do much good unless you wash them down with plenty of water. Vegetarians should have four to six glasses a day, meat-eaters at least eight.

Ironically, constipation is sometimes caused by consuming *too* much dietary fiber. If you suspect this is your problem, cut back on raw produce. Continue to eat whole grains—especially brown rice. It seems to be more easily digested than other high-fiber foods. And drink plenty of water.

COUGH

If you have a "wet" cough (one that produces phlegm), drink hot liquids—especially hot-and-sour soup or another spicy soup. Wet coughs should be encouraged—they are the body's way of expelling bacteria and other pathogens.

Also helpful: Hot apple or pear juice with cinnamon (from the Chinese medical tradition).

To stop a "dry" cough or a tickle in the throat, eat something salty—like *umeboshi plums.* These pickled plums are sold in health-food stores and Japanese groceries. Or—try licorice tea. It strengthens the lungs and is a traditional herbal remedy for asthma.

DIARRHEA

Mild diarrhea can often be controlled by eating small amounts of cooked white rice…or grated raw apple that is allowed to turn brown, so it develops the soluble fiber pectin.

Caution: Seek medical attention for severe, prolonged diarrhea or diarrhea accompanied by vomiting. That can signal dysentery, food poisoning or another life-threatening infection.

HEADACHE

Tension headaches are often triggered by insufficient food or insufficient fluids…or by prolonged exposure to summer heat.

Remedy: Two or more cups of cool juice. I've seen this "prescription" relieve headaches in as little as five minutes.

Fruit juice—especially apple or apricot juice —seems best. I don't know whether that's because of the pleasant flavor or because it gets carbohydrates and fluids into the system quickly.

For a headache caused by drinking too much alcohol or eating too much sugar, eat olives, anchovies or umeboshi plums.

You might also try steamed vegetables sprinkled with sesame salt. My father had an easy and delicious variation on this idea—eating a scallion that's been dipped in salt.

For a headache that stems from caffeine withdrawal, chew a piece of lemon. The strong, sour taste somehow counteracts the body's response to less caffeine. Drink plenty of water to prevent dehydration.

Over the years, I've noticed that migraines can be triggered by eating potato chips or another oily food on an empty stomach.

Remedy: "Spiked" lemon tea. Squeeze half a lemon into a cup. Dice the peel and simmer in 1¼ cups of water for 10 minutes. Strain into the cup. Add a pinch of cayenne or ½ teaspoon of grated fresh ginger—or ¼ teaspoon of powdered ginger. Sweeten with maple syrup or barley malt.

SORE THROAT

To soothe a sore throat, drink tea made from ginger or slippery elm (the latter can be found in health-food stores). Slippery elm lozenges are also effective.

Ginger tea is made by simmering three to four slices of fresh ginger in a cup of water for eight minutes. It is also good for coughs, chest congestion and motion sickness.

STOMACH UPSET

If you have heartburn or another form of *gastroesophageal reflux,* eat *cooked* food only —it's easier to digest.

Intestinal gas can often be relieved by an "antacid" made of *kudzu,* a starch made from the root of the kudzu plant. It's sold in health-food stores.

Dissolve one tablespoon of kudzu in a cup of cold water. Cook, stirring until thick. Then add a tablespoon of soy sauce.

To make kudzu pudding, dissolve two tablespoons of kudzu in a cup of apple juice. Add a teaspoon of vanilla if desired. Cook, stirring constantly, until thickened. Fold in a tablespoon of tahini (sesame paste). Eat hot or cold.

Soothing and very relaxing, kudzu pudding is an excellent remedy for stress or insomnia. Kudzu has also been shown to reduce cravings for alcohol.

RESPECT YOUR TASTE BUDS

Don't force yourself to eat foods you dislike. If you find a food distasteful, it probably isn't something that will help your body.

Fast Headache Relief Without Drugs

Art Ulene, MD, former medical correspondent for NBC's "Today" show and clinical professor of obstetrics and gynecology, University of Southern California School of Medicine, Los Angeles.

If you frequently get headaches, you should know about my natural self-treatment program. The program combines dietary strategies (identifying and avoiding "trigger foods") ...daily exercise and relaxation...plus visual imagery (creative visualization).

Imagery can be used anywhere, anytime. It's good both for warding off headaches...and for keeping them from getting worse.

My program is *very* effective. When I tested it with 19 headache sufferers, they reported 33% fewer headaches.

Their use of painkillers fell by 40%. That's important because while drugs do relieve pain, they can cause nausea and other side effects. In some cases, the side effects are worse than the headaches.

Caution: If you've just begun to get headaches, or if your pain is severe, consult a doctor. About 2% of headaches have an underlying cause that needs treatment—sinusitis, inflammation of a blood vessel or even a life-threatening problem like aneurysm or brain tumor.

But for tension-type and migraine headaches, imagery works very well.

What to do: Close your eyes and relax. Picture a red light attached to the part of your head that hurts. The light represents your pain.

Imagine slowly dimming and then extinguishing the light. This should take three to five minutes. As the light disappears, so should your headache.

If you're at home, use visualization along with a cold pack. A bag of frozen peas is good.

Natural Remedies For Fatigue

Adriane Fugh-Berman, MD, associate professor, complementary and alternative medicine, Georgetown University School of Medicine. She is author of *Alternative Medicine: What Works*. Lippincott, Williams & Wilkins.

Do you feel tired all the time? Do you lack the energy you used to have? Join the club. Chronic fatigue is an extremely common complaint—and one with many different causes. *Here's what you need to know to get to the root of your problem...*

- **Lack of sleep.** Although sleeplessness seems an obvious reason to be tired, it's often overlooked. These days, people like to brag about how little sleep they need. But there are actually very few people who truly need only five or six hours a night. Most of us need eight. Some of us need nine or 10. Just because you can get by on six or seven hours a night does *not* mean that's all the sleep you need. If you suffer from persistent fatigue, see how much better you'll feel with an extra 30 or 60 minutes of sleep each night.

Maximize the *quality* of your sleep, too. Never work or worry in your bedroom. Make your bedroom as quiet as possible—use earplugs if you must. If street lamps or other sources of light outside your window bother you, try heavy drapes or an eye shade.

- **Lack of exercise.** Too little exercise can cause fatigue—or make it worse. Of course, overexercising can also cause fatigue, but moderate exercise is actually an energizer. What's moderate? Twenty to 60 minutes three times a week is ideal. Do *not* exercise within two hours of bedtime. Doing so may interfere with your sleep.

•**Medication.** Sleeping pills can cause a sort of fatigue "hangover" in many people. That goes for *melatonin* as well as prescription sedatives like *diazepam* (Valium). Fatigue can also be a side effect of many other over-the-counter and prescription medications, including blood pressure drugs like *propranolol* (Inderal) and *atenolol* (Tenormin)…as well as many antidepressants and antihistamines. If you suspect your medication is making you tired, ask your doctor about alternatives.

•**Diet.** Heavy meals, especially late in the day, or particularly starchy meals can cause fatigue. If you insist on a heavy meal, have it early in the day. A hearty breakfast is less likely to sap your energy than a hearty lunch or supper.

What else can you do to boost your energy? Consider taking vitamin and herbal supplements. *B-complex* is especially effective—take this supplement once a day. *Vitamin B-12* is good, too. Take 1,000 micrograms a day. Since B-12 is found almost exclusively in meat and dairy products, many strict vegetarians suffer from B-12 deficiency—and from chronic fatigue as a result.

Vitamin B-12 may be better absorbed when it's injected, and some people swear by injections for an energy boost. I generally prefer B-12 tablets. They're far less costly and, I think, just as effective.

Coenzyme Q10 helps fight fatigue by maximizing the heart's pumping efficiency. Take 30 mg once or twice a day.

Ginseng tea, capsules or extract can be a potent source of energy. Be sure not to mix ginseng with caffeine or another stimulant. The combination can cause palpitations or irregular heartbeat.

Siberian "ginseng" isn't really ginseng at all, but another plant species called *Eleutherococcus*. It, too, has energizing qualities. Both herbs are *adaptogens*, meaning that they help the body to adapt to stress.

If these measures don't boost your energy, see a doctor. You may be suffering from depression, anemia, chronic fatigue syndrome or another disease that requires medical intervention.

Natural Alternatives to Common Medications

Michael T. Murray, ND, professor of botanical science at Bastyr University in Seattle. He is author of *Natural Alternatives to Over-the-Counter and Prescription Drugs.* Harper.

Conventional medications can be quite effective at controlling symptoms…but they can also cause nasty side effects.

Fortunately, there are natural alternatives to many of the most common prescription and over-the-counter (OTC) drugs. Available in health-food stores, these herbs, plant extracts, vitamins, etc., are often as effective as the medications they replace—and less likely to cause side effects.

If the idea of using natural remedies seems "flaky" to you, it's probably because mainstream doctors in the US tend to be strongly biased against them.

This bias is *not* shared by doctors elsewhere. In Germany, for example, the herb *St. John's wort* (Hypericum perforatum) is prescribed for depression eight times more frequently than synthetic antidepressants like *fluoxetine* (Prozac).

Here's a list of drugs you may be better off without, along with the natural alternatives with which to replace them.

Important: Choose products with labels specifying the concentration of active ingredients …and use them only under medical supervision.

HEADACHE REMEDIES

It's no secret that people with recurrent headaches tend to use lots of aspirin, ibuprofen and acetaminophen. Few people realize, however, that these OTC painkillers cause "rebound" headaches in 70% of the people who use them. That is, painkillers taken to stop pain wind up causing *more* pain.

Alternative I: Magnesium. Many tension-type and migraine headaches stem from a slight deficiency of this mineral. If your headaches do, magnesium oxide supplements should bring relief. Take 600 milligrams (mg) per day, divided into three 200-mg doses.

Alternative II: Feverfew. This herb is particularly effective against migraines. Take 80 mg of an extract containing at least 0.2% of *parthenolide*, the active ingredient in feverfew. No side effects have been reported.

ACID BLOCKERS AND ANTACIDS

Acid blockers like Zantac, Tagamet and Axid fight stomach upset and ulcers by blocking the release of stomach acid. But in doing so, they disrupt the digestive process. This can lead to nutritional deficiencies.

Acid blockers have also been linked to liver and kidney problems, yeast infection (*candidiasis*) and breast enlargement in men (*gynecomastia*).

Antacids like Tums and Maalox can cause a rebound effect, in which the stomach generates more stomach acid as the antacids wear off. Many antacids contain aluminum, which some suspect may be a cause of Parkinson's and Alzheimer's disease.

Alternative: Deglycyrrhizinated licorice (DGL). It promotes synthesis of the natural substances that line the intestinal tract, protecting it against acid irritation. In studies DGL has proven *more* effective than acid blockers and Maalox.

Typical dosage: Two 380-mg tablets, taken 20 minutes before meals.

Caution: If you have persistent stomach pain—especially pain that grows worse on an empty stomach—see a doctor. You may have a peptic ulcer.

ANTIHISTAMINES

Benadryl and other OTC antihistamines are effective at relieving nasal congestion, runny nose and other cold and hay fever symptoms. Some can cause dry mouth and drowsiness.

Alternative: Quercetin. This derivative of fruits and flowers keeps the body from releasing histamine and other compounds that trigger cold and hay fever symptoms.

Typical dosage: 200 mg, taken five minutes before meals.

SLEEPING PILLS

As many people suffering from insomnia have learned, sleeping pills can impair mental and physical function…and make it hard to "get going" in the morning.

Alternative: Valerian. This herbal sleeping aid works better than sleeping pills, without causing any morning "hangover."

Typical dosage: 150 mg, taken 45 minutes before bedtime. Look for a product that contains 0.8% *valerenic acid*, valerian's active ingredient.

ANTIDEPRESSANTS

All prescription antidepressants cause side effects. Almost half of all people who take fluoxetine or *sertraline* (Zoloft), for example, notice a decreased sex drive.

Alternative: St. John's wort. Double-blind studies have proven this herb to be *more* effective than prescription antidepressants. St. John's wort appears to be safe, though it can cause sun sensitivity and stomach upset.

Typical dosage: 300 mg, three times a day. Buy a product containing 0.3% of the herb's active ingredient, *hypericin*.

FINASTERIDE (PROSCAR)

Enlarged prostate (also known as *benign prostatic hyperplasia*, or BPH) affects 50% of men over age 60. Symptoms include frequent urination and a weak or uneven urine stream.

Doctors often treat BPH with *finasteride*. This drug blocks synthesis of testosterone, the hormone that fuels the growth of prostate tissue.

But finasteride can take up to six months to relieve symptoms. It can also cause depression and impotence.

Alternative: Saw palmetto. This herb, widely used in Europe, has proven effective against BPH in many studies. It causes no major side effects.

Typical dosage: 160 mg, twice a day. Expect improvement within four weeks. Buy a *fat-soluble* extract that contains 85% to 95% fatty acids and sterols.

Caution: Any man who thinks he has BPH should have a full physical. Urinary difficulties can be symptomatic of prostate cancer.

Natural Ways to Lower Your Blood Pressure

Stephen Fortmann, MD, professor of medicine at Stanford University School of Medicine, and director of the Stanford Center for Research in Disease Prevention, both in Palo Alto, CA. He is coauthor of *The Blood Pressure Book: How to Get It Down and Keep It Down.* Bull Publishing.

If your blood pressure is above 140/90, you may already know that taking steps to lower it will reduce your risk for heart attack, stroke, kidney failure and other serious ailments.

You might *not* know that the same steps are beneficial if your pressure is in the prehypertensive stage (120/80 to 139/89). *Even if your pressure is below 120/80, you'll enjoy long-term health benefits if you make certain lifestyle changes...*

LOSE WEIGHT

Not everyone with high blood pressure is obese, and not all obese people have high blood pressure. But for most people, losing weight reduces blood pressure.

Rule of thumb: A loss of one pound of body fat brings a one-point drop in systolic blood pressure (the upper number).

If you need to lose weight, set realistic goals. Plan to lose about one to three pounds a month.

EXERCISE REGULARLY

Exercise pumps up your metabolism, helping you burn more calories and preserve muscle tissue. Exercise seems to have a direct pressure-lowering effect, too.

Finding: When sedentary people began exercising regularly, their systolic pressure fell about 10 points.

Walking is an excellent form of exercise. *Here's how to pack more walking into your everyday life...*

● **Walk or bike to work, on errands, etc.** If it's too far to do so, consider parking your car a block away...or getting off one stop early on the bus or train.

● **Walk as much as possible while at work.** Take stairs instead of elevators. Walk to a coworker's office instead of telephoning. Take a brief walk at lunchtime...and during each work break.

● **At day's end, take a 15-minute walk** with a friend or family member. A late-afternoon walk helps you unwind...and takes the edge off your appetite.

REDUCE SODIUM INTAKE

The salt industry has been pushing the idea that only a minority of "salt-sensitive" people have to worry about the pressure-raising effects of sodium.

Reality: For most people, restricting sodium intake reduces blood pressure by two to three points.

Americans eat a great deal of salt without realizing it. Fast food—pizzas, hot dogs, hamburgers, etc.—are often loaded with sodium. So are canned foods, frozen dinners, prepared salad dressings and sauces, processed poultry and meat, pretzels, potato chips and smoked fish.

I tell my patients to avoid table salt and salty foods whenever possible. An adult needs only 200 mg of sodium a day. A single roast beef sandwich contains four times that amount.

In the supermarket, check labels for sodium content. When you cook, season with herbs instead of salt.

INCREASE POTASSIUM INTAKE

An analysis of 33 different studies by Paul K. Whelton, MD, of Tulane University in New Orleans, found that the systolic blood pressure of people who took potassium supplements dropped an average of five points.

Potassium supplements are okay, but it's better to get your potassium from foods. Potassium-rich foods include apples, melons, bananas, potatoes, tomatoes and nectarines.

Each day, have at least two servings of fruit and three servings of fresh vegetables. Juices are rich in potassium. Watch out for tomato juice, though. Most brands of tomato juice are sky-high in sodium.

REDUCE MEAT CONSUMPTION

Vegetarians tend to have lower blood pressure than nonvegetarians. Why? One possibility is that the antioxidants in fruit and vegetables help lower blood pressure.

Another is that the calcium in fruits and vegetables is easily absorbed. Calcium seems to help reduce blood pressure.

REDUCE ALCOHOL CONSUMPTION

In some individuals at least, regular drinking raises blood pressure. For these people, abstaining brings significant declines in blood pressure.

Example: A two-drink-per-day drinker who stops drinking might experience a 10-point decline in systolic pressure. Heavier drinkers who go on the wagon can experience a drop of up to 20 points.

DO RELAXATION EXERCISES

Psychological stress causes a transient rise in blood pressure, but doctors still don't know whether stress has any long-term effects.

It's clear, however, that relaxation exercises can bring lasting reductions in blood pressure. Many individuals who practice relaxation regularly experience as much as a five-point drop in systolic pressure.

What to do: Twice a week for 15 minutes—set an alarm clock so you won't have to keep track of time—sit on a comfortable chair in a quiet room.

Close your eyes. Relax your right arm until it feels warm and "floppy," then move on to your right thigh, calf, ankle and foot…left thigh, calf, ankle and foot…left arm…abdomen and buttocks…chest…neck…jaw and forehead.

Once your entire body is relaxed, envision ripples on a lake, soft breezes blowing through grass or another soothing scene.

SEVERE HIGH BLOOD PRESSURE

If your blood pressure is 140/90 or higher, your doctor will probably prescribe anti-hypertensive medication. Even so, lifestyle changes might enable you to get by on a lower dosage …or reduce your blood pressure to the point that drug therapy is no longer necessary.

Meditation Lowers Blood Pressure

Robert Schneider, MD, director of the Institute for Natural Medicine and Prevention, Maharishi Vedic Prevention Center, Hamden, CT.

In a study, patients with mild hypertension who practiced *transcendental meditation* (TM) twice a day had a greater drop in blood pressure than those who learned progressive muscle relaxation—tensing and relaxing muscles one at a time. They also had a greater drop in blood pressure than those who reduced salt and calorie intake and exercised regularly.

Also: The TM users' blood pressure reduction was about the same as that in people who take blood pressure medication.

In TM, you sit with your eyes closed and repeat a word or sound—a *mantra*.

Meditation and Pain Control

Amy Saltzman, MD, member of the board of trustees, American Holistic Medical Association, PO Box 2016, Edmonds, WA 98020.

Meditation helps control pain—and promotes general health. A series of studies published in prestigious medical journals over the past decade found that practitioners of meditation report significant decreases in pain, anxiety, depression, blood pressure and other physical symptoms—allowing doctors to decrease medication and doctors' visits.

The Benefits of Massage

Tiffany Field, PhD, director, University of Miami's Touch Research Institute, Dept. of Pediatrics, Box 016820 (D-820), 1601 NW 12th Ave., Miami 33101.

Massage promotes general good health, not just relaxation. It also strengthens the immune system by increasing the number of natural killer cells in the body.

Study: HIV patients who received regular massage showed reduced stress and improved immune function. Massage may soon be considered as basic a component of good health as diet and exercise.

Secrets of Self-Healing From Chinese Medicine

Roger Jahnke, OMD (doctor of Oriental medicine), an acupuncturist and Chinese medicine practitioner in private practice in Santa Barbara, CA. He is author of *The Healer Within: The Four Essential Self-Care Methods for Creating Optimal Health.* HarperSanFrancisco.

An avalanche of medical research shows that the human body is capable of remarkable feats of self-healing.

Self-healing happens automatically when you cultivate your body's innate self-healing powers.

How do you do that? *Chinese medicine makes use of four simple techniques...*

- **Deep breathing**
- **Gentle movement**
- **Self-massage**
- **Meditation**

Put these techniques to work for just 10 to 15 minutes a day, and you'll be more energetic and alert...and less vulnerable to illness and the negative effects of stress.

Although these techniques can be done as often as you like, it's a good idea to combine all four briefly first thing each morning.

DEEP BREATHING

Americans have forgotten how to breathe. We typically take very shallow breaths. This pattern of breathing constricts blood vessels, contributing to high blood pressure.

Shallow breathing also impairs immune function. It does so by slowing the circulation of antibodies and immune cells throughout the body.

By making a conscious effort to breathe slowly and deeply, you can counteract these physiological disturbances. *Try the following exercise right now...*

- **Take a slow, deep breath through your nose.** Allow the lower portions of your lungs to fill, then keep inhaling until your lungs are fully inflated.
- **Exhale slowly for 10 seconds.** You can exhale silently...or with an audible sigh of relief. Allow yourself to drift off into deep relaxation.

While even a single deep breath is beneficial, the accumulated effect of many such breaths is dramatic. Resolve to do two or three deep breathing sessions each day.

Do one session before getting out of bed in the morning, another just before you go to sleep at night.

Some people prefer to do deep breathing periodically throughout the day.

You might decide to take a deep breath each time the telephone rings...each time you stop at a red light...or each time you open the refrigerator. The point is to develop a habit of breathing deeply all day long.

GENTLE MOVEMENT

Research confirms that easy, low-intensity exercise provides virtually all the disease-fighting benefits of vigorous exercise—with far less risk of injury to both your muscles and joints. *The "flowing technique" is very popular in China...*

What to do: Stand with your feet shoulder-width apart and shoulders relaxed. Let your arms dangle at your sides. Bend your knees slightly...move your tailbone beneath your spine so as to "lengthen" your back...and lower your chin as if nodding "yes."

Rest briefly, begin to inhale slowly and turn your palms forward. Swing your arms forward and upward, slowly rising onto the balls of your feet as you do. Raise your hands (palms up) to shoulder height, keeping your elbows slightly bent. Turn your palms downward. Slowly lower your arms and exhale. Return your heels to the floor. As your hands pass your legs, allow them to swing back slightly while gently lifting your toes.

Repeat 10 to 15 times, developing a gentle rhythm.

SELF-MASSAGE

Self-massage has been a powerful healing tool in China for thousands of years...

•**Hand massage.** Using your left thumb, apply gentle pressure to the palm of your right hand. Place your remaining fingers on the back of the right hand for support.

Increase the pressure gradually until you're exerting about the same pressure needed to squeeze a new tennis ball.

Massage your hand all over, noting any areas of tenderness. Massage the fingers as well—all the way out to the tips. Finally, grasp each finger of your right hand on either side of the nail. Pinch gently.

Switch hands, and repeat. To conclude, return to any tender spots on either hand and knead them gently for a few additional minutes.

•**"Energizing" the internal organs.** Place your palms over the lower edge of your rib cage, near the sides of your body but still on the front. Rub your palms against your body in a circular motion, breathing easily and deeply as you do. Feel the warmth generated by your hands penetrating toward your organs.

Next, place one hand on your breastbone (sternum), the other on your navel. Rub in a circular motion with each hand.

Move both hands to your lower back, and repeat the process. The Chinese believe that sending warmth into the organs improves health and heals disease.

MEDITATION

Meditation reduces blood pressure, dilates blood vessels and stimulates the production of essential neurotransmitters and hormones.

One of the easiest and most powerful meditation techniques is *mindfulness*. Using this technique, you can free yourself of psychological and physical stress by focusing closely on a single bodily sensation.

Breath-awareness exercise: As you stand, sit or lie comfortably, focus all your concentration on the sensation of your breath as it passes through your nostrils. Your nostrils should feel cool as fresh air enters…and warm as you exhale.

You can do this mindfulness exercise for as briefly as a moment or as long as 20 minutes.

Notice that as long as you hold the focus on your breath, it's impossible to worry or think about stressful situations.

Ancient Chinese Secret For Relaxation and Better Health

Simon Wang, MD, PhD, professor of physiology at Guangxi Medical University in Guangxi, China. He is coauthor of *Qi Gong for Health & Longevity.* East Health Development Group.

Q*i gong* is the ancient Chinese art of relaxing, rejuvenating and healing the body and the mind. It consists of exercises that boost the flow of *qi* (pronounced chee), the universal life force within the body.

According to the principles of Chinese medicine, qi flows through the body along channels called *meridians.* As long as this flow is smooth, the body remains healthy. But any blockage or imbalance of qi quickly results in illness.

To learn more about qi gong and how to use it in our own lives, we spoke to Dr. Simon Wang, who has received a standard Western medical education, but has spent years studying and using qi gong…

No one knows exactly how qi gong works. My own hunch is that it affects the release of hormones in the body.

I could relate countless anecdotes about the effectiveness of qi gong. My 66-year-old father, for instance, has practiced it for years…and he never even gets a cold. *But qi gong has also been shown to be effective in many clinical studies…*

•**In a controlled study at the Shanghai Hypertension Research Institute,** subjects showed improved cerebral blood flow after 12 months of qi gong training. Headaches, high blood pressure and several other ailments are associated with reduced blood flow in the brain.

The same study showed reduced levels of blood lactate after qi gong training—suggesting a beneficial reduction in metabolic rate.

•**Studies conducted at the Traditional Medical College in Beijing** showed that people taught qi gong experienced a marked rise in alpha brain waves. Alpha waves are associated with a calm, alert state.

•**A study of 68 AIDS patients in San Francisco** showed that two months of qi gong training brought a 13% to 22% rise in the number of infection-fighting white blood cells.

HOW TO PRACTICE QI GONG

There are many types of qi gong. All involve manipulating the flow of qi via meditation, breathing exercises and self-massage.

Qi gong can be practiced while standing, sitting or lying down. It can be done anywhere you can find a little peace and quiet—at home or at work…or even while traveling.

Weather permitting, it's best to do qi gong outdoors. The flow of qi is stimulated by fresh air and close proximity to plants.

Qi gong works best if done every day, on a lifelong basis. Devote 20 minutes or so each morning to learning qi gong, and within two months you should feel calmer and more refreshed.

Here is my daily routine. *I do it every morning, immediately upon waking…*

RELAXING YOUR MIND

Lie in bed or sit cross-legged on a bed or the floor. Relax. Concentrate on breathing naturally for a minute or two.

Next, concentrate on "guiding" qi to an area deep within your brain, just behind your forehead. Imagine this "qi cavity" glowing with red or yellow light…or imagine that it's filled with ocean waves, a green meadow or another natural scene.

Concentrate on these images for five minutes. Gradually, a sense of calm will wash over you.

RUBBING YOUR HANDS

Now activate the qi cavities in your hands. Shift your focus from your head to your palms. Gently rub your palms together for a minute or two. Then use one palm to rub the back of the other hand for another couple of minutes.

Reverse hands and repeat, breathing naturally throughout.

RUBBING YOUR ARMS

Continue focusing on your palms. Close your eyes, and run your left palm up the outside of your right arm, from the wrist to the top of your right shoulder. Rotate your right arm outward, and run your left palm all the way down the inside of your right arm.

Do this 20 times, then switch arms and repeat.

BATHING YOUR FACE

Close your eyes. Gently press the tip of your tongue against the back of your upper teeth. Cover your face with your palms, with your fingers pointing upward. Using both hands, rub your face from forehead to chin. Then rub it again from chin to forehead. Repeat 20 times, until your hands and face feel warm.

RUBBING YOUR CHEST

Use your right palm to rub from the top of the right side of your chest, down and across your body to the lower portion of the left side of your chest.

Then take your left palm and rub from your upper left chest down and across to your lower right chest.

Repeat 20 times, concentrating on the center of your palms.

RUBBING *DAN TIAN*

Close your eyes. Using your right palm, rub your abdomen, just below the navel, in a tight, circular pattern. Repeat 20 times.

The lower abdomen contains the *Dan Tian* point, one of the most important of all qi cavities.

RUBBING *YONG QUAN*

Yong Quan is a qi cavity in the center of the sole of each foot.

Place the fingers of your left hand against the bottom of your right foot—at the point where the arch meets the ball of the foot. Rub rapidly in a circular motion 20 times, concentrating on the Yong Quan point. Then switch to your right hand and left foot, and repeat.

Some Medicinal Oils Are Very Good for You

Richard N. Podell, MD, clinical professor of family medicine at Robert Wood Johnson Medical School of the University of Medicine and Dentistry of New Jersey in New Brunswick. He is author of several books, including *Patient Power*. Fireside.

Conventional wisdom has it that oils are something to keep *out* of our diets. These liquid fats are just too laden with calories.

But there are certain oils that have great medicinal properties...

EVENING PRIMROSE OIL

Oil extracted from the seeds of the evening primrose plant *(Oenothera biennis)* is rich in *gamma-linolenic acid* (GLA).

Native Americans used the evening primrose as a medicine, and modern research has confirmed that its oil can help in a variety of conditions.

●**Diabetes.** Many people who have diabetes wind up with *neuropathy*, a form of nerve damage that causes pain and weakness. An impressive body of research shows that evening primrose oil can help diabetics guard against neuropathy.

In one 1993 study conducted in seven hospitals in England and Finland, 50 diabetic patients took 12 capsules of evening primrose oil daily for one year. Another 50 diabetic patients took an olive oil placebo for the same period of time.

Result: Those who took evening primrose oil experienced significant reductions in pain and weakness, and improvements in nerve function and reflexes. Those who got the olive oil experienced no such improvements.

BORAGE OIL

Borage *(Borago officinalis)* is a plant with blue star-shaped flowers. Oil extracted from its seeds contains an even higher concentration of GLA than evening primrose oil. Four standard capsules contain as much of the beneficial fatty acid as 12 evening primrose oil caps.

●**Psychological stress.** In a controlled study conducted at the University of Waterloo in Ontario, Canada, and reported in the *Journal of Human Hypertension*, 30 healthy college students were divided into two groups. The first group took nine borage oil capsules a day for 28 days. The second group took a placebo for the same time period. Before and after the supplement period, they were given a psychological test known to cause stress.

Result: The students in the borage oil group exhibited much less stress when they took the test the second time. Those in the placebo group exhibited no decline in stress the second time around.

FISH OIL

Salmon and other cold water fish are rich in *omega-3* fatty acids—substances the body uses to synthesize "good" prostaglandins.

A growing body of research suggests that fish oil is powerful medicine against a number of illnesses.

●**Crohn's disease.** This inflammatory bowel condition causes severe diarrhea and abdominal pain, and interferes with nutrient absorption. Crohn's disease often goes into remission only to flare up several weeks or months later.

One study done in Italy and published in *The New England Journal of Medicine* showed that fish oil supplements brought striking benefits to people with Crohn's.

In the study, 78 patients who were in remission took either nine fish oil capsules daily or a placebo.

Result: After one year, 74% of the control group had suffered relapses. Only 41% of those who took the fish oil relapsed.

USING MEDICINAL OILS

While there's little risk in taking a daily capsule of evening primrose oil, borage oil or fish oil on your own, be sure to check with your doctor first. He/she should be able to help you determine a dosage appropriate for you.

Certain risks are associated with use of natural oils.

Example: Fish oil can thin the blood enough to cause internal bleeding, especially when taken along with other "clot-busters" like garlic or aspirin. In some cases, it raises blood sugar and cholesterol.

Eat Away Arthritis

Lauri M. Aesoph, ND, a naturopathic physician in Sioux Falls, SD. She is author of *How to Eat Away Arthritis*. Prentice Hall.

Cayenne, ginger and turmeric can bring marked relief from arthritis pain. These spices work by blocking release of *substance P*, a brain chemical that transmits pain signals and activates inflammation in the joints.

Important: If you decide to begin "spice therapy," let your doctor know—so he/she can adjust your arthritis medication.

●**Cayenne.** Cayenne can be eaten as a spice …or applied in cream form to painful joints. In a study, up to 80% of arthritis patients were helped by an over-the-counter cream containing cayenne pepper extract *(capsaicin).*

Capsaicin cream is sold in drugstores under the brand names Capzasin-P, Pain Free and Zostrix.

Caution: Applying the cream to broken skin can cause pain. Also—don't eat cayenne if you have an ulcer.

●**Ginger.** In a study, ginger eased pain and swelling in 75% of arthritis patients. You can add fresh gingerroot to your cooking. Or take one to three gingerroot capsules a day.

Caution: Consuming more than 3 g of ginger at a time can cause stomach upset.

●**Turmeric.** This spice contains *curcumin,* a compound that reduces swelling. In one study, arthritis patients took either 1,200 mg of curcumin or 300 mg of the arthritis drug *phenylbutazone.* Both groups showed comparable improvement in symptoms, but the drug caused side effects.

Cook with turmeric…or take two curcumin capsules three times daily.

Caution: Limit daily turmeric consumption to one meal…or six capsules.

Natural Remedies for Impotence

Adriane Fugh-Berman, MD, associate professor, complementary and alternative medicine, Georgetown University School of Medicine. She is author of *Alternative Medicine: What Works.* Lippincott, Williams & Wilkins.

The first step in overcoming impotence is to find out which type you have. *Physical* impotence is caused by nerve damage (often as a result of injury or chronic conditions such as diabetes)…or poor circulation in the penis (often caused by fatty deposits in penile blood vessels). In addition, certain drugs can cause physical impotence. Nine out of 10 cases of impotence are of physical origin.

Psychological impotence stems from emotional stress, depression or strife within your personal relationship. If you have this form of impotence, your best bet is psychotherapy or couples counseling. About 10% of all cases of impotence have a psychological basis.

How can you tell physical from psychological impotence? Find out whether you have erections during sleep. There are fancy machines for measuring "nocturnal penile tumescence." But you don't need them. Here's a simple, inexpensive test you can do at home.

Just before going to bed, use tape to fasten a perforated strip of stamps around the base of your penis. Don't wrap your penis too tightly. You should be able to slip a coin between the stamps and your skin. In the morning, check to see if the strip of stamps has broken. Do this every night for a week.

If you're consistently breaking the stamps, odds are you have a psychological problem. Consider asking your doctor for referral to a therapist. If you're *not* breaking the stamps, your problem is probably physical. If so, your next step is to determine whether any medication you're taking is the culprit.

A variety of over-the-counter (OTC) and prescription drugs—and many herbal remedies—can cause impotence. These include decongestants containing pseudoephedrine… blood pressure medications, especially beta-blockers such as *propranolol* (Inderal) and *atenolol* (Tenormin)…and *selective serotonin reuptake inhibitor* (SSRI) antidepressants such as *fluoxetine* (Prozac) and *sertraline* (Zoloft).

If you suspect that your impotence is a side effect of a drug, ask your doctor about switching to another drug. If drugs *don't* seem to be causing your impotence, consider trying one of the natural remedies that are effective against impotence. *These include…*

●**Ginkgo biloba.** Good circulation to the penis is essential for good erections, and this potent blood thinner helps boost circulation throughout the body. In a study conducted by

Alan Cohen, MD, of the University of California at San Francisco, 32 of 37 patients with sexual problems (including impotence and inability to achieve orgasm) got better when they took 120 mg of ginkgo extract twice a day.

●**Ginseng.** Although it's best known as a mild stimulant, ginseng is also effective against impotence. Two varieties of ginseng are readily available—*Panax ginseng* and *Panax quinquifolius*. These can be taken as a tea, in capsule form (take one or two daily) or liquid extract (one or two dropperfuls a day). Be sure to take it in the morning. Taken in the evening, its stimulant properties can cause insomnia. Never combine ginseng with coffee or any other stimulant food or drug.

Made from the bark of a West African tree, *yohimbe* is often touted as a cure for impotence. Unfortunately, it can raise blood pressure and heart rate and cause anxiety, dizziness, headache and tremor. A pharmaceutical form of the herb, *yohimbine*, is available by prescription. However, I don't recommend either version of the herb because of these disturbing side effects.

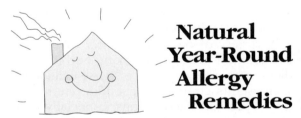

Natural Year-Round Allergy Remedies

Richard Firshein, DO, physician practicing complementary medicine in New York. He is author of *The Nutraceutical Revolution* (Riverhead) and answers health-related questions at *www.drcity.com*.

More than 20 million Americans suffer from springtime allergies. Over-the-counter and prescription antihistamines, decongestants and steroid nasal sprays may help—but they can cause drowsiness and nasal bleeding and may have other yet-unknown effects.

Here are some natural remedies that can often be used instead of—or in conjunction with—medications. Consult a doctor before trying any of these, especially if you are pregnant, planning surgery or taking other medications.

●**Quercetin.** This supplement is a *bioflavonoid*—the component in fruits and vegetables that gives them their vibrant color. It has natural antihistamine and anti-inflammatory effects.

Typical dosage: Start taking quercetin when spring weather begins, and continue through the end of June. Take 300 milligrams (mg) twice a day for one week. If that doesn't work, increase to 600 mg.

If you also suffer from fall allergies, begin again in mid-August and continue through the first frost. In hot climates, you may need to take quercetin year-round.

●**Stinging nettle.** Like quercetin, this plant extract is an excellent antihistamine and anti-inflammatory. It can be used in conjunction with quercetin or on its own.

Typical dosage: 400 mg twice a day during allergy season.

On-the-spot treatment: If you find yourself in the throes of an allergy attack despite taking quercetin and/or stinging nettle regularly, take an extra dose. I tell my patients to reach for these remedies whenever they would take an antihistamine.

Most allergy sufferers find quercetin and/or stinging nettle highly effective. But if they don't work for you, one of the following natural antihistamines and anti-inflammatories may help—either in conjunction with each other or alone. Try them in this order—but, of course, talk with your doctor first.

●**Vitamin C.** Take 1,000 mg once or twice a day during allergy season. This should be reduced or eliminated during the off-season. Recent studies suggest vitamin C in high doses may cause thickening of arteries and interfere with certain cancer therapy. Caution is advised for patients with these conditions.

●**Pycnogenol,** an antioxidant derived from the bark of pine trees. Take 50 mg twice a day.

●**Ginkgo biloba.** Take 60 mg twice a day. Once symptoms subside, stop taking this herb. Used in excess (more than 200 mg per day), it can cause diarrhea or sleeplessness.

Caution: People using blood thinners should avoid ginkgo biloba.

• **Feverfew.** Buy a product standardized to contain at least 0.7% *parthenolide*. That is the component of this herb that reduces swelling in the sinuses. Take 500 mg two or three times a day.

MORE ALLERGY DEFENSES

• **Rinse pollen out of your nasal passages before bedtime.** Use a saline nasal spray, or make your own nasal wash by dissolving one-half teaspoon of salt in one-half cup of water. Place a few drops of the solution in your nose with a dropper, then blow your nose.

• **Keep home and car windows closed—** to keep pollen outdoors. Run an air conditioner continuously to filter air and fight allergy-causing molds.

• **Run a HEPA filter all the time during allergy season—**to purify your air of pollen and other allergens. A HEPA vacuum cleaner may also help.

• **Shampoo your hair, eyebrows, eyelashes, mustache and beard** at bedtime and after outdoor activities. Dust mites and other allergens cling to hairs. Change clothes when you come inside.

• **Strengthen your immune system.** Better overall health means reduced allergy symptoms. Take a daily multivitamin/mineral supplement…eat healthfully…get adequate rest…exercise regularly…and don't smoke.

Natural Remedies for Pain Relief

Jamison Starbuck, ND, a naturopathic physician in family practice and a lecturer at the University of Montana, both in Missoula. She is past president of the American Association of Naturopathic Physicians and a contributing editor of The Alternative Advisor: The Complete Guide to Natural Therapies and Alternative Treatments. Time-Life.

For many people, reaching for pain relievers is as instinctual as eating. Hungry? Go to the refrigerator and grab a bite. Pain? Swallow a pill. But pain pills have their costs.

Acetaminophen (Tylenol, Panadol, etc.) can cause liver damage. Nonsteroidal anti-inflammatory drugs (NSAIDs), such as *naproxen* (Aleve) and *ibuprofen* (Advil, Motrin, etc.), can cause gastrointestinal bleeding and impaired kidney function. They can also inhibit cartilage repair in the knees, hips and other joints. In addition to being addictive, Lortab, Percocet and other narcotic painkillers can cause drowsiness and clouded thinking. The muscle relaxant *cyclobenzaprine* (Flexeril) has been linked with dizziness, rash, arrhythmia and even convulsions.

In certain cases, the risks posed by these adverse reactions are offset by clear benefits. When pain is especially severe, nothing can replace the merciful relief of medication. But for run-of-the-mill discomfort—tension headache, ankle sprain, joint stiffness, back pain and postsurgical pain—it's often better to skip drugs and opt instead for natural treatments.

Ice may seem old-fashioned, but it remains one of the best natural painkillers. It's great for back pain, aching, swollen joints and headache. It reduces congestion, improves blood flow and promotes healing. A bag of frozen peas works as well as an ice pack, and it can be refrozen and reused many times. Usually a 10-minute application, two or three times each hour, is effective.

If headaches are your problem, drinking lots of water is often all that's needed. In particular, tension headaches and "toxic" headaches from drinking too much alcohol or consuming too much caffeine respond well to "hydrotherapy." Have eight ounces of water every 10 minutes for one hour. Make sure a bathroom is handy before starting this remedy!

For acute sprains, strains and scrapes, bruises and other minor trauma, nothing beats *arnica*. This homeopathic remedy—available in health food stores and now many drugstores—reduces bruising and pain. Unless you are accident-prone, a single vial costing less than $10 should last several years. I recommend arnica in 30C potency—typically two pellets one to three times daily, for up to seven days.

For tendinitis and sciatica—and to speed recovery from surgery—I often recommend *bromelain*. This natural anti-inflammatory agent—an enzyme derived from pineapple—stimulates the breakdown of inflammatory compounds at the injury site. Bromelain is available in capsules at health-food stores and pharmacies. The typical dosage is 250 mg one to four times daily. Bromelain is off-limits for people with high blood pressure.

Boswellia serrata (frankincense) has a long tradition as an arthritis treatment in India and the Middle East. Though human studies on this herb are inadequate, the clinical experience of many practitioners—myself included—has been extremely promising. I routinely recommend Boswellia as a substitute for NSAIDs in cases involving back pain, arthritis, inflammatory joint pain and acute muscle and bone injuries. Even with long-term use, Boswellia does not seem to cause the gastrointestinal bleeding and pain that can be a problem with NSAID use.

Boswellia can be found in health food stores. Look for Boswellia alone, or combined with ginger and turmeric, two additional herbal pain relievers that are easy on the stomach. The typical dose is 300 mg of Boswellia, three times a day, as needed for pain.

Good Things About Ginkgo Biloba

The late Varro Tyler, PhD, ScD, former dean emeritus, Purdue School of Pharmacy, Purdue University, West Lafayette, IN.

Ginkgo biloba has long been known as a natural memory booster. But this herbal remedy is also effective against dizziness... ringing in the ears (*tinnitus*)...and the on-again, off-again leg pain called *intermittent claudication*. Each of these ailments can be caused by sluggish circulation.

How ginkgo works: It helps lower abnormally high levels of platelet activating factor (PAF), a natural body compound that promotes blood clotting, thus inhibiting circulation.

Ginkgo Biloba Trap

Marc Rosenblatt, MD, assistant professor of ophthalmology, Mount Sinai Hospital, New York City.

A 70-year-old man who had been taking 40 milligrams (mg) of the herb *ginkgo biloba* twice a day began experiencing blurred vision.

When doctors examined him, they found blood oozing down the iris of his eye.

Diagnosis: The bleeding was caused by the combination of *ginkgolide B*, a powerful blood thinner found in ginkgo, and aspirin, another drug with blood-thinning properties. The man was taking both.

Self-defense: Do not take ginkgo with another blood thinner unless your doctor says it's okay. Avoid ginkgo if you have a bleeding disorder.

Lavender and Insomnia

Alan Hirsch, MD, founder and neurological director, the Smell & Taste Treatment and Research Foundation, Chicago.

Lavender oil is a safe and effective remedy for insomnia sufferers.

What to do: Place several drops of essential oil of lavender on a cloth and leave it on your nightstand, or fill an electric diffuser with oil to disperse fragrance throughout the room... grow your own lavender and keep a basket of flowers at your bedside...or make an herbal pillow filled with these leaves (fill with fresh leaves every three weeks).

23

Health Care Smarts

Why Personal Medical Research Is So Important

Fred D. Baldwin, PhD

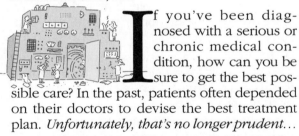

If you've been diagnosed with a serious or chronic medical condition, how can you be sure to get the best possible care? In the past, patients often depended on their doctors to devise the best treatment plan. *Unfortunately, that's no longer prudent...*

● **Medical knowledge is changing so rapidly** that few doctors can keep up. Each month, several hundred articles are published in medical journals—about cardiology alone.

● **Your doctor may be biased toward certain treatments** because of his/her training. Surgeons tend to favor surgery. Internists tend to recommend pills.

● **Your doctor may decide not to recommend a costly therapy** because of cost-cutting pressure from an HMO.

The truth is that you may never find out about a treatment that could cure you unless you do your own medical research.

Example I: A woman with a brain tumor was told by her doctor that her only option was surgery, which could leave her partially paralyzed. She contacted a support group and learned of a noninvasive alternative called the "gamma knife," a form of radiation therapy. Five years later, she's completely healthy.

Example II: Doctors told a woman with non-Hodgkin's lymphoma that her chances of survival were slim. Then her mother read about clinical trials of an extra-high-dosage form of chemotherapy known as *CHOP*. The woman has now been symptom-free for more than a year. Doctors say her prospects are excellent.

RESEARCH SERVICES

If you're low on time or energy—and don't mind paying for medical information—consider using a research service. For a fee of $150 to

Fred D. Baldwin, PhD, a Carlisle, PA, medical writer and coauthor, with Suzanne McInerney, of *Info-medicine: A Consumer's Guide to the Latest Medical Research*. Little, Brown.

439

$400, such services will scan huge medical databases and assemble a bound report containing copies of relevant articles.

Reputable research services include...

• **The Health Resource**, 933 Faulkner, Conway, AR 72034. 800-949-0090, *www.thehealth resource.com.*

• **Institute for Health & Healing Library**, California Pacific Medical Center, 2040 Webster St., San Francisco 94115. 415-600-3681.

• **Schine On-Line Services, Inc.,** 39 Brenton Ave., Providence, RI 02906. *www.findcure.com.*

DOING YOUR OWN RESEARCH

People are usually happy with the reports they obtain from these services. But by paying someone else to find out about their disease, they're missing out on self-education—a process many people find empowering.

Patients find that actively doing their own research helps allay their anxiety, making them feel hopeful instead of hopeless and helpless.

Good news: Doing sophisticated medical research has become easier than ever before. If you own a computer with a modem, you can do much of your work from home.

If you don't own a computer, see if you can use one at your local public or medical school library. To find a medical library near you, call the National Library of Medicine (NLM) at 888-346-3656, *www.nlm.nih.gov.*

• **Read about your ailment in consumer health guides.** Look it up in *Mayo Clinic Family Health Book* (Collins)...*The American Medical Association's Family Medical Guide* (Wiley)...and *The Merck Manual* (Merck Publishing Co.).

If you have trouble deciphering medical terminology, pick up a copy of *Mosby's Medical Dictionary* (Mosby).

• **Search out top specialists.** If you have a serious ailment, odds are your family doctor will urge you to see at least one specialist. But many doctors are obligated to refer you to a specialist whose name is on a list provided by an insurance company. This might not be the most highly skilled specialist.

Self-defense: Ask your doctor, "If this were your problem, whom would *you* consult?" As you contact the various experts, ask them the same question.

• **Put powerful databases to work for you.** Hundreds of health-oriented databases have been compiled by research facilities and libraries around the country.

The best is the online medical database provided by the NLM at *www.nlm.nih.gov.*

Medline contains references and abstracts from 4,600 medical journals.

Also on the NLM Web site, you'll find MedlinePlus for information on hundreds of diseases, conditions and wellness issues. Drug information, online medical dictionaries, a medical encyclopedia and links to other government health resources are available.

You can also do a search using *Index Medicus.* This vast *printed* index lists the same journal articles as Medline. It's available at most medical libraries.

• **Focus on the latest research.** Pay special attention to *review* articles. These summarize state-of-the-art treatments. They give a great overview and are usually written by top experts.

Note where these experts are, and contact them. If you have trouble getting through on your own, ask your doctor to arrange a consultation for you.

If you're using a print source like *Index Medicus,* look for articles whose titles contain the words "Current Trends," "Current Status" or "Review."

• **Look into clinical trials.** The National Institutes of Health (NIH) acts as a clearinghouse for information on clinical trials being conducted at research facilities around the country.

Their Web site, *www.clinicaltrials.gov,* provides information about government funded as well as privately funded clinical trials.

To find out about cancer trials, contact the National Cancer Institute at 800-422-6237. To find out about AIDS trials, contact the US Department of Health & Human Services at 800-874-2572, *www.hhs.gov.*

●**Look into alternative treatments.** A good place to start is Dr. Marc Micozzi's *Fundamentals of Complementary and Alternative Medicine* (Churchill Livingstone).

You can also contact the NIH National Center for Complementary and Alternative Medicine Clearinghouse (888-644-6226, *http://nccam. nih.gov*) to learn about alternative approaches for your ailment.

If you have computer access, check out alternative medicine resources at *www.healthfinder. gov* or *www.altmedicine.com*.

Beware: Some organizations listed on the Web are fronts for companies that sell rather dubious nutritional supplements.

●**Seek out others who have had your ailment.** They can be found via online discussion groups. Also, check out Medical Matrix at *www.medmatrix.org*. It lists medically oriented "newsgroups" on the Internet.

To find a support group: Contact the National Organization for Rare Disorders (800-999-6673, *www.rarediseases.org*). Or—consult *The Self-Help Sourcebook* (St. Clare's Health Services).

Making Sense of Medical News

Timothy McCall, MD, an internist, medical editor of *Yoga Journal* and author of *Examining Your Doctor: A Patient's Guide to Avoiding Harmful Medical Care*. Carol. *www.drmccall.com*.

Look beyond headlines. Media reports often exaggerate the importance of individual studies.

●**Consider the source.** Worry about ulterior motives if the study was sponsored by a pharmaceutical manufacturer or an industry association.

●**Were animals or humans studied?** Results from animal studies can't always be correlated to humans.

●**How many subjects were studied?** Too few means that the results are less likely to be valid.

●**Were the subjects like you?** A study of elderly men may mean little to you if you're a 35-year-old woman.

●**Don't overinterpret results.** Just because a study finds that garlic helps protect against some cancers, doesn't mean garlic is a cancer cure.

●**Don't change your lifestyle based on a single news report.** Stay with tried-and-true advice, such as sticking to a balanced, low-fat, high-fiber diet.

The Terrible Truth About Medical Misinformation

John Allen Paulos, PhD, professor of mathematics at Temple University, Philadelphia. Dr. Paulos is author of *A Mathematician Reads the Newspaper*. Anchor.

It seems you can't open a newspaper or turn on the TV these days without a dose of medical information—the latest risk to health, the newest treatment breakthrough, etc.

Unfortunately, much of what we read and see is grossly misleading. That can cause needless worry—or give needless reassurance. It can also lead us to adopt unsound health practices.

To guard against medical misinformation, keep in mind some basic facts about science, reporting and human nature...

SCIENCE VERSUS JOURNALISM

Scientific knowledge progresses *slowly* and *tentatively*. Most new studies add only a small piece to a very large puzzle.

On the other hand, reporters get paid for being dramatic. Pressure to produce an exciting story leads them to make studies sound more conclusive than they actually are. And bad news is inherently more compelling than good news.

Example: Finnish researchers found a higher rate of lung cancer among smokers who took beta-carotene supplements. Because many other studies have suggested that beta-carotene helps prevent cancer, this made for some pretty frightening headlines.

But the study wasn't all it was cracked up to be. The people in the study had been smoking heavily for an average of 36 years...and they continued to smoke during the six years of the study. Their experience was not necessarily applicable to others.

The researchers themselves conceded that the slight increase in cancer they found could have been simply the result of chance. That fact was ignored in most media reports.

READING BEYOND THE HEADLINES

Newspaper headlines are designed to grab the attention of readers. TV spotlights sensational sound bites and eye-popping visuals. But in science, the truth usually lies in the details—which are presented later, if at all.

Our emotions affect our interpretation of information presented to us. Once we see a picture of a child who is bedridden with leukemia, we're unlikely to pay much attention to how or why he/she got there.

Remedy: Recognize your tendency to jump to conclusions. Read the whole story. As you do, ask yourself the same questions a good journalist would ask—who, what, where, when, why, how and how likely.

If details are lacking, don't make any judgment until you get all the facts.

WHAT DO THE NUMBERS MEAN?

Statistics lend an air of authority to any health-related story. But what do the numbers refer to? Where did they come from? Reporters often ignore these all-important questions.

Example: It has been widely reported that condoms have a "16% failure rate." The figure came from a 1990 survey in which people were asked whether their birth control method had ever failed. Though 16 in 100 condom users surveyed said that condoms had failed, that does not mean that condoms fail 16% of the time.

Be especially wary of surveys in which people "self-report" complex information. People don't always tell the whole truth.

WHAT'S THE REAL RISK?

To judge by the media, virtually everything puts us at risk of some dread disease.

First question to ask: Just how big is the risk? We tend to overreact to threatening, unfamiliar things, particularly when they lie outside our control.

Try to look at risk-related statistics rationally, not emotionally.

Example I: Illicit drugs can indeed be deadly. But even the scourge of heroin (6,000 deaths a year) and cocaine (8,000 deaths) pale in comparison to the toll taken by tobacco (400,000 deaths) and alcohol (90,000 deaths).

Example II: To sound dramatic, a reporter might emphasize that 2,500 people die each year from a particular disease...and drive home the point with heart-wrenching interviews with their families.

But 2,500 deaths out of the total US population is not very significant.

Example III: Most of us have heard that "one woman in eight will develop breast cancer." But this figure is for *lifetime incidence*. It fails to take into account the fact that a woman's risk rises with age. It also assumes that all women will live at least to age 85.

In fact, fewer than one 20-year-old woman in 200 will develop breast cancer by the time she reaches age 40...and only one 40-year-old in 25 will develop breast cancer by age 60.

The reported rise in breast cancer risk sounds even less terrifying when you consider that much of the rise can be attributed to widespread screening, which has brought more cases to light...and that our ever-lengthening life spans are enabling more women to reach the age at which the disease usually strikes.

Bottom line: News reports often omit the context that gives meaning to statistics.

RESPECT THE POWER OF CHANCE

Ten people with advanced cancer receive a drug and have a dramatic remission? It *might* have been the drug...or they might have gotten better anyway.

When evaluating medical news, look for *statistical significance*. Statistically significant results are those that cannot be attributed to random chance.

The smaller the sample size (the number of people, animals, etc., participating in the study), the more likely that a dramatic result was due to chance.

When two things happen together, don't assume that one *causes* the other. A question that news reports often ignore is whether confounding variables may be responsible.

Example: A study found that people who drink wine have fewer heart attacks than those who drink beer or hard liquor. Does wine have a magic ingredient? Or is there another explanation?

One explanation researchers mentioned (but news summaries didn't) is that wine drinkers tend to be more educated and affluent than beer and whiskey drinkers. It's well known that wealth and education go hand in hand with greater health and longevity.

This is one reason why double-blind, controlled studies are more convincing than others.

In such studies, two matched groups are compared. One group receives a drug, for example, the other doesn't...and neither the experimenters nor the experimental subjects know which group is which. This makes it more likely that observed effects are due to the drug and not other factors.

On the other hand, be skeptical of anecdotal reports. Anyone can select a striking story. With no basis for comparison, however, even the most vivid event is meaningless.

Example: When a talk show guest blamed his wife's fatal brain cancer on her cellular phone, this caused panic among cellular phone users—and even sparked a decline in cellular phone stocks.

But about 10 million people now use cellular phones, and the overall brain cancer rate in this country remains at six per 100,000. By chance alone, you'd expect 600 phone users to develop the disease each year. Far fewer cases have been reported.

LOOK TO THE SOURCE

Any study appearing in a scientific journal like the *The New England Journal of Medicine,* the *Journal of the American Medical Association* or *The Lancet* has undergone a rigorous quality-control process known as peer-review.

Peer review means that experts in the field have judged the study to be of sufficient quality and importance to merit publication. An unpublished finding reported on TV has not been subjected to peer review—and is therefore less credible.

While "expert" commentary isn't foolproof, it's more reliable than a reporter's interpretation.

Of course, if you really want the details, you'll need to read the original journal article.

How Does Your HMO Stack Up?

The National Committee for Quality Assurance (NCQA) rates and accredits health-maintenance organizations.

Rated: The quality of an HMO's medical treatment...physicians' qualifications...preventive health services...medical record-keeping... the appropriateness of care...patients' rights.

While evaluations are paid for by participating HMOs, one in eight tested so far has received a failed rating. *www.ncqa.org.*

Picking an HMO

Susan Pisano, vice-president, communications, America's Health Insurance Plans, 601 Pennsylvania Ave., NW, Ste. 500, Washington, DC 20004.

Before enrolling in a health-maintenance organization, put these questions to the HMO representative...

●**Are there participating doctors near where I work or live?**

●**Where can I go for care at night or on weekends?**

●**Does the plan offer a choice of doctors?**

●**What percentage of participating doctors are board-certified?**

●**Does the member services department have useful information** about participating doctors?

Ask the HMO for references. Ask friends and family members about their experiences with HMOs, too.

The Value of Lab Tests

Marc Silverstein, MD, director, Center for Health Care Research, Medical University of South Carolina, Charleston. His study of lab tests in 531 patients, average age 63, was published in *The American Journal of Medicine,* 360 Park Ave. S., New York City 10010.

Routine lab tests are of little value for apparently healthy individuals. Many doctors order urinalysis, complete blood count, thyroid studies and blood chemistry as part of physical exams. But besides being costly, these four tests are unlikely to uncover a health problem in such individuals. If your doctor recommends the four tests as part of a routine physical exam, ask him/her to explain the health benefits of the information derived from these tests...and how the results will change his recommendations.

Avoiding Anxiety During an MRI

Helen Wahba, RN, staff nurse, department of radiology, MetroHealth Medical Center, Cleveland.

One in 10 people scheduled to undergo magnetic resonance imaging (MRI) find it impossible to do so.

Reason: Claustrophobia. MRI scanning involves lying down for 25 to 60 minutes in a very narrow tunnel for a very noisy exam.

Here's how to make the process much more bearable...

●**Ask your doctor to explain MRI testing procedures** well before your scheduled test. Pamphlets are provided by most scanning sites.

●**Have a family member or friend stay in the room with you during the scan.** If possible, ask this person to hold your ankle during the exam.

●**Make sure you are in a comfortable position before the exam begins.** A pillow under the knees reduces the strain on your back.

●**Keep your eyes closed throughout the procedure.** Drape a cloth over your eyes...

Editor's note: Less-confining "open" MRI machines are now available, but they may produce less-detailed images.

and imagine sitting on a beach or in your favorite chair at home.

●**Ask that the air conditioning be turned up.** That way, you can avoid the "closed-in" feeling of a too-warm room.

●**Wear prism eyeglasses.** These glasses let you see out of the tunnel while you're lying on your back. Ask loved ones to sit at the end of the tunnel so you can see them.

Ulcer Testing

A. Mark Fendrick, MD, professor of internal medicine, University of Michigan School of Public Health and School of Medicine, Ann Arbor.

Delay invasive tests for ulcers until you have tried drug therapy. Research shows that nearly all people with ulcers are infected with bacteria that are associated with ulcer recurrence. Medical guidelines now recommend using antibiotics to kill the bacteria.

Trap: Doctors may routinely order an initial uncomfortable endoscopy for patients suspected of having ulcers. *Better:* Have a blood test done to detect the antibodies. Consider antibiotic therapy if the test is positive. Have an endoscopy only if symptoms fail to disappear.

Genetic Testing Can Save Your Life...or Ruin It

Ellen Matloff, MS, a genetic counselor at the Yale Cancer Center in New Haven, CT. She specializes in counseling patients at high risk for certain forms of cancer.

Over the past 20 years, hundreds of diseases have been linked to mutations in certain genes. A growing number of these mutant genes can now be detected via a simple blood test.

How much influence does your genetic makeup have over your health? What can you do if a hereditary ailment runs in your family? Who should undergo genetic testing?

For the answers to these and other questions, we spoke with Yale genetic counselor Ellen Matloff...

●**To what extent is illness determined by "bad" genes?** We shouldn't really call these genes "bad." We all have genetic mutations. Each of us is probably predisposed to at least one disease—whether it's cancer, heart disease, high cholesterol or a blood disorder.

Having a mutation that has been linked to a specific illness doesn't *guarantee* that you'll develop that illness. It just means you're at high risk.

In many cases, you can minimize the risk by adopting a healthy lifestyle...and by keeping an especially close watch on your health.

With some genetic defects, including those causing certain types of thyroid and colon cancer, risk of developing the disease in question can be close to 100%. That means anyone with the mutant gene who lives to age 85 is almost certain to develop the cancer unless the organ is removed—no matter what other preventive measures are taken.

With other mutant genes, the risk is less certain. If you have one of the recently identified genes linked to breast cancer, for example, you have an 85% chance of getting breast cancer by age 85. The general population of women face a 10% risk of breast cancer.

These mutations are also associated with a 50% to 60% lifetime risk of ovarian cancer (versus a 1% lifetime risk for the general population).

●**For which diseases is genetic testing available?** Testing is now available for literally hundreds of diseases, including some hereditary forms of cancer of the breast and colon. That number is growing every year.

●**Who should undergo genetic testing?** For mutations associated with Huntington disease, muscular dystrophy and other *rare* illnesses, genetic testing is appropriate if the individual has already begun to show symptoms of the illness...or if he has a family history of the disease. The test results help the doctor confirm a suspected diagnosis.

Presymptomatic testing: Available for some forms of hereditary breast, ovarian, colon, thyroid and skin cancer—is appropriate only if...

●**One or more close family members** (parent, sibling, grandparent, aunt or uncle) has had the cancer in question.

●**A close family member had the cancer at an early age.** For breast cancer, early is considered to be age 40 or younger. Or, if the family member had the cancer more than once—in both breasts, for example. Consult your doctor.

●**What's involved in genetic testing?** Typically, a sample of blood or skin (cells scraped from the inside of the cheek) is required for testing.

The sample may be tested at the hospital—or sent out to an independent lab. Results are available within one to three months. Be sure to find a hospital that offers genetic counseling services along with testing. To find one, contact the National Society of Genetic Counselors (312-321-6834, *www.nsgc.org*) or the information desk of your local hospital.

●**What if I test positive?** For some diseases, there's nothing you can do to alter your fate. Take Huntington's disease. Even if you find out that you have the mutation linked to this fatal neurological disease, there's no way to prevent the nerve degeneration or slow its progress.

In such cases, one benefit to screening is the *elimination of uncertainty.*

Someone who tests positive for the gene for Huntington's might opt not to have children—for fear of passing on the mutation to them...or of being too ill to raise them.

Another person might choose to begin his family at a younger age, to use donor sperm or eggs or to do prenatal testing.

That person can now make meaningful plans for the future—make out a will, settle finances, even choose a nursing home. This may also be a time to consider spending more time with friends and family and to enjoy life to the fullest.

Many people find the reduced uncertainty to be positive—even if the news is bad.

With cancer-related mutations, the outlook is more positive.

Say you test positive for a mutation linked to breast or ovarian cancer. Your doctor may recommend that you have a mammogram or ultrasound scan more frequently than is ordinarily recommended. That way, you'll be able to detect any tumor at its earliest possible stage.

If you have the gene for colon cancer, you might have colonoscopies more frequently.

A more aggressive approach would be to take out the organ before it develops disease.

If you have your thyroid removed and take thyroid supplements, for example, your risk of thyroid cancer is almost zero.

A woman with a family history of breast cancer might opt to have her breasts removed. This approach, known as "prophylactic mastectomy," is an extreme step. But it can be a lifesaving decision.

Knowing you're at risk for a certain ailment can motivate you to stick to a healthy lifestyle —eating a low-fat, high-fiber diet, avoiding smoking, etc.

●**How should I go about deciding whether or not to get tested?** Discuss testing with a genetic counselor, your doctor—and your entire family. Consider what would happen if you were to test positive—or negative. Take time to think this over.

Many individuals who initially clamor to be tested ultimately decide not to—once they realize just what's involved.

In most cases, we recommend waiting until at least age 18 before getting tested for adult-onset disorders. Children should be tested only if there's a family history of a treatable childhood disease.

Easily Overlooked Medical Deductions

Nadine Gordon Lee, tax partner, Ernst & Young, LLP, 5 Times Sq., New York 10036.

Use this list as a reminder of some medical deductions you can easily overlook when you prepare your tax return…*

●**Alcoholism and drug abuse treatment.**

●**Contact lenses.**

*These expenses are deductible only to the extent that their total exceeds 7.5% of Adjusted Gross Income.

●**Contraceptives**, if they are bought with a prescription.

●**Hearing devices.**

●**Hospital services fees** (laboratory work, therapy, nursing services, and surgery).

●**Impairment-related work expenses** for a disabled individual.

●**Lead paint removal.**

●**Medical transportation**, including the standard mileage deduction.

●**Orthopedic shoes.**

●**Seeing-eye dog.**

●**Special equipment for the disabled.**

●**Special diet foods** prescribed by a physician and taken in addition to your normal diet.

●**Special schools for a handicapped child.**

●**Tuition fees** charged by a school for medical care.

●**Wigs** essential to mental health.

Refund Break for the Ill

Nicholas T. Scott, CA-9, No. 94-15321.

The statute of limitations for filing a return is temporarily suspended during a period when a person is incapacitated and unable to file a return. So when alcoholism rendered a person incapable of filing a return, the statute of limitations was *extended* and he could later file for a refund after the date on which the refund deadline normally would have expired.

Health Benefits Alert

Study by the Institute for Clinical Outcomes, 699 E. South Temple, Ste. 100, Salt Lake City 84102.

Be wary of insurance plans that severely limit the list of drugs for which they will reimburse you.

Reason: Forcing doctors to use a second-choice medication often leads to longer recovery times and may increase the cost of treating a particular illness.

Prostate Cancer Fact

American Institute for Cancer Research, Washington, DC.

About 90% of men who are diagnosed with prostate cancer before it has spread beyond the prostate gland—and who are then treated surgically—can expect to live at least another 15 years.

Cancer-Prevention Checklist

Hugh Shingleton, MD, former national vice president for cancer detection and treatment, American Cancer Society, 1599 Clifton Rd., Atlanta 30329.

• **Colorectal.** Men and women age 50 and older should have a sigmoidoscopy every three to five years and a fecal occult blood test every year.

• **Rectal/prostate.** Men and women age 40 and older should have a digital rectal exam every year, and men age 50 and older should have a prostate-specific antigen (PSA) test every year.

• **Cervical.** Women age 18 and older (or whenever sexual activity begins) should have a Pap test every year until age 39.

Exception for women 18-39: After three or more consecutive annual Pap tests with normal findings, the test may be done less often at the doctor's discretion.

Women age 40 and older should have a Pap test every year.

• **Uterine/ovarian.** Women between age 18 and 39 should follow the above recommendations for a Pap test. Women age 40 and older should have a pelvic exam every year.

• **Breast.** Women age 20 and older should self-examine their breasts at least once every month. Women between age 20 and 39 should have a manual clinical examination by a health professional every three years and a clinical exam every year once they reach age 40. Women between age 40 and 49 should have a mammogram every one to two years and every year once they reach age 50.

• **Other.** Both men and women between age 20 and 39 should receive health counseling and a cancer checkup every three years, and every year once they reach age 40.

Cellular Phones and Cancer Risk

Kenneth J. Rothman, DrPH, professor of epidemiology, Boston University Medical Center.

In a study of 250,000 cellular phone users, there was no increase in overall mortality. The study included "flip phones," which have antennas that must be held close to the head. It did *not* specifically address the question of whether these phones cause cancer.

You Can Catch Up On Sleep

Allan I. Pack, MD, PhD, director, Center for Sleep and Respiratory Neurobiology at the University of Pennsylvania, Philadelphia.

Recovery sleep need not be hour-for-hour, because sleep-deprived people go into deeper sleep more quickly and may need less recovery sleep than the sleep they lost.

Best Ways to Protect Your Lower Back

Natural Medicine for Back Pain: The Best Alternative Methods for Banishing Backache by Glenn S. Rothfeld, MD, founder and medical director of Whole Health New England in Arlington, MA. Rodale Press.

Anyone who sits for long periods of time each day is at high risk for developing lower back pain.

To reduce the risk: Cross your legs at the ankles, not the knees...stand up and walk around at least once every half hour.

Important: Your office chair should have a straight back...armrests...enough width and depth for you to move around...a back bulge that curves into the small of your back...seat padding that does not give more than half an inch.

If you do overstress your back and experience pain, apply cold as soon as possible. Continue the cold treatment periodically for one or two days.

Reason: Cooling the back helps prevent minute tears in the muscles from bleeding and reduces painful fluid accumulation.

After one or two days, switch over to heat treatments—two or three times a day, for 15 minutes at a time. This relaxes the muscles and reduces the pain. Moist heat—a hot water bottle wrapped in a wet towel—is better than dry heat from a heating pad.

Back Injury Study

Ann Myers, ScD, former faculty member, health policy and management, Johns Hopkins School of Public Health, Baltimore, and leader of a study of 600 city employees.

A study found that back injuries are twice as common among workers who have little control over their jobs as they are among workers who have a greater say in how they do the same kind of work.

The Benefits of Allergy Shots

Peter Creticos, MD, associate professor of medicine, Johns Hopkins University School of Medicine, Baltimore. His three-year study of 77 patients was published in *The New England Journal of Medicine*, 10 Shattuck St., Boston 02115.

Asthma attacks caused by exposure to pollen respond better to allergy shots than to oral allergy medication. The shots have long been used to control sneezing, runny nose and other *nonrespiratory* symptoms of ragweed allergic rhinitis (hay fever). But it's been unclear whether these shots are helpful to patients with ragweed-induced asthma.

Finding: Patients treated with allergy shots needed less medication, could breathe easier and were less sensitive to ragweed.

How to Tell if You Are Allergic to Nickel

James Marks, MD, chair of dermatology, Pennsylvania State University College of Medicine, Hershey.

Nickel is often overlooked as a cause of allergic reactions. The silver-white metal is found in everything from pierced earrings and keys to tools, zippers and, of course, nickel coins.

Symptom: An itchy, crusty and blistery rash.

Helpful test: Tape a nickel to your skin on a hot day. If your skin turns red, consult a dermatologist.

Lyme Disease Update

Charlene C. DeMarco, DO, a tick-borne disease specialist in private practice in Egg Harbor, NJ. Her study of 89 patients with late-stage Lyme disease was presented at the International Conference on Macrolides in Lisbon, Portugal.

Lyme disease responds well to the antibiotic *clarithromycin*. Of 28 patients who took 250 mg twice daily, 20 had moderate relief of the arthritis that's characteristic of the late stages of Lyme. Results were less dramatic in those who got once-a-day medication. Other antibiotics for late-stage Lyme disease must be injected. Late-stage Lyme disease occurs within 24 months of being bitten by an infected tick.

Lyme Disease Self-Defense

Allen C. Steere, MD, director of clinical research in rheumatology and immunology, Massachusetts General Hospital, Boston.

Remove the tick and save it in a vial…label the container with the date and location where you were likely to have been bitten…at the first signs of infection—rash, joint pain, fever, other flulike symptoms—take the tick to your doctor.

Reason: Knowing what kind of tick bit you helps the physician with diagnosis and treatment. It is not generally of value to analyze the tick itself for infectious agents.

Illness Can Be Good for You

Randolph M. Nesse, MD, professor of psychiatry, University of Michigan Medical School, Ann Arbor, and author of *Why We Get Sick: The New Science of Darwinian Medicine*. Vintage.

Some disease symptoms show that the body's natural defenses are working properly. Nausea and vomiting remove potentially fatal toxins from the body. Fever is a defense against infection. Coughing also removes toxins. Disease and health are more closely related than most people realize. The human body repairs damage by having cells divide—but the same mechanism gone awry can lead to cancer.

To Avoid Spreading Cold Sores…

Rodney Basler, MD, assistant professor of internal medicine and dermatology, University of Nebraska Medical Center, Lincoln.

Always use sunscreen on your lips when outdoors…keep blisters clean and dry…coat them with petroleum jelly or a similar substance to prevent cracking…do not share cups, straws, toothbrushes or towels during an outbreak. For people with frequent outbreaks, ask your doctor about taking low doses of the antiviral drug *acyclovir* to prevent outbreaks or lessen their severity. The medicine is sold by prescription under the name *Zovirax*.

Hooray!! Lower Cost Prescription Drugs

Charles B. Inlander, a consumer advocate and health-care consultant based in Fogelsville, PA. He was founding president of the nonprofit People's Medical Society, a consumer health advocacy group in Allentown, PA. He is author of numerous books, including *Take This Book to the Hospital With You*. St. Martin's.

To save money on medications that your doctor prescribes, you can…

- **Buy generics**—they can cost 70% less than virtually identical name brands.

- **Buy in bulk**—ask for a six-month prescription instead of a one-month supply that's renewable five times.

- **Play it safe with new medicines** by buying just a one-week supply until you find out about any possible side effects.

- **Shop around**—different drugstores price the same medicine differently.

• **Use mail order**—check with your employer or other services to find a good place to send for mail-order prescription drugs. Ordering through the mail will generally get you the lowest prices.

Help for Ex-Ex-Smokers

John Hughes, MD, professor, department of psychiatry, University of Vermont, Burlington.

Quitting smoking takes most smokers five or six tries. Very few people quit for good after the first time...but too many get discouraged when they can't quit and then don't try again.

Bottom line: Don't stop trying to quit smoking. Eventually you will be successful.

Heavy Smokers and the Nicotine Patch

Study of 522 smokers by Jorn Olsen, MD, PhD, University of Aarhus, Denmark, published in the *American Journal of Epidemiology,* 111 Market Pl., Ste. 840, Baltimore 21202.

Heavy smokers using nicotine patches to kick the cigarette habit should start out with the highest-strength patches and gradually taper off.

Reason: If the initial dose doesn't deliver enough nicotine, smokers may quickly stop the treatment. Over-the-counter patches currently available deliver from 21 milligrams (mg) to 7 mg of nicotine a day.

Cost: About $30 for one week's worth of patches.

24

Emotional Health Means a Happier You

How Your Emotions Affect Your Health... Proven Ways to Stay Well

John W. Travis, MD, and Regina Sara Ryan
Wellness Associates

The flood of news about health and fitness these days can be more confusing than helpful. If you've been exercising or eating "right" for years but still feel frustrated and unfulfilled, you are not alone.

There are ways to take charge of your health by tapping your inner resources effectively. The changes that we support are simple and are designed to increase self-awareness, since all aspects of life are interdependent.

Example: When you're worried about something, you're also likely to have an upset stomach.

What may appear to be individual events are really interconnected aspects of a larger, more complex system.

When you master small changes, you build a fortified base from which to take further steps on your healing journey toward wellness.

Although many people associate wellness only with fitness, nutrition or stress reduction, wellness is really much more. Wellness brings people into a domain of self-responsibility and self-empowerment.

SET GOALS FOR WELLNESS

Goals keep you on course. And more than that, goals are like magnets—they tend to attract people and resources that help get them accomplished. It's almost magical how this happens.

Often people set their sights too high and then quit completely when they don't make the grade. Approach these "impossible" goals by breaking them down into manageable parts.

BREATHING REDUCES STRESS

Stress is inevitable—you need it to warn you about the negative forces of life. But there are

John W. Travis, MD, and Regina Sara Ryan, coauthors of *Wellness: Small Changes You Can Use to Make a Big Difference.* Ten Speed Press. Dr. Travis is founder and codirector of Wellness Associates.

many forms of stress that wear you down and cause a variety of health problems.

You may not be aware of it, but every tense situation—or even memories of tense situations—causes a change in breathing. The more stressed you feel, the more shallow your breathing becomes. Consciously breathing deeply can relieve tension, quiet fear and relieve pain. So before you reach for aspirin or antacid tablets, do some breathing.

EMOTIONS AND HEALTH

There is a heavy price to be paid when feelings are denied or repressed. Lethargy, boredom and a lack of enthusiasm toward life may be the consequences. Those who are unaccustomed to dealing with feelings in healthy ways often seek out other means to cover up those feelings or distract themselves, such as alcohol, food, drugs, TV, unhealthy relationships or compulsive work.

Befriend your emotional self. Accept emotions as valuable signals that tell you something is in need of attention. *How to acknowledge emotions...*

- **Write an angry letter** and then tear it up.

- **Compose a poem** about your grief.

- **Draw, paint or even dance** to express your feelings.

- **Exercise vigorously.**

- **Talk about your feelings.**

- **Let fear be there.**

- **Let discouragement be there.**

Don't try to chase these emotions away. Look at them. Express them when it is appropriate to do so. Then move on.

SIMPLIFY YOUR LIFE

Becoming well in body, mind and spirit is not nearly as difficult as it may seem. Wellness is not a matter of accumulating something, like more research or experience.

Rather, wellness is realized by unburdening yourself of all those things that prevent the natural state of healthiness from being present. To become well is to appreciate simplicity. *Examples...*

- **One breath is precious**...one smile...one day of seeing the sun.
- **Simplify your life.**
- **Simplify your diet.**
- **Take time to rest your mind.**
- **See your loved ones as brand-new every single day.**

HONOR YOUR BODY'S WISDOM

Inhabit your body. Learn to start listening to what your body is saying to you and to trust what you hear.

Listening to others instead of yourself...or saying *yes* when you mean *no* are just two examples of the many ways you shortchange yourself. Wellness is about "coming home"—taking up residence inside your own body once again.

REPROGRAM YOURSELF

Current research in the field of psychoneuroimmunology verifies what folk healers have known for centuries—that thinking and emotions have a direct impact on the strength of the immune system.

The immune system is the first line of defense against disease. Strengthening your immune system consciously, through the use of imagery or nurturing self-talk, gives you a much better chance of maintaining whole-body health.

CONNECT TO THE EARTH FOR HEALING

When was the last time you sat on the ground or touched the earth in some way? This may seem silly, but physical contact with soil, natural waters, sunlight and fresh air is healing.

When stress has built up, a walk around the block is often all that is needed to restore perspective.

Beyond that, you connect with forces stronger than the individual self in nature, and this puts everything in perspective.

A PARTNERSHIP IN HEALING

There will be times in your life when you need the care and attention of a helping professional such as a doctor, psychologist, social worker, etc.

When you're looking for such professionals, it's important to find people willing to take the time to answer questions and listen to your concerns. If you find someone who is unwilling to do this, switch to someone who will.

BOTTOM LINE

Getting started on these small changes will help you make a difference in your life. We hope that you will experience increased self-awareness and self-appreciation…have a sense of greater inner strength…and, above all, live a healthier life.

The Truth… And Your Health

Brad Blanton, PhD, a psychologist in private practice in Washington, DC, and the author of *Radical Honesty.* Dell Trade Paperbacks.

Revealing your true feelings lowers your risk for cancer and heart disease. Dishonesty seems to weaken the immune system, raising the risk of infectious disease.

Helpful: Before responding to any question, ask yourself, *Is what I am about to say truthful? …Is it necessary?…*and *Is it kind?* By reflecting on these three questions, you'll be honest, while not hurting others.

All About Moods

Martin Groder, MD, a Chapel Hill, NC, psychiatrist and business consultant. He is coauthor of *Business Games: How to Recognize the Players and Deal with Them.* Boardroom Classics.

We are living in a time of great expectations and big disappointments. When things don't go our way or stress at work or at home gets us feeling down, we become uncooperative, grouchy and even angry.

Though feeling blue or cranky is perfectly normal and healthy, there are times when we would like a bad mood to lift more quickly than nature will allow it to do.

WHAT ARE MOODS?

Moods result from a complex interaction between the internal brain chemistry and the external events you experience.

In the brain, three major neurotransmitters affect the way we feel…

●**Serotonin,** which acts as a mood stabilizer.

●**Dopamine and norepinephrine,** which act as stimulants.

While the full extent of how these three neurotransmitters work is not very well understood, we do know that they are being generated all the time and they naturally move in their own cycles.

The chemicals are also affected by external stimuli—such as foods, drugs and smells—which can cause rapid changes in the production and balance of the neurotransmitters.

This helps explain why people can plunge into bad moods after hearing bad news. Likewise, a person in a bad mood can snap out of it instantly after getting a phone call from a beloved or humorous friend.

SHAKING A BAD MOOD

While feeling sullen is important to the development of a sense of critical self-analysis, there are steps you can take to trick your mind into letting go.

Important: If none of the strategies I'm about to recommend brings relief and your bad mood persists for more than two weeks, see your doctor. The problem may be depression, which must be addressed and treated more aggressively.

Strategies for pulling yourself out of a bad mood…

●**Trace the source of your bad mood.** Common sources of bad moods include recent illness…loneliness…boredom…unrealistic expectations…failure to accomplish a goal…catastrophizing by making mountains out of molehills…and unacknowledged disappointment, guilt or anger.

In these cases, taking the time to analyze what was happening in your life before the bad mood occurred is useful. Knowing where the negative feelings come from gives you some sense of control, and uncovering the cause of your bad mood may actually give you clues on how to remedy it.

Example: One of my patients felt anxious and irritable but didn't know why. We talked about what had been happening during the past few days and discovered the patient's spouse was the target of unexpressed anger. The spouse had been spending money with little regard to the fact that the couple was trying to get out of debt. Once the source of the bad mood was identified, the patient was able to talk directly about it and felt better immediately.

Another often overlooked source of bad moods is having been in a good mood for too long. People who are involved in highly intense projects at work find themselves disappointed when the projects end. In these cases, what feels like a bad mood is simply lack of rest or a neutral mood, neither good nor bad.

● **Make a list of all the positives in your life.** When you're in a bad mood, you view everything in a negative light. Setbacks and letdowns become magnified while positive things aren't recognized at all.

Helpful: If you make a quick list of all the positive factors in your life, your negative perception will likely shift.

● **Exercise.** Physical exertion produces endorphins—natural chemicals in the brain that are responsible for creating good moods. Depending on the individual, the physical activity doesn't have to be strenuous—even a brisk 20-minute walk is sufficient to combat a bad mood. Just being outdoors will expose you to sunlight—another natural antidepressant.

Over time, exercise will make you look better and improve your overall health. And by providing a steady stream of endorphins, regular exercise will actually help protect you from future bad moods.

● **Socialize.** One of the biggest mistakes we make when feeling blue is to isolate ourselves, which can make a bad mood even worse.

Helpful: Force yourself to call someone… or even throw a simple party—take-out pizza will do—and invite some people you haven't seen in a while.

● **Seek humor.** Nothing dissolves a bad mood faster than laughter. Go to a comedy club…rent a funny video…or call a friend who has a great sense of humor.

Helpful: Make a recording of your complaining, and listen to it. Even the most seemingly tragic *woe-is-me* complaint eventually sounds ridiculous.

● **Do something nice for someone else.** Forget yourself by concentrating on someone else. Buy a present for a friend. Call someone you haven't talked to in years. Volunteer at a hospital or nursing home, where you'll likely see others who have much more serious problems than yours.

● **Change your immediate environment.** The simple act of moving furniture around will help freshen your attitude. Hanging new curtains, switching lamp shades, changing your bedspread or rearranging pictures will also give you an immediate lift.

● **Enjoy the arts.** For centuries, the arts have been civilization's tonic. It's hard to stay in a bad mood when gazing at a magnificent painting or listening to music you love.

Even fooling around with paints or a piano will divert you from your woes and give you another way to express yourself.

● **Spend time in a natural setting.** Being close to nature makes us realize that no matter how we feel, the sun still rises and sets each day.

Sitting on a bench in a garden, strolling on a beach or lying on a hillside and gazing at the sky will remind you there is a larger world out there than your own.

Secrets of Inner Strength

Joan Borysenko, PhD, the noted lecturer on health and spirituality and president of a Boulder, CO, educational firm, Mind/Body Health Sciences. A former cancer cell biologist at Harvard Medical School, she is author of *Minding the Body, Mending the Mind* (Da Capo) and *A Woman's Book of Life* (Riverhead Books).

Ever notice how some people manage to stay on track despite suffering a serious illness, financial setbacks or other problems that would derail other people?

We spoke with Joan Borysenko, PhD, to learn more about such "emotionally resilient" individuals.

A cancer biologist turned mind/body researcher, Dr. Borysenko has spent decades studying emotional resilience. But her expertise on the subject also stems from personal experience.

She has flourished despite having had her share of misfortune—including a divorce, a near-fatal car accident and the suicide of her father, who was dying of leukemia.

How do emotionally resilient people differ from the rest of us? *Researchers have identified three key attitudes they all share...*

CHALLENGE

Emotionally resilient people view crises as opportunities for problem-solving—as challenges, not as threats to survival. I witnessed this phenomenon in my own life 14 years ago, when my three children and I ran aground while boating in Scituate, Massachusetts.

I immediately began to imagine the worst, thinking "We'll be stuck here all night."

But my 14-year-old son, Justin, was thrilled. "I'll rescue us," he said.

He had us step onto a sandbar, then began casting the anchor farther out in the river, pulling the boat along until we were afloat.

Justin's attitude was a wonderful example of emotional resilience. Mine was not.

CONTROL

Emotionally resilient people recognize that while they cannot control everything that happens to them, they can control their response to events.

They also know when to stop struggling... and when to just let things be. They personify Reinhold Niebuhr's famous serenity prayer: *God grant me the serenity to accept the things I cannot change, the courage to change the things I can and the wisdom to know the difference.*

COMMITMENT

Emotionally resilient people believe there is a higher purpose for even the most painful event.

That doesn't mean they view problems as intrinsically good. But they recognize that some good often does come from even the most traumatic events.

When my dad killed himself in 1975, I felt not only grief but also terrible guilt. As a cancer biologist, I felt I should have done a better job of helping him endure the difficult treatment process he was undergoing.

But I refused to give in to despair. I told myself that if I could help even one other family avert such a tragedy, my father's death would have meaning.

I quit my job at the lab and retrained as a behavioral medicine specialist. Then I founded a mind/body clinic at one of Harvard Medical School's teaching hospitals, beginning a new career helping patients and their families cope physically and spiritually with life-threatening illnesses.

A friend went through something similar when her son died in a car accident. To survive the wrenching pain, she forced herself to think about how her experience might help others.

She now volunteers as a support group facilitator, helping other parents who have suffered the loss of a child.

The late psychiatrist and Holocaust survivor Viktor E. Frankl maintained that it is the meaning that we ascribe to *negative* events that allows us to endure suffering without giving in to despair.

RESILIENCE CAN BE CULTIVATED

Emotional resilience doesn't always come naturally. It certainly didn't come naturally to me. *But it can be developed...*

●**Observe your usual response to emotional stress.** Do you "catastrophize?" Believe nothing you do will make a difference? Blame yourself?

Simply noticing these responses is often a starting point for change.

●**Learn more productive ways to respond to problems.** Whenever you feel worried or annoyed, ask yourself, "How does this situation challenge me? What can I learn from it?"

●**Take care of yourself.** When we're under severe emotional stress, we tend to abandon our healthful habits. But that is precisely when we need them the most.

No matter what else is going on in your life, always eat a balanced diet...exercise regularly ...and get plenty of sleep.

● **Feed your soul.** Each day, do something you find deeply pleasurable—whether it's walking in the park, listening to music or curling up with a book.

● **Find social support.** Sharing your problems with friends and/or family members is the best buffer against stress.

If you lack close relationships to call upon, join a support group. There's one for practically every crisis you may face.

To find a group in your area, consult a hospital social worker.

● **Practice gratitude.** In her best-selling book *Simple Abundance* (Warner), Sarah Ban Breathnach recommends spending a few minutes each morning and evening listing five things for which you are grateful.

This will help you focus more on life's gifts instead of its burdens. I think it's a great idea.

 Letting Go

Jim Spira, PhD, director of the Institute for Health Psychology, San Diego.

People who freely express negative emotions may live longer after heart attacks.

A Belgian study of 300 heart attack survivors found that those who held in their negative emotions—particularly anger and fear—were four times as likely to die within six to 10 years after their heart attacks than a group of survivors who spoke more freely.

Researchers speculate that the emotionally unexpressive types experience greater stress, which causes spasms in the arteries and increases the tendency of blood to clot—both of which contribute to heart problems.

A Survivor's Journey

Greg Anderson, founder and president of the Cancer Conquerors Foundation, Box 238, Hershey, PA 17033. He is author of *The 22 (Non-Negotiable) Laws of Wellness.* HarperOne.

In 1984, at the age of 38, I was diagnosed with lung cancer. After having one lung removed, I learned that the cancer had spread to the lymph system. My doctor gave me a month to live.

But I've been cancer-free since 1989.

What accounts for my survival? Good medical care, including radiation therapy, of course. But I'm convinced that much of the credit goes to my strict adherence to what I call the "laws of wellness."

I've identified 22 laws. *Here are the six most important ones...*

THE LAW OF THE BODY

The body component of wellness hinges on oft-heard advice—avoid tobacco and alcohol ...eat a variety of foods...minimize consumption of fat, salt and sugar...exercise daily... and avoid being overweight.

The latest research shows that eating a low-calorie diet that limits meats of all types adds to both the quantity and quality of your life.

Ideal: 1,500 to 2,000 calories a day for most people, depending on how much you exercise.

THE LAW OF EMOTIONAL CHOICE

Whether or not you realize it, you're capable of choosing which emotions you allow to affect your life. You also have the power to let go of negative feelings.

Problem: We tend to let our emotions dictate our behavior and experiences. We react to situations and to people around us instead of taking responsibility for our own feelings.

Example: If your boss criticizes you at a meeting, you can feel angry for hours...or you can follow the law of emotional choice. It says to let go of the emotion, forgive the transgressor and dismiss the behavior.

Casting off negative emotions does *not* mean that you condone bad behavior. It means you are aware of the stress you encounter on a daily basis—and refuse to let it ruin your life.

THE LAW OF WIN-WIN

Numerous studies illuminate the harm that comes from social isolation and the benefit that comes from belonging...

● **Heart attack victims face a greater risk of death if they go home to an empty house** than if they go home to a spouse or pet.

● **Breast cancer patients who join a support group live longer** than those who don't.

● **People with lots of close friends have stronger immune systems** than people with few friends.

Social wellness means more than simply belonging. It means getting along with others... and cultivating caring, supportive relationships.

Problem: Most people operate with a "win-lose" mentality. They unconsciously believe that in any given encounter, one person wins...and the other loses.

Better: Heed the law of win-win. This law says that it's better to find not *your* way, or *my way*, but a way that's *mutually* beneficial. You'll create allies, not adversaries.

THE LAW OF LIFETIME GROWTH

Most people view aging in terms of biology. In fact, 80% or more of the aging process can be attributed to our attitudes and expectations.

If you think you're too old to do something or to try something new, you are. If you think you're young, you are.

Our self-image is immensely powerful. Consider an acquaintance of mine. He started a new business—at age 96. He even took a 30-year mortgage on an office building. *That's* wellness.

Pursuing your interests prevents boredom and depression...keeps you healthy...and distracts you from physical discomfort. And preliminary data suggest that intellectual activity helps prevent Alzheimer's disease. Strive to grow each day.

THE LAW OF LIFE MISSION

In a survey, 75-year-olds were asked, "What makes life worth living?" The most frequent answer was, "Having a sense of purpose."

Serving others—the law of life mission—is essential for personal fulfillment. Unfortunately, many of us are so busy that we never sit down to consider our purpose in life.

Your purpose is more than your job. Before I fell ill, I lived the life of a fast-paced corporate executive—the classic workaholic. Cancer helped show me my mission—to create wellness for myself and others.

I can't say I'm happy that I got sick. But my illness was clearly filled with many surprise benefits.

How can you discover your life mission? Think. Reflect on your personal creed—your philosophy about why you were put on this earth. And write out a mission statement.

Most people have three distinct missions...

● **Inner mission**—What you want to achieve in personal growth. Look to become a more positive, loving influence in the world.

● **Shared mission**—What you want to achieve in partnership with someone else. Perhaps it's to help raise a child in a loving environment or to redeem an errant social condition.

● **Unique mission**—The mission only you with your unique talents and abilities can accomplish. This mission should involve helping others—doing volunteer work, for example.

THE LAW OF PERSONAL PEACE

Spiritual wellness involves focusing on a higher level of understanding of yourself and others.

I'm talking about learning to love and be loved unconditionally...to express gratitude for your life...to forgive yourself and others for past transgressions or perceived failures...and to let go of resentment and anger.

Achieve personal peace by quieting your mind and spirit. For a few minutes each day, meditate, perform deep breathing, take a bath, pet an animal or pursue another quiet, contemplative activity.

FOLLOWING THE LAWS

Incorporate these laws into your life one at a time. Today, focus on one law. Tomorrow, another. The next day, another—until you have fully incorporated the spirit of wellness into your life. You'll enhance your health, enrich your life...and change the world.

Acupuncture Can Help Depression

John J.B. Allen, PhD, distinguished professor of psychology, University of Arizona, Tucson. To find an acupuncturist near you, contact the American Association of Acupuncture and Oriental Medicine, PO Box 162340, Sacramento, CA 95816, *www. aaom.org.*

In a six-week study, patients given acupuncture experienced a 43% reduction in depressive symptoms. After treatment, more than half no longer met the criteria for clinical depression. That makes acupuncture just as effective as antidepressants and psychotherapy.

How to Put Much More Happiness in Our Lives

Bernie Siegel, MD, founder of Exceptional Cancer Patients in Middletown, CT, which provides information and therapeutic support to people with life-threatening and chronic illnesses. He is author of several books, including *Love, Medicine and Miracles* (Rider) and *Peace, Love and Healing* (Harper Paperbacks).

Each new year brings ambitious attempts to kick bad habits...live a healthier life ...and accomplish more at work.

But this year, instead of trying to reach many different and difficult goals, resolve to achieve just one—putting more happiness in your life.

Keep this resolution, and your life and immune system will improve, resulting in a healthier—and more prosperous—year. *Simple ways to put more happiness in your life...*

●**Change your attitude about your job and colleagues.** If you are stuck in a job you hate, explore your options for change and make an effort to switch to a career you will find more personally satisfying.

But if you can't change jobs—for financial or career reasons—change your attitude toward your job and the people with whom you work.

If you need motivation, listen to tapes...read uplifting books...and talk to inspiring people.

By behaving like the person you want to be, you can vastly improve your life.

The more you practice your new attitude, the better you'll become at reversing your bad moods and unhealthy feelings.

●**Make time for activities you enjoy.** Studies have shown that when people work on projects or hobbies that they enjoy, their blood chemistry is altered almost immediately in a positive way. When your blood chemistry is altered in this way, it increases your body's resistance to infections and life-threatening diseases.

Key: Engage in activities that make you lose track of time. Such activities depend on the individual—and can range from washing a car or painting a house to reading or exploring the Internet.

●**Change the way you think about failure.** Failure is a state of mind. When you fail to live up to your expectations or those of others, you can dwell on it until you feel terrible about yourself. Or you can choose never to feel this way again by thinking of failure as a redirection that leads to good things. Remember that "F" does not have to stand for *failure.* It can stand for *feedback.*

People who learn from upsetting events and then move on are happier and healthier than those who don't.

My wife has a wonderful saying—*Never consider yourself a failure. You can always serve as a bad example.* She knows that there is a use for everything—even failure—and that we can derive something good or beneficial from every unhappy life event.

●**Get fully in touch with your feelings.** Most of us are extremely adept at repressing issues with which we would rather not deal. We distract ourselves by cramming so many activities into our schedules that we never have time to get at the root of what is making us feel unhappy or anxious.

If you take the time to get in touch with your feelings, you can discover and heal the source of your psychological pain.

●**Keep a journal.** One of the best ways to get in touch with your feelings is to record them in a journal every day.·Carry a pad and pen with you, and jot down anything that moves you as each day progresses—whether the events are happy or upsetting.

At the end of each day, read over your notes so you can remember how you felt at specific times and what may have caused those feelings. You may also want to add to your notes.

Studies have shown that people who write regularly in journals feel less stressed and are less susceptible to various diseases.

●**Treat yourself as you would treat a beloved pet.** Many people have problems treating themselves well. They don't forgive themselves easily for making mistakes and do not give themselves permission to enjoy life.

I tell people to take care of themselves as they would a pet.

Examples: Would you allow your pet to smoke? Drink too much alcohol? Become obese? Of course not. You make sure it gets exercise, good food, occasional treats and enjoyable toys. And most important, you give it lots of hugs and express your love.

Do not resolve to eat a healthy diet and get plenty of exercise to avoid dying. Eat a healthy diet and exercise because you care enough about yourself to do it.

Love yourself enough to enjoy the beautiful things in life without feeling guilty. Buy a new outfit. Take a day off from work and go to the movies. Lighten up, and spend some time playing.

●**Make a difference.** Individuals who help others several times a week often live longer, healthier lives. When you volunteer to help other people, you feel better emotionally and physically. You achieve a natural high.

●**Develop a childlike sense of humor.** Just as children are able to see the silly side of almost everything in life, you can use humor to get through the ordinary hassles and crises you face. Watching humorous movies and TV shows can boost your physical immunity.

If you despise your job and hate going back to work on Monday...or you are scheduled for a medical treatment you dread, your body will start releasing stress-provoking chemicals before you get to the office or hospital. You can neutralize this reaction by reading an amusing book, listening to a funny tape or just looking for the humor in life.

Take charge of your life, and decide which labor pains you are willing to experience in order to give birth to yourself.

Gambling a Problem?

Eric Hollander, MD, professor of psychiatry, Mount Sinai School of Medicine, New York City. His study of 19 compulsive gamblers 22 to 57 years of age was presented at a meeting of the American Psychiatric Association.

Compulsive gambling can often be controlled with the antidepressant *fluvoxamine* (Luvox). Among 10 gambling addicts who took the drug for two months, seven said they no longer had the desire to gamble. Fluvoxamine is also effective against compulsive shopping.

The Smart Way to Handle Negative Emotions

David K. Reynolds, PhD, a leading expert on Eastern psychotherapies in Coos Bay, OR. He has trained numerous instructors in *Constructive Living* worldwide and is the author of more than 30 books, including *A Handbook for Constructive Living.* University of Hawaii Press.

Most people try to fix negative emotions like anxiety, anger or sadness. Instead of solving our problems, however, this approach inevitably leaves us frustrated and confused. It doesn't work because *feelings are uncontrollable.*

But we can control what we do. This simple fact is the basis of a way of life called *Constructive Living.* By helping us focus on what we can control (our behavior) rather than what we can't (our feelings, other people, the past), Constructive Living makes life more satisfying and meaningful.

ROOTS OF CONSTRUCTIVE LIVING

Constructive Living is based on two schools of Japanese psychotherapy...

● **Morita therapy** represents the action side of Constructive Living. Developed in the early 1900s by psychiatrist Morita Shoma, it has its roots in Zen Buddhism.

● **Naikan therapy** is the reflective side. It was developed in the 1930s by Yoshimoto Ishin, a businessman-turned-priest.

Despite its origins, Constructive Living is *not* a therapy. It's a way of living learned through daily practice and observation.

THE IMPORTANCE OF ACTION

Like the weather, feelings are unpredictable. Sadness and anger come and go. So do joy and excitement. The most sensible approach to handling such feelings is to accept them... and *continue doing what you need to do.*

Example: If you're nervous about starting a new job, do not fixate on your anxiety or try to eliminate it. Let it encourage you to learn as much as possible about your duties beforehand. Your performance will be enhanced...and you will probably find yourself feeling less anxious.

Bottom line: Trying to change the way you feel makes no more sense than trying to will a storm to stop. Just wait.

While you wait, take action toward your goals. Doing so prevents you from dwelling on things you cannot control and brings a sense of accomplishment—which should lead to greater happiness and satisfaction. Even if it doesn't, focusing on your *purpose* and *behavior* rather than your feelings will give you a sense of calm and contentment.

THE PROBLEM WITH WESTERN PSYCHOTHERAPY

Conventional psychotherapists have things backward. They try to help their clients feel better so that they can take steps to improve their lives.

You don't have to feel good about yourself to make changes in your life. In fact, things usually work the other way—we feel better as a *result* of having made constructive changes.

Feelings that are labeled "negative" in psychotherapy often have very useful roles.

Example: Fear helps us avoid physical danger...anxiety prompts us to organize our thoughts before making a speech.

Acknowledging these feelings doesn't mean you must submit to them. You can feel shy and still invite someone out to lunch. You can fear flying and do it anyway. You can feel sad about the end of a relationship and still go to work.

MORITA EXERCISES

Exercise I: Next time you find yourself brooding about someone who treated you badly, do something useful and vigorous. Wash your car, for instance, or vacuum the house.

By the time you're done, the troubling thoughts will probably have passed...*and* you'll have accomplished something.

Exercise II: List all the chores you have to do, then tackle them in alphabetical order. The point is to *do*—not agonize about what to do.

Exercise III: Over the next 24 hours, try several activities that you haven't tried before —knitting, cooking a new recipe, painting, etc. This teaches you not to let fear or other feelings keep you from trying something new.

THE ROLE OF REFLECTION

Balancing the *Morita* side of Constructive Living is *Naikan*, the reflective side.

Naikan teaches us to revere all the gifts we have been given. It shifts our focus from ourselves to other people.

When we fail to get what we want, it's easy to feel unhappy. We feel that we haven't gotten our fair share. But nothing we have is exclusively ours.

Our bodies are a gift from our parents, who got their bodies from *their* parents. We are sustained by food grown and processed by people we've never met. Even our ideas are based upon the wisdom of others.

Conventional therapy encourages people to review the bad things that happened to them in the past—all the ways others hurt or disappointed them.

How much time do you spend thinking about the ways *you* hurt other people?

Even if your parents were neglectful, you owe them a debt for giving you life. The fact that you reached adulthood means that *someone* in your past took care of you.

The proper response to recognizing all that we have been given is *gratitude.* Rather than focusing on how much the world owes us, focus on how much we have received from so many sources.

NAIKAN EXERCISES

Exercise I: At the end of the day, spend 20 minutes recalling what people did for you that day…what you did for others…and any trouble you caused others. *Don't* devote time to reviewing troubles others caused you. Most of us are already skilled at that.

Exercise II: Once a week, find something broken and fix it. *Examples:* A leaky faucet, a jammed copier, etc. This is a way of expressing gratitude to the things that support you every day.

Exercise III: Think of someone you haven't been getting along with—a coworker, for example. Say "thank you" to that person 10 times a day.

Exercise IV: Every day, secretly perform a favor for a family member. If anyone detects your "secret service," find another secret service to do.

Example: Shine your spouse's shoes and return them to the closet.

We tend to do things for others with the idea that we'll get something in return. This exercise reminds us that the world doesn't owe us anything.

Overcoming Fear of Failure

Arnold Fox, MD, a specialist in cardiology and internal medicine for more than 30 years and a former commissioner on the California State Board of Quality Assurance. He and his son, Barry Fox, PhD, are coauthors of several books, including *Beyond Positive Thinking: Putting Your Thoughts Into Action.* Hay House.

We generally understand that a chronic fear of failure can be detrimental to our careers or personal relationships. But recently, scientists have discovered that such negative feelings take a serious toll on our *physical* health, as well.

ADRENALINE AND CATECHOLAMINES

For better or worse, every thought in our head—positive or negative—affects our internal biochemistry. Fear, worry, self-doubt and other emotional "downers" do much of their behind-the-scenes damage by stepping up secretion of adrenaline and other hormones called *catecholamines.*

Even in individuals with perfectly normal hearts, catecholamines can trigger a condition called *paroxysmal tachycardia*—skipped or rapid heartbeat. This has been linked to sudden death.

Elevated catecholamines also boost cholesterol levels and blood pressure.

Result: Increased risk of heart attack and stroke.

Over time, chronically elevated levels of catecholamines raise the heart's metabolism, forcing it to work harder. The same chemicals reduce the body's output of insulin. Reduced insulin production raises the risk of both diabetes and atherosclerosis.

A steady flow of catecholamines also erodes the inner lining of small blood vessels. The vascular "potholes" resulting from this erosion fill up easily with platelets and cholesterol—even if cholesterol levels in the body are normal.

Our fear of failure can keep cholesterol at peak levels for long periods of time. *Illustration:* Cholesterol levels of medical students remain high even weeks after major exams.

Chronic worry also wreaks havoc on the immune system, reducing the effectiveness of our protective *T-cells.*

Anxiety can also stimulate the adrenal glands to secrete more cortisol, setting the stage for peptic ulcers.

CHANGING OUR PERCEPTIONS

To counteract the potentially deadly fear of failure, we must change our perceptions. *Key:* Realizing that failure itself is an unavoidable fact of life.

Each and every one of us has stumbled at some time or other. But that doesn't make us failures.

Even a long string of setbacks or mistakes doesn't qualify us for this sweeping, negative label. The scripts of our lives are filled with failures and unhappy scenes as well as successful and joyful ones.

Helpful: Replay and savor the positive scenes. Don't dwell on the negative scenes.

Review negative scenes only long enough to learn from them—and then move on.

People who view themselves as failures or chronic worriers are simply stuck in their negative scenes. They can't put the script down and move on to another page, so to speak.

A vicious cycle ensues, as the belief that they are failures and the constant fear of failing again discourage them from trying new experiences or persevering at tasks that can lead to more positive results. That holds true for their health, their careers and their relationships.

FINDING THE SILVER LINING

Mini-case study: Imagine two clerks in the same office, doing pretty much the same work.

One clerk thinks the work is beneath his talents and abilities. He resents having to take orders from a female boss and fears being viewed as a failure for having such a low-level job.

The other clerk, a child of recent immigrants, is glad to have a job that pays enough for her to attend evening classes and complete her college degree.

Although both clerks are performing the same tasks for the same pay, the first views the work as dreadful, the other as a great opportunity to get ahead.

To put it another way, the second clerk views her work as a *new, interesting* and *challenging experience* (NICE).

Clearly, the same stimulus can trigger NICE or negative feelings, depending on our perceptions. Positive perceptions allow us to control our world by altering our interpretations of situations and events. This helps us focus on our successes while gearing up for any difficult tasks that might lie ahead.

FOUR REASONS NOT TO GIVE IN TO FEAR

•**Internal messages**—*You can't do it...You're not good enough...You'll never make it...*and *You're going to fail*—whether intentional or not, verbal or otherwise, sap our confidence, energy and creative juices.

When we give in to fear and worry, our mental eye is fixed only on images of failure, weakness and embarrassment, blocking out positive, encouraging images.

•**We are often less worried about failure itself than about how we will look to others** if we do fail.

But excessive concern with appearances robs us of our initiative and of the freedom to take control of our lives. It programs us to behave according to others' expectations—setting us up for chronic anxiety.

•**Fear of failure, self-doubt and other "can't do" emotions** are what I call "master" addictions. They can lead to smoking, overeating, alcohol and drug abuse and other potentially deadly habits.

•**The word "worry" comes from the Old English *wyrgan*, meaning "to strangle."** That's what we do when we worry—we strangle our ability to think and perform effectively, along with our strength, flexibility, enthusiasm and belief in ourselves.

Concern—an awareness of problems and a desire to overcome them—spurs us on and helps us find solutions to our problems. By contrast, worry keeps us from taking any action at all.

TAKING POSITIVE ACTION

To free yourself from the stranglehold of fear, uncertainty and doubt...

•**Remind yourself that everyone makes errors.** More important is what we do with those errors. Don't allow your mistakes or failures to color your self-image.

Instead, say, *This led to results I really didn't want. Next time I'll avoid that...and look for another way of behaving.*

Helpful: Set clear goals. Know where you want to go, then divide your journey into small, manageable trips.

Follow these three easy rules...

•**Don't sweat the little things.**

•**Everything is little.**

•**If you can't flee, go with the flow.**

•**Almost every problem has a lighter side**—look for it! Humor is a great healer. It helps you avoid "sweating" the minor irritants and hurdles in your life and serves to put matters in perspective.

Try smiling especially when you don't feel like it. You may have to act at first, but the happy feelings will soon follow. Act confident and upbeat—and soon you will be.

●Take the focus of fear and worry off yourself. Use your talents and strengths to help someone else—a child struggling with homework, an elderly neighbor, a troubled friend. Often the best way to feel better about yourself and your life is to do something for others—even if that means simply offering your companionship and support.

●Don't wring your hands over the things you can't control. Focus only on those things you *can* control.

●Don't go it alone. If a task seems overwhelming, ask for help. Doing so is not a sign of weakness, but of resourcefulness and strength.

Make yourself part of a community. Whether it's a family, neighborhood, house of worship or any other caring group, feeling that you belong is an effective antidote to fear.

How to Overcome Emotions that Hold You Back

Marilyn Mason, PhD, associate professor at the University of Minnesota and a corporate consultant and lecturer in Minneapolis. She is author of several books, including *Seven Mountains: The Inner Climb to Commitment and Caring.* Plume.

Over the past 20 or more years, I have hiked up some of the world's highest peaks. When I started climbing many years ago, I wasn't much of an athlete. But over time, it was a thrill to see my stamina escalate…and my body strengthen.

More startling is how mountain climbing helped me gain greater control over my mind. I even learned to master my emotions—and anyone can do the same.

FACING YOUR FEARS

Fear is one of our deepest emotions. It can either motivate us or inhibit us from taking action. When fear overcomes us, it can cloud everything else we are experiencing or thinking. That can happen no matter how intelligent or well-balanced you are.

Fear helped our ancient ancestors recognize the danger of predators, inspiring them to flee and survive. Since we're rarely chased by lions today, fear has become a more complex emotion. Many times we are reacting to perceived dangers rather than real ones.

Fear can affect your thinking in many ways today—keeping you from pursuing an opportunity as well as telling you to flee danger.

Helpful: Whenever you sense that fear is preventing you from trying something new, ask yourself why you're afraid. Think about it. Write down your fear. Identifying your fears and recognizing when they are working against your best interests is a liberating experience.

Example: I was terrified before my first climb many years ago. Logic told me there was nothing to worry about—I knew the rope was more than strong enough to support my weight, and I had tremendous confidence in my climbing partner's ability to swing me back to the cliff if I slipped.

Getting ready, the more I thought about it, the more I realized that I wasn't scared of injury. I was scared that I wouldn't succeed—that I wouldn't be up to the climb. That surprised me—I never realized that I was so scared of failure. But as soon as I identified the fear, I was able to overcome it.

EMBRACING COMMITMENT

We live in a rapidly changing age, when technology permeates much of our daily existence. Technology has made us more productive and has increased the amount of information we experience and absorb.

But technology has also made us less patient. More and more happens in an instant today, so we become frustrated when phones are busy, ATM machines run too slowly or the checkout lines are long.

Our general impatience also prevents us from enduring temporary obstacles when pursuing larger goals. The easiest response to trouble at work or with a relationship seems to be giving up.

Helpful: Think about what really matters to you and remind yourself of its importance. Whenever you become frustrated with yourself or with forces you can't control, ask yourself if your goals are still desirable.

If the answer is *yes*, remind yourself that the greatest rewards are possible only if you're willing to stick it out through tough times. Life's greatest achievements are never reached without some struggle.

Example: Climbing Mt. Kilimanjaro taught me this. The mountain doesn't require a tremendous amount of technical climbing skills, just the desire to reach the top.

At first the climb is wonderful. The mountain is beautiful at low elevations. But before long, it's just volcanic rock with nothing to distract you from the next step in front of you except the increasing cold and thinning air. Succeeding requires stamina and focus on the result.

SEEKING SUPPORT

Despite the organizational shift at work from the individual to teams, the person who makes his/her own way is still greatly admired in our society. That's why many people feel like failures when they must ask for help.

But few people succeed on their own—even when it *seems* they did it alone.

Isolating yourself from others and being embarrassed to let others see the real you fosters dishonesty and limits your exposure to opportunity. You're more likely to cover up personal flaws than address them.

Helpful: Force yourself to open up by creating a personal board of directors. Speak with them individually twice a year—or when you need help or have a tough choice to make.

No one person has all the answers on his own. Good judgment depends on asking great questions of smart people.

Example: I've found that on difficult climbs, the encouragement of the group plays a big part in each individual's determination and success. I've come to realize that needing help now and then isn't a sign of failure. Climbing is a personal experience, but you can't do it alone.

DEALING WITH SETBACKS

We all suffer reversals now and then. That's part of life, and without them, we would never fully appreciate our triumphs.

But not everyone reacts the same way to setbacks. Some people see every failed expectation as a major failure, which causes them to belittle or berate themselves. This negative view can prevent you from taking actions or help you sabotage your efforts.

Helpful: Recognize that living life means taking chances. Taking chances, on occasion, means conceding defeat. When we have to make a decision, we do so based on the information available to us. Sometimes, we later find additional information which leads us to conclude our initial decision was incorrect.

When you suffer a setback, take a look at why you made the decision in the first place before labeling yourself a failure. Was it failure—or feedback?

Example: My first failure came on Devil's Tower, an almost mile-high rock monolith in Wyoming. I barely had been able to complete the first leg of the climb, and I knew more difficult sections lay ahead—so I turned back. I felt humiliated and defeated.

BOOSTING PERSONAL EXCELLENCE

Few things in life are as psychologically difficult as putting ourselves through an experience at which we failed in the past.

Revisiting a failed experience carries painful memories of personal failure. We automatically tell ourselves that we're bound to fail again, in many cases robbing ourselves of our best chance to succeed. Or we don't even bother trying at all.

Helpful: Prepare in advance for these apprehensions. Focus on what you learned on your first attempt, not how you were hurt.

Then consider how you've changed since your first try. Have you done additional research? Have you spent extra time practicing in preparation? Chances are, you're not the same person who failed the first time around.

Example: I returned to Devil's Tower a year later. There were still lingering doubts in my mind, but I had done a lot of climbing over the year, and I knew I was much more skilled than I was on my first attempt. I made it to the summit.

Extreme Shyness Is A Health Problem: How to Overcome It

Franklin Schneier, MD, research psychiatrist in the anxiety disorders clinic at the New York State Psychiatric Institute in New York City. He is coauthor of *The Hidden Face of Shyness: Understanding and Overcoming Social Anxiety.* Harper.

Everyone feels shy or anxious *sometimes*—whether it's butterflies in your stomach when you walk into a party or a cold sweat when it's your turn to give a toast.

Half of all people fear public speaking. Believe it or not, many say they would rather die than give a speech.

Social anxiety runs the gamut from occasional jitters to a disabling disorder that makes work and relationships impossible.

Wherever you fit in, taming those butterflies can vastly improve your quality of life.

WHERE BUTTERFLIES COME FROM

Anxiety is the body's automatic response to perceived danger. The brain signals the *hypothalamus*, a gland at the base of the brain that stimulates production of the adrenal hormones *cortisol* and *adrenaline*.

Once these "stress hormones" enter your bloodstream, your heart begins to race, your muscles contract and you break into a sweat.

Some people blush, as blood rushes into the capillaries in their cheeks. Others develop trembling hands or a queasy sensation in the stomach.

Many people escape these distressing sensations only by avoiding social situations. You may not even think of yourself as shy, just that you "don't like parties" or "don't enjoy making presentations."

Problem: Avoidance means missing out on opportunities for pleasure, satisfaction and career advancement.

It's *not* a matter of timidity or weakness. One of my patients had no trouble going into perilous situations in his work as a narcotics detective. But the need to testify in court left him paralyzed with fear.

WHAT ARE *YOU* AFRAID OF?

Two basic fears underlie most cases of social anxiety—the fear of embarrassment and the fear of being judged harshly. We're afraid we'll arouse anger, contempt or ridicule…say something that others will consider stupid…or just look foolish.

It's thoughts like these that give meetings and other social situations that have no physical risk a feeling of danger.

Making matters worse, we tend to become fearful of the bodily manifestations of anxiety. "I'll blush, and everyone will see it," we think …or, "My sweaty palms will reveal to everyone just how nervous I am."

Example: One of my patients, John G., was anxious about his upcoming wedding. Why? Because he would have to hold a glass of wine during the ceremony. He was afraid his hand would shake. The wedding guests would see he was a nervous wreck, he believed, and deem him a jerk.

TAMING YOUR BUTTERFLIES

The more you avoid situations that trigger anxiety, the more ingrained your fears become.

Avoidance is just the *opposite* of what you should be doing. To uproot your fears, you must confront them—by doing the very things that you find so frightening.

Helpful: Set reasonable goals, and take small steps toward those goals. If you're usually shy at gatherings, it's unrealistic—and counterproductive—to try to be the life of the party. Instead, aim simply to start a conversation or two.

OTHER HELPFUL STRATEGIES

•**Focus on your actions, not other people's reactions.** The person you try to engage in a conversation at a party may be receptive …or he/she may walk away. Either way, give yourself the credit you deserve for what *you* did—initiating the contact.

•**Become aware of the unrealistic thoughts that make you anxious.** Before making a toast or a business presentation, do you automatically shift into "low-confidence" gear? Do you think, "I'll mess up, and they'll laugh at me"?

In social situations, do you find yourself thinking, "I'll be tongue-tied and run out of things to say?"

In such cases, the best antidote is to think *realistically*. In your presentation, how likely are you *really* to mess up? Will people really laugh if you flub a line? Or will they appreciate your humanness and listen more closely?

Replace negative, anxiety-provoking thoughts with positive ones—"I've given presentations before, and they've been fine. If anything, I've gotten better since last time."

When my patient John G. contemplated his prenuptial jitters, he saw how unrealistic they were. If his hand did shake, he realized, his friends and family would not think he was a jerk. They would think he was moved by the occasion—and respect him all the more.

• **Rehearse situations that make you nervous.** If you're scheduled to give a speech, hone your talk beforehand using a tape recorder or a video camera. Stand in front of a mirror, or have a friend observe you.

In the case of John G., rehearsing his wedding with a family member helped him boost his confidence.

People who fear public speaking can gain priceless experience by participating (along with other fearful speakers) in programs offered by Toastmasters International. To find a chapter in your area, call 800-993-7732 or go online at *www.toastmasters.org*.

• **Develop skills that will give you confidence.** Read up on how to give an effective business presentation or speech. Observe people whose social graces you admire, making mental notes of what works for them.

Many adult-education centers offer courses in social skills. These classes teach you what to do at parties and on dates.

WHEN SELF-HELP FAILS

Many people who cannot control anxiety on their own benefit from cognitive-behavioral therapy. Via this form of therapy, you learn to identify and change negative, anxiety-producing thoughts...and to become more confident and outgoing.

In just a few months of individual or group therapy, you can learn skills that will help you for the rest of your life.

When cognitive-behavioral therapy isn't enough, I prescribe anxiety-reducing medication.

For *occasional* anxiety—if you have to give a talk once a month, for instance—the beta-blocker *propranolol* (Inderal) is often best. It blunts the body's reactions to adrenaline, helping to curb symptoms such as a pounding heart or queasy stomach.

Many musicians and other performers who suffer from stage fright get relief from propranolol.

When anxiety occurs on an everyday basis, I often prescribe *fluoxetine* (Prozac) or another *selective serotonin reuptake inhibitor* (SSRI). Anxious people who take SSRIs say they have fewer fearful thoughts and feel more comfortable in social situations.

If SSRIs fail—or if sexual problems or other side effects make them intolerable—I prescribe a tranquilizer like *clonazepam* (Klonopin)...or a monoamine-oxidase inhibitor antidepressant like *phenelzine* (Nardil).

Some people find that a few months of drug therapy is all that's needed. For others, long-term therapy is needed to maintain their improvement.

For a referral to a social anxiety specialist in your area, contact the Anxiety Disorders Association of America, 8730 Georgia Ave., Suite 600, Silver Spring, MD 20910. 240-485-1001, *www.adaa.org*.

25

New Ways for the 21st Century

Alternative Medicine Moves Mainstream

James S. Gordon, MD
Georgetown Medical School,
Center for Mind-Body Medicine

Americans' interest in alternative medicine and therapies has grown dramatically during the past few years. In the last year, more than one out of three people have used an alternative therapy to reduce stress and pain...and/or help cure an ailment.

The public's interest is so strong that the National Institutes of Health created the National Center for Complementary and Alternative Medicine, and many medical schools —including Harvard, Columbia and Stanford, as well as Georgetown, where I teach—now offer courses in alternative medicine.

As a physician, my concern is with finding the most effective synthesis of conventional and alternative medicines. Whenever I have

any doubt about my patient's condition, I always make sure a complete conventional diagnostic assessment is made before I begin a program of alternative therapies.

Among the alternative therapies that I have found particularly helpful...

RELAXATION THERAPIES

Many of these therapies can be self-administered and are extremely effective in reducing stress.

By reducing stress, you can lower blood pressure and improve your immune functioning. You may also be able to diminish the frequency and intensity of asthma attacks and migraine headaches and reduce chronic pain.

James S. Gordon, MD, clinical professor of psychiatry and of family medicine at Georgetown Medical School, Washington, DC. He is chairman of the Program Advisory Council, National Institutes of Health's Office of Alternative Medicine. Dr. Gordon is founder and director of the Center for Mind-Body Medicine, 5225 Connecticut Ave. NW, Washington, DC 20015, and author of *Manifesto for a New Medicine: Your Guide to Healing Partnerships and the Wise Use of Alternative Therapies*. Westview.

All relaxation therapies begin with the induction of a relaxed state. You can achieve this in many ways—through deep-breathing exercises, meditation and even physical exercise. Once you are able to achieve a feeling of relaxation, you can move on to more complex therapies such as imaging or hypnosis, which are directed at specific conditions or symptoms. *How they work…*

●**Deep breathing.** Sit in a comfortable chair with your feet on the floor. Breathe deeply into your abdomen. Put a hand on your belly, feeling it rise and fall. Let the belly be soft. (Remind yourself by saying *soft belly* as you breathe in and out.) Begin with five or 10 minutes of this, and do it once or twice a day. Increase the amount of time as it suits you. After a while, you'll find that a few deep breaths will be enough to create a feeling of relaxation.

●**Meditation.** One simple form is called concentrated meditation. As you breathe in, repeat a sound like *one* or a word or prayer that is meaningful to you. Focus your attention on the sound or word.

●**Imaging.** You can use your mind's eye to visualize a relaxing scene, such as a placid lake or a beautiful mountain. You can also use images to affect specific physical functions. For example, visualize your immune system's white blood cells fighting an infection or imagine more blood flowing to a stiff joint.

●**Hypnosis.** This state of deep relaxation can have an impact on both physical and psychological conditions. It is generally administered by a practitioner, who helps you enter a state in which you are detached from the world around you and have an increased capacity to focus. He/she can also teach you strategies for "self-hypnosis."

Hypnosis requires that you be "suggestible" —open to someone else's instructions or your own and willing to allow your imagination to take over so that you disassociate yourself from the outside world and focus intently on whatever thought, scene, feeling or smell you are asked to conjure up.

Either the practitioner can give instructions that you will come out of the hypnotic state after a period of time, or you can give them to yourself. Contrary to popular fears, a person who is hypnotized cannot be forced to do something he would not ordinarily do.

How to find practitioners: Deep-breathing and meditation classes are commonly offered at holistic education centers, stress management clinics, community centers, community colleges and some hospitals and medical centers.

NUTRITIONAL/HERBAL MEDICINE

●**Vitamins and minerals.** Specific nutrients, especially the antioxidants in vitamins A, C and E, beta-carotene and selenium, may be helpful in preventing some kinds of cancer or the recurrence of some forms of the disease. Some studies have also linked vitamin E to a reduction in the risk of heart disease.

What I recommend to my patients: Vitamin E/400 international units (IU), twice a day…vitamin C/l,000 milligrams (mg), once or twice a day…beta-carotene/a maximum of 25,000 IU once a day…selenium/50 micrograms, twice a day.*

I also urge my patients to consume 400 micrograms (0.4 mg) of folic acid a day. Folic acid is believed to prevent several birth defects and may reduce the risk of heart disease in men and women.

●**Herbs** contain ingredients that have specific pharmacological effects.

In both Western natural medicine and non-Western traditions, such as the Indian, Chinese and Native American, combinations of herbs are used to improve the functioning of various organs.

Keep in mind that herbs often take longer to work than traditional Western medicines. I advise my patients to look for improvements over a period of weeks or months.

It is important to work from an authoritative guide or herbal—a book about plants—especially with reference to their medicinal properties…and to take only the prescribed amounts. Herbs—like drugs—can have harmful side effects.

Good resources: *The New Holistic Herbal* by David Hoffman (Element Books) and *The Healing Herbs: The Ultimate Guide to the Curative Power of Nature's Medicines* by Michael Castleman (Bantam).

*Consult your doctor for the dosages that are appropriate for you.

Herbal therapies may treat everything from allergies to migraines and improve physical and mental functions.

How to find a practitioner: Since herbalists aren't licensed, your safest bet may be to find a physician, nurse or licensed nutritionist who uses herbs in his practice. You can also check with friends who have found someone who is competent.

ACUPUNCTURE

Acupuncture is a part of Chinese medicine. It dates back thousands of years and is often used in conjunction with herbal medicine, dietary changes and relaxation techniques.

How it works: The practitioner inserts fine needles at key points along the body that are believed to connect to organs and affect virtually all body functions.

During acupuncture, our bodies' natural painkillers, called *endorphins*, are released, along with other chemicals. Acupuncture has an antidepressant effect, improves lung capacity, boosts the immune system and may enhance circulation. It is often used to alleviate pain and may be used as anesthesia for surgery. In hundreds of sites around the country, acupuncture is used to treat alcoholism and drug addiction.

How to find a practitioner: There are four times as many qualified nonphysician acupuncturists as physicians who practice acupuncture. Licensing requirements vary by state. To locate a qualified medical acupuncturist in your area, contact your state licensing board or the American Academy of Medical Acupuncture (323-937-5514 or *www.medical acupuncture.org*).

HOMEOPATHY

Homeopathy originated in Germany and was brought to the US in the early 19th century. Homeopathic practitioners treat illnesses by prescribing small, highly diluted doses of natural substances, which, in larger, more concentrated doses, would actually cause the patient's symptoms.

Example: A tiny amount of an allergen, a substance that triggers an allergic response, would be used to treat an allergy.

I've found homeopathic remedies particularly useful in boosting immune systems and in treating nausea and vomiting, colds and flu and emotional or physical shock.

Studies suggest that homeopathic remedies may also be effective in the treatment of hay fever, arthritis and diarrhea.

How to find a practitioner: Homeopaths are not licensed, except in Arizona. Some physicians, nurses and physician assistants currently use homeopathy in their practices.

Ask the practitioner where he has studied, whether he has passed some type of certification exam and how long he has been practicing homeopathy. As with any practitioner, you might want to ask if you can speak with patients whom he has already treated.

MANIPULATIVE THERAPIES

• **Chiropractic and osteopathy.** In both of these therapies, practitioners use their hands to manipulate bones in the spinal column, the neck, the head and the joints. By manipulating bones, practitioners feel they alter the functioning of the nervous and circulatory systems. They believe that manipulation affects all the internal organs, not just the musculoskeletal system.

• **Doctors of Chiropractic** (DCs) are licensed by each state and must complete two years of undergraduate study and a four-year course at a chiropractic college.

• **Doctors of Osteopathy** (DOs) receive a four-year education similar to that of a doctor. They also must complete a year-long residency and take the same licensing exams. DOs can prescribe drugs.

• **Massage therapy** can reduce muscle tension and stress, improve joint mobility and promote healing of some injuries.

Some states require that massage therapists be licensed or certified while other states do not. Look for a therapist who has a certificate indicating that he has passed the national exam of the American Massage Therapy Association.

Some licensed physical therapists and registered nurses now practice massage therapy.

How to Get Your HMO to Cover Alternative Medical Treatment

Alan Raymond, vice president of marketing and communications for Harvard Pilgrim Health Care, an HMO, Brookline, MA, and author of *The HMO Health Care Companion*. Harper Perennial.

All HMOs rely on primary care doctors to provide or approve most care for their members. They also tend to cover only "medically necessary" and "nonexperimental" treatments.

Therefore, HMOs may not be willing to reimburse members for alternative medical treatments, such as acupuncture, biofeedback, massage therapy and chiropractic care.

But such treatments are growing in popularity. More than one-third of all Americans have already tried at least one of them.

Here's how to get your HMO to pay for alternative approaches…

●**Find out if the HMO must pay for the treatment in your state**, and under what circumstances. Some states now require that health insurers pay for certain treatments—especially chiropractic care. Your state's insurance department can fill you in.

●**Convince your primary care physician to recommend an alternative treatment.** Explain how it will likely succeed in treating your medical problem. Some HMOs will pay for alternative treatments—if you get a referral from your HMO doctor. Call the HMO to find out its policy.

●**Ask alternative treatment providers if they know of HMOs that cover their care.** Ask if they will allow referrals for alternative treatments. There may be limits—for example, chiropractic treatment for lower back pain may be covered, while the use of alternative therapies for chronic illness may not be.

●**Ask your employer to add alternative therapies to your benefits.** Some HMOs offer riders that expand coverage to include nontraditional therapies. It will cost your employer more, so you will probably see somewhat higher premiums as a result. The larger the number of your fellow employees who want such a benefit, the more likely it is your request will be granted.

●**If treatment is denied coverage, use tax-sheltered money.** Many employers offer flexible spending accounts, which permit you to set aside pretax dollars to pay for uncovered medical expenses.

Acupuncture and chiropractic care qualify, since the IRS has ruled that both are tax-deductible medical expenses. The IRS hasn't ruled on other treatments, so check with your employer. Also find out if you need a medical doctor's referral before getting your treatment.

Be careful when you set aside money in a flexible spending account. If you don't use all the money that is set aside by the end of the year, you forfeit the remaining amount.

Magnets Stop Pain… Ease Arthritis…Help Heal Broken Bones and More

Ron Lawrence, MD, a neurologist in private practice in Agoura Hills, CA. He is former president of the North American Academy of Magnetic Therapy, 2240 W. Agoura Rd., Ste. 202, Agoura, CA 91301.

In China, France, Japan and especially in India, magnetic therapy has long been used to speed the healing of broken bones and soft-tissue injuries.

In the US, magnetic therapy is sometimes considered a form of quackery. But following the publication of several "pro-magnet" studies in the *Journal of Electro- and Magnetobiology* and elsewhere, a few pioneering doctors in this country are starting to use magnets in their practices.

Already, magnetic therapy has proven effective at treating slow-healing fractures and arthritic knees and necks. Studies also suggest that regular use of magnets may reverse osteoporosis…prevent heart disease…slow tumor growth…and boost mental function in some Alzheimer's patients.

I know from personal experience that people sleep better and wake up feeling more refreshed after a night on a magnetic mattress. I sleep on one myself!

Is magnetic therapy safe? *Absolutely.* Magnetic resonance imaging (MRI) machines routinely expose patients to magnetic fields as high as 15,000 gauss—with no negative effects. It stands to reason that a medical magnet rated at 200 to 800 gauss poses little threat.

HOW MAGNETS WORK

Studies have demonstrated quite clearly that when placed directly on the skin, a simple, handheld magnet works by...

•**Increasing blood flow.** It does so by stimulating cellular activity through the so-called "Hall effect." This is general heating of the magnetized area.

Some scientists think magnets improve the functioning of the autonomic nervous system, which could also stimulate blood flow to the affected area.

•**Diminishing pain.** This occurs via a combination of the Hall effect and possibly some stabilizing influence on the autonomic nervous system.

•**Speeding up the healing process.** It does so by boosting the body's synthesis of *adenosine triphosphate* (ATP), the "fuel" that fires all cellular processes...and by enhancing the blood's ability to carry oxygen.

MAGNETS VERSUS ARTHRITIS

Magnetic therapy helps relieve arthritis pain *and* slows the deterioration of cartilage inside arthritic joints.

For my patients with arthritis, I recommend sleeping on a magnetic mattress pad...or wrapping a flexible, magnetic bandage around the affected joint. If you do sleep on a magnetic pad, remove it for a day or two, every two to four weeks. This seems to prolong the beneficial effects.

HEADACHES AND BACK PAIN

Magnetic pillow liners appear to be an effective treatment for chronic headaches and jaw pain.

People with chronic back pain have obtained significant relief from sleeping on magnetic mattresses, and/or using magnetic seat cushions.

SOFT TISSUE INFLAMMATION

Tennis elbow, carpal tunnel syndrome and other tendon or ligament problems heal faster when wrapped in magnetic bandages.

In most cases, the magnet is wrapped into place over the affected area—and left in place until the pain disappears.

BROKEN BONES

In some hospitals, powerful electromagnets are being used to speed healing of stubborn bone fractures. Magnetic therapy also seems to promote regeneration of spinal disk tissue.

ASTHMA

Regular use of magnets helps prevent the violent allergic reaction in the lungs that is characteristic of bronchial asthma.

Helpful: Sleeping on a magnetic mattress ...or wearing a magnetic bandage on your chest.

PUTTING MAGNETS TO WORK

The benefits of magnetic therapy are often apparent within the first hour of treatment. In others, three or four days of steady treatment are required.

For maximum benefit: Place magnets as close to your body as possible. The strength of the magnetic field drops off sharply with distance.

A variety of magnetic devices is now available—including mattress pads, seat cushions, pillow liners, magnet-studded bandages and simple handheld magnets.

Good source of medical magnets: Synergy for Life, Box 5962, Winston-Salem, NC 27113. 888-311-2963, *www.synergyforlife.com.*

Chinese Medicine Works Well on Americans, Too

James S. Gordon, MD, author of *Manifesto for a New Medicine: Your Guide to Healing Partnerships and the Wise Use of Alternative Therapies.* Westview. He is clinical professor of psychiatry and family practice at Georgetown University School of Medicine and director of the Center for Mind–Body Medicine, both in Washington, DC.

There's little doubt that Americans enjoy the most technologically advanced medical care in the world. Still, there's much we can learn from the Chinese system of medicine.

Scientific studies of China's ancient healing system are just beginning, and more are needed. But a growing body of research suggests that acupuncture, herbal remedies and other components of Chinese medicine do provide relief for many common ailments—even when Western medicine has failed.

Chinese medicine is helpful for everything from asthma and arthritis to migraines and menstrual cramps. It can help cure alcoholism and other addictions...and helps alleviate nausea and other side effects of cancer chemotherapy.

WHAT IS CHINESE MEDICINE?

The Chinese system of medicine is hard for Westerners to accept—or even grasp. More than a collection of exotic treatments, it's a unique way of looking at the world and the body.

The language Chinese physicians use to describe symptoms, diagnoses and physical processes is the language of the natural world. It uses terms like *earth, metal* and *fire* instead of the technical jargon familiar to most Western physicians and their patients.

Whereas Western medicine focuses on the specific disease entities and diagnostic categories, the Chinese system views the body as both expressing and fueled by a basic animating force called *qi* (pronounced *chee*).

This vital energy circulates constantly through *meridians*—lines along the body on which the acupuncture points lie. Chinese medical therapies are concerned with restoring the balance of qi.

Everything taking place in the organs and elsewhere in the body is considered to be interconnected to the individual's psychology, the time of day, season of the year—indeed, to *all* phenomena in the natural world.

The diagnostic techniques Chinese doctors use are alien to Western physicians. *They include...*

- **Touching and listening to the belly.**

- **Identifying imbalances in the body** by observing the patient's face and voice. For example, dark circles under the eyes might indicate a kidney ailment long before lab tests reveal it.

- **Observing not just one pulse**, but 12 different pulse points along the wrist.

- **Noticing the appearance, texture and moistness of the tongue.** A trembling tongue might suggest that qi is depleted.

ACUPUNCTURE

Acupuncture has proved helpful for a variety of ailments—irritable bowel syndrome... migraines...hot flashes...addictions. It can even serve as anesthetic during surgery.

The Chinese maintain that acupuncture redistributes the flow of qi, thereby affecting the activity of organs.

In Western terms, acupuncture induces the body to release natural anti-inflammatory substances and painkilling opiates.

To find a qualified acupuncturist in your area, ask your doctor or your friends for a referral. If your state requires licensing to practice acupuncture (about half of all states do), call the state medical board to make sure the person you're considering is licensed.

HERBAL REMEDIES

The Chinese use herbs...gold and other minerals...and animal products (such as dried fish, bile and bones) to restore balance to the body.

Example I: Ginseng eases stress, boosts immune function and enhances mood.

Example II: Certain mushrooms, including shiitake, strengthen the immune system.

Don't start taking massive doses of an herbal remedy just because you've read about it. That can cause dangerous—and perhaps fatal—side effects.

Chinese herbalists use *tiny* doses of many herbs. This strategy ensures maximum benefit while minimizing side effects.

If your doctor, acupuncturist or chiropractor is unable to recommend an herbalist, visit the nearest Asian-American neighborhood. The neighborhood pharmacist may be able to suggest someone. Many states require licensing of herbal therapists.

TAI CHI AND QI GONG

Tai chi (pronounced *tie chee*) consists of a series of smoothly connected postures. There are many different "forms," or sequences, of these movements.

Performed with rapidity, tai chi is a martial art. Done slowly and contemplatively, however, it increases energy, flexibility and mental clarity.

Tai chi instruction is offered at recreation centers, YMCAs, YWCAs and health clubs.

Qi gong (pronounced *chee gong*) is an integrated system of movement, breathing and visualization. It involves fewer movements than tai chi...and greater use of imagery.

In addition to its calming effects, qi gong seems to lower blood pressure...enhance immune function...and ease breathing in asthmatics.

Many Chinese medicine practitioners are trained in qi gong, as are a growing number of Westerners.

Placebo Power: How To Harness It

Howard M. Spiro, MD, professor emeritus of medicine and former director of the Program for Humanities and Medicine at Yale University School of Medicine in New Haven, CT.

Physicians have long observed that even very sick patients sometimes get better after taking a "sugar pill," or *placebo*.

For years, doctors viewed this placebo effect as an irrational element in an otherwise logical and systematic world of clinical medicine and medical research—a nuisance that needed to be explained away.

Now: Evidence is mounting that mental activity has a powerful effect on the body. Doctors are seeking ways to *exploit* the placebo effect for their patients' benefit.

We asked Dr. Howard M. Spiro, a nationally renowned gastroenterologist with a special interest in placebos, to tell us more about placebos and their expanding role in medical care...

●**What is a placebo?** Where treating patients is concerned, it's a pill that contains only inactive ingredients.

Prior to the 1960s, it was routine for doctors to give sugar pills to patients who complained of ailments that defied diagnosis. Patients were told, "Take this. It should help."

Anyone who got better after taking a placebo was assumed to be complaining of an ailment that didn't really exist.

Another important use of the placebo is in clinical trials of new drugs. Here the placebo gives researchers a way to "control" for nonmedical factors that could affect the outcome of treatment—a patient's greater attention to health care during a study, for example, or simply the passage of time.

●**Why do placebos work?** One theory is that placebos help boost the body's production of the natural painkilling compounds called *endorphins*.

Another is that placebos simply distract the mind, keeping patients from noticing pain.

A placebo might foster the body's innate self-healing power simply by bringing to mind the emotional comfort associated with childhood memories of going to the doctor.

It's also possible that placebos do *nothing*—that the patient would have gotten better anyway, regardless of treatment. Given a few weeks or months, for example, up to half of all peptic ulcers heal *by themselves*—no matter what treatment is given.

●**Do doctors still give out sugar pills?** No. Today it's considered unethical to give a patient a drug without telling him/her exactly what it is.

However, placebo-like treatments are still being given to patients. Vitamin B-12 injections, for instance, are supposed to help fight fatigue and weakness.

I myself offer the injections to some patients. It would be unethical for me to tell a patient, "This treatment will cure you."

What I say is, "I suggest you get this shot. I can't promise it will help, and I can't tell you how it works. But other patients say the shot made them feel better."

●**How can doctors exploit the power of placebos without deceiving patients?** Doctors who speak optimistically to patients help them *feel* better...and this optimism may be associated with *physical* improvement as well.

Sadly, many doctors have forgotten the healing power of comforting words.

Doctors have also forgotten how to listen. At one time, listening was central to medical practice. But to many doctors, listening to patients now seems old-fashioned. They tend to rush to offer pills and procedures that are often unnecessary.

●**Does the doctor's style tie in with the placebo effect?** Absolutely. A good doctor-patient relationship is integral to the placebo effect and to healing. It fosters *catharsis*—the emotional release a patient feels after telling a doctor his troubles.

Interview doctors until you find one who listens well...and who has the time to talk to you.

The Seven Simple Steps To a Century of Great Health

Robert D. Willix, Jr., MD, a traditionally trained physician and surgeon in a private alternative medicine practice in Boca Raton, FL. He is author of *Healthy at 100: 7 Steps to a Century of Great Health*. Shot Tower Books.

When Americans get sick, they go to the doctor and say, *"Fix me."* But— *only you* can fix *you*...and *you can!*

There is no biological reason we can't live to be a ripe old age, free of pain, illness and decay —still vital—and sexually active.

Working to balance modern scientific research and the ancient healing arts of India and China, I have developed a seven-step program to achieve that goal. Actively enhancing the link between mind and body will change the way you look, feel and live.

Follow my seven-step plan in any order you choose.

You start with the step that's least difficult for you and work on it as long as necessary— three months, six months, a year—until you're ready to try the next step.

As you move forward, reaping the benefits, observe the power you have gained in changing your life.

As with car repair and maintenance, the earlier you start my program, the more mileage you'll get. But it will definitely improve your health and outlook at any age.

***Step 1:* Perform your own health risk appraisal.** To learn whether you're at greater risk of developing certain diseases than the general population, know your risk factors. With your health provider's help, choose actions to take or avoid to reduce your risk.

●**Physical status.** Do you have high blood pressure or high cholesterol? Both increase the risk of heart attack, stroke and premature death.

●**Family history.** Ask your close blood relatives how long other family members have lived. Find out if any of them had major chronic illnesses or conditions such as cancer, heart disease, osteoporosis, diabetes and degenerative arthritis.

Mistake: People with short-lived families resign themselves to an early death. That's totally unrealistic. Heredity accounts for no more than 10% of the chance of death.

●**Lifestyle.** Do you exercise and stretch regularly? How healthfully do you eat? Do you get enough rest and make an effort to avoid stress? Do you drink too much alcohol or use tobacco products?

***Step 2:* Use antioxidants.** The most important medical discovery of the past 50 years is that antioxidants minimize the damage done by free radicals, agents in the blood that attack and weaken body tissues.

I am not impressed by a few imperfect studies debunking the remarkable effects of antioxidants. These studies do not refute 40 years of impressive research concluding that antioxidants help prevent heart disease, stroke, cataracts, skin wrinkling, senility and breast, lung and colon cancer—while slowing aging itself. For further proof, I could cite the remarkable positive effects that taking supplemental antioxidants has had on hundreds of my own patients.

The best source of antioxidants is organically grown fruits (three to five servings a day) and vegetables (three to four servings a day).

But if you're among the 90% of people who eat the typical American diet, which includes lots of meat and fat but few fresh foods, you need supplements.

Every day, take 500 to 2,000 milligrams of vitamin C, up to 10,000 international units (IU) of vitamin A, 400 to 800 IU of vitamin E* and 12,000 to 25,000 IU of beta-carotene, which the body converts to vitamin A.

***Step 3:* Practice some form of aerobic exercise to keep your heart healthy.** Exercise is a more powerful medicine than any drug. The evidence is overwhelming that people who exercise live longer and have less risk of death from heart disease. Exercise pumps oxygen through the body tissues. That's good for everyone and especially good for people with kidney disease.

Any exercise that is somewhat strenuous will do. Just be sure to raise your heart rate (you don't have to feel it pounding). You can ride a bike or walk. Do this for 30 minutes three times a week. After three months, you will feel better. Continue this regimen, working up to at least five days a week.

***Step 4:* Meditate for stress management and mind/body health.** Stress, which many experts consider the most common cause of disease in this day and age, can rob you of life. By relieving stress, regularly practiced meditation becomes rejuvenating.

None of my accomplishments has had a stronger impact on my life than using meditation to neutralize the effects of stress on my nervous system.

At least once, preferably twice, a day meditate for 10 to 20 minutes.

Consider *tai chi chuan*…centering prayer…transcendental meditation…intoning a mantra. The aim is to create a quiet space between your thoughts. It requires conscious effort and is not the same as relaxing.

No time? Think again. Meditation will *increase* your productivity for the rest of the day. Its impact on the ability to absorb knowledge is tremendous.

*Due to the possible interactions between vitamin E and various drugs and supplements, as well as other safety considerations, consult your doctor before starting a vitamin E regimen.

***Step 5:* Practice weight training for stronger bones.** Brittle bones (osteoporosis) lead to falls, broken hips and a susceptibility to pneumonia while bedridden. And older people tend to have weak legs in general.

I call one simple exercise "chair-ups." Sit in an armchair. Can you raise yourself repeatedly, without touching the arms? Keep practicing until you can. That will strengthen your legs a great deal.

***Step 6:* Stretch and strengthen your back.** Being supple will allow you to turn your head around while driving and not have a dangerous "blind spot." You can bend down to pick things up and stand up again without creaking and cracking.

Flexibility helps prevent the natural degeneration into stiffness that comes with aging… and helps prevent injury from accidents, the major cause of disability in older people, and back problems, suffered by 85% of American adults.

Stretch each and every day. Find a stretching routine you like and do it for two to five minutes shortly after getting up in the morning.

Keep trying to place your palms on the floor without bending your knees. The closer you can get, the more effective the stretch.

***Step 7:* Eat right.** In my view, all extremes in nutrition are to be avoided. Low-fat diets alone don't make a difference. Eliminating any single factor won't keep you healthy. What's crucial is to maintain a balance of proteins, carbohydrates (pasta, whole grains) and plenty of organically grown fruits and vegetables. Eat more vegetable than animal protein. Read labels carefully and choose natural foods.

Look at where the food came from. Oatmeal and cream of wheat are closer to nature than sugar-coated bran flakes. When you see a box of cereal growing from a tree, you'll know it's a good food.

All About Light Therapy

George Brainard, PhD, professor of neurology and director of the Light Research Program at Thomas Jefferson Medical College in Philadelphia. He is a consultant for NASA and the National Institutes of Health on the behavioral aspects and therapeutic effects of light.

Touted as a quick fix for everything from insomnia to low sex drive, melatonin has fast become one of the biggest-selling nutritional supplements in US history.

For some individuals, however, the problem is not having too *little* melatonin—but too *much*. As a result, many people may be "overdosing" on this hormone.

MELATONIN AND DAYLIGHT

Melatonin is a natural hormone produced by the pineal gland, a pea-sized gland located at the center of the brain.

Melatonin synthesis is governed by *circadian rhythms*—the daily cycles of light and darkness to which each of us is exposed.

During exposure to sunshine or another bright light, the pineal gland stops making melatonin. That makes you alert.

In dim light or darkness in the evening, melatonin production soars. That's why we tend to get sleepy at night.

Problem: For many individuals, this melatonin production cycle has been disrupted. That's because so much of our time is spent indoors, under *artificial* light.

DISTURBED RHYTHMS

If you're not exposed to enough bright light each day, circadian rhythms may fall out of whack. This phenomenon is called *circadian rhythm desynchronization.*

Circadian desynchronization can also be caused by taking melatonin supplements…by jet lag…or by working odd hours.

Heart disease is twice as prevalent among night-shift workers as among those who work a normal nine-to-five shift.

In addition to heart disease, circadian disruption has been linked to…

- **Insomnia and other sleep disturbances.**
- **Gastrointestinal problems.**
- **Persistent drowsiness or fatigue.**
- **Poor job performance.**
- **Menstrual irregularities.**

Light deprivation is also associated with a serious form of depression called *seasonal affective disorder* (SAD).

Psychiatrists now believe that SAD affects 10 million Americans (particularly during fall and winter, when time spent outdoors is at a minimum). Another 25 million are thought to have a milder, "subsyndromal" version of SAD called SSAD.

There have been hints that light deprivation may also be a factor in other disorders. Breast cancer, for instance, is far less prevalent near the equator—where the sun is brightest—than it is farther north or south. And breast cancer rates in the northern US are up to twice as high as rates in the South.

THE MODERN LIFESTYLE

Humans evolved to spend a great deal of time outdoors—and that meant lots of exposure to sunlight.

The electric light changed all that. Now our bodies are exposed mostly to artificial light… and most artificial light is far too dim to induce the pineal gland to stop making melatonin.

To stop making melatonin, the body needs about 2,500 lux (10 lux roughly equals the light shed by one candle).

Outside on a sunny day, light can reach 100,000 lux. By contrast, indoor lighting ranges from only 100 to 800 lux.

Implication: You may be working all day in light that's bright enough to see by—yet still be in "biological darkness" as far as your pineal gland is concerned.

THE NATURAL SOLUTION

Should you be worried about light deprivation? If you feel healthy, probably not. But if you are experiencing mood changes, fatigue, insomnia or daytime drowsiness, light deprivation might be an issue.

Simple solution: Get more natural sunlight. I urge my patients to take a 30-minute stroll outdoors each morning before work. Walking at lunch is good, too.

While indoors during the day, try to sit near a window in a well-lighted room.

BRIGHT LIGHT TREATMENT

Light deprivation can also be remedied with daily exposure to special artificial light (brighter than typical indoor lighting).

Typically, the minimum of 30 minutes up to two hours a day of "light therapy" will counteract light deprivation.

Especially beneficial: Exposure to bright light early in the morning, during the transition from sleeping to waking.

Various artificial light sources are now available. At present, most use white light—although other colors are under study.

• **Light boxes** consist of an array of fluorescent bulbs that collectively give off about 2,500 lux. The individual sits in front of the panel, about three feet away.

• **Work stations** are units angled overhead and placed closer to the eyes than a light box. They produce about 10,000 lux. They are comparable to light boxes in terms of effectiveness.

• **Light visors** are worn like a hat, with light shining onto the face. These devices permit mobility during light therapy.

• **Dawn simulators** slowly increase the light in your bedroom as you wake up. Several studies have shown this approach to be effective in relieving SAD.

For a list of light box manufacturers and treatment centers, contact the Society for Light Treatment and Biological Rhythms, 4648 Main St., Chincoteague, VA 23336. *www.sltbr.org.*

All About Prolotherapy

Robert G. Klein, MD, an internist and prolotherapist in private practice in Santa Barbara, CA...and Janice Guthrie, founder and director of the medical information and research firm, the Health Resource, 933 Faulkner St., Conway, AR 72034.

Chronic back pain, whiplash injuries to the neck and many other types of musculoskeletal pain that are not alleviated by physical therapy, painkilling medication or chiropractic manipulation can often be controlled via *prolotherapy.*

In this highly effective but little-known treatment, small amounts of an irritant solution—usually concentrated glucose—are injected into the painful area.

The resulting inflammation promotes growth of collagen, the protein that's a major component of ligaments, the cable-like structures that hold our joints together.

New collagen growth helps reduce pain and increases joint stability by strengthening the fibrous capsule around joints. It also brings significant improvement in joint mobility.

Many forms of chronic musculoskeletal pain are caused by ligament damage. Car accidents, falls or repetitive movements cause ligaments to loosen and/or tear. Prolotherapy is effective for most ligament-related pain.

SIDE EFFECTS

Prolotherapy patients generally feel fine for four to eight hours after the injections because a local anesthetic is given along with the irritant. The discomfort that usually follows slowly subsides over the next several days.

Many individuals who undergo prolotherapy experience pain, swelling, soreness, temporary stiffness and bruising at the injection site. Fortunately, discomfort can usually be minimized by medication, ice and massage.

Caution: Smoking makes the therapy less effective, as does use of aspirin and other anti-inflammatory drugs.

PRECISION COUNTS

Most patients need a series of injections over a period of several weeks or months. In some cases, prolotherapy is teamed with other forms of soft tissue treatment—such as physical therapy, joint manipulation or acupuncture.

Prolotherapy injections must be given *precisely* at the junction of a bone and a ligament. Misplaced injections are ineffective and possibly dangerous. If the irritant is inadvertently injected into the spinal canal, for instance, paralysis or even death could occur.

Consequently, prolotherapy injections must be administered only by a clinician thoroughly trained in the technique. Some say that orthopedic surgeons are ideal for administering prolotherapy injections. That's because they have a thorough knowledge of the location of ligaments and muscles.

FINDING A PROLOTHERAPIST

Only about 300 orthopedic physicians and osteopaths in the US and Canada currently use prolotherapy in their practices.

Among these practitioners is former Surgeon General C. Everett Koop, MD. He began using prolotherapy himself in the early 1960s, after another doctor used it on him to cure the once-intractable pain in his neck and arm.

For more information about prolotherapy, contact the American Association of Orthopaedic Medicine (800-992-2063, *www.aaomed.org*).

INSURANCE COVERAGE

One prolotherapy session costs $75 to $300. The number of sessions needed depends upon both the severity of the pain and the patient's response to the treatment.

Some major health insurance companies now cover prolotherapy. Others decline coverage because they consider it to be an "unproven" or "experimental" treatment.

How to Harness the Amazing Power of Your Immune System

Henry Dreher, a health and medical writer who specializes in mind–body and alternative medicine and author of *The Immune Power Personality: Seven Traits You Can Develop to Stay Healthy.* Plume.

The single best way to stay healthy is to strengthen your immune system. A strong immune system aggressively fights diseases ranging from common colds to arthritis and cancer. It can even prevent a wide range of ailments—particularly heart disease and cancer.

As the number of antibiotic-resistant bacteria increases, a strong immune system is your best defense against illness.

THE BODY'S POLICE FORCE

To help you understand your immune system, think of it as a police force of cells that conducts surveillance missions throughout the body. There are cells of different rank, and each has a different job to do. Like any good militia, all of the immune cells cooperate with each other to identify and arrest "invaders"—bacteria, viruses, cancer cells, etc. They also rush to each other's aid when necessary.

The cells' marching orders originate in the brain and certain organs, such as the thymus, a gland located behind the breast bone. The thymus acts as a "training school" for immature white blood cells.

Enemy viruses are captured by "field officers"—immune cells—including T-cells, B-cells and protein molecules called *antibodies*.

These immune "officers" communicate by spewing various "messenger" molecules that travel to other "troops" moving throughout your body.

When we don't have enough immune cells to conquer invading infections, we become ill. We can also become sick when our cells don't receive the proper messages because the different levels in the cell hierarchy fail to communicate with each other.

In the case of arthritis and other autoimmune diseases, our immune cells mistakenly attack our own cells, causing inflammation and crippling pain. Put differently, the police attack suspects who are really innocent.

SIZING UP YOUR IMMUNE SYSTEM

How can you tell if your immune system is dangerously weak?

Although there are numerous expensive tests that are used to diagnose immune deficiency, such specific conditions are rare. Most people have suboptimal immune function because they are run down.

An easier, more affordable way to assist your immune system's strength is to ask yourself a series of questions…

•**Am I constantly fighting bouts of colds,** the flu or bronchitis that last for two or more weeks at a time?

• **Am I fatigued throughout the day**…or on a regular basis?

• **Do I suffer from chronic conditions** such as allergies, asthma or arthritis?

If you answered yes to any of these questions, your immune system is probably flagging. Consult your doctor—but also consider taking several immune-boosting steps.

STRENGTHENING YOUR IMMUNITY

• **Improve the quality of your diet.** High-fat diets and a lack of vital nutrients compromise your immune system. That's because excessive intake of animal fats, such as red meats and whole-fat dairy products, trigger *free radicals*—unstable molecules that can harm immune cells.

Eating polyunsaturated vegetable oils, which are found in many snack foods, sauces, margarine and salad dressings, also produces free radicals.

• **To lower fat, cut back on red meats.** Instead, eat skinless chicken, fish and beans, which are excellent sources of protein.

• **Use moderate amounts of the safest oils**—olive and canola—instead of butter and other vegetable oils.

• **Eat more vegetables and fruits.** Nearly all are fat-free and contain nutrients that boost the immune system, such as vitamins A and C as well as phytochemicals. These compounds are found in plants and can fight disease.

Helpful: To get the proper amount of vitamins in your food each day, doctors advise that you eat a steamed vegetable side dish and a salad that includes dark leafy lettuce, peppers, bean sprouts, radishes and carrots at lunch and dinner. They also suggest you eat two to three pieces of fresh fruit each day.

• **Consider a vitamin/mineral supplement.** In a study of 96 people at the Memorial University of Newfoundland, some of the participants received a supplement with 18 nutrients while the other group received a pill with only calcium and magnesium in it. Those who received the larger supplement had fewer infections and half the number of sick days compared with others in the study. And… blood tests proved they had stronger immune responses to viruses.

Essential: Be sure that any multivitamin and mineral supplement contains the vitamins A, C, D and E…the B vitamins…beta-carotene…and the minerals zinc and selenium. Each nutrient plays a role in strengthening your immune system. Consult your doctor or nutritionist for doses.

Important: Avoid megadoses of specific vitamin supplements. Such doses can be dangerous —and won't boost your immune system any more than if you had taken the recommended amount.

• **Get into the habit of exercising daily.** Regular exercise has been shown to strengthen a particular group of immune cells that kills viruses and cancer cells. Researchers at the Harvard School of Public Health have shown that regular exercise can even prevent breast and gynecologic cancers among women.

Contrary to popular opinion, however, excessive exercise is not necessarily better for you. One study showed that excessive exercise— several hours a day of strenuous activity for five or more days a week—may actually dampen immunity, making you more susceptible to various ailments.

Better: Do about 30 minutes of aerobic exercise, such as walking, bicycling or swimming—three to five times per week. If that isn't possible, try a comfortable walking routine for 15 minutes a day.

• **Learn to reduce stress**—and control your emotional health. In a famous 1991 study published in *The New England Journal of Medicine*, scientists at Carnegie-Mellon University in Pittsburgh injected cold viruses into people and studied their stress levels. The researchers discovered that the chance of catching a cold was directly proportional to the amount of stress the volunteers had experienced.

Though most busy people can't avoid stress entirely, they can protect themselves from becoming consumed by it and learn to manage anxiety and pressure more efficiently. *Strategies…*

• **Write about your anxiety.** Holding in negative emotions has been shown to worsen stress levels and weaken immune cells.

James Pennebaker, PhD, of the University of Texas at Austin, has shown that one can bolster immunity and prevent illness by jotting down thoughts of fear, grief and anger about stressful events—both past and present.

Dr. Pennebaker suggests writing about such events for 20 minutes a day without stopping or censoring yourself.

By keeping a stress journal for three or four days, you will train yourself to identify toxic thoughts and unhealthy stress levels. You will develop a private way to release them and avoid letting them build up and aggravate and harm you.

●**Teach yourself to be more assertive.** Studies show that the patients who beat the odds against cancer and other serious illnesses are often assertive types who stand up for themselves and take charge of their own well-being. *Strategies for becoming more assertive…*

□ **Use quiet contemplation or meditation** to develop an awareness of your needs and rights versus those of everyone else.

□ **Engage in assertive communication** in which you clearly state your needs.

□ **Learn to say *no*.** Conquer the habit of saying yes to every request or obligation when your energy is at stake. Remind yourself that your health comes first and taking on too much can risk your immune system.

●**Practice relaxation.** A study at Ohio State University showed that people who practiced relaxation techniques had stronger immune system cells. Two relaxation techniques that are easy to practice any time of day are *meditation* and *deep breathing*.

Useful exercise: Sit in a quiet room. Close your eyes and breathe deeply. Say the word *om* in your mind as you breathe in…and say the word *sah* as you exhale.

If your mind wanders, gently bring your attention back to your breathing. Allow each exhale to be an opportunity to let go of tensions in your body and mind. Practice this at least once a day for 20 minutes or whenever you feel that stress and tension have risen to an uncomfortable level.

More About You… Your Immune System and Much Better Health

Henry Dreher, a health and medical writer who specializes in mind–body and alternative medicine and author of *The Immune Power Personality: Seven Traits You Can Develop to Stay Healthy.* Plume.

Conventional take-a-pill, have-an-operation medicine has largely failed to combat chronic, painful conditions such as arthritis, asthma and allergies. And conventional medicine does not always have adequate treatment against cancer, AIDS and heart disease. But we can help fight illness…*with our minds.*

Relaxation techniques, exercise and good nutrition can help a lot, but they're not enough.

Short-sighted: Most corporate-sponsored stress reduction programs concentrate on relaxation techniques rather than facing up to sources of stress and working to solve them. The pivotal psychological factor in illness is not whether we'll encounter stress. That is a given. It's how we cope with stress.

As we grow older, our bodies find it harder and harder to fight disease as our immune systems begin their natural decline. Yet by developing certain aspects of our personality, which I call *Immune Power traits*, we can help fend off disease or reduce its symptoms.

All seven traits described below are directly or indirectly linked to a vigorous immune system. All are backed by scrupulous research showing that the mind can contribute to our risk of, and recovery from, almost any disease involving a dysfunctional immune system, from migraines to rheumatoid arthritis.

A person with an *Immune Power Personality* finds joy and meaning, even health, in the challenges of life. Stressful events are handled with acceptance, flexibility and a willingness to learn and grow.

We are all born with the potential to have Immune Power traits and can reawaken them at any age. It doesn't mean you have to change certain fixed parts of your personality.

The point is to draw on the strengths of your own character to assume challenges and cope with losses and other stressful events that you can't control.

SEVEN IMMUNE POWER TRAITS

Explore one new trait per week, continuing the previous ones. You're likely to find many of your headaches, stomachaches, back pain or other symptoms fading away.

●*ACE factor:* **Attend, Connect, Express.** Awareness of your mind-body signals—the opposite of repression and denial—strengthens the heart and the immune system.

●**Attend** to your feelings.

●**Connect** feelings to your consciousness.

●**Express** feelings appropriately. You may find out that you haven't been paying attention to the real cause of your ongoing distress.

●**Capacity to confide.** Sharing your concerns with others actually enhances your immune response. It's the opposite of being bottled up—verbally and emotionally. *Helpful:* Ask the person to listen in silence.

Exercise: For 20 minutes on three to four consecutive days, write down your deepest thoughts and feelings about the most traumatic event you can remember. If nothing comes to mind, choose an event that symbolizes a set of emotions that had a long-lasting effect on you.

●**Hardiness.** Hardy individuals can resist the slings and arrows of life. They seek support to bolster their self-worth...not to reinforce the *poor me* syndrome. *The hardy share the following three major characteristics:*

●**Commitment** and wholehearted involvement in their work, relationships and activities.

●**Control** over their life circumstances, facing problems with creativity and confidence. (Control freaks manipulate others...completely different.)

●**Challenge** (that may be in the occasion when stressful events strike). People with a sense of challenge adapt well to change.

To develop the three *C*s, focus your awareness on the sources of stress, then develop an action plan to restore balance. Sometimes no amount of focusing can lead to positive change.

Alternative: Compensatory self-improvement. Identify a related problem that you can resolve.

●**Assertiveness.** Standing up for yourself reduces your sense of victimization. Being a martyr can be a destructive way to treat your mind and body. Passivity is unhealthful in the long term.

Example: In many cases, AIDS and cancer patients who actively participated in their own care lived longer than those who did not.

●**Affiliative trust.** The desire and capacity for a positive, loving relationship based on mutual respect and trust actually boosts your defenses against a whole range of physical symptoms. Unconditionally giving love relaxes you...and changes your outlook.

Example: A 42-year-old man with severe heart disease, tired of surgery, forced himself to suppress his chronically hostile behavior by thinking through situations before reacting to them. He began to spend more time with his family. His chest pain and shortness of breath were quickly relieved and eventually disappeared.

●**Altruism.** Assisting others provides a *helper's high*, which promotes both health and spirit. *Adopt four characteristics of healthy helping...*

●**Personal contact.** Writing a check isn't the same as connecting with someone. Teach someone to read...serve food to the homeless...volunteer at a day-care center...offer advice to new business owners.

●**Frequency.** *The ideal frequency is about the same as for meditation or exercise:* Roughly two hours a week. Following a schedule will help you maintain your commitment.

●**Helping strangers.** We exercise more freedom of choice in helping strangers than family members or close friends. Bonding with strangers helps get rid of a sense of isolation.

●**Letting go of results.** Like any gift, your time should be given with no strings attached. Helping must be its own reward.

●**Self-complexity.** We boost our physical health by being able to draw support from many vital selves to sustain our energy, well-being and sense of purpose through painful times. For a sense of balance, foster diverse interests. People with more self-complexity have less depression and illness when self-esteem in one part of their lives is temporarily drained.

DRAW A BLUEPRINT

Find your own path to each of these health-promoting traits. If one is entirely out of character and unappealing to you, you may decide to reject it. Keep in mind, though, that the interconnections between traits provide the fullest benefits and a balanced life.

A positive aspect of one trait offsets the negative in another.

Example: A person who asserts his needs can give openly to others without becoming a victim.

Focus on the Immune Power traits where you need the most help.

Example: Someone who constantly yells at people would benefit from affiliative trust.

If you feel set in your ways, go about the process gently and patiently. Recognize that you can heal some wounds—even lifelong ones—by confronting the aspects of your personality underlying them…gently and persistently.

Head Trauma Advance

Guy L. Clifton, MD, chairman of neurosurgery, University of Texas Health Science Center, Houston.

Neurosurgeons have turned to hypothermia as an important treatment for potentially deadly head injuries.

How it works: The patient is wrapped in cool packs containing ice water. Over an eight-hour period, body temperature is lowered to 90°F, slowing metabolism and blocking trauma-induced chemical reactions that cause irreversible brain damage. Once the immediate danger passes—usually after 48 hours—the patient's body temperature is returned to normal. In a pilot study, 52% of the patients given hypothermia recovered completely, versus only 36% who received "normo-thermia," in which the patient is maintained at normal body temperature.

Heart Failure and Biofeedback

Debra K. Moser, RN, DNSc, professor and Gill chair of cardiovascular nursing, University of Kentucky, Lexington.

Heart failure patients benefit from biofeedback training, in which they learn techniques to raise their finger temperature. (Increased finger temperature is a sign of relaxation.)

Study: After a single 30-minute session, patients' blood vessels opened wider and their breathing slowed.

For information on how to find biofeedback practioners in your area, visit the Association for Applied Psychophysiology and Biofeedback's Web site at *www.aapb.org.*

Electrostatic Massage

Milton Hammerly, MD, medical director of complementary and alternative medicine for the Catholic Health Initiatives' Centura Health facilities.

Did you know that *static electricity* is an effective remedy for headaches, arthritis and other common sources of pain?

Physicians have long recognized that the human body is pulsing with minute electrical currents. If this flow becomes disrupted, "normalizing" it may promote healing. In fact, doctors have been using low-voltage electrical current to mend broken bones.

A similar effect can be obtained using static electricity. Sweeping a charged object across a painful or injured region of the body attracts a flow of healing electric current to the area.

Doing so also speeds circulation of fluid away from the area, thereby reducing swelling.

To do "electrostatic massage" (EM), you'll need a one-foot section of polyvinyl chloride (PVC) pipe, 1.5 inches in diameter…plus an ordinary painter's mitt. These items are available at hardware stores.

What to do: Rub the pipe vigorously with the mitt for one minute, then slowly sweep the pipe over the painful area. Move in a head-to-toe direction—one-quarter to one-half inch away from the skin.

I've used electrostatic massage in my practice for more than two years now—with remarkable results.

Ninety-two percent of sinus headache sufferers benefited from EM, as did 81% of fibromyalgia sufferers…76% of tension headache sufferers…75% of muscular pain sufferers… and 72% of osteoarthritis sufferers.

I usually recommend two 15-minute electrostatic massage sessions each day for as long as pain persists.

Abdominal Aneurysm Treatment

Peter D. Fry, MD, clinical professor of surgery, University of British Columbia, Vancouver.

Abdominal aneurysms can be treated without surgery. Until fairly recently, these weakened blood vessels had to be removed through a large incision running from the breastbone to the pelvis. Now, doctors thread a woven polyester tube called a *stented graft* through a small incision in the groin. The tube becomes a lining for the blood vessel at the point where it threatens to burst. This less-invasive procedure typically involves only a two-day hospital stay. Traditional surgery usually involves a more lengthy hospitalization.

"Super Glue" vs. Sutures

James Quinn, MD, research director, division of emergency medicine, Stanford University School of Medicine, Stanford, CA.

Super glue may be better than sutures for closing many skin lacerations. In a study, doctors were able to close lacerations faster and with less pain when they used a medical version of the adhesive *octylcyanoacrylate* instead of sutures. The glued cuts healed just as well as cuts closed with sutures.

Bonus: Unlike sutures, which must be removed several days later, glue requires no follow-up care. It sloughs off in a few weeks.

Limitation: The glue is inappropriate for use on the hands, feet or joints.

Multiple Sclerosis Breakthrough

Todd Richards, PhD, professor of radiology, University of Washington, Seattle. His two-month study of 30 MS patients was published in the *Journal of Alternative and Complementary Medicine,* 140 Huguenot St., New Rochelle, NY 10801.

Multiple sclerosis (MS) symptoms can often be controlled with a wristwatch-sized device that emits brief magnetic pulses. MS patients who wore the *EnerMed* device for 10 to 24 hours a day for two months reported better bladder control, clearer thinking and more energy than similar patients who wore a placebo device.

Also: Hand function, mobility, sensation, muscle control and vision all improved for the Enermed group.

More information: Contact the manufacturer, Energy Medicine Developments, 888-363-7633, *www.enermed.com.*

Nausea Relief

Hillary Steinhart, MD, associate professor of medicine, University of Toronto, and head, combined division of gastroenterology, Mount Sinai Hospital, Toronto.

A battery-operated device worn on the wrist relieves seasickness, morning sickness, chemotherapy-related vomiting and post-surgical nausea. Called *ReliefBand*, the $130 device stimulates nerves in the wrist, keeping signals that trigger nausea from reaching the brain.

Only side effect: Tingling of the hand when the band is at higher settings.

Hidden Drug Dangers

Jack M. Rosenberg, PharmD, PhD, director of the International Drug Information Center at the Arnold and Marie Schwartz College of Pharmacy Health Sciences at Long Island University in Brooklyn, NY.

Over-the-counter (OTC) drugs can be purchased just as easily as a bottle of shampoo or a box of cereal—but that doesn't mean that they're harmless.

Few people realize that in some cases, OTC drugs contain the same amount of an active ingredient as that found in prescription medications. Using OTC drugs incorrectly—for example, taking them for too long or in excessive doses—can cause serious side effects.

Example I: People with arthritis often use OTC painkillers, such as *ibuprofen* (Advil) or *naproxen* (Aleve), for months or years—even though the label advises against taking these drugs for more than 10 consecutive days without consulting your doctor. The long-term use of such drugs greatly increases the risk for stomach bleeding as well as heart and/or kidney problems.

All OTC medications include a standardized "Drug Facts" label (on the outside of the packaging and also in an insert) that details the approved uses of the drug...active ingredients ...how to use it...and possible risks. The information is often confusing and printed in such small type that it's almost impossible to read.

Important: Read the OTC drug label *before* leaving the store. If you're purchasing from a drugstore, ask a pharmacist to explain any instructions that you don't understand.

What to look for...

ACTIVE INGREDIENT

This term refers to the medication that relieves symptoms. There might be dozens of drugs that have the same active ingredient.

What you may not know: Manufacturers occasionally change the active ingredients in OTC products.

Example: The antidiarrheal drug Kaopectate once contained *attapulgite*, a type of clay that is safe for patients taking blood-thinning medication. Kaopectate now contains *bismuth subsalicylate,* an aspirin-like ingredient that increases the risk for bleeding in patients taking blood thinners.

INACTIVE INGREDIENTS

This term refers to the chemicals that are used as preservatives, binders and colorants/flavors—but have no medical effects.

What you may not know: Some people are allergic to certain inactive ingredients.

Example: Hundreds of products, such as the OTC antihistamine *loratadine* (Alavert), contain the inactive ingredient lactose, which can trigger reactions in lactose-intolerant people.

USES

Known as "indications" on some labels, this term refers to the list of symptoms that a drug is designed to treat.

The US Food and Drug Administration (FDA) allows drug manufacturers to list only uses for which the medication has been proven to be safe and effective.

What you may not know: It can be risky to take drugs "off-label"—for uses other than the indications and/or directions found on the label.

Example: Taking high doses of the OTC B-vitamin niacin to lower cholesterol is an off-label use. Prescription niacin is approved for lowering cholesterol, but taking it without being monitored by your doctor can lead to liver damage.

WARNINGS

Many patients ignore the warnings on OTC medications because they assume the drugs must be safe or they wouldn't be sold without a prescription. Not true. OTC drugs can cause side effects that are just as serious as those caused by prescription drugs.

What you may not know: In addition to explaining the main risks of a medication, "warnings" may include information on who should not take the medication, when to consult your doctor if symptoms persist, when to take medications with foods (or when to avoid certain foods and beverages), whether it's safe to drive, etc.

Even if you've taken a particular OTC drug for years, check the warning label each time you purchase it. A drug that was safe when you first started taking it might cause problems if you now take other medications or if the ingredients or your health needs have changed. Always check the expiration date.

26

Stop the Presses

Nobel Prize Winner's Breakthrough—Prevent Heart Attack and Stroke With Nitric Oxide

Louis J. Ignarro, PhD
University of California at Los Angeles, School of Medicine

One tiny molecule produced by the body may do more than any drug to prevent heart attack and stroke. Nitric oxide, a gas that occurs naturally in the body, is critical for healthy circulation. It helps dilate blood vessels, prevent blood clots and regulate blood pressure, and it may inhibit the accumulation of arterial plaque.

HOW IT WORKS

Nitric oxide is a signaling molecule primarily produced by cells in the endothelium (inner lining) of blood vessels. A signaling molecule fits into docking sites (receptors) on cell walls and triggers biochemical reactions. *Nitric oxide helps prevent heart disease and stroke by...*

• **Expanding blood vessels.** Nitric oxide protects the blood vessels' smooth muscle tissue from harmful constriction, and this allows blood to circulate with less force. Some doctors report that elevating nitric oxide in hypertensive patients can lower blood pressure by 10 to 60 points.

• **Controlling platelet function.** Platelets, cell-like structures in blood that can clump up together, may form blood-blocking clots, the main cause of heart attack and stroke. A vascular network that is enhanced by nitric oxide sheds platelets and inhibits dangerous clots.

• **Reducing arterial plaque by 50%.** Arterial plaque, which consists of fatty deposits in the coronary arteries, is the underlying cause of heart disease. Nitric oxide is an antioxidant that inhibits the passage of monocytes, a type

---

Louis J. Ignarro, PhD, winner of the 1998 Nobel Prize in Physiology or Medicine for his research on nitric oxide. He is also a distinguished professor of pharmacology at the University of California at Los Angeles School of Medicine, and author of *No More Heart Disease*. St. Martin's.

of immune cell, into the artery wall. This in turn reduces the underlying inflammation that promotes plaque.

●**Lowering total cholesterol by 10% to 20%.** That's a modest decrease—but there's some evidence that nitric oxide is even more effective when combined with the cholesterol-lowering statins. Nitric oxide lowers cholesterol through its antioxidant activity. The preliminary research suggests that stimulating nitric oxide production in people who have elevated cholesterol makes it possible to lower their statin doses by at least 50%.

TO BOOST NITRIC OXIDE LEVELS

It is not yet known how much nitric oxide normally is present in the body or what levels are optimal. This gas is difficult to measure because it disappears almost instantly upon exposure to air. Research scientists can measure levels with electrodes inserted in blood vessels. Simpler tests are needed before doctors can measure nitric oxide as part of standard checkups.

Beginning in early adulthood, nitric oxide levels gradually decline, probably due to damage to the endothelial cells caused by such factors as a high-fat diet and a sedentary lifestyle.

Nitric oxide can't be taken in supplement form because it's a gas. However, patients can take other supplements that increase production of nitric oxide in the blood vessels. *These supplements, all available at health-food stores, have few if any side effects...*

●**L-arginine,** an amino acid found in meats, grains and fish, passes through the intestine into the blood. From the blood, it enters endothelial cells, where it is used to make nitric oxide.

A Mayo Clinic study found that people taking L-arginine showed significant improvement in endothelial function and blood flow compared with those taking placebos. It is hard to get sufficient L-arginine from food, so supplements are recommended.

Dose: 2,000 to 3,000 milligrams (mg) taken twice daily—for a total of 4,000 to 6,000 mg.

●**L-citrulline.** Supplemental arginine doesn't enter cells readily unless it is combined with L-citrulline, another amino acid. Melons and cucumbers are rich sources of L-citrulline, but

they don't provide high enough levels to significantly increase nitric oxide levels.

Dose: 400 to 600 mg daily.

●**Daily multivitamin that includes vitamin E.** Vitamin E helps reduce the assault of cell-damaging free radicals on the endothelial lining and may promote higher levels of nitric oxide. The amount of vitamin E that is in most multi-vitamin/mineral supplements is about 50 international units (IU), an effective dose.

Warning: Don't take the high-dose vitamin E supplements. Recent studies suggest that people who take daily doses of 400 IU or higher may be more susceptible to heart disease and other illnesses.

●**Vitamin C.** Like vitamin E, vitamin C will reduce oxidation in the blood vessels and may cause an increase in nitric oxide. People who consume high levels of vitamin C experience a reduction in arterial plaque, which is associated with higher levels of nitric oxide. You can get your vitamin C from food, but I recommend supplements because they are so convenient and easy to take.

Dose: 500 mg daily.

DIET AND EXERCISE

In addition to taking supplements, it is important to maintain a healthy lifestyle by watching what you eat and being active. *Try to...*

●**Do aerobic exercise for at least 20 minutes three days a week.** This stimulates endothelial cells to continuously produce nitric oxide, even on days that you don't exercise.

●**Minimize intake of saturated fat.** Saturated fat, found in such animal products as red meat, poultry, butter and whole milk, contributes to the accumulation of arterial plaque and impairs nitric oxide production.

Better: Olive oil, fish and flaxseed. The fats found in these foods help protect the endothelium by elevating levels of beneficial HDL cholesterol and lowering the harmful LDL form.

●**Eat more fiber.** The dietary fiber in grains, fruits and vegetables lowers blood pressure and LDL cholesterol and raises HDL, thereby protecting endothelial cells.

Bonus: Many of the foods that contain fiber also are rich in antioxidants, which inhibit the cell damage that lowers nitric oxide. Eat at least 25 grams (g) of fiber daily—and drink at least eight 8-ounce glasses of water each day to make sure that the fiber moves through your system properly.

How to Prevent a Heart Attack

Asim K. Duttaroy, PhD, professor of nutritional medicine, department of nutrition, University of Oslo, Norway.

People who ate two to three kiwi fruits daily for 28 days reduced their platelet aggregation response (potential for blood clot formation) by 18% and their blood triglyceride (fat) levels by 15% compared with people who ate no kiwi. The fruit is rich in polyphenols (antioxidant plant chemicals), vitamins C and E, magnesium, potassium and copper, all of which protect the blood vessels and heart. Kiwifruits are available in grocery stores year-round and can be peeled, sliced and added to green or fruit salads.

Five Little-Known Ways to Lower Heart Attack Risk

Michael Mogadam, MD, clinical associate professor of medicine at George Washington University School of Medicine in Washington, DC. He is author of *Every Heart Attack Is Preventable: How to Take Control of the 20 Risk Factors and Save Your Life*. New American Library.

Most Americans know all of the traditional heart disease risk factors—lack of physical activity, high cholesterol, high blood pressure, diabetes, obesity and smoking. Although these are important, there also are lesser-known risk factors. *Ways to avoid them...*

•**Boost your HDL level.** Though high LDL ("bad") cholesterol has long been considered the major culprit in heart attack risk, low HDL ("good") cholesterol actually is the bigger risk factor, especially in women. About 70% of women and half of all men with coronary artery disease (CAD) have low HDL cholesterol.

What to do: If you're a woman with HDL below 55 or a man with HDL below 45, take steps to boost your good cholesterol. Engaging in regular, vigorous exercise can raise HDL levels by 10% to 15%. Limiting carbohydrates to less than 45% of your daily diet and increasing monounsaturated fats (which are found in olive, canola and hazelnut oils) can raise HDL levels by 10%. Cholesterol-lowering statin drugs also may raise HDL levels by as much as 10%. Taking 1,500 milligrams (mg) of the B vitamin niacin under the supervision of a health-care provider can raise HDL by 25% to 30%.

Note: At high doses, niacin can cause side effects, such as flushing, liver problems and irregular heart rhythm.

Warning: Low-fat diets invariably lower HDL levels, which may actually *increase* heart attack risk. To ensure a healthy cholesterol ratio, don't simply eliminate fats from your diet. Monounsaturated and nonhydrogenated polyunsaturated fats should provide up to 30% of your total daily calories.

Good sources: Olive oil, canola oil, nuts and avocados.

•**Determine your LDL size.** LDL cholesterol particles come in two sizes—large (type A) and small (type B). A predominance of the type B particles increases risk of CAD by 300% to 500%, *even when LDL levels are normal* (less than 100).

Reason: Small LDL particles pass through the inner lining of coronary arteries more easily, possibly triggering a heart attack.

What to do: If you have low HDL cholesterol levels (below 45 for men and below 55 for women), particularly if any family members developed CAD before age 55, have your LDL particle size measured. This simple blood test is widely available, and many insurers now cover the cost.

The best way to decrease your type-B LDL count is to eat a healthful diet comprised of 30% fat, mostly in the form of monounsaturated fats, and limit carbohydrate intake to no more than 45% of total calories.

To boost your intake of beneficial omega-3 polyunsaturated fats, eat two to three seafood meals weekly. Choose the fattier fish, such as salmon and tuna.

Self-defense: Pregnant and lactating women should ask their doctors about limiting intake of fish due to its mercury content.

Avoid the trans-fatty acids and the omega-6 polyunsaturated fats found in margarine, fried foods, baked goods, corn and safflower oils.

●**Know your birth weight.** A low birth weight is a significant and independent risk factor for heart attack, hypertension and diabetes in adulthood. Research has shown that people who weighed less than 5.5 pounds at birth are three times more likely to develop CAD than people who weighed more than 7.5 pounds at birth.

What to do: Tell your doctor if you had a low birth weight (less than 5.5 pounds)—and show him/her this article. Many health-care providers are unaware of the increased risks associated with low birth weight.

If you were a very small baby, ask your doctor to test regularly for other coronary risk factors, such as hypertension, elevated cholesterol, diabetes and LDL particle size. These factors should be treated aggressively to offset the unalterable risk of low birth weight.

●**Choose heart-healthy beverages.** The heart-protective benefits of alcohol have been well-established. When consumed in moderation (one glass daily for women and no more than two glasses daily for men), wine, beer and mixed drinks reduce CAD by 30%.

Researchers now are discovering that water also may play a role in preventing heart attack. Physicians at Loma Linda University recently reported that drinking five or more glasses of water daily (versus two or fewer) reduces fatal heart attack risk in men by 51% and in women by 35%.

Water seems to protect against heart attacks by making blood less likely to clot. Minerals in hard tap water, such as calcium and magnesium, also may help guard against heart disease.

What to do: Drink from six to eight 8-ounce glasses of water daily. Ask your local water utility if your water is hard (mineral rich) or soft.

Even soft water from the tap may be a healthier choice than filtered bottled waters, which are generally stripped entirely of minerals.

Helpful: Consider installing a faucet-mounted home water filter that removes waterborne parasites from your water but doesn't filter out the beneficial minerals.

Good brands: Moen and Culligan.

●**Take folic acid.** This B vitamin has been shown to lower levels of homocysteine, a protein in the blood that significantly increases risk for cardiovascular disease when it is elevated. Folic acid also lowers the risk for heart attack and stroke.

In continuing research of more than 80,000 nurses, the risk for heart attack was reduced by about 6% for every additional 100 micrograms of folic acid in their diet.

What to do: Eat more folic acid-rich foods, such as spinach, asparagus, lima beans, wheat germ and fortified cereals. If your homocysteine level is greater than 9, you may need to take a folic acid supplement daily.

How to Predict Heart Disease

Karen L. Margolis, MD, associate professor of medicine, University of Minnesota, Minneapolis.

In a study of more than 72,000 women without infection, those who had the highest levels of white blood cells (WBCs)—6,700 to 15,000—were twice as likely to die from heart disease as women with the lowest levels. Researchers believe this link also applies to men.

Theory: WBC levels, which typically rise in response to infection, also can be a marker for inflammation, which weakens blood vessels and may trigger blockages leading to heart attack or stroke.

Self-defense: Request a WBC count with your next blood test. A level above 6,700 may indicate increased heart disease risk.

Cheap, Safe and More Effective than Statins

Jay S. Cohen, MD, adjunct associate professor (voluntary) of family and preventive medicine, University of California, San Diego. He is author of *What You Must Know About Statin Drugs and Their Natural Alternatives* (Square One) and *Over Dose: The Case Against the Drug Companies* (Tarcher-Putnam). *www.medicationsense.com.*

First it was on the market, then it was off the market, now it's back on the market. In recent years, the cholesterol-lowering natural supplement *red yeast rice* has sparked many battles among the pharmaceutical companies, the US Food and Drug Administration (FDA) and supplement manufacturers. But in the face of the ongoing controversy regarding statin drugs and how low cholesterol should be, it is good to know about all the options. Red yeast rice is one worth considering.

ABOUT THE CONTROVERSY

In 1998, the FDA yanked red yeast rice, or *monascus purpureus*, from supplement shelves because it contains a natural form of *lovastatin*, the same active ingredient in the patented drug Mevacor. The issue was supposedly one of safety, with prescription statin manufacturers claiming that red yeast rice was an unapproved drug rather than a dietary supplement.

The truth, according to Jay S. Cohen, MD, adjunct associate professor (voluntary) of family and preventive medicine at the University of California in San Diego, is that red yeast rice can naturally lower cholesterol levels in the body with fewer side effects and at a considerably lower cost than prescription statins.

However, the FDA didn't see it that way and got onboard with the drug companies. Was red yeast rice taken off the market because of the health risk or because of pharmaceutical company pressures? Or both? Only the FDA knows for sure.

Although the FDA removed it from the market ostensibly to protect the public, critics charge that it really was the pharmaceutical industry that was being protected from competition from a safer and less-expensive product.

In 1999, a federal judge lifted the ban on red yeast rice products, and today they are available at quality health-food stores.

ASIA'S NATURAL CHOLESTEROL BUSTER

Red yeast rice is made simply by fermenting red yeast on rice. It is commonly consumed as part of the traditional cuisine in China as well as other Asian countries, where people have long believed that it strengthens the heart and circulatory system. Used as a natural food flavoring and coloring agent, it is the ingredient that gives Peking duck its deep red color.

A study at UCLA School of Medicine confirmed red yeast rice's natural cholesterol-busting abilities. In a rigorous double-blind, randomized trial, this supplement significantly reduced total cholesterol compared with a placebo. Among 83 people who took red yeast rice for 12 weeks, total cholesterol dropped by an average of 16% (from approximately 250 to 210)...cholesterol remained at about 250 in the 41 people who were given a placebo. There also was a positive impact on LDL cholesterol and triglyceride levels.

A SAFER ALTERNATIVE

Red yeast rice is a good alternative for people who need mild to moderate cholesterol control but don't want to take statin drugs, says Dr. Cohen. It contains a wide array of cholesterol-lowering compounds, including lovastatin, but all in tiny amounts. This can make it safer than statin drugs and their array of potentially serious side effects, such as liver problems, muscle damage, joint pain, abdominal discomfort and even cognitive or memory problems. According to Dr. Cohen, these effects generally are underestimated and downplayed by the pharmaceutical companies.

EXERCISE CAUTION

Although the amount of lovastatin in red yeast rice is small, it still requires monitoring. Don't take red yeast rice without telling your doctor, and while you are taking it, get checked regularly for liver or muscle problems. Red yeast rice is available in different dosages. The usual recommendation is 1,200 milligrams (mg) daily, divided into two doses. Do not take more than 2,400 mg daily. To reduce the risk for digestive disturbance, take with food.

Some recommendations from the informative manual, *The Physicians' Desk Reference* (*www.pdrhealth.com*)...

●**Do not take red yeast rice if you have liver disease** or are at risk of developing it, or if you drink more than two alcoholic beverages a day.

●**Do not take this supplement if you are pregnant** or breast-feeding.

●**Do not take red yeast rice if you have a serious infection** or after major surgery.

●**If you develop any muscle pain,** tenderness or twitching, stop using it and consult your doctor.

●**Do not combine red yeast rice with prescription cholesterol-lowering drugs.**

The bottom line? Statins have powerful side effects. Red yeast rice may be a safer alternative for people with mild to moderately high cholesterol. Should you want to try it, it is best to do it under the watchful eye of a physician trained in herbal remedies.

There are many other natural supplements that are helpful for high cholesterol, including plant sterols, inositol hexaniacinate (no-flush niacin), fiber, policosanol, guggulipid, soy and garlic.

The Supplement that Slashes Cholesterol 54% Better than Statins

Bottom Line's Prescription Alternatives by Earl L. Mindell, RPh, PhD. Bottom Line Books.

Supplements containing policosanol have been found to work well to balance cholesterol counts. Biochemically speaking, policosanol is made up of a series of what's known as fatty alcohols. If you want to know what these *fatty alcohols* naturally look and feel like, scrape a little bit of the waxy film off the leaves of a tree or the peel of a citrus fruit. Commercially sold policosanol supplements are usually made from either sugarcane or beeswax. Citrus peels, wheat germ and caviar are other rich sources of policosanol.

Policosanol has been shown to lower LDL cholesterol levels by up to 20%, and it raises HDL by an average of 10%—without the side effects caused by statins. As a matter of fact, in a study of nearly 28,000 people who used policosanol for two to four years, less than half of 1% of the subjects experienced notable adverse effects from their daily dose.

In one study, published in a recent issue of the journal *Gynecology and Endocrinology*, researchers enlisted 244 menopausal women for whom six weeks on a conventional cholesterol-lowering diet did no good. The women were given either a placebo pill or 5 milligrams (mg) of policosanol each day for 12 weeks. The women given policosanol were then given 10 mg for 12 more weeks. By the end of the study, the policosanol users had some amazing changes in their cholesterol levels: Their LDL fell by 25.2%, their total cholesterol fell by 16.7% and their ratio of total cholesterol to HDL fell by 27.2%!

Another study—this one from the *International Journal of Clinical Pharmacology*—compared the effects of policosanol with those of pravastatin, a commonly used statin drug, in elderly patients with high cholesterol and high risk of heart attack. These patients took 10 mg of policosanol or pravastatin for eight weeks. Those who took policosanol lowered their LDL by an average of 19.3%...their total cholesterol by an average of 13.9%...and their ratio of total cholesterol to HDL by 24.4%. Pravastatin reduced LDL by only 15.6% and the total cholesterol to HDL ratio by 15.9%, but didn't raise levels of artery-cleaning HDL. In this study, policosanol also stood out for its ability to inhibit the tendency of blood to clot together and clog blood vessels.

Policosanol causes none of the adverse effects statins can cause. It appears to work by slowing the production of cholesterol in the liver while increasing the liver's ability to reabsorb LDL. The most frequently cited side effect? Weight loss—not exactly an undesirable side effect for most people at risk of developing heart disease. Unlike statins, policosanol causes no decrease in libido, and there's a hint of evidence from an animal study that it may actually *increase* libido slightly! Policosanol also inhibits the oxidation of LDL cholesterol, the free radical attack that makes LDL so much more dangerous to blood vessel health. In animal studies, it decreased the uncontrolled inflammation and cell growth known to lead to artery disease. Policosanol also helps to thin the blood, decreasing the chances of a clot forming to plug up an artery and cause a heart attack or stroke.

Levels of a specific type of proinflammatory biochemical called *thromboxane* can rise too high as a direct result of a poor, refined-food diet, and can cause artery walls to clamp down tight, decreasing blood and oxygen flow to the heart and elsewhere. Some studies have shown a decrease in levels of this type of thromboxane with policosanol.

Breakthrough Therapies For Heart Disease, Cancer —and Varicose Veins

Jeff Geschwind, MD, associate professor of radiology, oncology and surgery at Johns Hopkins University School of Medicine, and director of cardiovascular and interventional radiology at the Johns Hopkins Hospital, both in Baltimore.

Heiko Schöder, MD, assistant attending physician at Memorial Sloan-Kettering Cancer Center and assistant professor of radiology at Weill Medical College of Cornell University, both in New York City.

Sheldon Sheps, MD, cardiologist and emeritus professor of medicine at the Mayo Clinic College of Medicine, Rochester, MN.

Sophisticated radiologic treatments—like high-speed computed tomography (CT) scans—now are being used both as an alternative to traditional surgery and as a new diagnostic tool for a number of common ailments.

Typically administered by interventional radiologists, these treatments are available at most medical centers across the US.*

Three leading experts discuss these new therapies below...

*Interventional radiologists specialize in minimally invasive treatments that use image-guided techniques. To find such a specialist in your area, consult the Society of Interventional Radiology (800-488-7284, *www.sirweb.org*).

CANCER TREATMENT
Jeff Geschwind, MD

When surgical removal of a malignancy of the liver, kidneys, bone or other organs is not an option, due to the size or location of the tumor, patients may now receive a new therapy called *radiofrequency ablation.*

What's involved: An interventional radiologist uses an ultrasound to locate the tumor. A needle is then placed through the skin directly into the malignancy. A radiofrequency current is emitted through the needle to burn away the tumor without damaging any surrounding tissue. The treatment typically takes one to three hours and can be performed as an outpatient procedure, without general anesthesia.

Typical cost: $13,000 to $20,000.

Important: Radiofrequency ablation is only appropriate for the smaller malignancies— that is, tumors no larger than 3 to 4 centimeters (cm) in diameter. This procedure is not a cure for cancer but can be used to help control it.

VARICOSE VEINS

Approximately 25% of all American women and 10% of American men suffer from varicose veins. These will occur when a vein's emptying mechanisms malfunction, resulting in reflux (the pooling of blood), most often in the legs or pelvis. Besides being unsightly, varicose veins also can lead to chronic pain.

A new image-guided technique called *vein ablation,* done with radiofrequency or laser heat, now makes it easier to destroy varicose veins without surgery or the injection of chemical solutions.

What's involved: Guided by ultrasound, the radiologist threads a small catheter into the varicose vein. The laser is then fired briefly, which heats and seals the vein. The treatment takes less than an hour, and the patient is up and walking 20 minutes later.

Typical cost: $2,000 to $3,000 per leg.

Another new technique uses image-guided therapy to eliminate varicose veins in the pelvis. Some nine million American women suffer from unexplained chronic pelvic pain.

Pelvic congestion syndrome is a condition that has traditionally been very difficult to diagnose and thought to be untreatable. Doctors now believe that many of these cases are caused by varicose veins in the pelvis.

A *venogram* allows doctors to identify varicose veins in the pelvis. During this procedure, a catheter is inserted and threaded through the affected vein, and an X-ray dye is injected to highlight the vein. An X ray is then taken. Next, small steel coils are implanted to block blood flow through the abnormal vein. This causes the varicose veins to shrivel and disappear.

Typical cost: $7,000.

MALIGNANCY DETECTION
Heiko Schöder, MD

A new technology, known as PET-CT fusion, allows doctors to pinpoint the precise location of cancer cells in the body (for all types of cancer) without having to rely on additional imaging procedures and examinations. The positron emission tomography (PET) locates the small lesions, and the CT scan then precisely pinpoints them.

What's involved: The patient first undergoes a CT scan, a computer-enhanced X-ray study that produces two-dimensional images. Then the patient undergoes a PET scan. For this test, a radioactive substance that's called a "tracer" is injected into a vein. The patient next is placed inside a ring-shaped PET scanner, which detects radiation and records sites of high activity, where cancer is likely to be present. The two tests take about one-half hour to perform. Afterward, the radiologist "fuses" the results of a PET scan with the detailed anatomical images of a CT scan.

Typical cost: $2,000 to $4,000 for both.

A study at Memorial Sloan-Kettering Cancer Center found that the use of combined scans improved accuracy by 42% when diagnosing the location of tumors of the head and neck.

CORONARY ARTERY DISEASE
Sheldon Sheps, MD

A new five-minute, noninvasive imaging test known as an *electron beam* CT (EBCT) heart scan assesses the amount of calcium in your coronary arteries. Because calcium is a major component of arterial plaque, a high coronary calcium level indicates significant plaque buildup in the blood vessels.

What's involved: A cardiologist or radiologist uses the recently developed ultrafast-CT scanner that provides detailed pictures of your heart. The procedure exposes the patient to relatively low levels of radiation.

Typical cost: $400.

A heart scan provides a quick and accurate assessment of heart attack risk without the potential risks associated with an angiogram, in which a catheter is used to inject a dye into the heart that can be seen on X rays.

Surprising Stroke Risks Even Doctors Overlook

Gregory W. Albers, MD, professor of neurology and neurological sciences at Stanford University Medical Center and director of the Stanford Stroke Center. He also is chairman of the American College of Chest Physicians' expert panel for both stroke and atrial fibrillation, cochairman of the National Stroke Association's Stroke Center Network and chairman of the American Heart Association's Metro Stroke Task Force.

Stroke is the second most common cause of brain damage (after Alzheimer's disease) and the third most common cause of death (after heart attack and cancer).

Most of us know that risk of stroke can be reduced by controlling high blood pressure and cholesterol, eating a well-balanced diet and exercising on a regular basis. But it is what you may *not* know about this disabling disorder that could save your life.

Often overlooked stroke risks...

PREHYPERTENSION

Until just recently, blood pressure less than 140/90 was considered normal. However, studies now indicate that a reading of 120/80 or higher raises the risk for stroke and should be treated with a combination of exercise, diet and medication, if needed.

What you may not know: Although diuretics, beta blockers and ACE inhibitors have long been utilized to lower blood pressure, recent research reveals that a newer class of antihypertensive medication, called angiotensin II receptor blockers (ARBs), may provide unique protection against stroke.

Recent study: An ARB known as *losartan* (Cozaar) reduced stroke risk by an additional 25% over the beta blocker *atenolol* (Tenormin). Several large trials are under way to further study ARBs. If the results are as promising as this preliminary one, ARBs could become the antihypertensive medication of choice for preventing stroke.

Bonus: ARBs cause fewer side effects than other blood pressure medications.

Self-defense: If you take blood pressure-lowering medication, ask your physician if an ARB would be appropriate for you.

ATRIAL FIBRILLATION

This heart rhythm disturbance affects two million Americans. With atrial fibrillation (AF), the upper chambers of the heart quiver rapidly or irregularly and fail to pump efficiently.

What you may not know: Each year, up to 70,000 strokes are caused by AF. During AF, some patients experience a racing heart, palpitations or a fluttering in their chest, dizziness and/or shortness of breath. For other patients, the first symptom of AF may be a stroke.

Self-defense: To determine if you may have AF, put your index finger on your wrist and check your pulse for an irregular or random rhythm. AF can be confirmed with a routine electrocardiogram (EKG).

If you are diagnosed with AF, your doctor may prescribe an antiarrhythmic medication, such as *digoxin* (Lanoxin) or *amiodarone* (Cordarone), or a type of electric shock, known as cardioversion, to correct the arrhythmia.

However, the recurrence rate for AF is high with these therapies. It is usually preferable to choose a treatment that prevents blood clots, rather than focusing on the heart rhythm disturbance. Lifetime use of anticoagulants can reduce stroke risk in AF patients by 68%.

The most frequently prescribed anticoagulant, *warfarin* (Coumadin), is extremely effective at preventing clots and reducing stroke risk in people with AF. Unfortunately, it has a narrow "therapeutic index"—slightly too much in your system can cause bleeding…slightly too little will permit stroke.

Warfarin also interacts with other drugs, supplements and even foods.

Example: Vitamin K, which is found in the leafy greens and margarine, counteracts the effects of warfarin.

Because warfarin interferes with so many common substances, people taking it need to undergo monthly blood tests…and physicians must adjust the dosage frequently. As a result, less than half of AF patients who should take Coumadin actually do.

The anticoagulant called *ximelagatran* (Exanta) looked promising as a way to revolutionize stroke and blood clot prevention. However, it was recently withdrawn from the market due to reports of serious liver problems in a clinical trial.

LEG PAIN

Just as atherosclerosis can narrow blood vessels to the heart and brain, it also can block arteries in the extremities, causing peripheral artery disease (PAD). Leg pain—especially in the calves—is the chief symptom. Known as intermittent claudication, the pain typically begins with walking and ends when you stop. PAD affects up to 20% of Americans who are age 65 or older.

What you may not know: If you have PAD, you also may have atherosclerosis elsewhere in the body, such as the heart or the brain. This puts you at increased risk for stroke. What's more, you also can have "silent," or asymptomatic, PAD. Risk factors for PAD are the same as those for cardiovascular disease—high blood pressure, high cholesterol, diabetes, smoking, age, etc.

Self-defense: PAD is easily and painlessly diagnosed with an ankle brachial index test, which measures the ratio of blood pressure in the arm and ankle.

If you're diagnosed with PAD, your physician might prescribe an antiplatelet medication, such as aspirin or *clopidogrel* (Plavix). Moderate exercise to reduce leg pain and blood pressure or cholesterol-lowering medications also may be recommended.

SLEEP APNEA

This disorder occurs when breathing is temporarily interrupted during sleep. An estimated 24% of men and 9% of women suffer from significant sleep apnea.

What you may not know: People with sleep apnea are three to six times more likely to suffer a stroke. Their blood pressure increases dramatically during the night, which can raise the risk for atherosclerotic blockages of the carotid—or neck—arteries, and this is a chief cause of stroke.

In one recent study involving men ages 45 to 77, more than 21% of patients with sleep apnea had calcified plaques, which block blood flow, in their carotid arteries. Only 2.5% of the healthy control patients had calcified plaques.

Self-defense: Obesity is the leading risk factor for sleep apnea...and loud snoring and excessive daytime sleepiness are telltale signs. If you suspect you may have sleep apnea, consult your physician about diagnosis and the best treatment options.

Caution: It's important for AF patients who have symptoms of sleep apnea to undergo sleep apnea screening. Mayo Clinic researchers recently reported that AF is twice as likely to recur in patients with untreated sleep apnea.

Latest Developments In Stroke Rehab

Michael Reding, MD, associate professor of neurology at Weill Medical College of Cornell University, New York City. He is director of stroke rehabilitation at the Burke Rehabilitation Hospital, White Plains, NY.

Most stroke patients require rehabilitation to recover their physical skills and to regain the ability to live independently. Recent developments in stroke rehabilitation are helping patients recover better and faster, sometimes even several years after the stroke.

The following therapies are the latest approaches to stroke recovery. Check with the stroke centers located in your area about what is available.

ARMS AND LEGS

Stroke patients often require physical therapy for arm or leg weakness or immobility. Repetitive physical movements prevent muscle atrophy and enhance the brain cells in the area surrounding the stroke damage. *Breakthrough therapies...*

•**Robotic therapy.** MIT researchers have developed the tabletop robot MIT-Manus, which significantly improves arm mobility—and may be more effective than conventional physical therapy.

How it works: The patient puts his/her lower arm and wrist into a brace attached to the robot. A video screen prompts the patient to perform arm exercises, such as connecting dots on the screen. The robot monitors movement and increases or decreases resistance as required—and even moves the arm if the patient is unable to do so. The robot can move the arm thousands of times in a single session and detects (and responds to) movements and muscle tension that are too subtle for the patient to notice.

Patients who use robotic therapy have muscle strength scores that are about twice as high as those undergoing traditional physical therapy.

Most patients enjoy the interactive nature of this "video game" therapy. It gives immediate feedback and boosts their motivation to keep trying. Between 18 and 36 sessions are needed.

•**Bilateral arm training with rhythmic auditory cueing (BATRAC).** When patients move both the damaged arm and the healthy arm together (bilateral movement), the healthy side of the brain promotes better functioning in the side damaged by stroke.

How it works: The patient works with an occupational therapist for about an hour several days a week. He performs movements to the beat of a metronome or other auditory device. He moves both arms simultaneously—for example, moving arms away from the body, then moving them back in. Early studies indicate that patients treated with BATRAC have greater improvements in upper-extremity motor function than those who are treated with conventional therapy.

●**Constraint-induced movement therapy.** When a stroke victim has trouble moving a limb, damage to the brain's sensory cortex may cause him to lose awareness of that hand, arm or leg—and he stops moving it entirely.

How it works: In constraint-induced therapy, placing the healthy limb in a sling forces the patient to use the disabled limb, thereby facilitating the regaining of movement control. This approach requires the patient to practice for up to six hours a day for several weeks. He might be asked to pick up a block of wood, sweep floors, throw balls or draw pictures repeatedly.

The therapy is performed in a clinic setting, often in groups to encourage participation and enhance motivation.

Studies show that this approach results in improvements in motor function and muscle strength.

WALKING

Patients who are in conventional rehabilitation programs typically use canes or leg braces for support.

For safety reasons, they walk slowly, and they may not reach their optimal level of recovery.

●**Body weight support.** With body weight support, patients can more than double their speed. Faster walking hastens recovery and prepares patients for the types of movements they will need in daily life, such as quickly crossing a street.

How it works: The patient is suspended in a harness attached to a weight-support system. The harness prevents the patient from falling, so he can increase the speed of the treadmill and push himself harder. The harness adjusts to support more or less of the patient's body weight, depending on his progress.

SWALLOWING

Many patients experience difficulty swallowing (dysphagia). Traditionally, speech therapists teach patients how to initiate normal swallowing movements.

●**VitalStim therapy.** Electrical stimulation applied to the neck causes the muscles that are involved in swallowing to activate at the appropriate times. This approach is effective in as little as one week.

How it works: Electrodes are placed on the neck. Electrical currents stimulate muscles in the throat to contract. The treatment, lasting 20 to 30 minutes, may be repeated 10 or more times over a week. It retrains the brain to stimulate involuntary swallowing movements.

Drawbacks: This does not work for all patients. Many require speech therapy sessions. Also, the treatment may be uncomfortable—it causes a feeling of tightness in the neck, as though one is being grabbed by the throat.

VISION

●**Visual retraining.** Stroke victims who experience vision damage can gain significant improvement from a technique called visual retraining, or vision restoration therapy.

How it works: The patient fixes his eyes on a spot on a monitor, then clicks a button when he becomes aware that another dot has appeared in the periphery. This stimulates neurons in the visual center of the brain. Sessions usually are 30 minutes, twice daily, for six months.

A study presented at the American Stroke Association International Conference reported that patients were able to detect 62% of the peripheral dots after six months, compared with 54% when they began. Follow-up studies show that 70% of patients maintain the improvement more than a year later.

BEWARE OF DEPRESSION

Depression is common in stroke patients in the first year.

One study found that patients who suffer poststroke depression are 3.5 times more likely to die within 10 years than those who aren't depressed.

Stroke patients should be evaluated for depression and, if diagnosed, given appropriate treatment, which can include psychotherapy and/or antidepressants. Treatment can greatly improve patients' motivation and increase their rate of recovery.

Cancer Vaccines Offer New Hope

Michael Morse, MD, associate professor of medicine in the division of medical oncology at the Duke University Medical Center, Durham, NC. He is editor of *Handbook of Cancer Vaccines* (Humana) and has published more than 150 scientific papers, book chapters and abstracts on immunotherapy and has developed several cancer vaccinations.

Until recently, cancer treatment was limited to three options—surgery, chemotherapy and/or radiation.

Now: Cancer *vaccines* are a promising new treatment for virtually all types of malignancies.

To learn more, we spoke with Michael Morse, MD, a medical oncologist and leading authority on cancer vaccines…

●**Is the idea of cancer vaccines new?** Not at all. In the 1700s, it was observed that people with tumors occasionally improved after they experienced an infection. Then, more than a century ago, William Coley, a New York surgeon, identified a patient who had an incurable sarcoma (cancer of the bone, muscle or other supportive tissue) but who experienced a significant reduction of the sarcoma after contracting a skin infection.

Coley then tried treating some patients by injecting them—and their tumors—with a fluid in which two types of bacteria were grown. This was called Coley toxin, which artificially induced inflammation in cancer patients and resulted in an improvement in 40% of patients and a cure in 10%. This treatment, nonspecific *immunotherapy*, activates the immune system in a general way.

In the last 20 years, immunotherapy for cancer, using vaccines to activate the immune system in a specific way, has become an important field of cancer research.

●**How do cancer vaccines work?** Cancer vaccines aren't like vaccines for viral diseases, such as influenza. Although they do not currently *prevent* cancer, we do hope that one day they will. Rather, they use various methods to stimulate the cells of the immune system to attack cancer cells.

A cancer vaccine uses an *antigen*, a protein-based derivative from a tumor. Once inside the body, the antigen is taken up by *dendritic cells*, sentinel-like immune cells that break up the antigen and represent it in a form that T-cells can recognize. These T-cells are stimulated by the dendritic cells to then divide into large numbers and to acquire the capacity to recognize and destroy harmful tumor cells.

Our goal is to trigger the immune system to produce an abundance of these "smart" T-cells that can work to eliminate the malignancy.

●**What kinds of cancer can the vaccines fight?** Virtually every type of cancer has been studied in a clinical trial, including brain cancer. Many of these trials have been conducted with patients who have metastatic, or advanced, disease.

Vaccines also are being used in "adjuvant" settings—in a person who has had a tumor and has a high risk of recurrence. For example, a patient who has been surgically treated for breast cancer may subsequently receive chemotherapy, hormonal therapy *and* a cancer vaccine in a clinical trial to discover if immunotherapy helps make the other two treatments more successful in preventing a recurrence.

Many of these adjuvant studies are focused on melanoma, a deadly skin cancer, because it is thought to be more susceptible to the immune system's attack.

●**How successful are cancer vaccines?** Studies show that 3% to 5% of solid tumors, such as those found in the lung, breast or prostate, shrink after the use of a cancer vaccine.

In nonsolid, or hematological, cancers, such as leukemias and lymphomas, the response rate is slightly higher, because of the unique antigens in these types of cancers.

These success rates may sound low, but there's reason to be optimistic. Many studies report that a patient whose immune system is successfully activated by the vaccine either lives longer or experiences slower growth of the cancer than someone whose immune system is not successfully activated.

A recent study of the vaccine Theratope, used for breast cancer, did not show a positive result overall but did show benefit in a subgroup of women who were taking hormone therapy, mostly the drug *tamoxifen* (Nolvadex). The median overall survival for patients taking hormonal therapy who received Theratope was 36.5 months, compared with 30.7 months for those who received the control vaccine. Further clinical trials will focus on the effectiveness of cancer vaccines in these and other subgroups.

Before long, we may learn the best way to give dozens of specifically targeted vaccines to help many kinds of patients.

Researchers also have reason for cautious optimism because these vaccines do work—they generate T-cells that recognize and fight cancer. Before cancer vaccinations, there were fewer such T-cells.

Even when tumors do not significantly shrink, cancer patients who have an immune response to vaccines have had longer periods before the cancer worsened than non-vaccine patients, and they have survived longer.

●**Are cancer vaccines toxic?** No, not in the same way that chemotherapy can be toxic. Using a vaccine to stimulate the immune system might be thought of as a "natural" way to treat cancer. It does not have the same side effects as those caused by chemotherapy and radiation, but it can cause fevers, allergic reactions and autoimmune disorders.

Cancer patients consider vaccines non-toxic, and that's one reason why they are so excited about the prospect of this treatment.

●**How can people with cancer find out** about the availability of cancer vaccines? Cancer vaccines are being tested but are not yet available as part of the standard treatment regimen offered by cancer specialists.

However, there are more than 150 ongoing clinical trials involving cancer vaccines. Talk to your oncologist about cancer vaccines to see if this treatment might be available and right for you.

For more information on clinical trials for cancer vaccines, contact the National Cancer Institute, 800-422-6237, *www.cancer.gov/clinical trials.*

Skin Cancer: Debunking the Myths

Barney J. Kenet, MD, a dermatologist specializing in skin cancer. Dr. Kenet is a dermatologic surgeon at New York–Presbyterian Hospital/Cornell Medical Center in New York City, and is coauthor (with Patricia Lawler) of Saving Your Skin—Prevention, Early Detection, and Treatment of Melanoma and Other Skin Cancers. *Four Walls Eight Windows.*

Everyone knows that excessive sun exposure is dangerous, yet up to 50% of people over age 65 are diagnosed with melanoma or some other type of skin cancer.

Why? Even health-savvy individuals remain confused about the best ways to adequately protect their skin.

Most dangerous myths…

Myth #1: **A beach umbrella keeps you safe from the sun.**

Reality: When you're at the beach, a large percentage of ultraviolet (UV) light bounces off the sand onto your skin, even when you are beneath an umbrella. Water and snow have the same reflective effect.

When boating or sitting beneath a beach umbrella, apply a sunscreen to all the exposed areas, including your face and neck—even if you're wearing a brimmed hat. When skiing, apply sunscreen to your face and neck.

Myth #2: **Sunscreen with a sun-protection factor (SPF) of 45 is three times more effective than SPF 15.**

Reality: Most doctors recommend using a sunscreen with an SPF of at least 15. A higher SPF will not give you much additional protection. A sunscreen that has an SPF of 45 is only about 5% more protective than an SPF 15 sunscreen. The higher-rated sunscreen doesn't last any longer, either.

All sunscreens need to be reapplied every two hours—and whenever you're exposed to water. This includes "waterproof" sunscreens, which provide some protection while swimming but still must be reapplied.

Make sure your sunscreen is labeled "broad spectrum"—meaning that it blocks both ultraviolet A (UVA) and ultraviolet B (UVB) rays. Look for titanium dioxide or Parsol 1789 in the listing of ingredients.

Myth #3: **Sunscreen provides complete sun protection.**

Reality: While sunscreen is essential, there are other steps you also should take. The most important is to minimize sun exposure between 10 am and 4 pm, when the sun's rays are most intense. Hit the beach in the early morning or late afternoon instead.

To protect the commonly neglected areas, be sure to wear…

• UV-protective lip balm with an SPF of 15 or higher.

• A hat with a three-inch brim. Baseball caps don't protect the ears or the back of the neck—common skin cancer sites, especially for golf and tennis players.

• UV-protective sunglasses. UV exposure can cause cataracts.

• Sun-protective clothing. UV rays can pass through many fabrics, including cotton. If you hold a garment up to a light and can see the shape of the bulb shining through, it's not providing adequate sun protection.

Many companies offer lightweight, tightly woven garments designed for comfort and maximum protection.

Example: Solumbra 30+ SPF sun protective clothing (800-882-7860, *www.sunprecautions.com*).

If you will be outdoors and don't have special clothing, be sure to wear sunscreen under your shirt.

Myth #4: **Family history is the best indication of skin cancer risk.**

Reality: A family history of skin cancer is a major risk factor—but the most important factor is your own skin type. People who have light-colored skin and eyes (blue or green) and freckles are at highest risk for all types of skin cancer and sun-related skin damage, such as wrinkles.

People with many moles, freckles and spots have the next-highest cancer risk, followed by individuals with a family history of skin cancer. If you have any of these risk factors, you need to carefully monitor your sun exposure.

When the skin is exposed to sunlight, it increases the body's production of *melanin*, the main skin pigment. This results in tanning, in which a brown color is imparted to the skin.

The more difficult it is for you to tan, the more vulnerable you are to skin cancer.

If you're dark-skinned, tan easily, don't have many moles and have no family history of skin cancer, your risk is low but you should still protect yourself from the sun.

Myth #5: **Building a "base" tan protects against sunburn.**

Reality: There is no such thing as a "safe" tan. UV exposure increases lifetime risk of skin cancer and other skin damage. Rather than expose yourself to those pre-vacation rays, protect yourself by following the rules described in this article.

Myth #6: **"Self-tanning" products help protect against sunburn.**

Reality: Self-tanning products are perfectly safe and are a good way to appear tan without any sun exposure. However, the dyes in these products do not offer UV protection. Some of these products do contain sunblock—but this provides only two hours of protection following application.

Myth #7: **Melanoma occurs only where the skin has been exposed to the sun.**

Reality: Sun exposure is just one of the potential causes of melanoma. For unknown reasons, cancerous moles can also develop under the arm, between the buttocks or toes or on the bottom of the foot. If you have a mole, spot or freckle *anywhere* on your body that shows a sudden change in size, shape or color, get it checked by a dermatologist.

Myth #8: **Melanoma is always deadly.**

Reality: When limited to the top layers of the skin, melanoma has a cure rate of 100%. That's why it's important to do a monthly self-exam of all skin surfaces, using a full-length and a handheld mirror.

You should also get screened annually by a dermatologist (twice a year, if you have skin cancer risk factors). During the screening, the doctor should use *epiluminescence microscopy* (ELM). This new technique, which involves examining moles with a handheld microscope, detects melanoma earlier than ever.

Prostate Cancer Fighter

Peter J. Ferguson, PhD, research associate, London Regional Cancer Program, London, Ontario, Canada.

In laboratory experiments, disease-fighting flavonoids found in cranberries destroyed human prostate cancer cells.

Theory: Flavonoids interfere with the signals that tell cancer cells to proliferate. More research is under way to confirm these findings.

In the meantime, eat homemade cranberry sauce, snack on whole dried cranberries (sold in supermarkets) and/or drink 100% cranberry juice.

Best Herb for Male Urinary Tract Problems

Andrew L. Rubman, ND, director, Southbury Clinic for Traditional Medicines, Southbury, CT, and consulting medical editor for *Bottom Line's Daily Health News*.

Whole saw palmetto extract might work even better than standard saw palmetto extract for male urinary tract problems. But, be sure to see a doctor formally trained in botanical medicine before trying any of the herbal medications.

Recommended: The Eclectic Institute's fresh freeze-dried berry extract, Serenoa serrulata (800-332-4372, *www.eclecticherb.com*).

Longevity Boosters From the World's Longest-Lived People

Bradley J. Willcox, MD, principal investigator of geriatrics, Pacific Health Research Institute, Honolulu, HI and assistant professor of geriatrics, University of Hawaii. He is also coauthor of *The Okinawa Program: How the World's Longest-Lived People Achieve Everlasting Health—and How You Can Too*. Three Rivers Press.

The residents of Okinawa, an island chain of Japan, are among the healthiest and longest-lived people in the world. Okinawa has more 100-year-olds than anywhere else—33.6 per 100,000 people, compared with approximately 10 per 100,000 in the US.

The 25-year Okinawa Centenarian Study discovered that, compared with Americans, Okinawans have...

●**80% lower risk of breast and prostate cancers.**

●**50% lower risk of colon and ovarian cancers.**

●**40% fewer hip fractures.**

●**Minimal risk of heart disease.**

What is the secret to the Okinawans' longevity—and what can we do to achieve the same healthful vigor? *The following factors are especially important...*

ACCEPTING ATTITUDE

While many Americans have Type A personalities, Okinawans believe that life's travails will work themselves out. The average American might be said to suffer from *hurry sickness*. Okinawans prefer to work at their own pace, referred to locally as *Okinawa Time*. They don't ignore stress...but they rarely internalize it.

Stress signals your body to secrete large amounts of *cortisol* and other stress hormones. That damages the heart and blood vessels and accelerates bone loss.

To reduce stress: Don't take on more than you can handle...take advantage of flextime at work...don't get worked up about things you can't change, such as traffic jams or rude behavior...practice deep breathing and meditation.

LOW-CALORIE INTAKE

Okinawans consume an average of 1,900 calories a day, compared with 2,500 for Americans. Studies have shown that animals given a diet with 40% fewer calories than the diets of free-feeding animals live about 50% longer.

Reason: Harmful oxygen molecules (free radicals) are created every time the body metabolizes food for energy. Because the Okinawans take in fewer calories, their lifetime exposure to free radicals—which damage cells in the arteries, brain and other parts of the body—is reduced.

499

PLANT-BASED DIET

About 98% of the *traditional* Okinawan diet consists of sweet potatoes, soy-based foods, grains, fruits and vegetables. This is supplemented by a small amount of fish (and lean pork on special occasions). These plant foods contain *phytonutrients*—chemical compounds that reduce free radical damage. A plant-based diet is also high in fiber, which lowers cholesterol and reduces the risk of diabetes, breast cancer and heart disease. The *current* Okinawan diet is about 80% plant food.

Wok advantage: The Okinawans' style of cooking is high-heat stir-frying in a wok, which requires little oil. They typically stir-fry with canola oil, which is high in heart-healthy monounsaturated fat and omega-3 fatty acids. These fatty acids lower levels of LDL (bad) cholesterol while increasing levels of HDL (good) cholesterol.

SOY FOODS

Elderly Okinawans eat an average of two servings of soy foods daily—such as tofu, miso soup and soybean sprouts. Soy is rich in flavonoids, chemical compounds that reduce the tendency of LDL to stick to arteries, thereby reducing the risk of heart disease or stroke. Soy foods may also protect against cancer…menopausal discomfort (such as hot flashes)…and osteoporosis. You don't have to eat a lot of soy foods to get similar benefits. One daily serving of tofu (about three ounces) or soy milk (eight ounces) may be protective.

FISH

Fish harvested from the waters surrounding Okinawa is an integral part of the residents' daily diet. The omega-3 fatty acids in fish "thin" the blood and reduce the risk of clots—the main cause of heart attack.

Omega-3s also inhibit the body's production of inflammatory chemicals called *prostaglandins.* That may lower the risk of inflammatory conditions, such as arthritis and the bowel disorder Crohn's disease.

Americans can get similar benefits by eating fish at least three times a week. Cold-water fish —salmon, mackerel, tuna—contain the largest amounts of omega-3s. Fish oil supplements are a worthwhile alternative for people who are "fish phobic."

HEALTHY WEIGHT

The traditional Okinawan diet is low in fat and processed foods, as well as calories—so obesity is rare in elder Okinawans. This means their risk of weight-related health problems, such as diabetes, heart disease and cancer, is much lower than that of Americans. This is in stark contrast to younger Okinawans, who eat a more Westernized diet and have the highest obesity levels in Japan.

Postmenopausal bonus: After menopause, a woman's main source of estrogen is no longer the ovaries, but extraglandular tissues, mainly body fat. Women who maintain a healthful weight produce less estrogen, which reduces the risk for breast cancer.

JASMINE TEA

Okinawans drink about three cups of jasmine tea daily. It contains more antioxidant flavonoids than black tea. Those antioxidants may reduce risk for heart disease as well as some cancers.

NOT SMOKING

In the US, hundreds of thousands of people die from smoking-related diseases annually. Few elderly Okinawans have ever smoked… although one man interviewed for the study took up smoking when he was 100. He got bored with it and quit the next year. About 60% of younger Okinawan men now smoke.

EXERCISE

People are healthiest when they combine aerobic, strengthening and flexibility exercises. Okinawans often get all three by practicing martial arts or a traditional style of dance that resembles tai chi. *Smart regimen…*

• **Swimming, biking, jogging, etc.** for at least 30 minutes three times weekly.

• **Lifting weights** at least 20 minutes twice a week.

• **Flexibility exercises**—yoga or stretching —whenever you can and certainly after each aerobic or strength-training session.

SOCIAL LINKS

Moai is the Okinawan word that means "meeting for a common purpose." Groups of friends, colleagues or relatives get together at least once a month to talk…share gossip…and provide emotional or even financial support.

People who maintain active social networks live longer and are less likely to get sick. When they do get sick, they recover more quickly if they have the support of friends.

SPIRITUALITY AND RELIGION

People who have spiritual or religious beliefs live longer than those who don't. Spirituality and religion are a part of daily life in Okinawa. People pray daily for health and peace. They look out for one another in a "help thy neighbor" ethic called *Yuimaru.* Moderation is a key cultural value.

Women are the religious leaders in Okinawa. They also tend to have very high levels of life satisfaction and respect as they age.

Stop Memory Loss Before It's Too Late

Zaldy S. Tan, MD, MPH, director of the Memory Disorders Clinic at Beth Israel Deaconess Medical Center and instructor in medicine at Harvard Medical School, both in Boston. He is author of *Age-Proof Your Mind: Prevent, Detect, and Stop Memory Loss—Before It's Too Late.* Warner.

Alzheimer's disease, the dread destroyer of memory, doesn't happen all at once. Like heart disease and many other serious ailments, it's years in the making.

Only recently have medical researchers nailed down the early warning signs of Alzheimer's. People who have a condition known as mild cognitive impairment (MCI), which marks the transitional stage between normal aging and dementia, are highly likely to develop Alzheimer's. According to a Mayo Clinic study, 15% of people with MCI have Alzheimer's one year later, compared with 1% to 2% of those without MCI. Within four years, 50% of people with MCI will have Alzheimer's…after five years or longer, it's 80% to 90%.

Can this downward spiral be stopped? As yet, the jury still is out, but there is reason to be hopeful. After all, 10% to 20% of people who have MCI do *not* fall victim to Alzheimer's. What protects them?

A growing body of scientific evidence suggests that staying mentally active, exercising regularly and eating well can help preserve memory—and slow or perhaps even halt the progression of MCI.

NORMAL AGING OR MCI?

People with MCI have the same kind of lapses in short-term memory—forgetting facts, names, appointments, etc.—that most of us experience as we progress through our 50s, 60s and beyond…but many more such instances.

They still remember how to perform everyday activities, such as driving, reading, typing and cooking. Their ability to reason, solve math problems and control emotions also is left intact.

A key criterion for identifying MCI is "subjective" memory loss—that is, the person notices the lapses and thinks that they are troublesome and too frequent. Still, people differ widely in their sensitivity to their own memory performance. Often, friends and family become aware of memory problems before the person experiencing them does. Perhaps the most reliable indicator is performance on memory tests administered by a psychologist, psychiatrist, geriatrician or neurologist. Should you be tested? To find out, try the exercise on pages 502-503.

BRAIN TO SPARE

MCI progresses to Alzheimer's disease when enough brain cells are affected to seriously compromise the brain's ability to function. The more densely interconnected your brain cells are, the greater your "brain reserve." This allows your brain to keep on working well even if some cells have been affected.

Researchers now know that new *synapses*—connections between brain cells—can be formed throughout life.

Mental activity builds synapses the same way physical activity builds muscle. If you are concerned about your memory, it's critical to challenge your mind.

Self-defense: Spend at least one hour daily performing rigorous mental activity. Read books on subjects that demand concentration…do crossword puzzles at a level you find difficult…take an adult education course in a new discipline…work conscientiously to master a foreign language.

YOU CAN HALT MENTAL DECLINE

Mental activity is only part of the story. The same lifestyle and diet changes that are recommended to reduce the risk for heart attack, cancer and other serious diseases maximize brain reserve as well by maintaining brain cells and stimulating the connections between them.

•**Exercise.** Physical activity keeps brain cells well nourished and supplied with the oxygen they need to survive.

A six-year study of 345 Californians age 55 or older found significantly less mental decline among those who were more physically fit than the others.

Self-defense: Any regular exercise you enjoy, even 30 minutes of brisk walking daily, will help.

Ideal: Physical activities that also challenge your mind, such as ballroom dancing or learning a new sport.

•**Limit calories.** One source of free radicals (high-energy oxygen molecules that are known to damage brain cells) is the conversion of food to energy. The more you eat, the more toxic molecules are created.

Human population studies have linked calorie restriction to slower aging. In one study conducted at Columbia University, those who ate the fewest calories had the lowest risk of developing Alzheimer's.

Self-defense: If you're moderately active, aim for 1,800 to 2,200 calories per day.

•**Get your fruits and vegetables.** Foods rich in antioxidant vitamins and similar plant-based chemicals appear to protect brain cells against harmful free radicals.

In a Dutch study, people who consumed more than 23 international units (IU) daily of vitamin E had a 43% reduction in Alzheimer's risk. Similar protection was found in those who consumed 133 mg or more daily of vitamin C.

Self-defense: Include in your daily diet antioxidant-rich foods, such as spinach (one cup provides 10 IU of vitamin E)…or frozen peaches (one cup contains 235 milligrams [mg] of vitamin C).

There is less evidence that antioxidant supplements are protective.

•**Eat fish.** Like the heart, the brain benefits from the omega-3 fatty acids found in fish.

In a Rush University study of more than 800 older adults, the Alzheimer's risk in those who ate fish at least once weekly was 60% lower than in those who did not.

Self-defense: Eat cold-water fish that is high in omega-3 fatty acids—halibut, mackerel or salmon, for example—at least once weekly.

PROTECTIVE MEDICATION?

Research suggests that inflammation—the same process that causes many diseases, such as rheumatoid arthritis—destroys brain cells. Inflammation-fighting drugs may protect against Alzheimer's disease.

Studies from the Mayo Clinic have found a significantly lower incidence of Alzheimer's among people who took nonsteroidal anti-inflammatory drugs (NSAIDs), such as *ibuprofen* (Advil), regularly for at least two years.

Other studies suggest that people who take cholesterol-lowering statin drugs are also less likely to develop the disease.

The evidence is still too weak to justify regular use of NSAIDs or statins for everyone. These drugs have risks—NSAIDs can cause gastrointestinal bleeding and statins can cause side effects, such as muscle pain and liver problems.

If you have MCI, however, the drugs' potential benefits may outweigh the risks. Talk to your doctor.

Test Your Memory

Zaldy S. Tan, MD, MPH, director of the Memory Disorders Clinic at Beth Israel Deaconess Medical Center and instructor in medicine at Harvard Medical School, both in Boston. He is author of *Age-Proof Your Mind: Prevent, Detect, and Stop Memory Loss—Before It's Too Late.* Warner.

Ask someone to read aloud a list of four unrelated words, pausing for one second between each.

Examples: Freedom, strawberry, tiger, north …flower, truck, valor, dentist.

After memorizing the list, perform an unrelated task. Five minutes later, say the words out loud to your companion.

If you missed some, have him/her read them to you again. Five minutes later, repeat the words out loud again and note your score. Do the same 20 minutes after that. Most people will remember all or three of the words.

Because inborn memory ability varies and is influenced by age, education and other factors, there's no "passing grade" on this test. Take the test again four to six months later. If your ability to perform the test declines—particularly if you're aware of memory problems in the meantime—seek an evaluation.

You Can Prevent Alzheimer's Disease

Majid Fotuhi, MD, PhD, assistant professor of neurology at Johns Hopkins University School of Medicine and director of the Memory Disorders Unit at Sinai Hospital, both in Baltimore. He also is clinical instructor in neurology at Harvard Medical School, Boston, and author of *The Memory Cure: How to Protect Your Brain Against Memory Loss and Alzheimer's Disease.* McGraw-Hill.

The scientists who research Alzheimer's disease (AD) have yet to discover what causes the formation of abnormal protein structures (called plaques and tangles) that destroy brain cells.

However: It's now clear that certain lifestyle practices can guard against the inexorable memory loss and personality changes associated with this dreaded disease.

Evidence: In a landmark study of 678 Midwestern nuns, autopsy reports found that the brains of one-third of the 251 nuns who died in the course of the study had the plaques and tangles of AD but did *not* show symptoms of the disease. On the other hand, some nuns who had *fewer* plaques and tangles had experienced AD symptoms.

ASSAULTS ON THE BRAIN

AD gets the lion's share of attention, but it's just one of many enemies that menace the brain as we grow older. *Among them…*

•**Inflammation.** This is a normal defense mechanism in which the immune system destroys foreign molecules, such as viruses, by releasing high-energy molecules, including free radicals.

With aging, a mild degree of inflammation occurs in joints, skin and the brain, causing arthritis, skin wrinkles and memory problems.

•**Ministrokes.** Each ministroke (blockage of tiny blood vessels within the brain) may kill too few cells to have any noticeable impact, but when ministrokes occur hundreds—or even thousands—of times, they take their toll.

It's the *cumulative* impact that counts—the plaques and tangles of AD, plus all the other sources of damage.

Anything you do to promote the overall health of your brain may delay—or even prevent—memory loss and other AD symptoms.

PROTECT YOUR BRAIN

Many of the same practices that lower your risk for heart attack and stroke also reduce the chances that you will develop AD.

•**Control blood pressure.** High blood pressure can contribute to the narrowing of blood vessels and reduces blood flow to the brain, depriving it of oxygen and nutrients. This makes brain cells more vulnerable to AD damage and raises the risk for ministrokes.

Scientific evidence: Many studies have linked rising blood pressure with declining memory. A Scandinavian study of 1,449 middle-aged volunteers, reported in the *British Medical Journal,* found that those with mild hypertension—130 to 140 systolic (top number)—had twice the chance of having AD 20 years later. Those who had more severe hypertension—141 to 160 systolic—had nearly three times the risk.

Self-defense: Keep your blood pressure at 115/75 or less. If it exceeds 130/90 despite your efforts to bring it down—losing weight, exercising and quitting smoking—you may need medication, such as diuretics, beta-blockers or calcium channel blockers.

• **Lower cholesterol.** High cholesterol levels cause narrowing of blood vessels, which impairs circulation in the brain and may lead to ministrokes. Some research suggests that high cholesterol promotes the development of AD plaques.

Scientific evidence: The same Scandinavian study found that people with total cholesterol above 250 mg/dl were more than twice as likely to develop AD in later life than those with normal levels.

Self-defense: Aim for total cholesterol under 150 mg/dl. A healthy diet, exercise and smoking cessation can help bring it down. If your cholesterol remains above 150, talk to your doctor about medication.

Statins, such as *pravastatin* (Pravachol) and *atorvastatin* (Lipitor), are the drugs of choice for elevated cholesterol. Several studies have found that individuals taking these drugs have 60% to 80% less risk of developing AD than those not taking them.

DIET FOR A HEALTHY BRAIN

Like the rest of your body, your brain must be well fed to function optimally and stay healthy.

• **Eat at least five servings of fruits and vegetables daily.** They contain antioxidant vitamins and phytochemicals that protect brain cells from damage by free radicals.

Best antioxidant food sources: Blueberries, pomegranates, carrots and green, leafy vegetables.

One antioxidant that deserves particular attention is vitamin E.

Scientific evidence: A Dutch study of 5,395 people, age 55 or older, published in the *Journal of the American Medical Association,* found that those consuming the most vitamin E in foods and supplements had 43% less chance of developing AD than those consuming the least.

Boost your intake of vitamin E–rich foods, such as whole grains, avocados and olive oil.

• **Have fish twice weekly.** Cold-water fish, such as wild salmon and mackerel, contain omega-3 fatty acids that function as antioxidants as well as counter inflammation that can damage brain cells. Fish consumption also has been linked to improved circulation.

Scientific evidence: A study of 815 people, ages 65 to 94, found that those who consumed fish once or more weekly had 60% less risk of developing AD than those who did not.

• **Drink in moderation.** Temperate consumption of alcohol—two glasses of wine, two beers or one drink containing hard liquor daily—keeps brain cell membranes more flexible, which lets them function better.

Caution: Consuming greater amounts of alcohol, especially as you grow older, has been shown to impair memory and damage brain and other tissues.

Scientific evidence: A Dutch study published in *The Lancet* found that older adults who consumed mild to moderate amounts of alcohol daily had a 42% lower risk for dementia.

ACTIVITY FOR THE BRAIN

Brain function has been shown to improve in people who are active—both mentally and physically.

• **Stay mentally active.** Mental workouts stimulate the release of growth factors—chemicals that spur brain cells to forge a rich network of cells that can compensate if some cells are disabled by AD.

Scientific evidence: A study of 801 Catholic priests and nuns, age 65 or older, found that those who spent the most leisure time in activities that demanded thinking—reading books, playing cards, solving crossword puzzles—had half the AD risk of those who spent the least time involved in such pursuits.

Self-defense: Read books that make you think...follow political developments around the world...learn a foreign language...play games, such as chess, that require cognitive skills.

• **Get regular exercise.** Physical activity stimulates brain growth factors, improves circulation and reduces the risk for ministrokes.

Scientific evidence: A University of California at Los Angeles study that followed 6,000 women, age 65 or older, for six to eight years found that the more miles they walked daily, the lower their risk for dementia. Other studies that included men had similar results.

Self-defense: Just a little exercise makes a lot of difference. Do something active—brisk walking, tennis or dancing—for at least 30 minutes each day.

The Truth About Brain Food

Mark A. Stengler, ND, a naturopathic physician in private practice at La Jolla Whole Health Clinic, La Jolla, CA. He is associate clinical professor at both Bastyr University, Kenmore, WA, and the National College of Naturopathic Medicine, Portland, OR. He is author of numerous books on natural healing, including *The Natural Physician's Healing Therapies*. Bottom Line Books.

Everyone forgets something from time to time. Some people have trouble remembering names. Others can't keep track of their car keys. Whether we suffer everyday absentmindedness or moments of real memory loss, all of us are concerned about keeping our brain power intact.

In recent years, a great deal of research has focused on the most severe kinds of memory loss—senile dementia and Alzheimer's disease. In the US, these closely related conditions affect up to 10% of people over age 65 and nearly half of those over age 85.

Many studies have identified ways to lower risk of these age-related problems. Popular methods include stress-reduction strategies, such as daily exercise, positive mental imagery, biofeedback and close personal relationships, to prevent spikes in the memory-draining stress hormone *cortisol*..."brain workouts," including crossword puzzles, word games and challenging card games...and eight to nine hours of sleep each night. Good nutrition—and the right kind of supplementation—also can help protect our brains and safeguard our memories at any age. The sooner you get started with a brain-protecting regimen, the more you'll benefit.

For optimal brain function, your diet should be well-balanced with carbohydrates (40%), protein (30%) and fats (30%). You can accomplish this by eating meals that include whole grains, fruits and vegetables (for complex carbohydrates)...fish, poultry, lean meats, legumes, nuts and seeds (for protein)...and fish oil, olive oil, avocados, almonds, walnuts and ground flaxseed (for fats). Steer clear of dairy products and packaged and processed foods, such as cookies, white bread and pasta, which are packed with simple carbohydrates that wreak havoc on glucose levels, contributing to diabetes, stroke/vascular disease and dementia.

THE VALUE OF FISH

Fish provides *docosahexaenoic acid* (DHA) and *eicosapentaenoic acid* (EPA), the most plentiful fatty acids in the brain. DHA, an omega-3 fatty acid, is found in abundance in cold-water fish such as mackerel, sardines, salmon and herring. You also can get it from fish-oil supplements, egg yolks, DHA-enriched eggs and some algae supplements, such as Neuromins, a product that is available at most health-food stores.

Foods such as walnuts...leafy, green vegetables...and supplements including flaxseed and hemp oil contain *alpha-linolenic acid*, an omega-3 fatty acid that can be converted by the body into DHA and EPA.

How essential is DHA to memory? It has been known for some years that people have a higher risk of Alzheimer's if they have low blood levels of DHA. A study in *Archives of Neurology* revealed that people who ate fish one to three times a month had a 40% lower risk of Alzheimer's than those who never ate fish. Those who consumed fish once a week or more had a 60% lower risk. Fish may be baked, broiled or grilled.

It also makes sense to take a fish-oil supplement daily. I suggest 1,000 milligrams (mg) of combined DHA and EPA. Good brands are Nordic Naturals (800-662-2544, *www.nordicnaturals.com*) and Carlson Laboratories (888-234-5656, *www.carlsonlabs.com*), both available at health-food stores.

Caution: Fish oil can thin blood, so check with your doctor before using it if you take blood-thinning medications such as *warfarin* (Coumadin).

GLA IS ESSENTIAL

Omega-6s make up another class of essential fatty acids that are necessary for good brain function. Omega-6 is found in vegetable oils, including safflower, sunflower and corn oils. Most American diets contain too much of these oils due to consumption of packaged and fried foods. However, the most important omega-6 fatty acid is *linoleic acid*, which is converted in the body to *gamma-linolenic acid* (GLA). This essential fatty acid plays a big role in the formation of healthy brain-cell membranes, the part of the cell that stores information. Taking borage oil or evening primrose oil are healthful ways to increase GLA intake—hempseed and hempseed oil also are good sources. Another way to get GLA in the diet is by consuming flaxseed (with water to prevent constipation) or flaxseed oil.

COUNT ON CHOLINE

Just as a car needs spark plugs, an active brain needs quick-firing neurotransmitters. As the name implies, a neurotransmitter sends a signal—one that jumps from one brain cell to another. Substances that act as neurotransmitters—the most important of which is a brain chemical called *acetylcholine*—are vital components of the brain's communication system.

There's one hitch. In order for your body to manufacture enough *acetylcholine*, you need to get a closely related nutrient called *choline*. The best source of choline is *phosphatidylcholine* (PC), which occurs naturally in fish, egg yolks, legumes, nuts, meat and vegetables. It also is found in breast milk. To help prevent memory problems, you can boost your PC intake by taking a 1,500- to 2,000-milligram (mg) PC supplement daily. (Doses of more than 3,000 mg can cause digestive upset, including diarrhea, nausea and stomachache.)

PC is only part of the neurotransmitter equation. To turn PC into brain-friendly *choline*, you also need to get healthy doses of vitamin C and certain B vitamins. You can get plenty of these vitamins in your diet by eating red, yellow and green peppers, citrus fruits and cantaloupe for vitamin C and sweet potatoes, tuna and avocados for B vitamins. Also, I recommend taking a balanced daily multivitamin/mineral supplement.

Deficiencies of folic acid and other key B vitamins have been associated with an increased risk of Alzheimer's disease. These nutrients help to lower levels of *homocysteine*, a harmful by-product of protein metabolism that is increased in people who are genetically susceptible. That's why it is important to have your blood levels of homocysteine, folic acid and B-12 tested by your doctor to see if you need additional supplementation of folic acid and/or B-12.

THE EUROPEAN CURE

For years, European doctors have recommended a supplement called *L-alpha-glycerylphosphorylcholine* (GPC) to promote mental acuity (the ability to respond quickly and appropriately to mental challenges). GPC actually is used by the brain more effectively than PC to form *acetylcholine*—but it costs twice as much and is less widely available in the US. A good GPC supplement by Source Naturals is sold in some health-food stores under the brand name Alpha GPC. Take two 300-mg capsules twice daily for the first four weeks, then two 300-mg capsules once daily as a maintenance dosage. Side effects are rare, but take GPC with a meal if it seems to interfere with your digestion.

PS: BE SURE TO GET MORE

Phosphatidylserine (PS) is a fat that the brain needs to preserve the key brain chemicals *serotonin* and *dopamine*. It also has been shown to reduce levels of the stress hormone cortisol. PS is found in fish, soy and leafy, green vegetables. As we age, PS levels in the body start to decline, so most people need to take a supplement once they're past age 50.

A normal daily diet has about 70 mg of PS. You need about four times that much if you have memory problems. Nearly anyone can benefit from a 300-mg daily supplement of PS. You're likely to notice improvements in mental alertness after four to eight weeks. A small percentage of people have digestive upset, such as bloating and diarrhea, but you can reduce the dosage if this is a problem. PS is available at health-food stores and pharmacies. Make sure you buy a product that lists "phosphatidylserine" on the label. (Some supplements contain "phosphorylated serine," a nutrient complex that doesn't provide the same benefits as PS.) A high-quality PS supplement is made by Jarrow Formulas (to find a retailer, call 800-726-0886 or go to *www.jarrow.com*).

HELP FROM ALC

When taken as a supplement, a nutrient known as *acetyl-L-carnitine* (ALC) has been shown to improve cognitive function and memory in older adults. Researchers also have found that ALC slows the progression of early-stage Alzheimer's disease. By improving communication between the two main hemispheres of the brain, ALC helps enhance the interplay of creative and cognitive brain activity.

For people with mild memory problems, I recommend taking 500 mg of ALC daily on an empty stomach. For those with more severe problems such as dementia, I suggest the same dose three times daily. Cut back if you have digestive upset. Most health-food stores carry a reliable ALC formula produced by Now Foods (888-301-1336, *www.thecatalog.com*).

ADD ANTIOXIDANTS

In all likelihood, Alzheimer's disease and other types of dementia are related to excessive damage by free radicals (normal by-products of metabolism that can destroy cells, organs and tissues). Free radicals irreversibly injure our cells and contribute to accelerated aging, but studies have shown that this damage can be warded off by getting enough antioxidant nutrients to help guard our brain-cell membranes.

There's ample evidence that a daily dose of 2,000 international units (IU) of the powerful antioxidant vitamin E can slow the decline of cognitive function in people who have moderate to severe Alzheimer's disease. There have been controversial vitamin E studies that seemed to show a link to worsening chronic disease. However, I don't have much confidence in those studies because they were performed on unhealthy people. When it comes to Alzheimer's, results of vitamin E studies have been quite good.

All fresh fruits, vegetables and other plant foods provide multiple naturally occurring antioxidants. Juices are an especially concentrated source of antioxidants. In fact, a study of nearly 2,000 Japanese Americans found that those who reported drinking fruit and vegetable juices at least three times a week had a 75% lower risk of developing dementia than those who drank juices less than once a week. The most nutritious fruit juices include cranberry, pomegranate, apple and blueberry. I also like mixed vegetable juices containing any combination of spinach, celery, lettuce, parsley, watercress, carrot and tomato.

If there is a strong family history of dementia or you have beginning signs of it, take up to 2,000 IU of vitamin E daily. Green tea also is an excellent source of antioxidants. I recommend drinking two to four cups of green tea daily and eight ounces of fresh juice.

GINKGO—THE BRAIN PLEASER

Ginkgo biloba is an herbal remedy that has been shown to improve memory and cognitive processing by promoting blood flow to the brain. I recommend a 24% *flavoglycoside* extract. Start with a dose of 120 mg to 240 mg daily, and increase to 360 mg daily over a four-week period. Some people begin to see results in four to eight weeks. If you're already taking a blood-thinning medication such as aspirin or *warfarin*, consult your doctor before taking ginkgo.

Common Drugs Fight Alzheimer's

Gary Small, MD, professor of psychiatry and biobehavioral studies, director of the University of California at Los Angeles' Center on Aging, and leader of a study of Alzheimer's plaque buildup in brain tissue, reported in *Neuroscience*.

Nonsteroidal anti-inflammatory drugs such as *ibuprofen* and *naproxen* seem to help dissolve the brain lesions that occur in Alzheimer's patients, which are caused by plaque buildup. The drugs bond to and help dissolve the plaque, which also prevents new lesions from forming. This suggests that anti-inflammatories may be useful in lowering a person's risk of developing Alzheimer's, but more research is needed.

Natural Healers

Shari Lieberman, PhD, adjunct assistant professor of nutrition at the University of Bridgeport's Nutrition Institute, Bridgeport, CT. A member of the American Academy of Anti-Aging Medicine and the New York Academy of Sciences, she is author of *The Real Vitamin & Mineral Book*. Avery.

Most health-conscious individuals do their best to eat plenty of fruits and vegetables. But that's not enough.

Problem: Few people consider the nutrients that are lost after produce is harvested. For example, green vegetables lose almost all of their vitamin C after just a few days of storage at room temperature. What's more, cooking can deplete up to 50% of a variety of vitamins.

Solution: Many doctors now recommend vitamin and mineral supplements to compensate for dietary deficiencies and help prevent chronic diseases, such as heart disease, macular degeneration and osteoarthritis.

Everyone should take a daily multivitamin that provides all of the essential minerals and B vitamins, along with antioxidants, such as vitamins C and E.

Good brands: Solgar and Enzymatic Therapy. Unfortunately, once-a-day supplements provide only *minimal* levels of some important nutrients.

If you have—or are at risk for—one or more of the conditions listed below, you may benefit from taking, in addition to your multivitamin, the following supplements in higher-than-normal "therapeutic" doses.*

DEMENTIA/MEMORY LOSS

Millions of Americans age 65 or older suffer from Alzheimer's disease or age-related memory loss. Many of these older adults are deficient in B vitamins, especially B-12.

Key supplements…

• **B-complex supplement** provides the full complement of B vitamins, including B-1, B-2, B-3, B-6 and B-12.

Typical daily therapeutic dose: 50 to 100 milligrams (mg) of B-complex…plus 500 to 1,000 micrograms (mcg) of B-12 in a separate supplement.

• **Alpha-lipoic acid** improves brain function by slowing or stopping the death of nerve cells.

Typical daily therapeutic dose: 600 mg.

• **Vitamin E** protects brain cells from damage caused by disease-causing molecules known as free radicals.

Typical daily therapeutic dose: 1,200 international units (IU).**

• **Ginkgo biloba** improves brain circulation, reduces free-radical damage and may slow the onset of Alzheimer's.

Typical daily therapeutic dose: 240 mg.

Warning: If you are taking a blood-thinning medication, such as *warfarin* (Coumadin), consult your doctor before taking vitamin E or ginkgo biloba. Both have a mild blood-thinning effect.

HEART DISEASE

The standard drugs—such as nitroglycerin for treating angina and statins for lowering cholesterol—mainly manage heart disease symptoms, not the underlying causes. Statins lower levels of harmful LDL cholesterol, but they also deplete coenzyme Q10 (CoQ10) from heart cells. This naturally occurring enzyme is believed to strengthen the heart muscle.

Key supplements…

• **CoQ10.** All people with heart disease should ask their cardiologist about taking it. Studies have demonstrated that CoQ10 improves symptoms associated with congestive heart failure, angina and other heart disorders. In some cases, people who take the enzyme are even able to reduce their doses of heart medications.

Typical daily therapeutic dose: 50 to 300 mg. Start with the lower dose and gradually

---

*Supplement doses listed here are higher than the recommended daily intake. Because such doses may have unwanted effects, check with your doctor before trying any of these regimens. In rare cases, they may interfere with standard drug treatment.

**Choose natural vitamin E (d-alpha tocopherol), which is more effective than the synthetic version.

increase it until you notice a reduction of symptoms. Do *not* stop taking CoQ10 abruptly. Doing so can cause a rebound of symptoms.

•**Fish oil** lowers levels of C-reactive protein, a "marker" for artery inflammation that accompanies heart disease.

Typical daily therapeutic dose: 3 to 6 grams (g).

Helpful: Enteric-coated fish oil capsules dissolve in the intestine and are less likely than other products to cause a fishy taste when you burp.

Warning: Fish oil capsules can have a blood-thinning effect.

•**Antioxidant supplements** prevent cell damage in artery walls and reduce inflammation.

Typical daily therapeutic dose: 400 to 1,200 IU vitamin E...1 to 4 g vitamin C...and 25,000 IU natural beta-carotene.

•**Niacin** works as well as some statins at lowering total cholesterol—and it increases levels of beneficial HDL cholesterol. Combining niacin with a statin may allow you to take a lower dose of the statin drug. Because niacin can cause flushing, look for a "flush-free" product. At high doses, niacin can also cause liver problems, so use it only under a doctor's supervision.

Typical daily therapeutic dose: 2 g.

MACULAR DEGENERATION

Macular degeneration is caused by a breakdown of the *macula*, the part of the retina that is responsible for central vision. It's the main cause of severe vision loss in people age 50 or older. *Key supplements...*

•**Carotenoids**, especially beta-carotene and lutein, are used by the eye to build and repair damaged cells.

Typical daily therapeutic dose: 25,000 IU natural beta-carotene and 10 to 15 mg lutein.

•**Vitamin E** reduces oxidative stress in the eye and prevents further damage.

Typical daily therapeutic dose: 800 IU.

•**Zinc** is used by the eye to manufacture chemical compounds that aid vision.

Typical daily therapeutic dose: 22 to 50 mg.

OSTEOARTHRITIS

Osteoarthritis is the most common form of arthritis and the leading cause of pain and disability in older Americans. Anti-inflammatory analgesics, such as *ibuprofen* (Advil), are effective but often cause side effects, such as gastrointestinal bleeding.

Key supplements...

•**Fish oil** reduces levels of *arachidonic acid*, a fatty acid that forms inflammatory, joint-damaging chemicals known as prostaglandins.

Typical daily therapeutic dose: 3 to 6 g.

•**Vitamins C and E** block the effects of inflammatory free radicals in the joints. They work synergistically with fish oil to enhance its effects.

Typical daily therapeutic dose: 4 g vitamin C...and 400 to 1,200 IU vitamin E.

•**Quercetin**, a plant-based flavonoid, relieves pain as well as ibuprofen does.

Typical daily therapeutic dose: 2 to 4 g.

The Oxygen Cure

Daniel Hamner, MD, sports medicine physician and owner and founder of the Peak Energy Program in New York City. He is coauthor of *Peak Energy: The High-Oxygen Program for More Energy Now.* St. Martin's.

Every cell in the body needs oxygen to function properly. The brain alone uses at least 12% of the total oxygen that people inhale.

Problem: The breathing habits of most people *don't* always provide all the oxygen that the brain and body need.

Oxygen deprivation is a leading cause of persistent fatigue—a condition that accounts for up to 15 million doctor visits annually, making it one of the most common health problems in the US. It also causes mental fogginess and, in some cases, depression.

My story: For years, I barely had enough energy to get through my workdays. I started reading about energy-building techniques—

everything from yoga to the latest research in exercise physiology. I quickly realized that all of these techniques aim to increase oxygen levels in the body.

At the age of 47, I developed—and began practicing—a high-oxygen program. Within a matter of months, my oxygen usage rose from 42.7 milliliters of oxygen per kilogram of body weight per minute to 55 milliliters—a 30% increase. At the same time, my energy levels rose dramatically.

7 STEPS TO BETTER OXYGENATION

Nearly everyone can increase oxygen levels and experience a significant boost in energy in as little as two weeks. *Here's how...*

●**Step 1: Take a pro-oxygenator.** The herbal supplement ginseng enhances the body's ability to utilize oxygen. A four-week study of oxygen utilization found that people taking ginseng experienced a 29% improvement in oxygen transportation to tissues and organs.

Typical dose: 400 to 600 milligrams (mg) once daily.

Caution: Do not take ginseng if you have high blood pressure. If you are taking medication, consult your physician before trying ginseng.

●**Step 2: Stand straight.** Poor posture—rounding the shoulders, stooping forward, etc.—can inhibit oxygen intake.

People who stand straight, roll back their shoulders, push their chests out while squeezing their shoulder blades together and keep their chin up can increase lung capacity by 5%.

Helpful: To ensure proper form, practice this while looking in a full-length mirror.

●**Step 3: Exercise.** Aerobic exercise increases pathways in the body that carry oxygen to cells. People who start an aerobic exercise program experience an immediate increase in oxygen usage and energy.

My recommendation: Walk fast, run, swim, bike, etc.—for a minimum of 60 minutes three days a week.

Resistance training increases strength and endurance. Consult a physical trainer or other exercise professional for a strength-training regimen that works the muscles in your upper and lower body and your core (trunk).

My recommendation: Twenty to 30 minutes of strength training at least three times a week.

●**Step 4: Eat "charge-up" foods.** A diet high in complex carbohydrates—fruits (such as apples and oranges)...vegetables (such as carrots and spinach)...whole grains...legumes (such as black beans)...etc.—significantly improves the blood's ability to transport oxygen to cells. A high-fat diet does the opposite—it reduces the blood's oxygen-carrying capacity.

●**Step 5: Practice instant-energy breathing.** You can reverse fatigue almost instantly with a yoga breathing technique that floods cells with oxygen and boosts energy for 15 minutes or more. *What to do...*

●Sit up straight and take 20 to 30 quick, panting breaths. Only your belly should move, not your chest.

●Take a deep breath, filling your lungs with air...and hold for 30 seconds. If you can, gradually work up to holding your breath for 60 seconds.

●Exhale completely. Press your hand down against your belly. This puts pressure on your lungs and forces out more of the used air.

After completing the exercise, walk briskly for 10 minutes, if possible. This will pull additional air into your lungs and increase the circulation of oxygen-rich blood cells.

●**Step 6: Stop smoking—and avoid secondhand smoke.** Smokers tend to have less energy and more depression than nonsmokers, in part because they get less blood and oxygen to the brain.

Smoking—as well as exposure to secondhand smoke—increases blood levels of carbon monoxide, a waste chemical that increases fatigue. It also causes higher levels of arterial plaque—fatty accumulations that inhibit circulation.

People who attend smoking cessation programs, such as SmokEnders, or use stop-smoking products, such as nicotine patches, are about twice as likely to quit the habit as those who try to stop on their own.

Important: Take 1,000 mg of vitamin C daily when trying to quit smoking. Each cigarette inactivates 25 mg of vitamin C in the body.

●**Step 7: See a doctor if you have low energy.** Fatigue is a common first symptom of hundreds of medical conditions, including iron-deficiency anemia, food allergies, heart problems and cancer. Consult your doctor if you experience mental fogginess or low physical energy for more than a few weeks.

ARE YOU GETTING ENOUGH OXYGEN?

Most people can check their own oxygen levels with this simple test…

●**Stand in front of a step.** Relax for a moment, then check your resting heart rate. *To do this:* Place the tips of your index and middle fingers on the thumb side of your wrist. Count your heartbeats for 30 seconds, then multiply by two.

●**Rapidly step onto and off of the step for one minute.** Check your heart rate again. It probably has risen quite a bit—from, say, 80 beats to 120 beats per minute.

●**Rest for one minute, then check your heart rate again.** If it returned to the resting level, your blood is carrying adequate oxygen. If it stayed elevated above the resting level for more than one minute, your heart is trying to compensate for low blood levels of oxygen.

Vibrant Health via Nutraceuticals

Mary E. O'Brien, MD, a board-certified internist in Myrtle Beach, SC. She is cochair of the medical advisory board of the American Nutraceutical Association, *www.americanutra.com*, and coeditor of *Nutraceuticals: The Complete Encyclopedia of Supplements, Herbs, Vitamins and Healing Foods.* Perigee.

Echinacea, St. John's wort and other supplements have become big sellers in this country. But most Americans have yet to discover the full array of herbs, vitamins and minerals that can be used to relieve—or prevent—many health conditions.

Known as *nutraceuticals,** these supplements are derived from—or, in some cases, mimic—chemically active compounds found in plants.

Unlike over-the-counter or prescription drugs, which typically treat specific symptoms, some nutraceuticals may reduce oxidative damage by free radicals, which can contribute to heart disease and other chronic conditions. For some ailments, they can be just as effective as drugs but usually cause fewer side effects and cost less. Ask your doctor which products might be appropriate for you.

FATIGUE

A century ago, the average American slept 10 hours a night. Now the average American gets only seven hours of sleep each night. *To curb fatigue, try…*

●**Coenzyme Q10 (CoQ10).** 30 milligrams (mg) twice daily. It plays a vital role in the production of *adenosine triphosphate* (ATP), a molecule that is used throughout the body as a source of energy.

Helpful: Combine CoQ10 with 60 mg of the amino acid *carnitine* twice daily. This regimen activates energy-producing components (mitochondria) inside cells, which may boost energy and stamina.

●**Ginseng.** Begin with 100 mg once a day. The dose can be gradually increased up to 300 mg twice daily. Ginseng may function as a mild stimulant and has been used in Asian cultures to increase stamina and enhance well-being.

Caution: Ginseng can be harmful for people with high blood pressure, angina, headaches or hyperthyroidism.

HIGH BLOOD PRESSURE

Several of my patients have tried as many as four blood pressure drugs without being able to control their condition. *Ensuring adequate levels of certain nutrients may improve blood pressure control…*

●**Essential fatty acids (EFAs).** Found in salmon and other cold-water fish, flaxseed, walnuts and other nuts, EFAs may help prevent

*The US Food and Drug Administration (FDA) does not regulate supplements or herbs. Always check with your doctor before taking any of these products. They can interact with prescription medications.

arterial damage caused by high blood pressure. Sprinkle flaxseed on salads and cereals. Eat cold water fish at least twice a week.

●**Magnesium.** 750 mg daily. It helps regulate the relaxation and constriction of blood vessels. This may lower blood pressure.

●**Potassium.** 2,000 mg daily. It is essential in regulating heartbeat. It can lower systolic pressure (upper number) by four points and diastolic pressure (lower number) by three points, according to a recent study.

Caution: Limit supplemental potassium to 500 mg daily. Get the remainder of your daily intake from potassium-rich foods—apricots, bananas, cantaloupe, potatoes and spinach.

MEMORY PROBLEMS

●**Docosahexanoic acid (DHA).** 3 to 6 g daily. DHA is the most abundant fatty acid in the brain, but the modern diet may not provide enough. Foods that are rich in DHA include eggs, organ meats, cold-water fish and wild game.

●**Folate.** 800 micrograms (mcg) daily. It lowers levels of the blood protein *homocysteine*, reducing the risk for stroke and other vascular events that can lead to dementia. Recent research suggests that low levels of folate may be linked to Alzheimer's disease.

●**Ginkgo.** 60 mg twice daily. It increases blood flow to parts of the brain that lack sufficient circulation. It has no effect when blood flow is normal.

Caution: Ginkgo interferes with blood clotting. It should *not* be used by people taking nonsteroidal anti-inflammatory drugs (NSAIDs), such as aspirin, ibuprofen, etc., or prescription blood thinners, such as *warfarin* (Coumadin).

●**Vitamin E.** 100 to 400 international units (IU) daily. This antioxidant blocks the oxidation of LDL (bad) cholesterol and may slow the progression of Alzheimer's disease.

OSTEOARTHRITIS

It's been called "wear-and-tear" arthritis—but research suggests that the disorder results from poor cartilage regeneration. *To curb osteoarthritis, try...*

●**Glucosamine.** 500 mg three times daily. It may improve cartilage thickness and help repair existing damage. For many people, pain relief begins in four weeks.

●**Vitamin C.** 100 mg twice daily. The Framingham Heart Study showed that vitamin C can slow the progression of pain due to osteoarthritis of the knee.

PROSTATE ENLARGEMENT

More than half of men age 60 and older suffer from prostate enlargement. Benign prostatic hypertrophy (BPH) can result in urinary frequency, irritation or difficulty urinating. *To curb symptoms of prostate enlargement, try...*

●**Pygeum africanum.** 100 to 200 mg daily. This African herb contains *pentacyclic triterpenes*, chemicals that shrink prostate tissue. It also reduces prostate irritation.

●**Saw palmetto.** 160 mg twice daily. It may reduce prostate irritation within four weeks. *Finasteride* (Proscar), a prescription drug often prescribed for BPH, generally takes up to four months to work.

Caution: Taking saw palmetto may mask a high prostate specific antigen (PSA) level. Before taking saw palmetto, see your doctor for a baseline PSA test.

●**Zinc.** 15 to 30 mg daily. It is important for normal prostate health and boosts immune function.

Good food sources: Pumpkin seeds, red meat, shellfish, oysters, nuts and wheat germ.

Scents to Boost Energy, Mood, Memory and More

Alan Hirsch, MD, founder and neurological director of the Smell & Taste Treatment and Research Foundation in Chicago. He is a neurologist and psychiatrist, and author of Life's a Smelling Success *(Authors of Unity) and* What Flavor Is Your Personality? *(Sourcebooks).*

Scents stimulate important mental and physical functions. They trigger the release of neurotransmitters, chemicals that send signals to the brain. *Here is a sampling of what scents can do for you…*

CONTROL APPETITE

In a study of 105 people, we found that those who inhaled a chocolate-like aroma whenever they felt like eating lost nearly three pounds in two weeks. One study of 3,193 volunteers found that sniffing banana, green apple or peppermint scents resulted in an average weight loss of 30 pounds in six months.

Sniff the above scents often, and remember to smell every food before you eat it. Your brain will perceive that you're eating more, thus suppressing your appetite.

INCREASE ENERGY

These odors stimulate the part of the brain that promotes wakefulness…

• **Jasmine** causes an increase in beta waves in the brain, a sign of alertness. Jasmine tea is a great pick-me-up.

• **Strawberries** and buttered popcorn will cause exercisers to burn more calories.

• **Peppermint** works on sensory nerves and increases alertness. Try a peppermint candy or chewing gum.

• **Freshly brewed coffee** is very stimulating, probably because we associate the aroma with the energizing effects of caffeine.

BOOST ROMANCE

Both men and women are sexually stimulated by scents, but the odors that arouse them aren't the same.

For men: The smell of lavender or pumpkin pie increases blood flow to the penis by about 40%. The smell of doughnuts, black licorice, vanilla or women's perfume (any scent) also is sexually stimulating to men.

For women: The odors of cucumber and licorice are stimulating. Women are turned off by the smells of cherries, barbecued meat and men's cologne.

REDUCE ANXIETY

Fresh, natural scents, in general, induce calm. In one study we conducted, volunteers became extremely anxious when they were confined in coffin-like tubes, but then calmed down when the tubes were infused with the smells of green apple and cucumber. These odors seem to have an impact on the limbic system, the emotional center of the brain.

If you anticipate a situation in which you will feel anxious, wash your hair that morning with a green-apple–scented shampoo and/or put a dab of the shampoo in a cloth to take with you.

IMPROVE MEMORY

People who sniff floral scents increase retention of new material by 17%.

Sniff a floral odor when learning new material, then smell it again when you want to recall it. This is known as *state-dependent learning.* The material you learn in one state—while smelling roses—will be more accessible when you replicate that state in the future.

Healing Herbs

Mark Blumenthal, founder and executive director of the American Botanical Council (ABC), *www.herbal gram.org*, an Austin, TX-based independent, nonprofit organization dedicated to disseminating reliable information about herbs and medicinal plants. He is senior editor of the English translation of *The Complete German Commission E Monographs—Therapeutic Guide to Herbal Medicines*, a clinical guide on the safety and efficacy of herbal medicines, and senior editor of *The ABC Clinical Guide to Herbs,* both from ABC.

It was headline news when *The New England Journal of Medicine* published a study that cast doubt on the effectiveness of echinacea. The message to the countless consumers spending more than $300 million annually on the purported cold-fighting herb? *Save your money.*

University of Virginia School of Medicine researchers had found echinacea to be no more effective than a placebo at combating cold and flu symptoms. But don't clear out your herbal medicine chest just yet.

What went largely unreported was that study participants received only 900 milligrams (mg) of echinacea daily—less than one-third of the dose recommended by the World Health Organization for combating upper-respiratory infections. That's akin to expecting one-third of a dose of aspirin to relieve a headache.

What's the other side of the story? Dozens of clinical studies point to echinacea's effectiveness, including an August 2004 Canadian trial in which volunteers who took echinacea at the onset of colds experienced 23% milder, shorter symptoms, such as sore throat, stuffy nose, chills and headache, than those taking a placebo—a benefit that researchers linked to a marked increase in circulating white blood cells and other cells of the immune system.

More work is needed to identify the optimal echinacea species (supplements are commonly derived from *E. purpurea*, *E. pallida* or *E. augustifolia*) and the most potent plant parts (roots, stems, leaves or flowers).

Meanwhile, best results have been achieved by taking 3,000 mg daily of an echinacea product that combines one of the above-mentioned species and parts at the first sign of cold or flu until symptoms resolve.

Caution: If you're allergic to ragweed, avoid echinacea supplements derived from stems, leaves or flowers—they may contain pollen and trigger a reaction. Use an echinacea root supplement.

Five other herbs with scientific evidence on their side...

GARLIC

What it does: Helps prevent and possibly reverse arterial plaque buildup (atherosclerosis), a major risk factor for heart attack and stroke...reduces risk for stomach and colorectal cancers...and acts as a blood thinner to reduce the risk for blood clots.

Scientific evidence: In a recent German study, 152 patients with advanced atherosclerosis who took 900 mg daily of garlic powder for four years experienced a 3% decrease in existing arterial plaques in their neck (carotid) and thigh (femoral) arteries. Those taking a placebo experienced more than a 15% *increase* in arterial plaques.

Potential side effects: Bad breath and indigestion. Because garlic has a blood-thinning effect, it should not be used if you take aspirin regularly or an anticoagulant drug, such as *warfarin* (Coumadin). To minimize bleeding risk, ask your doctor about discontinuing garlic

supplements at least one week before undergoing elective surgery.

Typical dose: One clove of fresh, minced garlic daily, or 200 to 300 mg of standardized garlic powder, taken in pill or tablet form, three times daily.

GINKGO

What it does: Improves memory and concentration in people with early-stage senile dementia or Alzheimer's disease, as well as in healthy adults, by increasing blood flow to the brain. May also relieve tinnitus (ringing in the ears), vertigo and altitude sickness, as well as vascular problems such as intermittent claudication, a painful calf condition caused by decreased circulation to the legs.

Scientific evidence: An overwhelming majority of ginkgo trials have shown positive results. At least 33 randomized, controlled trials have shown this herb to enhance mental functioning or slow cognitive deterioration in older patients with dementia, while another 13 controlled studies have shown ginkgo to boost memory and cognitive performance in healthy adults.

Potential side effects: Stomach upset, headache, rash and/or dizziness. Like garlic, ginkgo should not be taken with aspirin or a prescription blood thinner such as warfarin. The herb was previously believed to increase the effects of *monoamine oxidase inhibitor* (MAOI) antidepressants, such as *phenelzine* (Nardil), but this has been refuted.

Typical dose: 120 mg daily. Nearly all positive ginkgo trials have used one of three formulations that are produced in Germany and sold in health-food stores in the US under the brand names Ginkoba by Pharmaton Natural Health Products...Ginkgold by Nature's Way...and Ginkai by Abkit Inc.

MILK THISTLE

What it does: Because of its strong antioxidant activity, milk thistle detoxifies the liver and may help regenerate liver cells. It may be appropriate for patients with alcohol-related liver damage or infectious or drug-induced hepatitis, as well as anyone who is regularly exposed to industrial pollutants.

Scientific evidence: At least 19 out of 21 clinical studies (a total of 2,200 people out of 2,400) have shown milk thistle to protect the liver against invasive toxins and possibly even stimulate the generation of new liver cells.

Potential side effect: Loose stools.

Typical dose: Take 140 mg of milk thistle three times daily.

SAW PALMETTO

What it does: Relieves the symptoms of benign prostatic hyperplasia (BPH), a noncancerous swelling of the prostate gland, which causes frequent and/or weak urination and is common in men over age 50.

Scientific evidence: In nearly two dozen clinical trials, saw palmetto has proven almost equal to prescription drugs, such as *finasteride* (Proscar) and *terazosin* (Hytrin), for relieving the symptoms of BPH. Unlike prescription prostate medications, which can cause side effects, including diminished libido, saw palmetto causes only minor adverse effects. Saw palmetto does not inhibit the production of prostate specific antigen (PSA), a protein that, when elevated, serves as an early warning for prostate cancer. (Conventional BPH drugs suppress PSA, complicating prostate cancer screening.)

Potential side effects: Stomach upset or nausea if taken on an empty stomach.

Typical dose: 320 mg daily. It requires four to six weeks to take effect.

VALERIAN

What it does: The root combats insomnia and acts as a mild sedative to relieve anxiety or restlessness.

Scientific evidence: All of the nearly 30 clinical studies to date have shown the herb to be effective against insomnia and anxiety. In a recent German trial, taking 600 mg of valerian root extract daily proved as effective as the prescription tranquilizer *oxazepam* (Serax) for improving sleep quality, but with fewer side effects. Unlike prescription sleep aids, valerian isn't habit-forming, won't leave you feeling groggy the next morning and doesn't diminish alertness, reaction time or concentration.

Potential side effects: None known. It is best to avoid combining valerian with conventional sedatives, such as *diazepam* (Valium), since the herb may exacerbate the drug's sedating effects.

Typical dose: 2 to 3 grams (g) of the dried crushed root, infused as a tea…or 400 mg to 800 mg in supplement form, taken one-half hour before bedtime.

Natural Sex Boosters

Ray Sahelian, MD, a board-certified family-practice physician and nutritional consultant in private practice in Marina del Rey, CA. He is the author of *Natural Sex Boosters* (Square One) and *Mind-Boosting Secrets* (Bottom Line Books, *www.bottomlinesecrets.com*).

The drug *sildenafil* (Viagra), introduced in 1998, revolutionized the treatment of sexual dysfunction. However, it and related drugs, such as *vardenafil* (Levitra) and *tadalafil* (Cialis), have significant limitations.

Although these impotence medications work well at promoting blood flow to the penis, they have little or no effect on libido or sexual sensation in men—or in women.

These drugs also have potentially serious side effects, such as vision problems, and some doctors believe that they may be dangerous for men who have cardiac conditions, such as irregular heart rhythms, history of heart attack or heart failure.

However, sex-boosting herbs have been used successfully for hundreds of years in Brazil, China, India and parts of Africa.

The following supplements, available at most health-food stores, can improve virtually all aspects of sexual performance, including increased desire, improved genital blood flow in men and women, and stronger erections.*

Start by choosing one herb that seems to best fit your needs. After one to two weeks, you can combine it with another supplement

*Check with your doctor before taking any of these products.

to enhance the effect. Or simply use a formula that combines these herbs.

Important: When combining herbs, cut the recommended dose of each in half to avoid potential side effects, such as restlessness.

HORNY GOAT WEED

This herb increases energy and libido in both men and women...and may produce firmer erections in men.

Horny goat weed reportedly got its name when a Chinese herder noticed that his goats became more sexually active after eating the plant. It's thought to influence levels of *dopamine* and other neurotransmitters that affect libido and mood. It also contains flavonoids, plant chemicals that dilate blood vessels and promote erections.

Scientific evidence: A study conducted in Beijing on 34 patients receiving dialysis for renal failure found that horny goat weed enhanced sexual activity in the patients taking it.

Typical dose: 500 to 2,000 milligrams (mg) daily. Start with 500 mg and increase, if needed. Side effects include restlessness and insomnia.

MUIRA PUAMA

This herb increases libido...orgasm intensity...and skin and genital sensitivity in men and women.

The bark and roots of this Amazon tree, sometimes known as "potency wood," increase sexual desire and sexual fantasies in men and women, and also facilitate a woman's ability to have an orgasm. It appears to work by promoting blood flow to the genitals in men and women.

Scientific evidence: A clinical study of 262 men, conducted at the Institute of Sexology in Paris, found that taking muira puama for two weeks improved libido in 62% of those studied.

Typical dose: 500 to 1,000 mg in capsule form three consecutive days each week.

Important: Muira puama should be taken in the morning. That's because it can cause insomnia when taken in the afternoon or at night. Muira puama may cause restlessness in some people during the daytime.

TRIBULUS

This herb increases energy and libido in both men and women...and it also improves erections in men.

This common roadside weed contains *protodioscin*, a chemical compound that is thought to increase production of the sex hormone testosterone in both men and women. It also dilates blood vessels in the penis, promoting firmer erections.

Scientific evidence: An animal study conducted at the National University Hospital in Singapore showed that rats that were given tribulus for eight weeks were found to experience firmer erections.

Typical dose: 500 to 1,000 mg daily. Take tribulus for one week, then stop for one week, and so on. This minimizes the risk for potential side effects, such as restlessness and increased body temperature.

ASHWAGANDHA

This herb increases mood and sexual desire and function in men and women. It can improve sex drive in both sexes by acting as a relaxant, and it also assists men in maintaining an erection.

Ashwagandha produces a calming effect by mimicking the action of GABA, a neurotransmitter in the brain that promotes relaxation. It also boosts nitric oxide production. Nitric oxide is known to enhance penile erection and vaginal sensitivity by increasing engorgement of the genital organs through blood vessel dilation.

Scientific evidence: A laboratory study conducted at the University of Texas Health Science Center found that ashwagandha inhibits the number of nerve cells that fire in the brain, much like the neurotransmitter GABA, resulting in an antianxiety and mood-enhancing effect.

Typical dose: 300 to 500 mg one to two times daily.

Important: For better absorption, take ashwagandha on an empty stomach.

Caution: Ashwagandha may cause drowsiness in some individuals. Do not drive after taking this herb.

Alleviate Neck and Back Pain with Fish Oil

Joseph Maroon, MD, vice chairman of neurological surgery, University of Pittsburgh.

When neck and back pain sufferers took a fish-oil supplement (1,200 milligrams [mg] daily) for 75 days, 60% reported significant pain relief that allowed them to decrease or discontinue use of painkillers.

Theory: The omega-3 fatty acids found in fish oil block the inflammation that can lead to neck and back pain. Fish oil also may help relieve joint pain.

If you have neck or back pain: Ask your doctor about taking fish oil. Do not use fish oil if you take *warfarin* (Coumadin) or another blood thinner.

Drug-Free Ways To Treat Pain

Norman Marcus, MD, director of the Norman Marcus Pain Institute, New York City. He is clinical associate professor in anesthesiology and psychiatry and director of Muscle Pain Research at New York University School of Medicine, and author of *Freedom from Pain*. Fireside.

More than 50 million Americans suffer from chronic pain—much of it untreated. But when pain sufferers do get medical care, they often receive *overtreatment*. Why is that?

Insurance companies and Medicare reimburse doctors for surgery and other invasive procedures—so that's what doctors are likely to provide. Insurance doesn't pay doctors to counsel patients about low-tech remedies, such as exercise and stress relief—even though these sometimes are the best ways to deal with persistent pain.

Here's how pain problems are frequently misdiagnosed and mistreated—and what you can do to get effective, commonsense pain relief...

BACK PAIN

Up to 80% of Americans suffer from low back pain at some point in their lives. Medical treatment for this chronic problem is based on the assumption that anatomical problems, such as herniated discs, cause the pain. A standard treatment is to operate, sometimes by surgically fusing the vertebrae (bones of the spine).

In reality, bones and discs usually don't cause low back pain. Sprained or strained muscles, ligaments and tendons—soft tissue made vulnerable to injury by overexertion and lack of exercise—underlie most cases.

Scientific evidence: In a study published in *Spine*, orthopedic surgeons treated 64 patients, ages 25 to 60, who had low back pain that had lasted one year or longer. X-rays showed degenerated discs. Half the group received surgery (fusion of the lumbar vertebrae). Half got nonsurgical treatments, including counseling and exercise.

A year after treatment, researchers evaluated both groups for pain, use of pain medication and other factors indicating treatment success or failure. The nonsurgery group had a *higher* success rate—76% compared with 70% of the surgery group (a clinically significant difference). And the nonsurgery group hadn't been subjected to the pain, risk and inconvenience of surgery.

NECK PAIN

In patients over age 40 who suffer from neck pain, a magnetic resonance imaging (MRI) scan or X-ray usually reveals degenerative changes in the vertebrae of the neck. Surgery may be recommended, but these changes are not the cause of most cases of neck pain.

A classic cause of neck (and shoulder) pain is working at a computer where the keyboard is too high or the chair too low—forcing the forearms into a position that creates a less than 90-degree angle in the elbow. This raises shoulder muscles, causing tension and pain in the neck and shoulders. Other common causes of neck pain are reading or watching television in bed and cradling the telephone on your shoulder.

SHOULDER PAIN

Shoulder pain and stiffness frequently are diagnosed as a rotator cuff tear, adhesive capsulitis (frozen shoulder) or "impingement syndrome" (a narrowed space between two rotator cuff muscles).

Your doctor may recommend surgery, followed by painful rehabilitation that may last as long as five months. Pain is generally relieved, but in some cases, patients never regain full function. Nonsurgical treatment to restore strength and flexibility to shoulder muscles can work as well as surgery—and there's no harm in trying it first.

Scientific evidence: Six months after "conservative" treatment for shoulder pain—shoulder exercises, physical therapy, ultrasound and pain-relieving steroid injections—64 out of 82 patients had significant pain relief and increased function, according to a study published in *Archives of Physical Medicine and Rehabilitation.*

HEADACHE

People with chronic migraine or tension headaches or both (mixed headache syndrome) usually are prescribed pain medications—which are costly and can damage the stomach, liver and/or kidneys with long-term use. But chronically tense midback, neck and shoulder muscles are a common cause of headache—and muscle tension can be treated without drugs.

Scientific evidence: A study published in *Cochrane Database of Systematic Reviews* analyzed 22 other scientific studies on headache treatments, with a total of 2,628 participants. Nondrug therapies, such as spinal manipulation, were as effective as medications—or even more so—for reducing the incidence of migraine or chronic tension headaches.

BETTER WAYS TO REDUCE PAIN

● **Find a pain specialist.** Your first stop should be your primary care physician, who can refer you to a pain specialist. He/she can perform a physical examination that evaluates muscles surrounding the painful joint for strength and flexibility as well as for spasm and trigger points (a tender muscle that refers pain to another part of the body)—an assessment that will show if muscles are causing the pain. If you need help locating a pain specialist, consult the American Academy of Pain Medicine, *www.painmed.org.*

● **Exercise.** Inactivity is the number-one cause of pain. Perform aerobic exercise daily.

Example: Brisk walking—fast enough to break a sweat—two to three miles a day. Most people who also perform the following exercises daily will notice improvement in the first three weeks, with additional results in six months.*

BEST EXERCISES FOR LOW BACK PAIN

Perform four repetitions of each of the following basic lower-body exercises daily…

1. Diaphragmatic breathing. Lie on your back, arms at your sides and knees bent. Slowly inhale through your nose, rounding out your belly. Then exhale through your mouth.

2. Shoulder shrug. Pull your shoulders up toward your ears as you inhale through your nose. Then exhale through your mouth as you let your shoulders fall back down.

3. Leg slide. Lie on your back, arms at your sides and knees bent. Slide your right leg down until it is flat on the floor. Relax the right leg for three seconds. Slide your right leg back to bent position. Repeat with your left leg.

4. Head rotation. Lie on your back, arms at your sides and knees bent. Drop your head to the left side. Return your head to center. Then drop your head to the right side.

5. Single knee to chest. Lie on your back, arms at your sides and knees bent. Bring your left knee to your chest as far as you comfortably can. Return your left leg to bent-knee position, then let it slide down until it is flat on the floor. Relax the left leg for three seconds, then slide it back to the bent-knee position. Repeat with your right leg.

*These exercises were created by Hans Kraus, MD, former associate professor of clinical physical medicine and rehabilitation at New York University Medical College. Dr. Kraus, who died in 1996, was national chairman of the medical committee for the YMCA's exercise program for back pain and personal physician to former President John F. Kennedy. For a copy of the complete Kraus Exercise Program, visit Dr. Marcus' Web site at *http://backpainusa.com*, or send a self-addressed, stamped envelope to Norman Marcus, MD, "Pain Exercises," 30 E. 40 St., New York, NY 10016.

6. Side-lying knee to chest. Lie on your left side, knees bent, head resting on your elbow. Bring your right leg toward your chest, letting the knee drop toward the floor. Then slide your right leg back, extending the knee until your leg is straight. Bring your leg back to the starting position. Roll onto your opposite side and repeat.

7. Buttocks squeeze. Lie on your stomach and place a pillow under your belly. Tighten your buttocks muscles and hold for two seconds. Relax the muscles.

BEST EXERCISES FOR
NECK PAIN, SHOULDER PAIN AND HEADACHE

Perform four repetitions of each of the following basic upper-body exercises daily. Begin with lower-body exercises 1, 2 and 4 (under "Best Exercises for Low Back Pain").

4. Elbow bend. Lie on your back, arms at your sides and legs extended. As you slowly inhale through your nose, close your fists and bend your elbows. Bring both arms toward your head. As you slowly exhale through your mouth, relax your arms and hands and let your arms drop back to your sides.

5. Chicken wings. Lie on your back, arms at your sides and legs extended. Rest your hands on your chest, elbows at your sides. Keeping your elbows down as much as possible, move them so they are pointing behind you. Return to the starting position.

6. Horizontal abduction–adduction. Lie on your back, hands at your sides and legs extended. Extend your right arm out to the side. Bring your right arm across your chest. Then return it to the extended position. Repeat with your left arm.

7. Shoulder rotation. Lie on your back, arms at your sides and legs extended. Extend your right arm out to the side. Bend your elbow and point your fingers behind you, getting your arm as flat on the floor as possible. Keeping your elbow on the floor, raise your arm 90 degrees so that your fingers are pointing toward the ceiling. Repeat. Then move your arm toward the floor, palm down, placing your arm as flat on the floor as possible. Raise your arm 90 degrees, fingers pointing toward the ceiling. Repeat. Perform the entire sequence with your left arm.

8. Shoulder bend. Lie on your back, arms at your sides and legs extended. As you slowly inhale through your nose, extend your arms behind your head, arms as flat on the floor as possible. As you slowly exhale through your mouth, return your arms to the starting position.

Illustrations by Shawn Banner.

Duct Tape Really Can Cure Warts

Dean R. Focht III, MD, fellow, division of gastroenterology, hepatology and nutrition, Cincinnati Children's Hospital Medical Center.

Placing duct tape (or other tape) over warts to get rid of them is not just an old wives' tale. A recent study found that placing tape over warts is more effective at eliminating them than standard medical therapy.

The study: Participants who had warts on fingers, palms, heels or soles of the feet were divided into two groups. One group put tape on warts for six days, then soaked the warts and scraped them with emery boards, waited 12 hours and reapplied the tape, repeating the process. The other group had their warts frozen off by a doctor, which is standard therapy.

Result: After just two months, 85% of those using the tape had gotten rid of their warts, versus only 60% of those who had received the standard freezing treatment.

Mighty Matcha

Science News, 1719 N St. NW, Washington, DC 20036.

The type of green tea used in Japanese tea ceremonies provides 200 times more *epigallocatechin gallate*, a potent anticancer chemical, than the green tea that's served in the US. Known as matcha, the Japanese tea is powdered before steeping—a technique that is believed to release more of the active compound than crumpled leaves. Matcha is available in some health-food stores and on the Web at *www.stashtea.com*.

Amazing! Salsa Stops Disease

Isao Kubo, PhD, professor, department of nutritional science and toxicology, University of California, Berkeley.

Salsa is not only a favorite tasty food, but it turns out to be a healthy one, too. It can actually *protect* and prevent you from getting sick. Cilantro, one of the common ingredients in this popular Mexican condiment, contains a compound that kills *Salmonella* bacteria, a frequent and sometimes lethal cause of food-borne illness, according to results of a study reported in the *Journal of Agricultural and Food Chemistry*.

EAT YOUR SALSA

Isao Kubo, PhD, lead researcher at the University of California, Berkeley, says that *dodecenal*—a compound that can be isolated from cilantro leaves—is the key Salmonella killer. Researchers were surprised to learn that dodecenal is the only natural antibacterial agent thus far known to be more effective than *gentamicin*, a powerful antibiotic medication that used to be prescribed by doctors to combat Salmonella.

In fact, in laboratory tests, dodecenal has proved to be twice as potent as gentamicin. Cilantro seeds have actually been used by traditional "food as medicine" practitioners to prevent dysentery for years.

Dr. Kubo explains that many compounds in cilantro show similar activity, and these may act synergistically. There may also be more antibacterial components in other salsa ingredients, which include tomatoes, onions and green chilies. The study suggests that people should eat more salsa with their food, especially fresh salsa.

NEW FOOD CURE?

In reality, it is probably impossible to eat as much cilantro as you would need to offer practical protection against food poisoning. However, Dr. Kubo notes that these new findings may lead to the expanded use of dodecenal as a safe, natural food additive to help prevent food-borne illness. Researchers speculate that the food industry may try to develop and market some form of dodecenal, and it may one day show up as a protective coating for meats or as a disinfectant to be used in cleaning and hand-washing.

In the meantime, some cilantro is better than none. Enjoy your salsa and continue to follow the rules of safe handling, cooking and storage of food.

Supercharge Your Immunity with Just A Few Herbs

James A. Duke, PhD, botany, and adjunct faculty at Tai Sophia Institute, a center for patient care and graduate education in complementary medicine, Laurel, MD. He is a leading authority on medicinal plants and former chief of the US Department of Agriculture Plant Laboratory. He is author of *Dr. Duke's Essential Herbs: 13 Vital Herbs You Need to Disease-Proof Your Body, Boost Your Energy, and Lengthen Your Life*. Rodale.

Medicinal herbs are rich in antioxidants that maintain health and slow the aging process. They also can prevent or alleviate age-related problems, such as arthritis, high blood pressure and failing vision.

We questioned world-renowned botanist James A. Duke, PhD, about which herbs are essential to healthy aging. Dr. Duke has a half-acre medicinal herb garden on his six-acre homestead in Fulton, Maryland.

While these herbs have few significant side effects and are far safer than most synthetic drugs, it is always wise to consult your doctor before treating a medical problem yourself.

Some herbs can interact with prescription and nonprescription drugs, magnifying or weakening their effects. In addition, some people may be allergic to herbs. Be alert to symptoms, such as a rash, when taking any herb.

With your doctor's approval, you can take these herbs all at the same time, along with vitamins, if you wish. Here are eight potent herbs that Dr. Duke uses himself. Follow the dosages suggested on the labels.

BILBERRY: VISION DISORDERS

Bilberry is rich in *anthocyanins*, chemicals that keep the capillary walls strong and flexible. It also is loaded with antioxidants that defend delicate tissue against free-radical damage.

In particular, bilberry protects the retina and its blood supply, preventing and improving vision disorders, such as macular degeneration.

Bilberry can ward off other eye problems, too, including cataracts, glaucoma and poor night vision.

CELERY SEED: GOUT AND ARTHRITIS

I have a special fondness for this herb, which has protected me from agonizing attacks of gout for the last seven years. It lowers blood levels of uric acid as effectively as *allopurinol*, the drug commonly prescribed for gout.

Celery seed, available in capsule form, also contains 25 anti-inflammatory compounds that can reduce the pain and swelling of arthritis. It has chemicals that make blood vessels relax and open, helping to alleviate high blood pressure and angina (chest pain caused by deficient blood flow to the heart).

In folk medicine, celery seed is reputed to be a digestive aid. It is used to relieve gas as well as heartburn, though this has yet to be clinically proven.

ECHINACEA: COLDS AND FLU

This popular herbal medicine is a powerful ally against colds and flu. The purple coneflower from which it comes has been used medicinally by Native Americans for centuries. At least three of the chemicals it contains—*caffeic acid, echinacoside* and *cichoric acid*—have known antiviral properties. In addition, echinacea boosts the body's own infection-fighting powers.

Take echinacea at the first sign of an upper-respiratory infection or flu. I also take it when I know I'll be in crowds or around other sources of infection.

This is not an herb for everyday use—the immune system eventually could stop responding to it. I don't take it for more than eight weeks in a row.

GARLIC: BLOOD PRESSURE AND CHOLESTEROL

This pungent bulb was prescribed by Hippocrates, the fifth-century BC Greek physician, and cited as a cure-all in an ancient Sanskrit manuscript. Today, we attribute its medicinal powers to a high concentration of sulfur compounds.

Garlic lowers blood pressure and cholesterol. There also is evidence that it can reduce the risk of cancer, particularly in the gastrointestinal tract.

Garlic contains at least 25 germ-killing compounds and fights bacterial, viral and fungal infections.

Eat at least one raw clove or four cooked cloves daily…or take garlic capsules.

HAWTHORN: POTENT HEART DRUG

An extract made from this flowering shrub can be useful against irregular heart rhythm, angina and shortness of breath. Hawthorn contains seven compounds known to prevent dangerous clotting and three that lower blood pressure. One study at University of Madras in India suggests that hawthorn also may reduce cholesterol.

MILK THISTLE: LIVER PROTECTION

The liver, the organ vital to detoxifying the blood, is under constant assault by pollution. Alcohol, also, is bad for the liver. Milk thistle, a relative of the artichoke, appears to protect the liver. It contains *silymarin*, which strengthens cell membranes and boosts the organ's ability to repair itself. Milk thistle even has been used to treat hepatitis A and C.

I take milk thistle capsules when I'm traveling and will be exposed to smog. If I lived in a major city with pollution problems, I would take it every day.

I also take it before a celebration, when I may be drinking a bit more alcohol than usual.

You can take silymarin capsules or eat milk thistle seeds, available in health-food stores, as you would sunflower seeds.

SAW PALMETTO:
PROSTATE PROBLEMS

At least half of men over age 50 have difficulty urinating because benign prostate enlargement chokes off the flow. An extract of saw palmetto, a tropical shrub, has been used for years to treat this problem. A review in the *Journal of the American Medical Association* concluded that saw palmetto facilitates urination in men with prostate problems about as well as medication. Natural chemicals in the herb appear to block a testosterone-type hormone that promotes prostate growth. Men without prostate problems may choose to take it as a preventive measure.

Saw palmetto also may slow down male pattern baldness.

TURMERIC:
HEART AND ARTHRITIS

This spice, made from the root of the tropical plant *Curcuma longa*, is a common ingredient in mustard and Indian food—it's what makes curry bright yellow. Turmeric is packed with antioxidants and contains powerful anti-inflammatory compounds called COX-2 inhibitors—the power behind arthritis drugs like Celebrex.

Some research suggests turmeric can stop inflammation about half as effectively as steroids such as cortisone—but without the troubling side effects. This makes it a valuable ally against arthritis. In addition, turmeric protects the heart. It makes blood platelets less likely to clump and form dangerous clots. It also fights cholesterol buildup in the arteries.

Turmeric is available as an herbal preparation. You also can add turmeric to your diet when cooking. I like to use it to make a curried celery soup.

WHICH BRANDS TO BUY

Herbal products are sold by many manufacturers, but there is no federal regulation to ensure quality control.

To be safe, select major brands, such as Nature's Herbs, Nature's Way and Solgar. These are available at most supermarkets, drugstores and health-food stores. Buy preparations that clearly indicate on the labels the exact amounts of active ingredients.

Nature's Virus Killers for Colds And Flu

Mark A. Stengler, ND, a naturopathic physician in private practice at La Jolla Whole Health Clinic, La Jolla, CA. He is associate clinical professor at both Bastyr University, Kenmore, WA, and the National College of Naturopathic Medicine, Portland, OR. He is author of numerous books on natural healing, including *The Natural Physician's Healing Therapies*. Bottom Line Books.

Do you have to get a cold or the flu this coming season? No! This year can be different. With the right preparation, quick intervention and a lineup of powerful, natural virus fighters, there's a good chance that you can enjoy fall and winter without getting sick. *Here's how...*

RELY ON NATURE'S VIRUS KILLERS

If you start to come down with a cold or the flu, my first recommendation is to change your diet. Eat lightly so that your body can focus on healing. For the first 24 hours, consume filtered water, broths and soups with lots of garlic, onions and spices, such as turmeric and cayenne, which relieve congestion, promote circulation and have a natural anti-inflammatory effect. Herbal teas (especially ginger, cinnamon and peppermint) and steamed vegetables also are good choices. When you're feeling better, move toward a more normal diet.

I have found several supplements to be effective for treating colds and flu. Consider taking these when people around you are sick or when you first feel symptoms. You can use one or any combination until you feel better. These also are safe for children when given in dosages of one-quarter to one-half of what I recommend for adults. The bigger the child, the higher the dose you can use.

• **Lomatium dissectum** is a plant once used by Native Americans to fight Spanish flu. Preliminary research shows that lomatium has the ability to prevent viruses from replicating and to stimulate white blood cell activity.

With colds and flu, I often see improvement within 24 hours. In my experience, the only side effect has been an allergic reaction in the form of a measles-like rash in a small percentage of users. This rash disappears a few days after lomatium is discontinued.

Eclectic Institute makes a potent product called Lomatium-Osha (800-332-4372, *www.eclecticherb.com*), which soothes the respiratory tract. This product is 50% alcohol, so take only the dosage recommended on the label. For children, add one-quarter of the adult dosage to hot water and let it sit for five minutes so that the alcohol evaporates.

Women who are pregnant or nursing should not use lomatium.

• **Elderberry,** as shown by research in Israel, can stimulate the immune system, enhance white blood cell activity and inhibit viral replication.

Flu patients have reported significant improvement within 48 hours of taking elderberry. It also helps with colds.

The elderberry used in research studies is Sambucol Black Elderberry Extract from Nature's Way (to find a retailer, call Total Health Discount Vitamins, 800-283-2833). Adults should take two teaspoons four times daily...children, one teaspoon four times daily.

• **Echinacea.** Contrary to recent media reports, extracts from this plant can be effective for treating colds and flu. Echinacea makes the body's own immune cells more efficient in attacking viruses.

The key is using a product that has been processed to contain a high level of active constituents. Ground-up echinacea root or leaves won't do much. The use of alcohol and water by the manufacturer to extract active components is critical to the product's potency.

Also, be sure to use enough (many people don't). Two potent, well-researched products are Echinamide: Fresh Alcohol-Free Echinacea Extract, Natural Berry Flavor...and Echinamide Anti-V Formula Softgels, both by Natural Factors (to find a retailer, call 800-322-8704 or go to *www.naturalfactors.com*). This echinacea has been shown to reduce the length and severity of the common cold.

If you feel a cold or the flu coming on, take 20 drops of liquid extract or two capsules every two waking hours for 24 hours, then cut back to every three waking hours until the illness has passed.

The same company makes a liquid preparation called Anti-V Formula, which contains Echinamide, lomatium and other virus fighters. It is the most aggressive product for cold and flu from the Natural Factors line and can be used instead of the other supplements. Take 1.5 milliliters (ml) every two waking hours for the first 48 hours and then every three waking hours until the illness is gone.

• **Homeopathic influenzinum** is an intriguing remedy that I have used with success.

Made from active flu strains, it stimulates the body's own defense system to resist infection. It works along the same lines as an oral vaccine, but since it is homeopathic, none of the flu particles are left in the preparation. It can be used for the prevention or treatment of flu and has no side effects.

Take two 30C-potency pellets twice daily for two weeks at the beginning of flu season (in early November). Take two pellets four times daily when exposed to flu sufferers or if you start to have symptoms.

It is available from health-food stores and The Vitamin Shoppe (866-293-3367, *www.vitaminshoppe.com*).

• **Oscillococcinum** is another great homeopathic remedy for flu, which is also available from The Vitamin Shoppe, health food stores and pharmacies or by calling 800-672-4556 or visiting *www.oscillo.com*.

It can be taken at the first sign of flu and is the number-one–selling homeopathic flu remedy in the US.

●**N-acetylcysteine (NAC).** This nutrient helps thin the mucus that may accompany a cold or the flu. In addition to making you feel better, NAC helps to prevent sinus and more serious chest infections.

A study at University of Genoa, Italy, showed that NAC, when taken as a supplement, could help prevent as well as treat flu. The nutrient increases levels of the powerful antioxidant *glutathione* in the body, which, in turn, improves immune function. NAC is available at any health-food store and many pharmacies.

If you tend to get the flu every year, take 600 milligrams (mg) twice daily when you are around people who have the flu or if you start feeling sick yourself.

●**Vitamin C** enhances the activity of white blood cells. I have found that taking 3,000 to 5,000 mg daily helps fight viral infections. However, some people get diarrhea from this amount. For immediate treatment of symptoms, start with 5,000 mg in divided doses. If loose stools occur, cut back to 3,000 mg (or even less).

Shorter Flu Recovery

Vivian Barak, PhD, head of the immunology lab for tumor diagnosis, Hebrew University-Hadassah Medical School, Jerusalem.

A new study found that flu patients who were given elderberry extract four times daily for five days recovered in four days compared with a recovery that took eight days for those given a placebo.

Theory: Elderberry prevents the flu virus from attaching to cells, which stops it from replicating.

Self-defense: Take four tablespoons of elderberry extract or four elderberry lozenges daily at the onset of flu symptoms and for the duration of the illness.

What You Need to Know To Protect Yourself from The Deadly Bird Flu

William Schaffner, MD, chairman of the department of preventive medicine at Vanderbilt University Medical Center, Nashville. He is a fellow of the Infectious Diseases Society of America, a liaison member of the Advisory Committee on Immunization Practices of the Centers for Disease Control and Prevention and an associate editor of *The Journal of Infectious Diseases.*

If you follow the news, you already know there's a chance that a flu pandemic (a global epidemic) is coming and that it may bring death on a massive scale. Federal, state and local agencies already are working up plans for prevention and treatment.

We can't—individually or as a nation—stop such a disease from reaching the US, but we *can* make ourselves safer by taking some smart precautions.

William Schaffner, MD, chairman of the department of preventive medicine at Vanderbilt University Medical Center and one of the world's top experts on infectious diseases, explains how a pandemic might occur and how to build up our defenses…

UNDERSTANDING THE DANGER

There's no way to predict exactly when the feared pandemic might occur—it could be years away. Based on the recent cases of Avian flu in humans in Asia and in birds in Europe and the Mideast, it might be as soon as next year—it could even be this year. A pandemic can occur at any time of the year, but it is more likely during the traditional flu season and could last a few years.

How the danger started: Eight years ago in Hong Kong, a deadly flu strain that normally affects birds began infecting a few humans as well. According to the World Health Organization, at least 116 people have been infected since 2003, mainly in Thailand and Vietnam. About half of them have died. Avian flu is no longer just Asia's problem—Romania, Turkey and Greece have just confirmed that avian flu has been found among birds there as well.

CHILLING DISCOVERY

Scientists recently discovered that the flu virus that ravaged the world in the 1918 Spanish flu pandemic also was derived from a bird flu virus. That devastating global outbreak killed 50 million people.

Unlike the 1918 virus, the current avian virus is not easily transmitted from person to person. With only a few exceptions, its victims have been infected by coming in direct contact with live infected birds, typically chickens or waterfowl, such as geese or ducks. But influenza viruses have a remarkable ability to mutate. The avian flu virus could change into something much more contagious to humans, then start spreading—within days, thanks to airplane travel. A deadly pandemic then could hit within weeks or months.

WHAT TO DO TODAY

Important steps that you can take to protect yourself against a flu pandemic…

•**Quit smoking.** If you needed one more reason, this is it. Smoking irritates the bronchial tubes, making them more vulnerable to any germs that find their way into the throat, including those that can cause avian flu. Smokers also have a harder time fighting any diseases that they do contract.

•**Maintain a healthy weight.** Carrying extra pounds puts unnecessary stress on your heart and lungs, making you more vulnerable to contracting avian flu.

•**Get vaccinated** with a flu shot or the nasal-spray vaccine. The current generation of flu vaccine provides no specific protection against avian flu, but it will help keep your body as strong as possible, improving your odds of survival in case avian flu does strike. Should the pandemic come, those who have been vaccinated but still come down with a flu will know right away that they probably have avian flu. (If you have egg allergies or have had serious reactions to flu shots in the past, talk to your doctor about whether a flu vaccine is safe for you.)

There is a prototype avian flu vaccine that appears to be doing well in clinical trials. Should an avian flu pandemic strike soon, it's possible that this prototype could be rushed into use—but at this point, we don't know how such a vaccine would be distributed… how big a dose would be needed…and how successful it might be against a mutated form of the virus.

•**Take vitamin C.** Some studies suggest that consuming vitamin C supplements and/or foods rich in vitamin C (such as oranges, grapefruits, bell peppers and tomatoes) might help the body avoid viral infections.

•**Stockpile emergency rations.** There would probably be a run on supermarkets at the first sign of a pandemic. Maintain a two-week supply of canned foods and water so that you don't have to leave home. This should be enough to last you until a government food-distribution plan is in place, should one be necessary. *Other items to have on hand:* Medications that you take regularly…alcohol wipes…surgical masks.

IF THERE IS AN OUTBREAK…

Should an avian flu pandemic reach the US, stay tuned to TV or radio news for instructions from your health department. There might be quarantines, evacuations or mass vaccination plans in your area.

•**Avoid crowded places.** The best way to remain safe during a pandemic is to limit your exposure to other people. All family members should stay at home as much as possible, avoiding unnecessary trips and visitors. Avoid airplanes, movie theaters and other places where large groups are in close proximity.

It's likely that some employers will tell workers that they can stay home for a time, though other people might have to choose between keeping their jobs and staying home. Local or state governments might close schools.

•**Take precautions** if you must go out during a pandemic. Stay away from anyone who is coughing or sneezing…wash your hands frequently with soap…and carry alcohol wipes to clean your hands after touching anything that has been handled by others.

Many people have asked about wearing cotton surgical masks. There's no evidence that they prevent viral infection, but they're cheap and available at many drugstores. They *might* help, so there's no reason not to wear one.

•**Get to a health-care provider** if the avian flu is in your region and you believe that you're coming down with flulike symptoms—chills, fever, sore throat, fatigue, cough, runny nose, headache or muscle aches. Antiviral drugs are effective only when taken within 48 hours of the onset of your first symptoms.

If possible, obtain your antiviral medication through your doctor's office or a public health office rather than from a hospital. (Your doctor might designate special hours for people with flu symptoms.) During a pandemic, hospitals are likely to be packed with infected people. Your flulike symptoms might mean you just have a cold—but your odds of actually getting avian flu will skyrocket once you enter a hospital handling lots of flu victims.

Are Antibacterial Soaps Making You Sick?

Michael Carlston, MD, former assistant clinical professor of family and community medicine, University of California, San Francisco, School of Medicine.

Consider a mother and a father with four children during the cold and flu season. Inevitably, when one child gets sick, the entire family does. The question is, how do you keep the germ of the day from knocking out the whole household?

According to Michael Carlston, MD, former assistant clinical professor of family and community medicine at the University of California, San Francisco, School of Medicine, the best advice is age-old advice—wash your hands. Wash your hands before eating, before leaving the bathroom and anytime they are dirty, he says. *But, here's the fascinating part of his advice...*

DON'T WASH WITH ANTIBACTERIAL SOAP!

Dr. Carlston's objections to using antibacterials is not that these products don't work, but that they work too well.

Dr. Carlston explains that antibacterials get rid of the "friendly" bacteria that humans need. What's left are the more virulent strains that can harm us, minus a lot of the "friendlies" that protect us from the dangerous ones. The use of antibacterial soap actually puts people at a disadvantage. In a study published recently in the *Annals of Internal Medicine*, researchers found that subjects who used antibacterial soap got just as many runny noses and upper respiratory illnesses as those who did not.

GETTING SICK CAN BE GOOD FOR YOU

Dr. Carlston cautions about becoming overly "germphobic" as the cold and flu season wears on, and wants you to realize that if you do get sick, it is not a totally bad thing. "There is a utility to getting sick," he says. When you get a little illness, such as a cold, it gives your immune system a chance to exercise its illness-fighting ability just as exercising your muscles does. Like muscle, if you don't use it, you lose it. An immune system that never gets the chance to respond to a challenge will not grow stronger.

Of course, he is not recommending that people go out looking for illnesses. It is instinctual and correct to avoid being near very sick people. (And, if you must be near them, don't forget to wash your hands!) It's just that a little sickness can make us stronger overall.

BUILDING YOUR IMMUNITY

Dr. Carlston notes that the average child will get about 10 colds in the first 18 months of life, but then he/she will get far fewer after that. This is because his immune system has learned how to respond. As adults, he says, our immune systems still need the exercise. Of course, this does not apply to those who are immunosuppressed by HIV or other illnesses —they must be extremely careful about avoiding germs.

For the rest of us, though, taking care of ourselves overall (eating nutritious food, exercising regularly, drinking plenty of water and washing our hands) plus catching a cold once in a while may be the best prescription for on-going health.

Sinus Infection Relief

Winston C. Vaughan, MD, director and founder, California Sinus Institute, Palo Alto, CA.

Anew sinus mist reduces repeat sinus infections. SinuNEB uses an inhaler called a nebulizer to convert antibiotics into a fine, inhalable mist that coats the lining of the sinus cavities.

Recent study: Patients with chronic sinusitis remained infection-free an average of 17 weeks after treatment, compared with only six weeks for patients who had undergone surgeries and were treated with antibiotics. SinuNEB also caused fewer side effects, such as upset stomach and diarrhea, than commonly prescribed antibiotics.

How to Eat Fruits and Vegetables Safely

Marion Nestle, PhD, is the Paulette Goddard professor of nutrition, food studies and public health at New York University in New York City. She is author or editor of five books, including *What to Eat*. North Point.

In the wake of the recent *Escherichia coli* (E. coli) outbreak from contaminated spinach, many Americans stopped eating spinach or became more rigorous in washing it. However, there are probably few people who adopted long-term strategies to protect themselves against dangerous contaminants that could be found in any fruits or vegetables.

WHY OUR FOOD IS AT RISK

Concern about safety should not prevent you from eating fruits and vegetables—the health benefits of produce far outweigh the risks. Nevertheless, health officials estimate that each year, foodborne bacteria, parasites and viruses sicken 76 million Americans, resulting in 325,000 hospitalizations and 5,000 deaths.

Contaminated fresh produce is the number-one cause of individual cases of foodborne illnesses, according to the Washington, DC–based consumer-advocacy group Center for Science in the Public Interest.

In the US, the safety of fruits and vegetables falls under the jurisdiction of the Food and Drug Administration (FDA). However, typically less than 2% of imported food products is inspected by the FDA, and domestic produce is rarely inspected at all.

FDA and US Department of Agriculture (USDA) guidelines for the safe handling of produce—known as "Good Agricultural Practices"—suggest methods to help prevent contamination with dangerous microorganisms from water, soil, manure or unhygienic food handlers.

However, these guidelines are voluntary—fruit and vegetable companies do not have to follow them. What's more, the reality is that the FDA does not have the financial resources or personnel to effectively monitor industry practices or the safety of the 741 pounds of produce that are consumed, on average, by every person in the US each year.

Fruits and vegetables are grown in what the FDA typically calls "nonsterile environments"—that is, they grow in dirt. If they come in contact with feces of grazing cattle, wild animals or birds, farm workers or any other source, they can become contaminated with potentially harmful microorganisms. This is clearly unappetizing, and fecal contamination causes health problems if the microorganisms are dangerous types.

BEST SELF-DEFENSE STRATEGIES

Most produce is safe to eat, but regardless of where you shop, there's no way to be 100% certain that the fruits and vegetables you're buying are free of contamination from dangerous microbes.

To do the best you can to protect yourself and your family from unsafe produce, follow these simple steps…

•**Be sure to remove the outer leaves of leafy greens.** That's the area that is most likely to come in contact with manure or other sources of dangerous contamination while leafy vegetables are growing in soil or processed after harvesting.

Caution: The FDA does not require food safety procedures to be followed for most produce, and this includes leafy greens, such as spinach and lettuce, as well as tomatoes and carrots.

Sprouts are an exception. They must be grown under strict safety rules, and problems with them have declined since those precautions went into effect.

●**Store produce in the refrigerator, and wash it before eating.** Harmful microorganisms can multiply on fresh fruits and vegetables, especially when they are transported great distances, sit in supermarket produce bins for extended periods and are not kept cold enough.

Best way to wash produce: Thoroughly rinse produce under running cool tap water. In addition, carefully scrub firm-skinned fruits and vegetables, such as apples and cucumbers, with a clean vegetable brush.

Be sure to clean the vegetable brush, utensils and other kitchen tools in hot water (or the dishwasher) after each use.

Caution: It is a good idea to wash bagged lettuce, spinach and other vegetables—even if the bag says the contents have been "triple washed." If the bags were not kept cold, bacteria could have multiplied inside the package.

To be extra safe, rinse off the inedible rinds of fruits, such as cantaloupe and avocados. If microbes are on the rind, the fruit inside can become contaminated when the rind is pierced.

Helpful: Don't splurge on expensive fruit and vegetable washes sold in the supermarket. There is no evidence that these special washes are more effective than chlorinated tap water.

Important: Although washing helps protect against foodborne illness from produce, the only way to guarantee that fruits and vegetables do not contain harmful microbes is to cook them in boiling water.

●**Buy certified organic.** Studies show that certified organic produce, which is grown in composted manure instead of chemical fertilizers, is no more likely to be contaminated with microbes than conventionally grown produce. That's because, to obtain organic certification, farmers must follow strict rules to ensure that harmful microbes in manure are destroyed (typically through a high-heat decontamination process). Growers of conventional produce are not required to follow such rules.

Organic produce is also a good option if you want to avoid synthetic pesticides and other chemicals that are typically used to kill insects in conventionally grown crops. These chemicals do not reduce your risk for contamination with bacteria and other microbes.

In addition, some research shows that organic produce may be superior to conventionally grown produce in its nutritional value.

Important: When buying organic produce, be sure that it is labeled with a "USDA organic" seal. This means that the producers follow organic growing rules established by the USDA Organic Standards Board and have been inspected by agencies licensed by the USDA to make sure the rules are followed.

Because organic produce is usually more expensive than nonorganic varieties, most people don't buy organic all the time. The Environmental Working Group (EWG), a Washington, DC–based, nonprofit environmental research organization, recommends buying organic varieties of produce whose nonorganic counterparts are typically highest in pesticides.

These include peaches, apples, sweet bell peppers, celery, nectarines, strawberries, cherries, pears, imported grapes, spinach, lettuce and potatoes. For a list of other fruits and vegetables evaluated by the EWG, go to the group's Web site, *www.foodnews.org*.

●**Buy from local farmers.** When food is shipped from far away and/or stays in the supermarket for long periods, there is more time for microbes to multiply.

Better Weight Loss

Barbara Rolls, PhD, professor and Guthrie Chair in Nutrition, the Pennsylvania State University, University Park. She is author of *The Volumetrics Eating Plan.* Harper.

In a study of 147 men and women who ate a reduced-calorie diet for a year, those who consumed 10.5 fluid ounces of low-fat, low-calorie soup twice a day lost 50% more weight than those who ate healthful but carbohydrate-rich snacks, such as baked chips or pretzels.

Theory: Although the soup had the same number of calories as the other snacks, the soup's greater weight and volume made study participants feel full enough to eat less for the rest of the day.

Self-defense: Consume a large mugful of a broth-based, low-fat, low-calorie, low-sodium soup rich in vegetables and/or beans as a first course twice daily.

The Calcium Diet

Michael Zemel, PhD, professor of nutrition and medicine and director of the Nutrition Institute, University of Tennessee, Knoxville. He is coauthor of *The Calcium Key: The Revolutionary Diet Discovery That Will Help You Lose Weight Faster.* Wiley.

Why are two out of three Americans overweight? Certainly we're eating more and exercising less. But there is another cause—a lack of the mineral calcium in our diets.

If you are among the Americans getting the lowest average level of calcium—255 milligrams (mg) per day—you are 84% more likely to be overweight than if you are among those getting the highest average level—1,346 mg per day—according to an analysis of data from the government's Health and Nutrition Examination Survey.

Simply by getting adequate calcium in our diets, as many as four out of five of us could lose the extra weight.

CALCIUM AND YOUR FAT CELLS

Calcium does far more than just keep your skeleton strong. Without enough calcium circulating in your bloodstream, your heart wouldn't beat, your blood wouldn't clot, your hormones wouldn't regulate your metabolism and your nerves wouldn't transmit signals.

If calcium levels fall—if you eat a low-calcium diet, for example—the body releases more of the hormone *calcitriol.* Calcitriol increases absorption of calcium in the intestines, so you get the most calcium possible from food.

In addition, it increases reabsorption through the kidneys, so that you lose as little calcium as possible through excretion.

Calcitriol also controls how fat cells work. When you get too little calcium and more calcitriol is released, your fat cells make and store more fat, causing weight gain.

MORE PROOF

In a study we conducted at the University of Tennessee, overweight people were put on one of three eating plans for six months.

●**Group 1** ate a diet that was 500 calories below maintenance level—the level at which you neither gain nor lose weight—and had no more than one serving of dairy a day for a total of 400 to 500 mg of dietary calcium.

●**Group 2** ate the same calorie-restricted diet but took an 800-mg calcium supplement for a total of 1,200 to 1,300 mg of calcium.

●**Group 3** also ate the calorie-restricted diet but included three servings of low-fat dairy a day, bringing their total calcium intake to 1,200 to 1,300 mg.

Results: Group 1 lost 6% of total weight …Group 2 lost 7.5%…and Group 3—the low-fat dairy group—lost 11%. Group 3 also lost more body fat than the other groups, particularly around the waist area. This is an important finding because a slimmer waist is associated with a lower risk of heart disease, stroke, diabetes and cancer.

This means that adding three servings of low-fat dairy to your diet can…

●**Increase the amount of weight you lose by 70%.**

●**Increase the amount of body fat you lose by 64%.**

●**Help you lose 47% more fat from your belly.**

Other studies have replicated these findings as well. In a 10-year study of 3,000 people ages 18 to 30, researchers at Harvard University found that people who ate three servings of dairy a day had a 60% lower risk of being overweight than those who consumed less calcium.

FOOD VS. SUPPLEMENTS

Studies show that calcium from dairy foods is more effective for weight loss than supplements. Why? Food is a complex mixture of known and unknown components. There is a cooperation among the components that can't be reproduced in a nutritional supplement.

Dairy contains calcium and a host of other biologically active components, including the amino acid *leucine*. Recent research reveals that leucine may increase the ability of muscle to use fat.

WHAT TO DO

To lose an average of one pound per week, you need to cut calorie intake and increase calorie burning by about 500 calories per day, or 3,500 calories per week. To boost the loss to 1.5 to two pounds, you need three or four servings of dairy a day, for a total of 1,200 to 1,600 mg of calcium. The easiest way to get that is with three servings of non-fat (skim) or low-fat milk (8 ounces per serving), yogurt (8 ounces) or cheese (1.5 or 2 ounces, processed).

Strategy: Have milk before a meal. Studies show that getting a liquid form of dairy before eating helps you feel full sooner at that meal and eat less at the next meal.

If you're lactose intolerant, try yogurt with live cultures or cheese (it has very little lactose) or take a lactose supplement when consuming dairy.

To cut 3,500 calories a week: One brisk, hour-long walk burns about 250 calories. If you do that four times a week, you still need to cut 2,500 calories per week, or about 350 calories a day. Look for one or two high-calorie items to eliminate from your daily diet.

Examples: A 12-ounce cola has 150 calories…two tablespoons of full-fat salad dressing, 150 …a glazed doughnut, 250…a 4-ounce bagel, 300.

Just eliminating these items will help you lose weight, but boosting calcium will help you lose more.

Weight-Loss Secret

Michael Zemel, PhD, professor of nutrition and medicine and director of the Nutrition Institute, University of Tennessee, Knoxville. He is coauthor of *The Calcium Key: The Revolutionary Diet Discovery That Will Help You Lose Weight Faster*. Wiley.

Yogurt helps you lose weight while protecting muscle.

Recent study: Overweight people who ate three servings of yogurt daily for 12 weeks lost 22% more weight, 61% more body fat and 81% more abdominal fat than people who ate a similar number of calories but no dairy products.

The TV Workout

Linda Buch, American Council on Exercise certified fitness trainer based in Denver, and coauthor of *The Commercial Break Workout: Trim and Tone Two Minutes at a Time*. Prime Lifestyles.

Exercising while watching TV can help keep you healthy. Whenever a commercial comes on, sit up in your chair with abdominal muscles tight and chest high (avoid arching your back). Keeping your feet shoulder-width apart, lean forward slightly and exhale while pushing up through your heels to a standing position. Then inhale as you slowly sit back down—using your leg muscles for control. Repeat this "sofa squat" throughout the entire commercial break.

A Stronger Body in Only 30 Minutes a Week

Fredrick Hahn, president and cofounder of the National Council for Exercise Standards, an organization of exercise, medical and scientific professionals. He is owner of Serious Strength, Inc., a Slow Burn strength-training studio in New York City, and coauthor of *The Slow Burn Fitness Revolution* (Broadway). *www.seriousstrength.com*.

We know the benefits of strength training. It will restore muscle…increase bone density…improve balance, decreasing the likelihood of falls…and promote weight loss and cardiovascular fitness. But the conventional strength training requires several hours a week and frequently causes injury.

New, better way: Slow Burn, in which the weights are lifted and lowered with incredible slowness—about 10 seconds up and 10 seconds down. *The benefits…*

•**It's safer.** Slow lifting reduces injury-causing stress on ligaments, tendons and joints. This means that even the elderly can do it safely.

•**It's more effective.** Without the aid of momentum, more muscle fibers are exercised.

•**It's more efficient.** You can get a complete workout in about 30 minutes each week —compared with at least three hours for conventional lifting.

HOW TO DO IT

In a Slow Burn workout, you complete a set of three to six repetitions of each exercise in 60 to 90 seconds. If you perform 10 exercises, you can complete your workout in approximately 10 to 15 minutes. Two workouts a week are all you need.

To obtain the best results, raise and lower weights at the rate of about one inch per second. Allow a total of about 100 seconds for all repetitions of each exercise—push-ups, leg curls, etc. Breathe normally.

Helpful: Use a metronome to maintain the one-inch-per-second rhythm.

Repeat each exercise until the muscles are fatigued and you can't do another repetition in perfect form. If you pass the 90-second point and feel as though you could keep going, the weights are too light. If you cannot complete three repetitions in 90 seconds, the weights are too heavy. Experiment to find the right weight.

The following program stimulates all muscle groups. Do three to six repetitions of each exercise. For exercises that require switching arms or legs, do three to six repetitions with each arm or leg. You will need adjustable hand and ankle weights. Look for sets that adjust from one to 20 pounds.

•**Push-ups.** Kneel on a towel with both your hands flat on the floor in front of you, shoulder-width apart. Keep your back straight—don't let it sway or arch.

Take three seconds to lower yourself the first inch and at least seven seconds to lower yourself all the way, until your forehead almost touches the floor. Without resting at the bottom, reverse direction. Don't lock your elbows at the top. Just as soon as your arms are almost straight, reverse and go back down. If kneeling push-ups are too easy, do the regular push-ups, with your toes on the floor.

•**Doorknob squats.** Open a door halfway so that you can grip both knobs. Place a stool or chair about two feet from the edge of the door. Stand arms' length away from the door. Then, lightly grasp the knobs for balance, and slowly bend your knees and lower your body as though you were sitting down. Take three seconds to lower yourself the first inch and seven seconds to go all the way down, until your bottom just touches the stool. Then reverse and rise back up. Be careful not to pull yourself up with your arms—use the muscles of your buttocks and thighs.

•**Side-lying leg lifts.** Try this exercise without ankle weights at first. If it's too easy, start with five-pound weights. Lie on your left side with your head propped on your left hand. Bend your left leg slightly so that your right leg rests on top of the calf. Slowly raise your right leg up toward the ceiling, moving from the hip. Take three seconds to move it the first inch and seven seconds to raise it all the way. Pause at the top, tightly squeeze the hip and buttock muscles for a few seconds, then slowly lower the leg back down. Repeat with the other leg.

•**Single-leg curls.** Attach one five-pound weight to your right ankle. The weight may be too light, but it's a good place to start. Lean forward and put both hands on a stool or chair...keeping your right knee slightly bent and spine straight.

Curl your right leg so that the heel nears your bottom. Take three seconds to curl the leg the first inch and seven seconds to curl it the rest of the way. Pause at the top, squeeze the muscles in the back of your thigh, then slowly reverse direction. Repeat with the other leg.

•**Side shoulder raise and overhead press.** This movement combines two exercises. Start with five-pound dumbbells. With a dumbbell in each hand, sit on a chair with your back straight and your feet flat on the floor. Slowly raise the weights away from both of your sides, taking three seconds to move them the first inch and seven seconds to raise them until they're parallel to the floor. Pause at the top for a few seconds, then slowly lower the weights.

Without resting, move to the second phase of the exercise. Elbows bent, hold the weights at shoulder height, then slowly raise them overhead, taking three seconds to move them the first inch and seven seconds to go all the way up. Pause for a second, then gradually lower the weights until they're back at shoulder height. Do not lock your elbows at the top. Let your muscles support the weights.

●**Single-arm back pull-ups.** You need a stool or chair and a six- to eight-pound dumbbell. Hold the dumbbell in your right hand…then face the stool with your left leg forward…and support yourself with your left hand on the stool. Let your right arm hang beside the stool.

Slowly pull the dumbbell back and upward, taking three seconds to move it the first inch and seven seconds to raise it all the way. Your right elbow will be facing up and behind you. Pause at the top, squeeze the arm and back muscles for a few seconds, then lower the weight back down. Don't let your arm hang down at the end of the movement. Keep tension on the muscles all the time. Repeat with the other arm.

●**Biceps curls.** Sit on a stool or straight-back chair with a five-pound dumbbell in each hand. Tuck your elbows into your sides, and keep them there throughout the exercise. The only thing that should move is your lower arm.

Curl the dumbbells toward your shoulders, taking just three seconds to move them the first inch and seven seconds to curl them all the way. Squeeze the muscles in the forearms and upper arms for a few seconds at the top of the movement, and then slowly lower the weights back down.

●**Shoulder shrugs.** Sit on a stool or straight-back chair with a 10-pound dumbbell in each hand. Let your arms hang down away from your hips, with the elbows slightly bent.

Then, raise up the tops of your shoulders as though you're trying to touch them to your earlobes. Sit up straight. Don't slouch forward or backward. Take three seconds to move your shoulders the first inch and seven seconds to raise them as far as they'll go. Pause at the top to squeeze the muscles in your shoulders, then lower them back down.

●**Abdominal crunches.** Lie on your back with your feet flat on the floor and your knees bent at a 90° angle. Tuck a rolled towel under your lower back…hold your arms straight in front of you…and keep your chin tucked into your chest. Curl your torso upward and forward, taking three seconds to move the first inch and seven seconds to move forward. Do not try to sit all the way up. Keep your lower back in contact with the towel. Pause and squeeze abdominal muscles at the top of the movement, then slowly lower your torso down. Don't rest your shoulders on the floor at the end. As soon as they brush the floor, repeat the exercise.

Slow Burn illustrations by Shawn Banner.

Exercises That Help With Everything You Do

Larkin Barnett, adjunct professor of exercise science at Florida Atlantic University in Boca Raton, and author of *Functional Fitness: The Ultimate Fitness Program for Life on the Run*. Florida Academic.

Functional training is a form of exercise that strengthens the muscles that we use in everyday activities, such as standing, walking, sitting, doing chores and carrying packages.

How it works: Functional training helps integrate the limbs and the trunk muscles for fluid, powerful movements…puts your body into proper alignment…improves posture and balance…and promotes deep breathing for relaxation.

A functional fitness routine can be incorporated into cardiovascular and strength-training workouts. *The exercises described below are designed for people of all fitness levels and should be performed daily…*

SIT UP AND TAKE NOTICE

Benefits: Corrects trunk alignment, including weak abdominal muscles that don't provide sufficient support for the lower back …and enhances stamina and endurance.

Good for: Carrying objects…walking and running…and relieving muscle tension caused by working at a desk or a computer.

What to do: While sitting in a straight-backed chair, scrunch your shoulders up toward your ears, then relax them. Inhale slowly while you raise your shoulders, then exhale slowly as you lower them. Do this three to five times, feeling tension drain out of your shoulders and neck.

Next, sit tall, perched on your sit-bones (you can find these by rocking side-to-side) and concentrate on stacking your hips, ribs, chest and head on top of each other like building blocks. Exhale powerfully while pulling your abdominal muscles inward toward your spine. Then pull your shoulders back gently. Take several deep breaths.

Finally, sit up tall, while picturing the tops of your ears stretching upward. This elongates the spine and improves respiratory function. Tighten your abdominals inward and upward toward your spine while exhaling forcefully three to five times.

THE COMPASS

Benefits: Strengthens your postural muscles (to improve coordination and balance)… and reduces fatigue and stress on the legs, hips and back.

Good for: Relieving muscle soreness from extended standing as well as improving performance in all sports and physical activities.

What to do: With your feet flat on the ground about 12 inches apart, pretend you're standing in the middle of a large compass. With exaggerated movements, shift your entire body toward each of the four main points on the compass—north (forward), south (backward), east (to the right) and west (to the left)—pausing momentarily at each point. Do this three to five times. Contract your abdominal muscles and notice how your control improves.

Gradually make your movements smaller and smaller. Do this for 30 seconds. End by standing still and feeling your body weight evenly distributed.

THE PELVIS AS A FISH BOWL

Benefits: Centers the hips and places the pelvis in neutral alignment, reducing stress on the legs, back and neck.

Good for: Lifting…getting in and out of bed …and swinging a golf club or tennis racket.

What to do: Standing with your feet about 12 inches apart, contract your stomach muscles and draw them inward and up toward your spine. Picture your hips as a fish bowl filled with water, with the bowl's rim at your waistline.

Now tip your hips forward slightly and visualize water spilling out of the front of the fish bowl. Next, tip your hips backward slightly and visualize water sloshing out of the back of the bowl. Finally, balance the fish bowl so that the rim is perfectly level. This is your pelvis's "neutral" position. Throughout the day, assume this position as you stand up, walk and sit.

Illustrations by Shawn Banner.

Vinegar May Help Fight Diabetes

Carol S. Johnston, PhD, professor of nutrition, Arizona State University East, Mesa.

In a recent study, healthy patients and patients with a prediabetic condition known as insulin resistance drank a vinegar drink (⅛ cup of vinegar, diluted with ¼ cup of water and sweetened with saccharine) or a placebo drink before a high-carbohydrate meal.

The vinegar treatment improved insulin sensitivity by up to 40% in both groups.

Theory: Vinegar inhibits the breakdown of carbohydrates, thereby decreasing the blood glucose spikes that occur in people with diabetes.

If you are diabetic or insulin resistant: Talk to your doctor about drinking diluted vinegar before meals.

Reduce Diabetic Nerve Pain

Mark A. Stengler, ND, a naturopathic physician in private practice at La Jolla Whole Health Clinic, La Jolla, CA. He is associate clinical professor at both Bastyr University, Kenmore, WA, and the National College of Naturopathic Medicine, Portland, OR. He is author of numerous books on natural healing, including *The Natural Physician's Healing Therapies.* Bottom Line Books.

Researchers evaluated the effects of the nutritional supplement acetyl-L-carnitine (ALC) on diabetic neuropathy, a condition that occurs when diabetes damages the nerves, especially those in the hands, legs and feet. Symptoms include numbness, tingling and/or pain.

New study: In two clinical trials, 1,257 people with diabetes took 1,500 milligrams (mg) of ALC, 3,000 mg of ALC or a placebo pill daily for one year.

Those who took 3,000 mg of ALC daily experienced a significant reduction in pain.

My view: While ALC often is prescribed for those with age-related cognitive decline (poor memory) and early-stage Alzheimer's disease, it now should be considered a primary form of treatment for diabetic neuropathy.

Take 1,000 mg of ALC three times daily (the same dosing schedule used in the study).

ALC has a blood-thinning effect, so check with your doctor before using it if you take a blood thinner, such as *warfarin* (Coumadin).

Are You Taking Too Many Medications?

John Abramson, MD, clinical instructor in primary care at Harvard Medical School, Boston. He is author of *Overdosed America: The Broken Promise of American Medicine* (HarperCollins) and coauthor of "The Effect of Conflict of Interest on Biomedical Research and Clinical Practice Guidelines: Can We Trust the Evidence in Evidence-Based Medicine?" in the September–October 2005 issue of the *Journal of the American Board of Family Practice.*

With our national pharmacy bill now topping $200 billion each year, and recent disclosures about harmful and ineffective drugs, more people are asking: *Are all those pills really necessary?*

To learn more, we talked with John Abramson, MD, a Harvard Medical School clinical instructor who is widely recognized for his in-depth research of the drug industry…

● **Are most Americans overmedicated?** They sure are. Americans take many drugs unnecessarily, and when drugs *are* needed, people often take the wrong ones. For example, before *rofecoxib* (Vioxx) was withdrawn from the market because it was found to cause heart attacks and strokes (and was discovered to provide no better relief of arthritis symptoms than older, much less expensive anti-inflammatory drugs), about 80% of the Vioxx that was prescribed worldwide was used in the US.

● **Are doctors to blame?** The vast majority of physicians prescribe medication because they think it's in their patients' best interest. But there have been radical changes in the way that our medical knowledge is provided. Prior to 1980, most clinical research was publicly funded, but now most is funded directly by the drug and other medical industries, whose primary mission is to maximize the return on investments for investors.

Ninety percent of clinical trials now are commercially funded—as well as 75% of published clinical research. When a pharmaceutical company sponsors a study, the odds are five times greater that the findings will favor its product.

Drug and medical industries fund 70% of continuing education lectures and seminars, which are among the activities that doctors are required to attend to maintain their licenses to practice. Wherever doctors turn for sources of information, drug companies dominate.

● **Who should be monitoring doctors' relationships with drug companies?** The real failure is on the part of government agencies, such as the US Food and Drug Administration (FDA) and the Agency for Healthcare Research and Quality. Medical journals and academic researchers have become dependent on drug company money and/or are vulnerable to drug company lobbying. Doctors and the public still trust these institutions to independently oversee the integrity of the medical knowledge that informs our medical care, when they simply are not able to do this anymore.

● **We all know that cholesterol-lowering statins are widely prescribed. Are they unnecessary?** Despite being on the market for 18 years and becoming the best-selling class of drugs, statins have never been shown in randomized, controlled trials to provide a significant health benefit when used by women of any age without heart disease or diabetes. The same is true for men over age 65 without heart disease or diabetes. Even so, millions of people in both groups now are taking a statin drug.

● **Is it ever advisable to take a statin?** Yes, there is good evidence that statins are beneficial for people who already have heart disease and for at least some people who have diabetes. A good case also can be made for men who are at very high risk for heart disease (LDL "bad" cholesterol approaching 200 and other risk factors).

● **What other drugs do you think are being prescribed because of drug company influence?** Antihypertensives—drugs used to treat high blood pressure—are good examples. Newer medications, such as calcium channel blockers and angiotensin converting enzyme (ACE) inhibitors, are among the most popular. One of them, *amlodipine* (Norvasc), was the second most commonly prescribed drug for older adults in 2003. But a study funded by the National Heart, Lung and Blood Institute found that diuretics, which have been around for decades, are as good or better than Norvasc in protecting against complications of hypertension, such as heart attack and stroke. A diuretic might cost $29 per year, compared with $549 to $749 for Norvasc, depending on the dose. The patents for diuretics expired decades ago, so drug companies don't profit much from them.

● **Should everyone who has high blood pressure just take a diuretic?** High blood pressure is a complex problem. Some people respond to one drug, some to another, and some need more than one. It would make sense, though, to start with a diuretic, and use expensive drugs such as Norvasc only when other alternatives haven't worked.

● **Are natural therapies a better alternative to some drugs?** If you look at the data rather than listen to the drug ads, you see that natural alternatives, such as improved diet and routine exercise, often are far more effective than drugs at achieving real health improvements, such as less heart disease and longer life.

Probably the most important test of a healthy diet's effect on heart disease is the Lyon Diet Heart Study conducted in Lyon, France. Heart attack patients were randomly counseled to eat a Mediterranean diet (high in unprocessed grains, fruits, vegetables and olive oil…very low in red meat, dairy fat and cholesterol) or a "prudent" post-heart attack diet (no more than 30% of calories from total fat and no more than 10% from saturated fat).

The people counseled to eat the Mediterranean diet developed 72% less heart disease than those in the prudent diet group over the next four years. There were 56% fewer deaths in the group counseled to eat the Mediterranean diet—that's two to three times the benefit achieved with statin drugs.

The same holds true for exercise. A study conducted at the Cooper Institute for Aerobics Research in Dallas followed 25,000 men who had undergone physical exams. Over the next 10 years, the men whose exercise endurance (as measured on a treadmill) was in the lowest 20% of the group were at a much higher risk of dying than those with high total cholesterol levels (above 240)—confirming that exercise is even more important than cholesterol control.

●**But many patients prefer pills because they're easier.** There is no question that many of us would rather take a pill than change our lifestyle. If the pills worked, it would simply be a question of how we want to spend our money. The problem is that the pills often are closer to folk medicine—empowered by our cultural beliefs but without a genuine scientific basis. About two-thirds of our health is determined by the way we live our lives, and—for better or worse—no pills can change that.

●**What's the solution?** Most doctors don't invest much time or energy helping patients to make healthy changes in diet and exercise or teaching stress reduction. If you are willing to consider these approaches before trying drug treatment, tell your doctor.

When medication is necessary, ask your doctor if a generic drug is just as effective as the expensive brand-name product. Remember, drug ads that tell you to "ask your doctor" about a particular drug have a single purpose—to sell more drugs, not to improve your health.

Prescription drug ads have become a normal part of our cultural landscape, but the US and New Zealand (with less than 4 million people) are the only two industrialized countries that allow them. The rest of the industrialized countries feel that assessment of the scientific information about prescription drug treatment should be left to doctors, who should work in a partnership with each patient to determine optimal medical care based on his/her individual situation.

How Safe Are Your Vitamins and Minerals?

Tod Cooperman, MD, president and founder of ConsumerLab.com, White Plains, NY, which provides the latest testing results and issues warnings and information about recalls approximately every two weeks. He is an editor of *ConsumerLab.com's Guide to Buying Vitamins & Supplements.* ConsumerLab.com.

The FDA requires nutritional supplement labels to state exactly what's contained in the package. But government inspectors rarely check.

Result: Many supplements contain too little or too much of the active ingredient...are contaminated with pesticides or heavy metals (arsenic, cadmium, lead)...or aren't properly absorbed by the body.

ConsumerLab.com, an independent evaluator of nutritional and vitamin/mineral supplements, recently tested more than 500 products in laboratories throughout the country to determine if their ingredients matched what was listed on the label. Products also were tested for contamination and their ability to dissolve in the body.

Best choices...*

MULTIVITAMINS/MINERALS

Most people use multivitamins and minerals as "nutritional insurance" to compensate for gaps in their diets.

Test results: Of the 27 products tested, nine failed. The most common problems were related to vitamin A. Some of the products contained more than 150% of the amount listed on the label.

Excessive vitamin A can cause headache, anemia and bone and liver damage. Other multivitamin formulas contained lower-than-listed levels of beta-carotene and folic acid, an essential nutrient for preventing birth defects.

Reliable products include...

●**Geritol Complete.**

●**Life Essentials Dietary Supplement.**

●**Nutrilite Daily Multivitamin and Multimineral Dietary Supplement.**

●**Ocuvite Zinc with Key Antioxidants Vitamin and Mineral Supplement.**

B VITAMINS

The eight B vitamins are involved in all aspects of metabolism, but your body can't produce them. B vitamins are available only through food or supplements. Some supplements contain a single B vitamin, while others contain all eight.

Test results: Of the 21 products tested, nine listed doses on their labels that were in excess of the safe upper limit (UL) for vitamin B-3

*Other approved products may display a seal of approval from ConsumerLab.com, the US Pharmacopeia (USP) or NSF International. All of these organizations evaluate supplements.

(niacin), as established by the Institute of Medicine of the National Academies.

High doses can be taken under a doctor's supervision to safely lower cholesterol. But people who take a B-complex supplement that contains 35 milligrams (mg) of niacin or more may experience side effects, such as facial flushing and skin tingling. At very high doses, niacin can cause liver damage.

Reliable products include...

• **Nature Made Balanced B-150 B-Complex Supplement Time Released**

• **Nutrilite Natural B Complex Dietary Supplement**

• **Stresstabs High Potency B-Complex with Antioxidants C & E & Folic Acid + Zinc Dietary Supplement**

• **Vitamin World B-100 Ultra B-Complex, 100 mg**

VITAMIN C

It's an antioxidant that may boost immune function, reduce cataracts and other eye diseases and protect against cancer.

Test results: Of the 26 products tested, one failed to dissolve properly and three didn't contain enough vitamin C.

Reliable products include...

• **Kirkland Signature Vitamin C with Rose Hips, 1,000 mg**

• **Nature Made Vitamin C, 1,000 mg**

• **Nature's Bounty Natural Vitamin C, 1,000 mg**

• **Nutrilite Bio C Plus, 250 mg**

Helpful: Don't spend extra money for natural forms of vitamin C. Synthetic and natural forms have the same effects in the body.

VITAMIN E

The amount needed for daily nutrition is easily obtained from foods (nuts, grains, oils, etc.). Higher doses are thought to be beneficial in preventing and/or treating prostate and other cancers, as well as Alzheimer's disease.

Test results: Of the 28 products tested, two had less vitamin E than listed on the label, and one product labeled as "natural" contained synthetic vitamin E.

Important: Natural vitamin E, listed on labels as d-alpha-tocopherol, works more efficiently in the body than the synthetic dl form.

Reliable products include...

• **Brite-Life Natural Vitamin E, 400 international units (IU)**

• **Carlson E-Gems Vitamin E, 400 IU**

• **Solgar Natural Vitamin E, 400 IU**

• **Twinlab E-400 Caps, 100% Natural, 400 IU**

CALCIUM

Most people take this mineral to strengthen their bones, but studies have suggested that it also may reduce the risk for colon polyps.

Test results: Of the 35 products tested, four contained less calcium than the amount that was listed on the label.

Reliable products include...

• **Citracal Ultradense Calcium Citrate, 200 mg**

• **GNC Calcimate Plus 800, 200 mg**

• **Nature's Bounty Calcium Citrate, 200 mg**

• **Puritan's Pride Calcium Citrate, 200 mg**

 # Do Your Supplements Really Work?

Tod Cooperman, MD, president and founder of ConsumerLab.com, White Plains, NY, which provides the latest testing results and issues warnings and information about recalls approximately every two weeks. He is an editor of ConsumerLab.com's *Guide to Buying Vitamins & Supplements.* ConsumerLab.com.

Vitamin and mineral tablets sometimes fail to dissolve in the body, usually because of poor manufacturing practices. *If you want to test the tablets yourself...*

• **Heat one cup of vinegar** (any type can be used) to about 100° F, keeping the liquid warm and at a steady temperature.

• **Place one vitamin or mineral pill in the cup.** For 30 to 45 minutes, stir the liquid periodically. Try to avoid hitting the pill.

• **If the pill doesn't dissolve within 45 minutes,** it may not dissolve completely when it is in the intestine, which diminishes its effectiveness.

Note: This test does not work for timed-release products and is not necessary to perform on chewables.

Emergency Room Self-Defense

Ted Christopher, MD, chairman, department of emergency medicine at Thomas Jefferson University Hospital in Philadelphia.

Hospital emergency departments (EDs) are busier now than ever. Because of decreasing health-care budgets, examining rooms and equipment are in short supply. Doctors, nurses and technicians are overworked. No wonder the average wait to see a doctor is 49 minutes—with many ED patients waiting hours.

For better emergency care…

• **Call 911 or an ambulance if you suspect heart attack or stroke,** two "time-dependent" conditions that can quickly worsen. Ambulance technicians will begin your care on the way …and you're more likely to be seen by a doctor as soon as you arrive at the hospital.

If your condition isn't truly an emergency, arriving by ambulance won't make a difference, and you could get stuck with paying the bill. The sickest patients always get taken care of first.

• **Go to the closest hospital if you think you have an emergency.** The majority of all hospital EDs are now being staffed with board-certified emergency physicians. Teaching hospitals are staffed with attending emergency physicians and many residents and interns. In nonteaching hospitals, there will be only one or two doctors on staff. You may spend time waiting in either setting.

• **Don't wait for a referral from your doctor.** It is no longer necessary to bring a referral or get prior approval from your doctor before going to the ED.

Everyone who comes to the ED undergoes *triage.* That's the process by which each patient is evaluated by a nurse to determine how serious his/her condition is and who is to be seen first by a doctor.

• **Know the names and phone numbers of all your doctors**—especially your primary-care physician, but also any specialists you may have seen. Your private doctors often possess medical information that can assist the emergency physician in treating you.

• **Bring all of your medications.** ED staff will learn a lot about your health history simply by reading the labels. If you're going to need drugs, it's vital that the doctors know what medications you're taking.

Helpful: Keep a list of all your medications, along with the details of other health information (serious allergies, for example), on the refrigerator door. If you're unable to talk, the ambulance crew can take the list to the ED.

Even better: Bring the actual bottles—the printed labels are easiest to read.

• **Report changes in symptoms immediately.** Don't suffer in silence in the waiting room. You'll see a doctor more quickly if you inform the staff that your symptoms are getting worse. You should be given medication, if necessary, even before you see a doctor.

Important Medical Tests Doctors Don't Tell You About

Leo Galland, MD, director of the Foundation for Integrated Medicine in New York City. His latest book is *The Fat Resistance Diet.* Broadway. *www.fatresistancediet.com.* Dr. Galland is a recipient of the Linus Pauling award.

The special screening tests—for discovering heart disease, aneurysms, lung cancer and ovarian cancer—could save your life. But there's a good chance that your physician won't order them because insurance companies rarely pay for them.

Reason: Insurance companies typically pay for tests only when you have been diagnosed with a particular condition or when there is a high likelihood that you might have it. With some exceptions, such as mammograms, insurance rarely pays for screening tests aimed at early detection.

Ask your doctor if you should have any of the following tests, even if you have to pay for them yourself. They are available at most diagnostic and medical centers around the country. Ask your doctor for a referral.

These tests aren't appropriate for everyone, but early research suggests that they could be lifesavers for those with key risk factors...

CHOLESTEROL TEST

Traditional cholesterol tests only measure HDL ("good") cholesterol and triglycerides. The formula used to calculate levels of harmful LDL cholesterol isn't always accurate. This partly explains why half of people who have heart attacks have cholesterol levels that appear normal.

Better: Expanded cholesterol tests measure LDL specifically, giving more accurate readings. About 40 million American adults have hidden heart disease. Expanded cholesterol tests could identify 95% of these patients before a heart attack occurs.

The tests also look at individual HDL and LDL particles and determine how helpful—or harmful—they are likely to be.

Example: HDL protects against heart disease, so high levels are desirable. But some people who appear to have high levels actually have a subtype of HDL that isn't very helpful. Also, though all LDL particles are bad, the smaller ones are more dangerous than the bigger ones. These kinds of differences just aren't detectable with the conventional tests—but they can be detected with the expanded tests.

Who should consider them: Patients with mildly elevated cholesterol levels—200 to 230 milligrams per deciliter (mg/dl)—who smoke or who have cardiovascular risk factors, such as heart problems, high blood pressure or a family history of heart disease.

Cost: $75 to $175.

ANEURYSM TEST

Aneurysms are bulges in artery walls. They can be deadly when they rupture, killing 80% to 90% of people who have ruptured aneurysms. About 30,000 Americans die from this annually.

Better: An aneurysm scan uses an ultrasound wand to detect aneurysms in the abdominal aortic arteries. It's the only noninvasive test that allows doctors to identify aneurysms before they rupture. Surgery to repair aneurysms can increase survival rates to 99%.

Who should consider it: Anyone over age 60 who has cardiovascular risk factors, such as high blood pressure, or who smokes...as well as anyone over age 50 who has a family history of heart disease.

Cost: $60 to $200, depending on the extent of the scan.

HEART DISEASE TEST

Current methods for detecting heart disease risk, such as checking blood pressure, miss up to 75% of patients who later on develop heart problems.

Better: The electron beam tomography, or EBT, heart scan is the first direct, noninvasive way of identifying atherosclerosis, the primary risk factor for heart disease. The patient lies in a doughnut-shaped machine while the electron beams map out calcium deposits in the arteries. The buildup of calcium indicates the presence of plaque—fatty deposits that hamper blood flow to the heart and increase risk of blood clots. The patients who are found to have early signs of heart disease can take the appropriate steps—such as lowering cholesterol, controlling blood pressure, stopping smoking, etc.—to prevent problems from progressing.

Drawback: Calcium deposits don't always indicate an elevated risk of heart attack. The deposits may be harmless. On the other hand, a person who has a clear scan could actually have dangerous levels of plaque.

Patients with high calcium levels also may have to take a follow-up stress test. If this test is positive, the patient may have to undergo an angiogram—an invasive procedure. If the angiogram shows no heart disease, the patient has undergone these extra tests unnecessarily. Still the EBT is considered useful because traditional tests don't catch most heart problems.

Who should consider it: All men over age 45 and women over age 55. If you have heart disease risk factors—smoking, a family history of heart disease, etc.—consider having an EBT 10 years sooner.

Cost: About $400.

LUNG CANCER TEST

Lung cancer rarely causes symptoms until it reaches an advanced stage. The five-year survival rate is about 15%. Conventional X-rays may fail to detect early-stage tumors.

Better: The spiral CT scan can detect cancerous tumors as small as one grain of rice. Eighty percent of lung cancers spotted in scanning studies were caught at a potentially treatable stage.

Drawbacks: The test can result in false-positives—findings that indicate cancer when none is present. This could lead to unnecessary and risky lung biopsies. The false-positive rate improves when patients have follow-up scans.

Who should consider it: Smokers as well as former smokers age 50 and over who have smoked at least one pack daily for 10 years or two packs daily for five years.

Cost: $300 to $500.

OVARIAN CANCER

More than 14,000 American women die from ovarian cancer every year. It is one of the deadliest of female cancers. Like lung cancer, it often has no symptoms until it reaches an advanced stage of development.

Better: An ultrasound device inserted into the vagina allows doctors to inspect the ovaries for any malignant changes. University of Kentucky researchers used this test on 23,000 women. Twenty-nine showed cancerous ovarian tumors, 76% of which were detected at an early, more treatable stage. Typically, only 25% of ovarian cancers are caught early.

Drawback: The test isn't able to differentiate between malignant and benign growths—so positive test results could result in unnecessary procedures.

Who should consider it: Women age 45 and older with risk factors, such as a family history of ovarian, breast or colon cancer...or a history of fertility or hormone-replacement treatment...or who never have been pregnant.

Cost: About $250.

Nobel Prize Winner Who Discovered Real Cause of Ulcers Tells All

Barry J. Marshall, MD, senior principal research fellow, School of Biomedical, Biomolecular and Chemical Sciences, University of Western Australia, Perth. He is the winner, with J. Robin Warren, MD, of the 2005 Nobel Prize in Physiology or Medicine and the editor of *Helicobacter Pioneers*. Blackwell Scientific.

When two Australian physician-researchers first suggested that ulcers might be caused by a stomach bug, the medical establishment scoffed.

For decades, doctors had believed that emotional stress prompted the stomach to churn out acid to the point that it literally ate a hole in the stomach lining. Doctors treated the resulting ulcers with antacids—and even psychotherapy to help sufferers relax.

Gastroenterologist Barry J. Marshall, MD, and pathologist J. Robin Warren, MD, speculated that a bacterium, later named *Helicobacter pylori,* or *H. pylori*, was the real culprit.

In 1984, they published their H. pylori report in the British medical journal *The Lancet*. The two doctors won the 2005 Nobel Prize in Physiology or Medicine for their discovery.

To learn more about ulcers, we interviewed Dr. Marshall shortly after he won the Nobel Prize...

•**What made you persist in an area of research that contradicted conventional medical treatments?** After Dr. Warren completed research showing that about half of the patients who underwent stomach biopsies had bacteria that created inflammation in the stomach lining, it was natural for us to continue investigating the role that the bacteria was playing.

Once the connection with ulcers was made, we saw that antibiotics cured 92% of patients no matter how severe their disease. In fact, we found such a high cure rate versus no "cures" in the standard treatment group that we only needed to treat a small number of patients from the standard group to convince ourselves that we were correct.

●**How do you think your winning the Nobel Prize for research on H. pylori will affect ulcer treatment?** Very conservative doctors who do not ordinarily look for H. pylori now may be forced to do so, because their patients may have read about our research in news reports on the Nobel Prize.

●**Why do some individuals with H. pylori develop ulcers and others don't?** You catch H. pylori from family members or contaminated water in developing countries.

For an ulcer to develop, the patient must be able to produce high levels of stomach acid. When H. pylori is present, infection-fighting white blood cells attack the bacteria. In doing this, the cells damage the stomach lining, causing inflammation (gastritis) and, years later, an ulcer. Because H. pylori bacteria produce varying levels of toxins, some do not damage the stomach wall enough to cause an ulcer.

●**Aren't some ulcers caused by the use of stomach-irritating painkillers?** Yes. Aside from H. pylori, many aspirin-type drugs, called nonsteroidal anti-inflammatory drugs (NSAIDs), usually taken for arthritis, can lead to ulcers. Approximately 40% of ulcers result from NSAID use. The remainder are due to H. pylori.

●**Does H. pylori ever cause anything more serious than an ulcer?** Yes. The inflammation produced by H. pylori also can lead to stomach cancer.

●**Who should be tested for H. pylori?** Anyone with stomach symptoms, such as pain or burning in the upper stomach, nausea or vomiting. Also, if you have a family history of stomach cancer—in a parent or sibling—you should be tested. The test itself involves drawing a blood sample to test for antibodies or a breath test.

●**If a person tests positive for H. pylori, what's the best treatment?** The best treatment is acid reduction—with proton-pump inhibitors, such as *esomeprazole* (Nexium), *pantoprazole* (Protonix) or *rabeprazole* (AcipHex) —combined with an effective antibiotic. Usually taking an antibiotic, such as *clarithromycin* (Biaxin) with *amoxicillin* (Amoxil), for 10 to 14 days will work.

●**Does eliminating the bacterium pose any risks?** No. However, paradoxically, H. pylori does lower stomach acid levels in some people. In these people, H. pylori protects them somewhat against acid-stimulated diseases in the esophagus, such as gastroesophageal reflux disease (GERD), and, as a result, esophageal cancer. That's because stomach acid leaking up into the esophagus increases cancer risk in that location. However, this should not stop us from treating H. pylori, because both the bacteria and GERD are easily treatable.

●**Some studies have shown that cranberry juice may help fight ulcers. Is this an important discovery?** It is likely that many food products do inhibit H. pylori and, as a result, help ulcers heal. In most cases, however, the effect is not very strong.

●**What areas of research do you think hold the most promise for a cure or new treatment for disease?** Many aspects of H. pylori colonization still are not understood. For example, at least 30% of H. pylori genes have no known purpose. Deciphering these genes will provide important insights into the functioning of the gastrointestinal system. My lab at the University of Western Australia is performing molecular studies to discover new useful genes in our H. pylori strains.

●**Did you or Dr. Warren have any idea that you might win the Nobel Prize?** We knew immediately that we had made an important discovery. In such an underpopulated area as Western Australia, however, we could not imagine how many millions of people would benefit. We dreamed of winning the Nobel Prize but always thought that other recipients over the years were worthy laureates.

You May Have this Stomach Bug and Not Even Know It

Martin J. Blaser, MD, the Frederick H. King professor of internal medicine and chairman and professor of microbiology in the departments of medicine and microbiology at New York University School of Medicine, New York City. He is president-elect of the Infectious Diseases Society of America and a member of the editorial boards of various medical journals.

Twenty years ago, in a report published in the prestigious British medical journal *The Lancet*, scientists from Australia announced that they had isolated a microorganism that lives on the thick mucous lining of the stomach. They theorized that the bacterium might play a role in chronic active gastritis, a persistent inflammation of the stomach.

Over the next two decades, research into the bacterium—named *Helicobacter pylori*, or *H. pylori*—led to a new era in gastrointestinal medicine. The bacterium was found in the stomachs of more than half the world's population—70% to 90% in developing countries, and about 30% in the US. H. pylori also was discovered to be a leading cause of ulcers and stomach cancer.

These days, a doctor who finds a patient infected with H. pylori attempts to eradicate it. But is that treatment always helpful? Or, as newer studies suggest, is the eradication of H. pylori creating an unexpected and unprecedented epidemic of diseases of the esophagus, the tube that connects the back of the throat to the stomach?

To answer these and other questions, we spoke to Martin J. Blaser, MD, a renowned authority on H. pylori.

●**Billions of people worldwide are infected with H. pylori. Is this a normal condition or a disease?** The most recent evidence strongly suggests that H. pylori was once even more common than it is now, perhaps found in everyone. In other words, it is probably a normal part of the bacterial environment, or flora, of the stomach, much like the so-called friendly bacteria in the intestines.

Our industrial, postmodern society is not conducive to H. pylori. Studies show that in populations that have better hygiene and sanitation as well as smaller families, there is a lower incidence of colonization with H. pylori. (Scientists don't know exactly how the bacterium spreads from person to person.) With the widespread use of antibiotics and the concerted efforts of physicians to remove H. pylori from large numbers of people, the bacterium is disappearing in developed countries, particularly in the US.

●**Is the disappearance of H. pylori a positive development?** Yes and no. Everybody who has the organism has a condition called *chronic superficial gastritis*—a mild inflammation of the stomach that has no symptoms. However, having that condition increases the risk of developing an ulcer by approximately three- to fourfold and stomach cancer by tenfold.

This is especially true for people who carry a strain of the bacterium called *CagA+*, one of a number of types of H. pylori. Where H. pylori is disappearing, ulcers and stomach cancer are disappearing as well. And that's good. More and more cases of ulcers are being caused by the chronic intake of non-steroidal anti-inflammatory drugs (NSAIDs), such as aspirin and *ibuprofen* (Advil).

But as these diseases have gone away, other diseases have become more common—particularly gastrointestinal reflux disease (GERD), commonly referred to as heartburn. In some people, GERD leads to a condition called Barrett's esophagus (abnormal changes in the cells lining the esophagus), which in turn can lead to esophageal cancer.

In the US, the rate at which esophageal cancer is increasing is one of the fastest for all malignancies. The same is true in other developed countries, such as England, Norway and Australia.

●**Why would a decrease in H. pylori cause an increase in GERD and esophageal cancer?** With aging, there is a normal diminution in the production of stomach acid. Eradicating the CagA+ strain of H. pylori creates a biochemical process that allows the stomach to generate full levels of acid, even at age 50 and older. And it's the regurgitation of stomach acid into the esophagus that causes GERD.

Additionally, studies show that there is an inverse relationship between the level of the CagA+ strain of H. pylori and esophageal cancer—those without CagA+ have a four- to five-fold higher risk of developing esophageal cancer.

•In light of these findings, who should be treated for H. pylori? If somebody has an ulcer, there is no question—get rid of H. pylori. The benefits far outweigh the risks. And if someone has a rare form of stomach cancer called gastric lymphoma, eradicating H. pylori is a standard part of treatment.

Otherwise, there is no reason to remove the bacteria—even though removing it, in cases of indigestion, is standard practice for many physicians. H. pylori is not a pathogen. Studies show that removing it does not improve the symptoms of indigestion.

New studies show that the stomachs of people who have H. pylori produce more *leptin*, a hormone that inhibits appetite. As H. pylori is being eradicated, obesity is increasing. Is there a link? Many scientists think this is a possibility.

•If a person should be treated for H. pylori, what is the best method? The best therapy is the simultaneous use of three or four medications, usually two antibiotics, such as *amoxicillin* (Amoxil), *metronidazole* (Flagyl), *tetracycline* (Achromycin V) or *clarithromycin* (Biaxin), an acid inhibitor (such as a proton-pump inhibitor or H2-blocker) and/or bismuth salts. The use of this combination regimen for seven to 10 days has eradication rates of higher than 90%.

Asthma Breakthrough

Thomas Casale, MD, chief of allergy and immunology and director of clinical research at Creighton University, Omaha.

The medication *omalizumab* (Xolair) reduces asthma attacks by more than 50% and also allows patients to reduce use of inhaled corticosteroids, which can cause side effects. The drug, which is injected once or twice a month, is for patients with moderate to severe allergic asthma that can't be adequately controlled by other drugs.

Caution: Patients given omalizumab in clinical trials had slightly higher cancer rates than placebo patients, but the difference was not statistically significant. Patients with a personal or family history of cancer should discuss risks with their doctors.

New Treatment for Incontinence

Farnaz Alams Ganj, MD, assistant professor, obstetrics and gynecology, Akbarabadi Hospital, Iran University of Medical Sciences, Tehran.

Urinary urge incontinence, a condition that results in urine loss before being able to get to the toilet, can be greatly eased by Milk of Magnesia.

Recent finding: Women who took one teaspoon of magnesium hydroxide—the active ingredient in Milk of Magnesia, Mylanta and Maalox—twice a day had significantly fewer episodes than those taking a placebo.

Theory: Magnesium hydroxide minimizes contractions of the bladder muscle that is responsible for an overactive bladder.

Can Earwax Removal Help Hearing Loss?

David Memel, MD, senior teaching associate, division of primary health care, University of Bristol, England.

Earwax removal via a syringe can improve hearing—but not always. In a new study of more than 100 patients who visited a doctor for earwax removal, two-thirds did *not* experience better hearing after the procedure. However, in patients who did benefit, hearing improved significantly, by up to 35 decibels. Patients who do not benefit from earwax removal may be hearing impaired. They should see an audiologist for testing.

Index

A

ABCD method of weight loss,
 339–340
Abdominal exercises, 13
Abortions, breast cancer and,
 128
Absentmindedness, cures for,
 289–290
Acetaminophen, 6, 116, 119
Acetyl-L-carnitine in protecting
 brain, 507
Achilles tendinitis, 29
Acid blockers, alternatives for,
 428
Acne
 laser therapy for scars from,
  22–23
 medications for, 304
Acquired immunodeficiency
 syndrome (AIDS) virus. *See
 also* Human immuno-
 deficiency virus (HIV)
 killing of, 310
Acupuncture, 469, 472
 for depression, 458
Acyclovir, genital herpes and, 260

Adalac, 83
Adalat (*nifedipine*), 112
Adrenaline, 461
Adrenal insufficiency, 38
Advice, giving, to others, 14–16
Advil, 113
Aerobic exercise, 76, 475, 486
Aggression, curing, 291
Aging
 alpha hydroxy acid and,
  305–306
 antioxidant vitamins and, 306
 doctor's mistakes and, 270–271
 dog ownership and, 273
 eldercare and, 281
 fiber and, 269
 flavonoids and, 269
 healthy, 268–269
 key to successful, 265–267
 maintaining mental ability in,
  273–274
 metabolism and, 332
 moisturizers and, 306
 shoes and, 278
 skin and, 297–299
 strength training and, 273
 sunscreens and, 305–306

 tretinoin and, 306
 vitamin E and, 275
Ailments, water therapy for, 50
Air filters
 in controlling indoor pollution,
  355
 natural, 62
Air freshener, dangers in, 316
Airplane travel
 earaches on, 367
 jet lag in, 6–7, 50
 staying healthy on, 49–50
Alcohol
 in ales, 231
 aspirin and, 66
 avoiding, in fighting jet lag, 6
 in beer, 231
 cancer and, 282
 dehydration and, 313
 diabetes and, 282
 drowning and, 320
 social drinking, 234
Aldactone (*spironolactone*), 113
Alendronate
 as alternative to hormone-
  replacement therapy, 124
 hip fractures and, 291

Ales, alcohol in, 231
Aleve (*naproxen*), 113
Allergies. *See also* Asthma; Hay fever
  asthma and, 224
  benefits of shots for, 448
  causes of hidden, 233–234
  environmental control of, 356
  fighting, with stinging nettle, 422
  food, 39, 223–224, 314
  ingredients in remedies for, 113
  migraines and, 224
  natural year-round remedies for, 436–437
  to nickel, 448
  osteoarthritis and, 224
  to peanuts, 155–156
  pet, 57
  reactions to, 43–44
  spring, 153–154
Alopecia areata, 195
Alpha-blockers, 205
Alpha hydroxy acids
  aging and, 305
  skin care and, 293
Alprostadil for impotence, 199
Alternative therapies, 417–418
  See also Herbs; *specific*
  acupuncture as, 458, 469, 472
  Chinese medicine, 471–473
  finding, 441
  HMO coverage for, 470
  magnets, 470–471
  move to mainstream, 467–469
  Qi gong as, 432–433, 472–473
  referral to doctors in, 96
  relaxation as, 467–468
Alzheimer's disease
  causes of, 266
  diagnosis of, 266–267
  diets and, 234
  exercise versus, 276
  medications in fighting, 507–508
  mild cognitive impairment and, 501–502
  preventing, 503–505
  relief from, 280
  statins and, 106–107
Amalgam (silver) fillings, dangers of, 371
Amitriptyline (Elavil)
  for fibromyalgia, 322
  GERD and, 149
Anaphylaxis, 314

Androgenic alopecia, 195, 196
Anemia, pernicious, 325
Anesthesia
  local, 191
  regional, 191
  surgery and, 191
Aneurysms
  abdominal, 483
  brain, 323
  tests for, 539
  treatment of, 483
Anger, aspirin and, 83
Angina pectoris, symptoms of, 70
Angiography, 86
Angioplasty, 74–75, 76
  saving your heart without, 79–80
Angiotensin-converting enzyme (ACE) inhibitors, 41, 76
Anorexia
  older women and, 136
  vegetarianism and, 217
Anosmia, 341
Antacids, 6, 113
  alternatives for, 428
Antiaging supplements, 286–287
Antianxiety medications, effect on sex, 259
Antiarthritis exercises, 381
Antibacterial soaps, 526
Antibiotics, 6, 107–108
  blood thinners and, 113
Antidepressants, 419–420
  alternatives for, 428
  dangers from, 118–119
  effect on sex, 258
  for narcolepsy, 326
Antiglare filters on computer screens, 347
Antihistamines, 6
  alternatives for, 428
Antioxidants, 474–475
  aging and, 306
  asthma and, 147–148
  benefits of, 219–220
  in boosting memory, 291
  free radicals and, 236–237, 274
  in protecting brain, 507
  sources of, 219–220, 238
  as supplement, 509
  taking, 66
  vitamins and, 64
Antiperspirants, mammograms and, 132
Antiplaque rinse, 371

Anxiety, 349–350. *See also* Stress
  avoiding, during magnetic resonance imaging (MRI), 444
  scents in reducing, 513
Anxiety disorders, 161
Aphrodisiacs, 256
Apomorphine, 201
Appetite, scents in controlling, 513
Apple cider vinegar bath, 50
Arterial plaque, nitric oxide in reducing, 485–486
Arteries, vitamin C and, 247
Arthritis
  celery seed for, 521
  chores in the kitchen and, 60
  dressing and, 148
  driving with, 60
  herbs and, 434–435
  in knee, 228
  magnets for, 471
  mind/body approach to, 276–278
  turmeric for, 522
  vitamin C and, 246
Arthritis pain
  beating, 27–29
  diet for relief of, 209–210, 229–231
  sex and, 260
Ashwagandha as sex booster, 516
Aspirin, 6, 64, 76, 85, 115–116
  alcohol and, 66
  anger and, 83
  as blood thinner, 83
  in reducing risk of colon cancer, 34
  stomach problems and, 120
  taking with vitamin E, 248
Assertiveness, 171
Asthma. *See also* Allergies; Hay fever
  allergies and, 224
  causes of, 146
  declaring war on, 146
  exercise for, 381
  glaucoma and, 362
  inhalers and, 120
  magnets for, 471
  omalizumab (Xolair) for, 543
  peak flow meter and, 318
  prevention of, 217–218
  self-test for, 146–147
  thunderstorms in triggering attacks of, 317
  vitamin C and, 246
Ataxia, 24

Athlete's foot, 55
  remedy for, 6
Athletic shoes, 56
Atorvastatin (Lipitor), 106
Atrial fibrillation, as stroke risk,
  493
Attention deficit/hyperactivity
  disorder (ADHD), relief from,
  161–162
Auditory habituation, 368
Autologous blood donation,
  190, 312
Automatic Teller Machines
  (ATMs), protecting yourself at,
  288–289

B

Babies
  diet of, 155
  music and, 155
Back
  best ways to protect lower,
    448
  stretching and strengthening,
    475
Back injuries
  preventing, 146
  study on, 448
Back pain
  drug-free treatment of, 517
  fish oil in alleviating, 517
  lower, 9
  magnets for, 471
  preventing on airplane, 49–50
Bacteria, information on, 49
Bacterial meningitis, 317
Balloons, dangers from, 158
Bananas, frozen, 220
Bandage removal, painless
  adhesive, 62
Barbecues, nutrition and, 227
Basal energy expenditure, 344
Basil for hay fever, 423
Bay leaf, benefits of, 414
Bed-wetting
  prevention of, 161
  stopping, 161
Beef frankfurters, dangers in,
  316
Beer
  alcohol in, 231
  size of stomach and, 329
Bee sting, first aid for, 58
Behavior, sleep and, 157
Belief, lifesaving power of,
  393–394

Benign paroxysmal positional
  vertigo, 24
Benign prostatic hyperplasia
  (BPH), 428
  diagnosing, 205
  treatment for, 203–204
Benzene, 39
Benzoic acid, 233
Beta-blockers, 41, 76, 113
  effect on sex, 259
  heart attacks and, 87
Beta-carotene
  facts on, 249
  need for, 243
  research on, 239–241
  sources of, 219–220, 243
Beverages
  choosing heart-healthy, 488
  sports, 381
Bicycling
  helmet for, 62
  stationary, 382
Bifidobacteria, refrigeration of,
  245
Bifocals in children, 363
Bilateral arm training with
  rhythmic auditory cueing
    (BATRAC) for strokes,
    494–495
Bilberry for vision disorders,
  521
Biofeedback
  for incontinence, 53
  for tinnitus, 368
Biopsy for prostate cancer, 35
Bird flu, protecting yourself
  from, 524–526
Birth control
  emergency, 140–141
  safest pills, 141
Birth defects, vitamins versus,
  248
Birthmarks, skin cancer and,
  299
Birth weight, as risk factor for
  disease, 488
Bladder
  pain relief, 135–136
  remedies for infection of, 420
  training of, for incontinence,
    53
Bladder cancer, vitamin C and,
  247
Blood-boosting medications,
  312–313
Blood circulation, ginger for,
  415

Blood clots, 65, 67
  foods and, 226
Blood pressure. *See also*
  Hypertension
  benefits of pills for, 275
  borderline risk, 74
  congestive heart failure and,
    280
  controlling, in protecting
    brain, 503–504
  garlic for, 521
  kidney damage and, 318
  lower your, 64
  meditation in lowering, 430
  natural ways to lower your,
    429–430
  taking your own, 74
Bloodshot eyes as sign of
  diabetes, 359
Blood thinners, antibiotics and,
  113
Blood transfusions, 311–313
  autologous donation, 190, 312
  reducing risks, 191
Blood vessels
  helping work properly, 84
  nitric oxide in expanding, 485
Body
  decoding language of, 8
  energy and biological clock of,
    225–226
  health risk and shape of, 336
  reading messages of, 7–9
Body weight support therapy
  for strokes, 495
Bone density, 136
Bones
  fractures of, 44
  magnets for broken, 471
Bone thinning, 136
Botox, 22
Bowel movements, better, 122
Bowel trouble, 8–9
Bra, breast cancer and, 130–131
Brachytherapy, 35
Brain
  activities for, 504–505
  aneurysm in, 323
  diet for healthy, 504, 505–507
  protecting, 503–504
Bran bath, 50
Breakfasts, better, 222
Breast cancer. *See also*
  Mammograms
  abortions and, 128
  bras and, 130–131
  in men, 208

milk and, 130
promising technologies, 130
screening breakthroughs, 128–130
support group for, 45
Breast cysts, strategies for avoiding troublesome, 127–128
Breast-feeding, 134
Breast implants, 132
Breast lumps
evaluating, 128
normal, 131–132
Breasts, enlarged, in men, 23
Breath
avoiding bad, 61
sweeter, 372
Breath-awareness exercise, 432
Breathing, elevation and, 57
Broken bones, magnets for, 471
Bug killer, dangers in, 316
Bunions, 54
Bupropion (Wellbutrin), 419–420
Burning mouth syndrome (BMS), 372
Butter, mixing with olive oil, 213
B vitamins, 67–68
benefits of, 536–537
Bypass surgery, 76, 77–79
dangers from, 81
saving your heart without, 79–80

C

Caffeine
in children, 157
facts on, 222–223
limiting your consumption of, 6
stress and, 354
sudden cut backs in, 315
withdrawal, 223
Calcitonin-salmon for osteoporosis, 124
Calcium
benefits of, 537
constipating effect of, 151
controversy over, 241–242
getting more, 65
increasing, 64
magnesium and, 151–152
osteoporosis and, 240–241
sources of, 231, 243; 245
women and, 136–137

Calcium channel blockers, 41, 76, 83, 149
Calcium diet, 529–530
Calcium supplements, 241–242
Calendula officinalis, 417
Calories
counting, 227
Harris-Benedict equations for determining, 344
restriction of, 212
sipping ice water in burning, 333
Camps
having fun at, 159–160
safety standards at, 160
Cancer. *See also* Bladder cancer; Breast cancer; Colon cancer; Colorectal cancer; Esophageal cancer; Lung cancer; Ovarian cancer; Prostate cancer; Skin cancer; Testicular cancer
alcohol and, 282
channel blockers and link with, 120
checklist for prevention of, 447
chemotherapy and, 133
diet and, 235–236
living longer with, 405–406
radiofrequency ablation for, 491
reducing your risk of, 57
selenium versus, 250
self-defense, 226
statins and, 107
unfaithful husbands and, 140
vaccines for, 496–497
Capoten (*captopril*), 113
Carbidopa (*Sinemet*) for fibromyalgia, 323
Carbohydrate addict, 343
Carbohydrate-rich foods, 343
Carbohydrates, 212
insulin and, 342–343
managing your intake of, 343
mood and, 215
sources of, 215
trouble with, 211
Carbon monoxide poisoning on pleasure boats, 313
Cardiomyoplasty, 78–79
Cardiopulmonary resuscitation (CPR), 56
Car-jacking, protecting yourself from, 288
Carotenoids, 68, 236, 237
for macular degeneration, 509

Carpal tunnel syndrome, 29
prevention of, 345–346
Cataracts
obesity and, 361
prevention of, 218, 360
surgical options for, 194, 361
timing in treating, 360–361
Catecholamines, 461
Cat litter, dangers of, 316
Cayenne
arthritis and, 435
benefits of, 414, 421
Celery seed
benefits of, 414
for gout and arthritis, 521
Cellular phones, cancer risk and, 447
Cereal, finishing your, 218
Cerebellum, stimulating, 400
Cervix-sparing hysterectomy, 139–140
Chagas, 312
Chamomile, benefits of, 416
Channel blockers, cancer link and, 120
Cheese, healthier cooking with, 232
Chemical peels, skin care and, 294
Chemicals, toxic, 319
Chemotherapy, cancer and, 133
Chestnuts, fats in, 236
Childbirth, episiotomy during, 139
Children
bifocals in, 363
caffeine and, 157
camps for, 160
choking and, 158
dehydration and, 158
foods to be avoided by young, 155–156
helping them relax, 161
secondhand cigarette smoke and, 157
sex and, 153
skin care for, in puberty, 158
sunglasses and, 156–157
ulcers in, 155
warts and, 160–161
what you need to know about health care for, 143–144
Chinese medicine, 471–473
secrets of self-healing from, 431–432
Chiropractic, 469
Chitosan, 238

Choking, children and, 158
Cholesterol
  coffee and, 314
  control of, 81–82, 117
    without medication, 220–222
  controversy over, 117
  diet for reducing, 63–64
  differences in test results, 85
  garlic for, 87–88, 521
  medications for, 76, 83–84, 85,
    106–107, 117
  nitric oxide in lowering, 486
  policosanol in lowering,
    490–491
  psyllium in lowering, 238
  red yeast rice in lowering,
    489–490
  stress and levels of, 173
  tests for, 539
Choline in protecting brain, 506
Chondroitin, 27–28
Chromium, 68
  supplements and weight loss,
    241
Chromium picolinate
  controversy over, 241
  danger of, 250
  kidney failure and, 250
Chronic fatigue, causes of,
  38–40
Chronic illness, importance of
  support groups for, 45–46
Chronic pain
  causes of, 26
  origins of, 25–26
  reducing, 26
Cigars, health risks of, 318
Circadian rhythms, 476
  desynchronization, 476
Cisapride (Propulsid), 149
Citrus fruits, 235
Clinical trials, 440
Clomipramine (Anafranil), 260
Clonazepam (Klonopin) for
  narcolepsy, 326
Clopidogrel, 83
Cochlear implant, 365, 366–367
Coenzyme Q-10, benefits of,
  427, 511
Coffee
  cholesterol level and, 314
  in controlling hay fever, 58
  surgery for drinkers of, 194
Cognitive-behavioral therapy, 3
  in controlling tinnitus, 368
Coital alignment technique
  (CAT), 253

Colchicine, 122
Cold feet, 8, 55
Cold hands, 8
Cold operating rooms, heart
  attacks and, 185
Colds. See Common colds
Cold sores
  avoiding spreading of, 449
  relief from, 165
Cold-water treading, 51
Collagen injections, skin care
  and, 22, 294, 298
Colon, herbs for, 424
Colon cancer
  aspirin in reducing risk of, 117
  detection of, 272
  irinotecan (Camptosar) for, 283
  preventing, 33–34
  reducing risk of, 57
  self-defense, 36–37
Colonoscopy, 33, 36
  need for, 37
Combined hyperlipidemia, 213
Comfrey, benefits of, 416
Common colds, 150
  airplane travel and, 49
  avoiding, 17–19
  echinacea for, 521
  food remedy for, 424–425
  ginger for, 415
  natural cures for, 522–524
  remedies for, 113, 166, 246, 420
  vitamin C and, 241
Communication, 261
  better, 392
  doctor–patient, 97, 98
  love and, 262
  sex and, 262
Compresses, 51
Compulsions, four-step plan for
  beating, 411–412
Compulsive gambling, 459
Computers
  antiglare filters on screens, 347
  eye exercise and, 363
Concentrated meditation, 468
Conferences, power eating at, 216
Congestive heart failure
  blood pressure and, 280
  prevention of, 218
Constipation
  avoiding, 151–152
  food remedies for, 425
  relief, 58
Constraint-induced movement
  therapy for strokes, 495
Constructive living, 459–460

Consumer health guides, 440
Corns, 54
Coronary artery disease,
  electron beam CT for, 492
Corticosteroids
  inhaled, 121
  for joint pain, 30
Cosmetic surgery, 22–23, 308
Cough, remedies for, 113, 425
Coumadin (warfarin), 112
Craving-reducing foods, 343
Cream, replacing in recipes, 222
Crime, staying safe and, 287–289
Crohn's disease, 37
Cryptosporidium, avoiding, 223
Cunnilingus, 256
Curcumin, 212
Curved penis, surgery for, 199
Cuts, 152
  vitamin E and, 248
Cutting boards, plastic versus
  wood, 320
Cystitis risk, diaphragms and,
  141
Cytomegalovirus (CMV),
  screening for, 312

D

D-alpha tocopherol, 274
Daily headache syndrome, 118
Dancing, for health, 385
Dandruff shampoo, 300
  better use of, 61
Death, domineering men and,
  197
Decongestant eyedrops,
  363–364
Deep breathing, 431, 468
Deep vein thrombosis (DVT),
  313
Deglycyrrhizinated licorice, 428
Dehydration
  alcohol and, 313
  kids and, 158
  preventing, 385
Dementia
  estrogen and, 275
  natural remedy for, 508
Dental care
  brushing in, 61, 369, 370–371
  easier visits in, 103
  floss in, 369
  preventing infant tooth decay,
    156
  professional cleaning of teeth
    in, 370

toothbrushes in, 369, 370–371
toothpaste in, 316, 371
vegetarian risk for periodontal
disease and, 369
X-rays in, 371
Dentist
stroke risk and, 281
telling good from bad, 103–104
Depression
acupuncture for, 458
exercise and, 388
osteoporosis and, 134
statins versus, 121
in stroke patients, 495
treating naturally, 418–420
vitamin B and, 245
Dermabrasion, skin care and,
294
Dextroamphetamine (Dexedrine)
for narcolepsy, 326
Diabetes, 38
alcohol and, 282
bloodshot eyes as sign of, 359
eye exams, 310
foot ulcers, 306
milk and, 320
misconceptions about two
kinds of, 163–165
reducing nerve pain in, 534
statins and, 107
vinegar in fighting, 533–534
vitamin D and, 247
Diabinese (chlorpropamide),
113
Diaphragms, cystitis risk and, 141
Diarrhea
food remedies for, 425
remedy for, 6
Diet. See also Nutrition
Alzheimer's disease and, 234
for arthritis pain relief,
229–231
baby's, 155
calcium, 529–530
cancer and, 235–236
cholesterol reduction, 63–64
dangerous, 228
eggs in, 213
exercise versus, 378
"fat banking" and, 333–334
for healthy brain, 504, 505–507
heart disease and, 87
immune system and, 236–238
for life, 336
low-fat, 237, 475
in men, 208

in reducing skin cancer risk,
295
in maintaining healthy lifestyle,
486–487
pills, 53
plant-based, in boosting
longevity, 500
power eating and, 225–226
problems with, 211–212,
332–333
reasons for failure of, 329–330
in reducing stress and
depression, 419
set point versus, 334–335
tricks, 228
vegetarian, 76, 336
Dietary fiber, sources of, 65
Diet doctors, weight-loss secrets
of, 337–338
Digestion, strengthening your,
390
Digital rectal examination, 35
Disaster training, 16–17
Disease. See also Infectious
diseases
benefits of symptoms of, 449
salsa in preventing, 520
stopping worry about, 3–4
Disinfectants, danger from,
310
Diuretics, 41
effect on sex, 259
Divorce, men and, 208
Dizziness, 23–25
Docosahexanoic acid
for memory problems, 512
in protecting brain, 505
Dr. Ruth's secrets of great sex,
260
Doctor-patient relationship,
getting most from, 90–91
Doctors. See also Pediatricians
continuing education and, 102
getting best care from, 91–92
getting information on,
182–185
listening by, 96
looking for new, 102
mistakes of, in treating elderly,
270–271
picking, 89–90
protecting yourself from
financial interests of, 99–100
recommendation of specialists
by, 95–96
referral to alternative, 96
talking to, 97–98

as up-to-date, 101–102
washing of hands by, 101
weight-loss secrets of diet,
337–338
women and, 102–103
Dogs, ownership and longer life,
273
Doxazosin (Cardura), 205
Drawstring, dangers of, 163
Driving with arthritis, 60
Drowning, alcohol and, 320
Drugs. See Medications;
Over-the-counter drugs;
Prescription drugs
Duct tape in curing warts, 519
Dust, controlling, in indoor
pollution, 356

E

Earaches when flying, 367
Ear infections, 162
chronic, 144, 366
Earlobes, creased, 367
Ear thermometer, 314
Earthquakes, surviving, 16–17
Earwax removal in hearing loss,
545
Eating plan, developing healthy,
329–330
Echinacea, 238
benefits of, 421
for colds and flu, 521, 523
Echocardiogram, 82
Egg donor, how to find, 262
Eggs, 213
substitute for, 228
Eicosapentaenoic acid, 229
in protecting brain, 505
Ejaculation, retrograde, 206
Elavil (amitriptyline), 113
Elderberry for colds and flu, 523
Eldercare, 281
Electric toothbrushes, 369,
370–371
Electrocardiogram, stress, 75
Electron beam CT (EBCT) for
coronary artery disease, 492
Electrostatic massage, 482–483
Elevation, breathing and, 57
Emergency room, 44
self-defense for, 538
Emotions
effect on health, 451–453
overcoming negative, 463–464
Empowerment, 401
Endoscopy, 191

Energy
    scents in controlling, 513
    secrets of having boundless,
        389–391
Entrainment, 2
Environmental control of
    allergies, 356
Environmental toxins, 39
Ephedrine, 113
Epigallocatechin gallate, 520
Epiluminescence microscopy in
    diagnosing melanoma, 498
Epinephrine, 314
Episiotomy, 139
Erotica, 256, 262–263
Erythropoietin (EPO), 313
Escherichia coli, 47
Esophageal cancer, *Helicobacter
    pylori* in, 542–543
Essential fatty acids, benefits of,
    511–512
Estrogen, dementia and, 275
Estrogen replacement therapy
    (ERT), 126. *See also* Hormone
    replacement therapy (HRT)
Exercise machines, overrated, 385
Exercise(s)
    abdominal, 13
    aerobic, 76, 475, 486
    Alzheimer's disease versus, 276
    antiarthritis, 381
    for asthmatics, 381
    benefits of, 156, 274
    in boosting longevity, 500
    breath-awareness, 432
    dangers of too much, 375–376
    depression and, 388
    developing as habit, 387–388
    dieting versus, 378
    Dr. Kenneth Cooper's plan,
        379–380
    eye, 363
    functional training, 532–533
    heart attack and, 85–86
    ideal, 26–27
    importance of, 335
    impotence and, 258
    in improving hearing, 276, 365
    incontinence and, 133
    insomnia versus, 382–383
    Jack LaLanne's plan, 373–379
    length of sessions, 380, 383
    longevity and, 379
    in lowering blood pressure, 429
    magic fives of, 374
    mood versus, 388
    Morita, 460

Naikan, 461
    in preventing heart disease, 84
    in reducing stress and
        depression, 419
    rehabilitation, 25
    for relaxation, 430
    sleeping and, 385
    smarter, more effective, 379
    stationary biking, 382
    sticking with, 381–382
    swimming, 386
    timing of, 379
    in treating pain, 518–519
    tubing in, 383–384
    videos in, 378
    vitamin E and, 248–249
    weight loss and, 386
External beam radiation (EBR),
    35
Eyedrops
    decongestant, 363–364
    vasoconstrictor, 364
Eyelashes, mites in, 363
Eyes
    exams
        need for annual, in diabetics,
            310
        timetable for, 362–363
    exercise for, 363
    laser surgery for, 191
    low-vision aids for, 280
    macular degeneration and,
        278–280, 509
    nutrition and, 210, 364–365
    protecting, with nutrition, 361
    reducing injuries to, 364
    secrets of avoiding serious
        troubles with, 357–359
    solutions for bloodshot, 359
    strain, computer use and, 347

F

Face-lift, 23
Failure, overcoming fear of,
    461–463
Fainting, dangers of, 278
Falls, avoiding disabling, 281
Famciclovir (Famvir), genital
    herpes and, 260
Familial adenomatous polyposis,
    37
Family and Medical Leave Act
    (1993) (FMLA), taking
    advantage of, 349
Family history, skin cancer risk
    and, 498

Family tree, creating your
    medical, 4–5
Fat, 212
    cutting, 229
    diets low in, 208, 237, 475
    eating less, 231
    minimizing intake of saturated,
        486
"Fat banking," 333–334
Fat-free foods, 232
Fatigue
    natural remedies for, 426–427
    nutraceuticals for, 511
Fears
    facing your, 463
    overcoming, 465
Feet
    diagnosing problems with, 320
    odor in, 55
    pain in, 307, 336
    prevention and treatment of
        common problems, 53–55
Fellatio, 256
Female athletes, knee injuries
    and, 136
Fennel, 413
    benefits of, 416
Fentanyl (Duragesic), 278
Fertility
    ovarian cancer and, 142
    treatment, 141–142
Fetal transplant, 272
Fever
    hospitalization and, 275
    pediatrician's home remedies
        for, 166
Feverfew, 428
    benefits of, 416
Fiber, 216
    aging and, 269
    benefits of, 486–487
    importance of, 235
Fibromyalgia, managing,
    322–323
Financial interests, protecting
    yourself from your doctor's,
    99–100
Finasteride (Proscar, Propecia),
    196, 205
    alternative for, 428–429
Finger dexterity, maintaining,
    274
Fish, 67
    benefits of eating, 66, 230, 505
Fish oil
    in alleviating neck and back
        pain, 517

in lowering C-reactive protein, 509

for osteoarthritis, 509

Fish oil supplements

benefits of, 230

heart attacks and, 87

Fitness. *See also* Exercise(s)

Jack LaLanne on, 373–375

5-alpha reductase inhibitors, 205

Flattery, learning art of, 10–11

Flavonoids, 226, 228, 235

aging and, 269

Flaxseed oil, benefits of, 230

Flea collar, dangers in, 316

Flexible sigmoidoscopy, 36

Floods, surviving, 16–17

Flossing, 370–371

Flu, 146

echinacea for, 521

food remedy for, 424–425

natural cures for, 522–524

protecting yourself from bird flu, 524–526

shorter recovery from, 524

shots for, 146

Fluoride rinse, 371

Fluoxetine (Prozac), 419

Fluvoxamine (Luvox), 419

Folate

for memory problems, 512

sources of, 283

Foldable intraocular lens (IOL), 194

Folic acid

benefits of, 249

dangers of, 249

in lowering levels of homocysteine, 488

need for and sources of, 243

pregnancy and, 135, 240

Foods

allergies, 39, 223–224, 233, 314

to be avoided in young children, 155–156

cancer-fighting, 235–236

cravings

controlling, 332, 341

freeing yourself from, 335

danger zones, 214

fat-free, 232

healing and, 424–426

heart-protective, 67

intolerance, 233

moods and, 214–216

poisoning, 47–48

preparing carefully, 47

soy, 67, 236

in boosting longevity, 500

statistics on wasted, 226

Forgetfulness, 58

Formaldehyde, 39

in controlling indoor pollution, 355

Fractures, 44, 471

hip, 134, 291

Free radicals, 236–237, 274

Friends

benefit of having, 70

healing power of, 401–403

value of imaginary, 157

Fruits

buying certified organic, 528

citrus, 235

getting kids to eat, 156

how to eat safely, 527–528

Functional incontinence, 52

Fundoplication, 149

G

Gabapentin (Neurontin), 277

Galanin, 333

Gallstones, prevention of, 218

Gambling, compulsive, 459

Gamma camera, 130

Gamma linolenic acid (GLA), 39

in protecting brain, 506

Gardening, maximizing workout, 331

Garlic, 67, 238

for blood pressure, 521

for cholesterol, 87–88, 521

health benefits of, 414, 421, 514

Gas appliances, controlling indoor pollution of, 355

Gas fumes, dangers from, 324

Gastritis, *Helicobacter pylori* in, 542–543

Gastroesophageal reflux disease (GERD), 20, 149

Helicobacter pylori in, 542–543

Genetic testing, 444–446

Genital herpes, 254

acyclovir and, 260

famciclovir (Famvir) and, 260

medications for, 260

Ginger

arthritis and, 435

for upset stomach, 415

Gingerroot, benefits of, 421

Gingivitis, 370

Ginkgo biloba

in boosting memory, 292, 512

health benefits of, 438, 514

for impotence, 435–436

problems with, 438

in protecting brain, 507

Ginseng

benefits of, 427, 511

for impotence, 436

Glaucoma, 358

asthma and, 362

preventing, 362

steroid inhaler use and, 362

testing for, 362

treating without side effects, 362

Globus pallidus, 272

Glucosamine, 27–28, 512

Glucose level, elevated, 317

Glucose-tolerance factor (GTF), 66

Glucose-tolerance test, 39

Glutamic acid, 236

Glutaraldehyde, 310

Gout, celery seed for, 521

Grapefruit, danger from, 112, 120

Green oat straw as aphrodisiac, 256

Green tea, 236

benefits of, 520

Group therapy, 76–77

Guided imagery

in controlling tinnitus, 368

for wellness, 394–395

Gums

preventing disease, 370

receding, 370

H

Habits, breaking bad, 51–52

Hair

conditioner, dangers in, 316

dye, dangers in, 316

making most of, 197

sun protection for, 295

Hair loss

causes of, 195–196

prevention of, 195–196

Hair weaves, 196

Halo effect, creating positive, 10

Hammertoes, 54

Hands

bath for, 51

washing of, by doctors, 101

washing your, 47

Hantavirus, 310–311

Happiness, putting in life, 458–459

Hawthorn for heart disease, 521

Hay fever. *See also* Allergies; Asthma
  alternative remedies for, 422
  coffee in controlling, 58
Headaches. *See also* Migraines
  avoiding triggers, 59
  food remedies for, 425
  magnets for, 471
  prevention of, 59
  rebound, 118
  relief without medications, 426
  remedies for, 59–60, 427–428
  sex and, 261
  treating, 518
Head trauma, 482
Healing
  food and, 424–426
  intentional, 406–408
Health
  effect of emotions on, 451–453
  needed information about child's care, 143–144
  sex and, 260–261
  time connection between time and, 1–2
  tips for improving, 13–14
  using mind in improving, 395–398
  walking your way to better, 377–378
Health clubs
  scams of, 378
  unhealthiness of, 378
Health maintenance organizations (HMOs)
  coverage for alternative therapies, 470
  evaluating, 443
  getting information from, 347–348
  getting most from, 93
  picking, 443
Health risk, body shape and, 336
Health risk appraisal, 474
Healthy, secrets to staying, while traveling, 5–7
Hearing
  cochlear implant for, 365
  exercise in improving, 276, 365
  free test for, 365
  preventing loss of, 365–367
  tinnitus and, 367–368
Hearing loss, earwax removal in, 545
Heart
  stress and, 173–174

taking care of, 63–65
Heart attacks, 43, 80
  beta-blockers and, 87
  cold operating rooms and, 185
  cutting death risks, 87
  dog ownership and, 273
  early treatment of, 88
  exercise and, 85–86
  fish oil and, 87
  getting right treatment, 284–285
  getting to the hospital quickly, 69
  iron supplements and, 240
  lowering risks of, 487
  nitric oxide in preventing, 485–487
  preparing for emergencies, 69–70
  preventing, 487
  reducing risk of, 232
  sex and, 259–260
  surviving, 68–70
  symptoms of, 68–69
Heartburn
  beating, without medications, 60
Heart disease
  beating, 75–77
  bypass surgery and, 77–79
  causes of, 65
  diet and, 87, 210, 213
  exercise in preventing, 84
  hawthorn for, 521
  height and, 85
  impotence in predicting, 202
  predicting, 70, 488
  preventing, 65–66
  protection from, 67, 282
  stroke and, 282
  tests for, 539–540
  treatment for, 84
  weight and, 68
Heart failure, biofeedback and, 482
Heart surgery
  new Brazilian procedure in, 86
  questions to ask if considering, 187–188
  recovery from, 190
Heating pad, homemade, 60
Heel pain, relief from, 55
Heel spurs, 54–55
Heel surgery, 190
Height, heart disease and, 85

Helicobacter pylori, 155
  as cause of ulcers, 540–541
  in gastritis, 542–543
Helmet, bike, 62
Hemorrhagic stroke, 42
Hemorrhoids, 8, 151
  preventing, 53
  stopping recurring, 165
Hepatitis A vaccine, 121
Hepatitis B
  screening for, 311
  vaccine for, 155, 319
Hepatitis G, screening for, 312
Herbal teas, 413–414
  making, 417
Herbs, 468. *See also specific*
  arthritis and, 434–435
  healing, 513–515
  immunity and, 520–522
  medicinal, 416–417
  as remedies, 420–422, 472
  value of ingredients, 242
Hernia
  hiatal, 20
  surgery for, 192
Herpes, update on, 254
Hexachlorobenzene, 317
Hiatal hernia, 20
Hiccups, cure for, 62
High blood pressure. *See* Blood pressure; Hypertension
High-density lipoproteins (HDL)
  boosting level of, 487
  triglycerides and, 82
High heels, 130
Hip fractures
  reduction of, 291
  weight loss and, 134
Histamines, 233
Home office, making safer, 356
Homeopathic influenzinum for colds and flu, 523
Homeopathy, 469
Homeowner's policy for national disasters, 17
Home security, 288
Home diagnostic tests, 58
Homocysteine
  folic acid in lowering levels of, 488
  test, 81
Honey as substitute for refined sugar, 390
Hormone replacement therapy (HRT), 124–126
  alternatives to, 124, 125
  debate over, 124–125

Hormones
  men's health and, 203
  therapy for prostate cancer, 36
Horny goat weed, as sex
  booster, 516
Hospitals
  common billing errors, 186
  controlling stays in, 179–181
  emergency room care in, 44,
    538
  getting information on,
    182–185
  having healthier and happier
    stays in, 177–178
  medication mistakes and, 186
  rankings of, 179
  reducing length of stay in,
    184–185
  shopping around for, 190
  shrewder stays at, 179
  signs of good, 179
  surviving stays at, 181–182
Hostility, disease and, 352
Hot flashes, relief for, 128
Hot weather, jogging in, 386
Household products, hidden
  dangers in, 315–317
Human immunodeficiency virus
  (HIV). See also Acquired
    immunodeficiency syndrome
    (AIDS) virus
  home test kits for, 261–262
  screening for, 311
Human T-cell lymphotropic
  virus type I (HTLV-I),
    screening for, 312
Humor in lengthening life, 171
Hunting, danger of, 86
Hurricanes, surviving, 16–17
"Hurry sickness," 499
Husbands, unfaithful, and
  cancer, 140
Hypertension, 40–41, 41. See
  also Blood pressure
  in doctor's office, 101
  information about, 71–72
  medication in lowering blood
    pressure, 430
  natural ways to lower blood
    pressure, 429–430
  nutraceuticals for, 511–512
  preventing, 72–74
Hyperthyroidism, 325
Hypnosis, 468
Hypochondria
  causes of, 3

effectiveness of medications
    for, 3
  therapy for, 3–4
Hypoglycemia, 39
Hypogonadism, 203
Hypothyroidism, 324
  treating, 325
Hysterectomies
  cervix-sparing, 139–140
  sex and, 261

I

Ibuprofen, 6, 85, 116
Ice water, sipping, in burning
  calories, 13, 333
Imaging, 468
Immune system
  diet and, 236–238
  harnessing amazing power of,
    478–480
  information on, 480–482
Immunity
  heightened, 46
  herbs and, 520–522
Immunizations. See Vaccines
Implantable defibrillators,
  effectiveness of, 75
Impotence, 255
  exercises and, 258
  medications for, 199
  natural remedies for,
    435–436
  in predicting heart disease,
    202
  snoring and, 199
  strategies for overcoming,
    199–200
  treatments for, 200–202
Incontinence
  exercise and, 133
  functional, 52
  overflow, 52
  simple solutions for, 52
  smoking and, 137
  stress, 52
  treatment for, 543
  urge, 52, 545
Inderal (propranolol), 113
Indigestion, eliminating, 20–22
Indole-3 carbinol, 235
Indoor pollution, 14, 354–356
Infections
  bladder, 420
  ear, 144, 162, 355
  infertility and, 198
  sinus, 527
  throat, 144–145

urinary tract, 140
  yeast, 141
Infectious diseases
  travel and, 7
  ultimate guide to, 47–48
Infertility
  infections and, 198
  tight underwear and male, 198
  unexplained, 198
Inhaled corticosteroids, 121
Inhalers, asthmatics and, 120
Injection therapy for impotence,
  201–202
Injuries
  back, 146, 448
  homeopathic remedy for,
    423–424
  in-line skating and, 315
  knee, 136
  soft-tissue, 29
In-line skating injuries, 315
Inner strength, secrets of,
  454–456
Insect repellent, 6
Insomnia
  exercise and, 382–383
  lavender and, 438
  music in fighting, 56
  painkillers and, 116
  smokers and, 318
Insulin, carbohydrates and,
  342–343
Insulin-dependent (Type 1)
  diabetes, 325
Insulin resistance, vinegar in,
  533–534
Insurance plans, medications
  reimbursed for, 446–447
Intentional healing, 406–408
Intermittent claudication, 309
Interstitial cystitis, 135–136
Irinotecan (Camptosar) for colon
  cancer, 283
Iritis, 363
Iron, 237
  controversy over, 241–242
  heart attacks and supplements,
    240
Irregularity, avoiding, 151–152
Irritable bowel syndrome (IBS),
  424
Itching, 301

J

Jasmine tea in boosting
  longevity, 500
Jaw pain, relief from, 62

Jet lag, 50
  fighting, 6–7
Job strain, 167
Job stress, reducing, 353–354
Jogging in hot weather, 386
Joint pain, beating, 29–31
Journal, keeping, in reducing
  stress, 353
Journalism, science versus,
  441–442
Jowls, sagging, 23
Juice, 231

K

Kegel exercises for incontinence
  in women, 53, 165
Keloids, help for, 295
Kidney damage, blood pressure
  and, 318
Kidney disease, protein and,
  213
Kidney failure, 116
  chromium picolinate and, 250
Kidney stone, cutting
  recurrence of, 229
Kitchen
  arthritis and chores in, 60
  disease-causing germs in, 311
Kitchen cabinet, effective
  remedies from, 420
Knee
  arthritis in, 228
  female athletes and injuries of,
  136
Kombu, 236

L

Lab tests, value of, 444
L-acetyl carnitine in boosting
  memory, 292
Lactobacilli, refrigeration of, 245
Lactose intolerance, 219
L-alpha glycerylphosphorylcholine
  (GPC) in protecting brain, 506
Lanoxin, licorice and, 113
Lapacho, benefits of, 421
L-arginine in boosting nitric
  oxide levels, 486
Laser eye surgery for age-
  related macular degeneration
  (AMD), 279–280
  Laser prostatectomy, 204
Laser treatments
  for skin, 294, 299
  for whitening teeth, 372
LASIK surgery, 191

Laughter, health benefits of, 391
  aging and, 269
Laundry detergent, dangers of,
  316
Lavender
  benefits of, 416
  insomnia and, 438
Laxatives, 6, 152
L-citrulline, 486
L-dopa
  for fibromyalgia, 323
  for Parkinson's disease, 271
Lead, 39
  dangers of, 313, 319
  obesity and, 156
  poisoning, 319
Leg cramps, 309–310
  nighttime, 309
  post-exercise, 309
Legionnaire's disease, 48
Leg pain as stroke risk, 493
Lemon balm tea, 413
Lemon grass for hay fever, 423
Leukocytospermia, 198
Licorice, benefits of, 415
  Lanoxin and, 113
Lidocaine for fibromyalgia, 323
Life
  creating healthy, 407–408
  happier, healthier, 392–394
  highest life expectancy, 146
  longer, 70
  secrets of winning the game
  of, 9–11
Lifestyles
  major changes in, 63–65
  modifications, 76
Light therapy, 13, 476–477
Lipitor (atorvastatin), 106
Lipoprotein (a) test, 81
Liposuction, 23
Liquid nutritional supplements,
  223
Liver protection, milk thistle in,
  521–522
Liver spots, 298
Living alone, nutrition and, 213
Local anesthesia, 191
Lomatium dissectum, for colds
  and flu, 523
Longevity
  exercise and, 379
  rural living and, 285
Lopressor (metoprolol), 113
Lovage, benefits of, 416
Love, communication and, 262
Lovemaking, 260

Low back pain, remedy for, 146
Low-density lipoproteins (LDLs)
  "bad" cholesterol, 65
  determining particle size,
  487–488
Low-fat diets, 237, 475
  men and, 208
Low-vision aids, 280
Lung cancer
  surviving, 456–457
  tests for, 539–540
Lungs, vitamin E in protecting,
  248
Lycopene, 236
Lyme disease, update on, 449
Lyming, 14

M

Macular degeneration, 358
  guarding against, 278–280
  natural remedies for, 509
Magnesium, 68, 428
  calcium and, 151–152
  in fighting migraines, 249
  poisoning from, 122
Magnetic resonance imaging
  (MRI), avoiding anxiety
  during, 444
  and breast cancer, 129–130
Magnets, uses of, 470–471
Makeup, dangers in, 316
Malignancy, PET-CT fusion in
  detecting, 492
Mammograms. See also Breast
  cancer
  antiperspirants and, 132
  computer-aided detection
  (CAD), 129
  how often, 128–129
  large women and, 132
  scheduling, 132
Manipulative therapies, 469
Manual dermasanding, 126
Marigold for hay fever, 423
Marijuana, as medicine, 107
Marjoram, benefits of, 417
Massages, 59
  benefits of, 430–431
  electrostatic, 482–483
  salt, 50–51
  self-, 431–432
  sensual, 262
  as therapy, 469
Masturbation, 256
Mayan medicine man, healing
  secrets from, 422–423

McDougall program, 80
Measles, vaccination for, 314–315
Meat
America's appetite for, 213
barbecuing, 227
safer marinating, 229
Medical care. *See also*
Alternative therapies; Health maintenance organizations (HMOs); Hospitals
getting best possible, 94–95
recommendation for specialist, 95–96
self-defense, 285–286
taking charge of, 100
Medical costs, controlling your, 100
Medical deductions, easily overlooked, 446
Medical emergencies
handling serious, 43–44
planning ahead for, 102
Medical hygiene, 101
Medical labs, mistakes made by, 317
Medical misinformation, the truth about, 441–443
Medical news, making sense of, 441
Medical records, privacy and, 321
Medical tests, 66
getting information on, 538–540
Medicated baths, 50
Medications. *See also* Over-the-counter drugs; *specific*
for acne, 304
for atrial fibrillation, 493
avoiding errors with, 108–112, 323–324
blood-boosting, 312–313
for blood pressure, 275
constipation and, 151
for controlling cholesterol, 76, 83–84, 85, 106–107, 117
dangerous interactions, 112–114
effectiveness of, for hypochondria, 3
effect of anti-anxiety, on sex, 259
effect of ulcer, on sex, 258
in fighting Alzheimer's disease, 507–508
for gastroesophageal reflux disease, 149
for genital herpes, 260

getting information on, 105–106
for heart disease, 75–76
for impotence, 199
for incontinence, 53
for infertility, and ovarian cancer, 142
insurance reimbursement for, 446–447
interactions with foods, 112
measuring dosages, 110
memory loss and, 502
for narcolepsy, 326
natural alternatives to common, 427–429
neuroprotective, 42
for peripheral artery disease, 493
for premature ejaculation, 260
for prostate cancer, 206
saving on, 115
side effects of, 232
taking too many, 534–536
Medicinal herbs, 416–417
Medicinal oils, 433–434
Medicine cabinet, what to keep in, 56
Meditation, 76, 406–407, 468
benefits of, 432
concentrated, 468
in lowering blood pressure, 430
pain control and, 430
for stress management, 475
Melanoma
facts on, 307–308
myths about, 498
reducing risks, 299
support group for, 45–46
Melatonin, 476
Memory
boosting flagging, 291–292
natural remedy for loss of, 508
nutraceuticals for problems in, 512
protective foods, 210–211
scents in improving, 513
stopping loss of, 501–502
testing your, 502–503
vitamin deficiency and, 272
Men
becoming fathers, 197
breast cancer in, 208
divorce and, 208
enlarged breasts in, 23
hair loss in, 195–197
herbs for urinary tract problems in, 499

hormones and health of, 203
impotence in, 199–202
infertility and, 197–198
low-fat diets and, 208
metabolism and, 197
potbellies in, 197
prostate problems in, 203–207
socially dominating, 197
testicular cancer in, 207
Ménière's disease, 24
Meningitis, bacterial, 317
Menopause
heart disease and, 278
secrets of happy, healthy, 123–124
Menstrual cramps, easing, 141
Mental abilities, 409
aging and maintaining peak, 273–274
cross-training, 13–14
using, 11–12
Mercury, 39
Metabolism
aging and, 332
men and, 197
Methylphenidate (Ritalin) for narcolepsy, 326
Midlife wisdom, 409–411
Migraines. *See also* Headaches
allergies and, 224
beating, 31–32
magnesium in fighting, 249
Mild cognitive impairment (MCD), 501–502
Milk
breast cancer and, 130
diabetes and, 320
Milk thistle
health benefits of, 421, 514–514
in liver protection, 521–522
Mind/body techniques
in controlling tinnitus, 368
for enhanced wellness, 391–392
made easy, 401
Mindfulness, 432
Minerals. *See also specific*
safety of, 536–537
Mineral supplements, 68, 468
getting enough, 137
need for, 244
recommendations on, 241
Minoxidil (Rogaine), 196
Mint tea, 413
Mites in eyelashes, 363
Mitoxantrone (Novantrone), 206

Modafinil (Provigil) for
  narcolepsy, 326
Moisturizers
  aging and, 306
  skin care and, 293
Mold as indoor pollution, 355
Monoamine oxidase inhibitor,
  113
Monosodium glutamate, 233
Moods
  bad, exercise versus, 388
  foods and, 214–216
  information on, 453–454
  scents in boosting, 512–513
Morita exercises, 460
Morning sickness, 135
Morphine (Duramorph), 278
Mosquito prevention, 152
Moth repellent, dangers in, 316
Motion sickness remedy, 6
Muira puama as sex booster,
  516
Multiple sclerosis, breakthrough
  in, 483
Multivitamins, benefits of, 536
Mumbling, cure for, 153
MUSE (Medicated Urethral
  System for Erection), 201
Mushrooms, 236
  reishi, 237
  shiitake, 237
Music
  babies and, 155
  in fighting insomnia, 56
  stress and, 174

N
N-acetylcysteine for colds and
  flu, 524
Naikan exercises, 461
Nail fungus, treatments for, 232
Narcolepsy, 326
Nardil (phenelzine), 113
Natural air filters, 62
Natural disasters, surviving,
  16–17
Natural-killer cells, 236
Natural remedies
  for dementia/memory loss, 508
  for heart disease, 508–509
  for impotence, 435–436
  for macular degeneration, 509
  for osteoarthritis, 509
  for pain relief, 437–438
Natural rhythms, keeping, 390
Nausea, relief from, 483

Neck-lift, 23
Neck muscles, keeping firm, 303
Neck pain
  airplane travel and, 49–50
  drug-free treatment of, 517
  fish oil in alleviating, 517
  relief from, 62
Neck wattles, 23
Nefazodone (Serzone), 419
Negative emotions
  expressing, 456
  handling, 459–461
Neighborhood disaster
  committee, organizing, 17
Neurology, stroke victims and,
  282
Neuronitis, vestibular, 24
Neuropeptides, 333, 397
Neuroprotective medications, 42
Neurotransmitters, 332
  release of, 512–513
Nickel, allergies to, 448
Nicotine
  gum, smokers and, 119
  patch, in quitting smoking, 450
  as therapy for ulcerative
    colitis, 119
Nighttime leg cramps, 309
Nitric oxide, preventing heart
  attacks and strokes with,
  485–487
Nitrogen dioxide, 39
Nitroglycerin, 75
Noise
  minimizing, at home and at
    work, 13
  white, 368
Non-Hodgkin's lymphoma, red
  meat and, 217
Nonsteroidal anti-inflammatory
  drugs (NSAIDs), 27
Nonulcer dyspepsia (NUD), 21
Nosebleed, stopping, 60
Nose piercing, 317
Nuprin (ibuprofen), 113
Nursing homes, transfer policies
  of, 275
Nutraceuticals
  benefits of, 511–512
  cooking with, 14
Nutrition. See also
  Carbohydrates; Diet; Protein
  as alternative medicine,
    468–469
  eyes and, 361, 364–365
  living alone and, 213

proper, for healthy heart and
  long life, 67–68
Nutritional supplements
  liquid, 223
  need for, 242–244
Nuts, 67

O
Oatmeal, high-fiber foods and,
  113
Obesity
  cataracts and, 361
  lead and, 156
  ultrasound liposuction and, 192
Obsessive-compulsive behavior,
  411–412
Okinawans, longevity of, 499–501
Older women, anorexia and, 136
Olive oil, 67
Omalizumab (Xolair) for
  asthma, 543
Omega-3 oils, benefits of, 230
One-breath meditation,
  practicing, 13
Open-heart surgery,
  breakthrough in, 79
Operations, anesthesia and, 191
Orbital cortex, 411
Oregano for hay fever, 423
Orthophenylphenol, 316
Orudis KT (ketoprofen), 113
Oscillococcinum for colds and
  flu, 523
Osteoarthritis
  allergies and, 224
  natural remedies for, 509
  nutraceuticals for problems in,
    512
Osteopathy, 469
Osteoporosis
  advances in, 133
  calcium and, 240–241
  depression and, 134
  risks for, 287
Outpatient surgery, preparing
  for, 188–189
Ovarian cancer
  family connection, 138
  fertility medications and, 142
  genetic testing for, 138
  protecting yourself from,
    138–139
  risk factors for, 137–138
  symptoms of, 138
  tests for, 540
  treatment for, 138, 142

Ovary removal, danger of, 142
Overactive thyroid, 325
Overflow incontinence, 52
Over-the-counter drugs
  dangers from, 484
  prescriptions versus, 114
Oxybutinin for incontinence, 53
Oxygenation, steps in better,
  510–511
Oxygen deprivation, 509–510

P

Pain
  arthritis, 27–29, 229–231, 260
  back, 9, 471, 517
  chronic, 25–26
  diabetic nerve, 534
  diary of, 276
  drug-free ways of treating,
    517–519
  foot, 307, 336
  heel, 55
  jaw, 62
  joint, 29–31
  leg, 493
  meditation in controlling, 430
  natural remedies for relief of,
    437–438
  neck, 49–50, 62, 517
  shoulder, 517–518
  specialist in, finding, 518
Painkillers, 113
  dangers from, 116
  insomnia and, 116
Paint stripper, dangers of, 316
Pallidotomy, 272
Pancake, nonfat recipe for, 219
Parasites, avoiding, in water, 48
Parkinson's disease, treatments
  for, 271–272
Parnate (tranylcypromine), 113
Paroxetine (Paxil), 419
Parsley tea for bladder infection,
  420
Pasta
  buying, 216
  spinach, 225
Patient-assistance programs, 45
Peak flow meter, for asthmatics,
  318
Peanuts, allergies to, 155–156
Pediatricians. See also Doctors
  home remedies of, 166
  taking caregiver to, 158
Pelvic congestion syndrome,
  491–492

Pemoline (Cylert), for
  narcolepsy, 326
Penciclovir (Denavir) for cold
  sores, 165
Pennyroyal, benefits of, 417
Pentosan polysulfate (Elmiron),
  135–136
Peppermint for irritable bowel
  syndrome, 424
Perfectionism, 171
Performance anxiety, 263
Periodontal disease
  treatment for, 369
  in vegetarians, 369
Peripheral artery disease (PAD),
  as stroke risk, 493
Periwinkle for hay fever, 423
Pernicious anemia, 325
Personality, Type A in heart
  patients, 86–87
Pessimism, 290
Pet allergies, controlling, 57
PET-CT fusion in detecting
  malignancy, 492
Peyronie's disease, 199
Phenol, 294
Phenylephrine, 113
Phosphatidylserine
  in boosting memory, 291–292
  in protecting brain, 506–507
Physical therapy for joint pain,
  30
Physicians. See Doctors,
  Pediatricians
Phytonutrients, 235
Piercing, nose, 317
Pine extract bath, 50
Placebo, power of, 473–474
Plantar fasciitis, 29
Plants, stress and, 174
Ploidy analysis for prostate
  cancer, 35
Poisoning, 157
  carbon monoxide, 313
  causes of, 157
  food, 47–48
  lead, 319
  magnesium, 122
Policosanol in lowering
  cholesterol, 490–491
Pollution, indoor, 14, 354–356
Polymerase chain reaction
  (PCR) test for prostate cancer,
  35
Positive thinking, 391
Positron emission tomography
  (PET), 75, 130

Post-baby blues, 135
Post-exercise leg cramps, 309
Postherpetic neuralgia (PHN),
  301
Posture, reading, 14
Potassium, 68
  getting more, 65
  increasing intake of, 64, 429
Potbellies, risk of stroke and, 197
Power eating, 225–226
Pravastatin (Pravachol), 83, 85,
  106
Pregnancy
  folic acid's role in, 135, 240
  reliability of ultrasound exams,
    136
  smoking and, 134–135
  thinking and, 135
Prehypertension, as stroke risk,
  492–493
Premature ejaculation, 198, 263
  medications for, 260
Premature labor, hot summer
  days and, 134
Prepatellar bursitis, 29
Prescription drugs. See also
  Medications; specific
  dangers of, 102
  finishing, 114
  getting lower cost, 449–450
  interactions of, 113
  over-the-counter drugs versus,
    114
  for psychiatric problems, 101
  risk from, 117
  saving money on, 44–45
  self-defenses, 115
  and sex, 258–259
  for stomach problems, 21
  tablets versus liquids, 117
Privacy, medical records and,
  321
Procaine for fibromyalgia, 323
Procardia, 83, 112
Progestin, as alternative to
  hormone-replacement
  therapy, 124
Prolotherapy, 477–478
Prostaglandins, 229
Prostate
  enlargement, 204
  nutraceuticals for problems
    in, 512
  treatments for, 204–206
  saw palmetto for problems of,
    522
  tests for problems of, 204

Prostate cancer
  facts on, 447
  fighting, 499
  information about, 34–36
  medications for, 206
  radiation for, 35, 206
  surgery for, 35, 205–207
  tomatoes and, 217
Prostate specific antigen (PSA)
  test, 35, 204, 205, 280
    problems with, 280–281
Prosthetic device for impotence,
  202
Protein, 212
  kidney disease and, 213
  mood and, 215
  sources of, 215
Pseudoephedrine, 113
Psychiatric medications,
  prescribing, 101
Psychodynamic therapy, 3–4
Psyllium, 152, 238
Puberty
  facts of, 163
  skin care for kids in, 158
Pulmonary artery
  catheterization, 190
Pulmonary embolism, 50
Pygeum africanum for prostate
  enlargement, 512
Pygeum extract, benefits of,
  421–422

Q

Qi gong, 432–433, 472–473
Quercetin, 236, 428
  for osteoarthritis, 509

R

Radiation for prostate cancer,
  35, 206
Radiofrequency ablation in
  treating cancer, 491
Rashes, pediatrician's home
  remedies for, 166
Rebound headaches, 118
Recovery sleep, 447
Red meat, non-Hodgkin's
  lymphoma and, 217
Red rose for hay fever, 423
Red wine, 67
  heart protection and, 282
Red yeast rice in lowering
  cholesterol, 489–490
Reflux, 20
Regional anesthesia, 191

Registered dietitian (RD), 341
Rehabilitation exercises, 25
Reishi mushrooms, 237
Relationships, sleep positions
  and, 264
Relaxation, 407
  as alternative to hormone-
    replacement therapy, 124
  in controlling seizures, 173
  exercises for, 430
  response, 276–277, 393
  techniques, 172
  therapies, 467–468
  yoga for, 408–409
Religion, in boosting longevity,
  501
Resectoscope, 205
Resilience, 455–456
Restenosis, 247
Restless legs syndrome, 162–163
Retin-A, 298
Retinal breaks, detachment and,
  358–359
Retrograde ejaculation, 206
Reversible predominantly
  posterior
  leukoencephalopathy (RPPL),
  315
Rheumatoid arthritis, relief
  from, 386
Robotic therapy for strokes,
  494
Rodent, danger from, 310–311
Romance, scents to boost, 513
Rosacea, 300
Rosemary, benefits of, 415
Rotator cuff tendinitis, 29
Rural living, longevity and, 285

S

St. John's wort
  as antidepressant, 428
  for irritable bowel syndrome,
  424
Salmonella, 311
Salsa in disease prevention, 520
Salt. See also Sodium
  eating less, 65
  facts on, 214
  massage with, 50–51
  substitutes for, 113
Saponins, 236
Saturated fat, minimizing intake
  of, 486
Saw palmetto, 428
  health benefits of, 203, 515

for male urinary tract
  problems, 499
  for prostate problems, 512, 522
Scams, health club, 378
Scars
  help for, 295
  skin cancer and, 299
Scents
  in boosting energy, mood and
    memory, 512–513
  inhaling energizing, 13
  in weight loss, 341–342
Science, journalism versus,
  441–442
Scrotum, varicose veins of, 207
Scrub, 302
Sea vegetables, 236
Seborrheic keratoses, 298
Secondhand smoke, avoiding,
  510
  in children, 157
  dangers from, 314
Seizures, relief from, 120
Selenium, 68, 237
  benefits of, 250
  cancer versus, 250
  need for and sources of, 243
Self-healing, spices and, 414
Self-help experts, advice from,
  403–405
Self-hypnosis, 277
  in controlling tinnitus, 368
Self-massage, 431–432
Self-medication, 118
Self-talk, 277
Self-tanning products in
  protecting against sunburn, 498
Senna, constipation and, 152
Sensory stimulation, 391
Sertraline (Zoloft), 419
Set point, dieting versus,
  334–335
Sex
  abuse, 263
  after 60, 256–258
  arthritis pain and, 260
  aversion to, 263
  boredom with, 255–256
  children and, 153
  communication and, 262
  desire, synchronizing, 264
  Dr. Ruth's secrets of great, 260
  frequency of, 261
  having great, 253–254
  headaches and, 261
  healing power of, 251–252

health and, 260–261
heart attacks, 259–260
hysterectomies and, 261
inhibition, 263
initiation of, and, 259
lovemaking, 260
natural boosters, 515–516
perking up, 254–256
prescription drugs that affect, 258–259
problems, 262–264
saying no to, 259
sleep and, 259
toys, 256
urinary tract infections and, 140
Shampoo, dandruff, 300
Shaving cream, dangers in, 316
Shiitake mushrooms, 237
Shingles, 300–301
treatment of, 121
Shin splints, 29
Shoes
athletic, 56
not wearing, in controlling indoor pollution, 355
for senior citizens, 278
Shortness of breath, 43
Shoulder bursitis, 29
Shoulder pain, drug-free treatment of, 517–518
Shyness, overcoming extreme, 465–466
Siberian ginseng, benefits of, 427
Sigmoidoscopy, 33–34
Sildenafil (Viagra), 201
Simvastatin (Zocor), 106
Sinus congestion, remedies for, 420
Sinus infection, relief from, 527
Sinusitis, 19–20
symptoms and causes, 19–20
treating, 20
Skin
aging and, 297–299
care of, 293–294, 302–304
collagen injections in care of, 22, 194, 298
dry and itchy, 298
keeping young, 305–306
for kids in puberty, 158
repairing damaged, 304
Skin cancer, 299
debunking myths of, 497–498
facts on, 308

protecting yourself from, 295–297
risks of, 295, 304
Sleep
behavior and, 157
catching up on, 447
disorders, 57
exercise and, 385
medications for narcolepsy, 326
pills, alternative for, 428
relationships and positions, 264
sex and, 259
in treating stress and depression, 173, 418–419
weight loss and, 336
Sleep apnea, as stroke risk, 494
Sleepiness, daytime, 326
Slouching as cause of carpal tunnel syndrome, 346
Smoking
effect of, on skin, 297
insomnia and, 318
nicotine gum and, 119
pregnancy and, 134–135
prohibiting, in reducing indoor pollution, 354
quitting, 63, 84, 283–284, 450, 500, 510–511
risks from cigar, 318
secondhand, 64, 157, 314
Snoring, 152
impotence and, 199
weight loss and, 344
Snow, shoveling wet, 318
Soaps, antibacterial, 526
Social drinkers, facts on, 234
Social links in boosting longevity, 500–501
Sodium. See also Salt
reducing intake of, 64, 429
Sodium benzoate, 233
Soft-tissue injuries, 29
magnets for, 471
Sore muscles, relief from, 386
Sore throat, 8
Sound masking, 368
Soy foods, 67, 236
in boosting longevity, 500
Sparkling waters, sugar in, 219
Sperm, 197
Sperm donor, how to find, 262
Spermatocele, 207
Spices, self-healing and, 414
Spinach pasta, 225
Spirituality, in boosting longevity, 501

Sports bra, buying, 131
Sports drinks, 381
Spring allergies, 153–154
Staphylococcus aureus, 311, 317
Statins
depression versus, 121
red yeast rice versus, 489–490
uses of, 106–107
Stationary biking, 382
Steroid inhaler use, glaucoma and, 362
Stimulants for narcolepsy, 326
Stomach
aspirin therapy and problems, 120
food remedies for upset, 425–426
ginger for upset, 415
size of, and beer drinkers, 329
Strength, turning stress into, 170–171
Strength training, 385–386, 475
aging and, 273
benefits of, 530–532
dangers in, 319
for incontinence, 53
walking in, 387
workouts in, 380
Strep-throat, 119
Stress
avoiding, 168–170
breathing, in reducing, 451–452
busters, 175–176
cholesterol levels and, 173
controlling, 274
coping with, 64–65
disease and, 352
fighting, 174
heart and, 173–174
job, 352–354
making work for you, 167–168
music and, 174
plants and, 174
reducing, 174, 390
relaxation therapy for, 172–173
sleep versus, 173
stretches, in reducing, 352–353
treating natural way, 418–420
turning into strengths, 170–171
writing in management of, 174
Stress electrocardiogram, 75
Stress incontinence, 52
Stretch marks, help for, 139
Strokes, 43
dentist and risk of, 281
diagnosis danger, 315

heart disease and, 282
hemorrhagic, 42
neurologist and, 282
nitric oxide in preventing, 485–487
potbellies and, 197
preventing, 274
rehabilitation following, 494–495
risks for, 88, 492–494
treatment of, 41–43
Sudden infant death syndrome (SIDS), 156
Sugar
chronic fatigue and, 39–40
honey as substitute for refined, 390
in sparkling waters, 219
Sulfacetamide (Klaron), 304
Sulforaphane, 235
Sun
blocking, 295, 305
dangers from, 301–302
spots, 299
Sunburn, pediatrician's home remedies for, 166
Sunglasses
kids and, 156–157
update on, 364
UV-blocking, 296
wraparound, 364
Sunscreens, 302–303
aging and, 305–306
applying, 296
danger of, 304–305
effectiveness of, 297, 498
recommendations on, 296
skin care and, 293
sun protection factor (SPF), 497
using, 297
Super glue, sutures versus, 483
Supplements, 66
antiaging, 286–287
antioxidant, 509
calcium, 241–242
chromium, 241
evaluation of, 537–538
fish oil, 87, 230
liquid nutritional, 223
mineral, 68, 137, 241, 244
nutritional, 242–244
vitamin, 67–68
Support groups
for chronic illness, 45–46
finding, 441
Surgery
anesthesia and, 191

bypass, 77–80, 81
cataract, 194, 361
for coffee drinkers, 194
cold operating rooms and, 185
cosmetic, 22–23, 308
for curved penis, 199
donating blood for, 190
heart, 79, 187–188, 190
heel, 190
hernia, 192
laser eye (LASIK), 191
outpatient, 188–189
for Parkinson's disease, 272
for prostate cancer, 35, 205–207
rapid healing after, 189–190
recovery time from, 186
super glue versus sutures in, 483
Sutures, super glue versus, 483
Sweets, craving, 62
Swimming for exercise, 386
Syphilis, screening for, 311

T

Tablets, liquids versus, 117
Tadalafil (Cialis), 201
Tai chi, 472–473
Talcum powder
dangers of, 142, 316
Taxes, medical deductions, 446
Teas
green, 236, 520
herbal, 413–414, 417
jasmine, 500
lemon balm, 413
mint, 413
parsley, 420
thyme, 413
Teeth, professional cleaning of, 370
Telangiectasia, 308
Telephones
cancer risk from cellular, 447
crime and pay, 288–289
Tennis elbow, 29
Tenormin (atenolol), 113
Terazosin (Hytrin), 205
Testicular cancer
self-defense for, 207
self-exam for, 207
treating, 207
Testosterone patch, 118
Tetanus booster, need for, 314
Thallium scans, 75
Theophylline, 149
Thermometer, ear, 314

Throat infections, recurrent, 144–145
Thromboxane, 491
Thunderstorms in triggering asthma attacks, 317
Thyme
benefits of, 417
for sinus congestion, 420
Thyroid
checking up on, 324–325
lumps and tumors in, 325
overactive, 38
underactive, 38
Thyroid-stimulating hormone (TSH), 325
Thyroxine (T4), 325
Tick bites, guard against, 48
Time
awareness, 1–2
connection between health and, 1–2
creating retreats from, 2
history of, 1–2
Timeshifting, 1
exercises in, 2
Tinnitus, 367–368
Tissue-type plasminogen activator (TPA), 42
Toenail fungus, 55
Tolinase (tolazamide), 113
Tomatoes, prostate cancer and, 217
Tongue scraping, 61
Toothbrushes. See also Dental care
electric, 369, 370–371
kinds of, 370
replacing, 370
Tooth brushing. See also Dental care
amount of, 369
better, 61
importance of, 370–371
Tooth decay, preventing infant, 156
Toothpaste. See also Dental care
best, 371
dangers in, 316
Toxic chemicals, 319
Tramadol for fibromyalgia, 323
Transurethral incision of prostate (TUIP), 205–206
Transurethral microwave thermal therapy (TUMT), 206
Transurethral needle ablation (TUNA), 206

Transurethral resection of prostate (TURP), 205
Trauma, head, 482
Travel. *See also* Airplane travel
infectious diseases and, 7
secrets to staying healthy while, 5–7
Trazodone, 201
Treadmill, calorie burning and, 338
Tretinoin, aging and, 306
Tribulus, as sex booster, 516
Trichloracetic acid, 294
Trichloroethylene, 39
Trigger foods, for asthmatics, 147
Trigger-point therapy, 14
Triglycerides
high-density lipoproteins and, 82
levels of, 88
Triiodothyronine (T3), 325
Trimethoprim sulfamethoxazole (Bactrim), 140
Trochanteric bursitis, 29
Tubing as exercise, 383–384
Tumescent liposuction, 23
Turmeric, 236
arthritis and, 435, 522
TV workout, 530
Type A personality, and heart patients, 86–87
Tyramine, 233

U
Ulcerative colitis, 37
nicotine therapy and, 119
Ulcers, 155
cause of, 540–541
in children, 155
diabetic foot, 306
effect of medications for, on sex, 258
risk of getting, 121
testing for, 444
vitamin C in preventing, 246
Ultrafast computed tomography scan, 81
Ultrasound exams, and
breast cancer, 129
pregnancy, 136
Ultraviolet light, dangers of, 304, 306
sunglasses to block, 296
Underwear, tight, and male infertility, 198

Urethral needle ablation (TUNA), 203–204
Urge incontinence, 52
Urinary incontinence, 52, 133
Urinary tract infections (UTIs)
saw palmetto extract for, in men, 499
sex and, 140

V
Vaccines
for cancer, 496–497
for hepatitis A, 121
for hepatitis B, 155, 319
for measles, 314–315
safety of, 144
up-to-date, 144–145
Vacuum device for impotence, 202
Vaginal douching, 140
Vaginal dryness, 255
Vaginal lubricants, as alternative to hormone-replacement therapy, 124
Valerian
as alternative for sleeping pill, 428
health benefits of, 515
Vardenafil (Levitra), 201
Varicose veins
of scrotum, 207
vein ablation for, 491–492
Vasectomy, alternative to reversal, 198
Vasoconstrictor eyedrops, 364
Vasomax, 201
Vegetables
cruciferous, 235
getting kids to eat, 156
Vegetarian diets, 76, 336
anorexia and, 217
periodontal disease from, 369
Vein ablation for varicose veins, 491–492
Venlafaxine (Effexor), 419
Venogram in identifying varicose veins, 492
Vertigo, 24
Vestibular neuronitis, 24
Vinegar in fighting diabetes, 533–534
Vision disorders, bilberry for, 521
Visual retraining following strokes, 495
VitalStim therapy for strokes, 495

Vitamin A derivative, skin care and, 293–294
Vitamin B, depression and, 245
Vitamin B-6, need for and sources of, 243
Vitamin B-12, 245–246
Vitamin C, 67, 237
aging and, 269
arteries and, 247
arthritis and, 246
asthma and, 246
benefits of, 537
bladder cancer and, 247
in boosting nitric oxide levels, 486
chewable forms of, 246–247
colds and, 241
need for and sources of, 220, 243
for osteoarthritis, 509, 512
in preventing ulcer, 246
in quitting smoking, 511
winter needs, 247
wrinkles versus, 295
Vitamin D
adults and, 247–248
diabetes and, 247
need for and sources of, 243
Vitamin E, 67, 237, 240
aging and, 269, 275
benefits of, 537
cuts and, 248
exercise and, 248–249
for memory problems, 512
need for and sources of, 220, 243
for osteoarthritis, 509
in protecting lungs, 248
taking aspirin with, 248
Vitamin K, clotting action of, 112–113
Vitamins, 468
birth defects versus, 248
memory and deficiency of, 272
need for, 244
safety of, 536–537
storing, 245
supplements, 67–68
timed-release, 245
Vitiligo, 325

W
Waist-to-hip ratio (WHR), 197
Wakame, 236
Walking, 341
benefits of, 133

for better health, 377–378
in stroke rehab, 495
with weights, 387
Warfarin (Coumadin), 42
Warts
  in children, 160–161
  duct tape in curing, 519
Water
  avoiding parasites in, 48
  drinking, to prevent jet lag, 6
  filter, in controlling pollutants, 355–356
  getting recommended intake of, 59
  need for, 320
  safety of distilled, 223
  therapy for ailments, 50
Weed killer, dangers of, 316
Weight
  birth, as risk factor for disease, 488
  heart disease and, 68
  keeping off, 330–331
  maintaining, 330–331
Weight lifting. *See* Strength training
Weight loss, 139
  better, 528–529
  chromium supplements and, 241
  diet doctors' secrets of, 337–338
  exercise and, 386
  hip fractures and, 134

in lowering blood pressure, 429
  proven methods of, 340–341
  reasons for problems with, 339–340
  scent therapy in, 341–342
  secrets of permanent, 334–335, 530
  secrets of successful, 327–328
  sleeping and, 336
  snoring and, 344
Wellness
  guided imagery for, 394–395
  mind/body techniques for enhanced, 391–392
Whitening, teeth, laser procedure for, 372
White noise generators, 368
Whole milk, dangers in, 317
Wisdom, midlife, 409–411
Women
  anorexia and older, 136
  calcium and, 136–137
  doctors and, 102–103
  initiation of sex and, 259
  Kegel exercises to beat incontinence, 53, 165
  mammograms for large, 132
Women's Health Initiative (WHI) on hormone replacement therapy, 124–125
Workaholism, 350–352
Work hours, hazards of, 83

Workouts. *See also* Exercise(s)
  gardening, 331
  getting most out of your, 384–385
  TV, 530
Wounds, preventing scarring, 166
Wrinkles, 298
  laser therapy for deep, 22–23
  removing, 126
  vitamin C versus, 295
Writing in stress management, 174

X

X-ray, child's need for, 143

Y

Yeast infection, relief from, 141
Yerba mate, benefits of, 422
Yoga, 76
  for deep relaxation, 408–409
Yogurt for yeast infections, 141
Yohimbine, 201

Z

Zinc, 237
  controversy over, 241–242
  for macular degeneration, 509
  for prostate enlargement, 512
Zolpidem (Ambien)
  for fibromyalgia, 322
  for narcolepsy, 326